Childhood Language Disorders in Context: Infancy through Adolescence

Nickola Wolf Nelson
Western Michigan University

Merrill, an imprint of
Macmillan Publishing Company
New York

Maxwell Macmillan Canada
Toronto

Maxwell Macmillan International
New York   Oxford   Singapore   Sydney

Cover art: Karen Guzak
Editor: Ann Castel
Production Editor: Jonathan Lawrence
Art Coordinator: Peter A. Robison
Text Designer: Jill E. Bonar
Cover Designer: Russ Maselli
Production Buyer: Patricia A. Tonneman
Illustrations: Maryland Cartographics, Inc.

This book was set in Meridien and Univers by V & M Graphics and was printed and
bound by R. R. Donnelley & Sons, Company. The cover was printed by Lehigh Press, Inc.

Macmillan Publishing Company
866 Third Avenue
New York, NY 10022

Macmillan Publishing Company is part of the
Maxwell Communication Group of Companies.

Maxwell Macmillan Canada, Inc.
1200 Eglinton Avenue East, Suite 200
Don Mills, Ontario M3C 3N1

Library of Congress Cataloging-in-Publication Data
Nelson, Nickola.
      Children with language disorders: infancy through adolescence/
    Nickola Wolf Nelson.
          p.   cm.
      Includes bibliographical references and index.
      ISBN 0-675-21203-0
      1. Language disorders in children. 2. Language disorders in
    adolescence.   I. Title.
    RJ496.L35N46 1993
    618.92′855—dc20   92-4781
                                                    CIP

Printing: 1   2   3   4   5   6   7   8   9   Year: 3   4   5   6   7

Photo credits: pp. 5, 25, 56, 78, 152, 187, 258, 324, and 393 by Jeremy K. Fair.

To my parents,
Betty Anderson Wolf
and the memory of
Lawrence Winton Wolf,
who provided the context for developing roots and wings,

And to my grandmothers,
Marjorie Waggoner Anderson,
who showed that education is where you find it,
and the memory of
Pauline Keimig Wolf,
who first made me think I could write

Preface

This book is for children with language disorders. Although the immediate audience comprises graduate students and upper-level undergraduate students preparing to serve children with language disorders, ultimately the book is for the children themselves.

As a textbook it will be more accessible to students who have some background in linguistics and in normal and disordered language acquisition. Although the book is introductory in breadth, it covers many issues with relative depth. I am a speech–language pathologist, and I have used the book in preliminary form with two classes of graduate students in speech–language pathology. I have also taught courses that included graduate students in special education who were majoring in other areas, and I have included some introductory material with those students in mind (particularly Chapter 2 and parenthetical explanations of terminology). I hope that the book will be useful to practicing professionals and to parents as well. My experiences with them have certainly helped me write it.

THE CENTRAL FOCUS

The book's central focus is the development of language and communication. It is not about a particular kind of child; it is about all kinds of children at all ability levels and ages from infancy through adolescence. The common factor is their difficulty in learning to communicate with language. That is not to say that the conditions that put children at risk for normal language learning are not important. I believe that they are, and the reader will find an etiological thread regarding theories about causes throughout the book. However, the book's ultimate purpose—and the primary reason for considering the nature of language

disorders—is to find ways to facilitate language learning when it does not proceed naturally. In fulfilling this purpose, the book focuses on communicative meanings, forms, and interactions that arise in the course of normal development from infancy through adolescence. It focuses secondarily on the causative conditions likely to limit that development.

PART ONE: TAKING A BROAD VIEW OF LANGUAGE-LEARNING SYSTEMS

A variety of pathways may be taken to facilitate positive change in language-learning systems. Viewed comprehensively, a language-learning system includes not only the developing skills, knowledge, and biological systems that children bring to the task, but also the contexts and communicative partners that contribute to the acquisition process.

Part One addresses these issues from varied perspectives. Chapter 1 sets the stage by presenting the conceptual framework for the book. It introduces the theme that *problems are not just within children, and neither are the solutions.* Readers are urged to ask insightful questions not only about children's language abilities and impairments, but also about the communicative needs and opportunities that arise in the important contexts of children's lives.

Chapter 2 provides background information about language, speech, and communication. Multidisplinary perspectives are introduced, and language, speech, and communication are defined. I emphasize the strong links among the three systems but also present evidence for their relative separability and argue for considering each during language assessment and intervention. Nonlinguistic and paralinguistic communication are also reviewed, as are the five systems of language—phonology, morphology, syntax, semantics, and pragmatics. Issues regarding bilingualism and dialect difference are introduced.

Because issues related to bilingualism and dialect difference cannot be isolated from broader issues of language learning and education, neither are they isolated in a single chapter of this book. Although most examples illustrate the acquisition of standard American English, this bit of ethnocentricity is countered by equal emphasis on the need for multicultural sensitivity. To exhibit multicultural sensitivity, language specialists must appreciate the richness of cultural variation, be familiar with language systems other than standard English, and recognize the need for modified language assessment and intervention strategies for children from varied language-learning communities. Guidance regarding such issues is provided thoughout the book.

Chapter 3 introduces six theoretical perspectives, which appear again in later chapters to organize discussions of causative factors (Chapter 4) and language assessment and intervention principles (Chapter 6). The six theories explain language acquisition alternatively by emphasizing biological maturation, linguistic rule induction, behaviorism, information processing, cognitivism, and social interaction.

Chapter 4 provides an overview of causes, categories, and contributing factors, including a discussion of the value of categorization. Causative conditions associated with language disorders are presented under three main headings: (1) central processing factors, (2) peripheral sensory and motor system factors, and (3) environmental and emotional system factors. Central processing categories include specific language disability, mental retardation, autism, attention-deficit hyperactivity disorder, and acquired brain injury. Peripheral sensory and motor system categories include hearing impairment, visual impairment, and physical impairment. Environmental and emotional system categories include neglect and abuse, and behavioral and emotional development problems. Mixed factors are also considered. Within each category, I present the available evidence for subtypes, for differentiating language disorder from delay, and for each of the six theories introduced in Chapter 3. Diagnostic features associated with categorical conditions are summarized in boxes. Chapter 4 concludes with a section on prevention.

Chapter 5 addresses the relationship between public policy and service delivery. As a result of federal mandates, individuals employed in school settings and other public agencies bear a major responsibility for language intervention with children. The text therefore emphasizes information about Public Laws 94–142, 99–457, and 107–476, now known collectively as the Individuals with Disabilities Education Act (IDEA). Chapter 5 also provides general information about service delivery settings, people, and scheduling.

Chapter 6 concludes Part One with an overview of issues related directly to language assessment and intervention. The chapter begins with a flowchart outlining decisions from the point a problem is suspected until a child or adolescent no longer needs special services. Again, the six theoretical perspectives introduced in Chapter 3 are used to organize discussion of assessment and intervention practices. Assessment and intervention are not viewed as separate, but as highly integrated processes. The remaining sections of the chapter extend discussions related to the assessment issues of team process—diagnosing disorder, determining eligibility for service, establishing prognosis, and outlining parameters of impairment, disability, and handicap.* The sections on intervention address processes for selecting goal areas and gathering baseline data, designing and implementing intervention plans, monitoring progress, using exit criteria, and judging program accountability.

PART TWO: BALANCING AGES AND DEVELOPMENTAL STAGES

Part Two is organized developmentally into three chapters addressing early, middle, and later stages of development. (Such an approach is not without drawbacks; these are discussed in the introduction to Part Two.) Historically, a developmental focus too often has meant that professionals have attempted to measure a child's current level of functioning relative to quantitative norms for variables such as vocabulary size and mean length of utterance. Based on such

---

*Terminology continues to develop. As this book goes to press, there is a movement away from using the term *handicap* because of its negative social connotations, but it still conveys an important distinction in this book. *See* Pope, A. M., and Tarlov, A. R. (Eds.). (1991). *Disability in America: Toward a national agenda for prevention.* Washington, DC: National Academy Press.

standards, programs have been devised and implemented, often in separate, specialized settings, to teach children discrete language structures that normally developing children would learn at about the same stage. Aspects of this approach are still pertinent, but the narrowness of its focus has been recognized, and it is now being replaced by more comprehensive approaches and a broader perspective of "normal." Newer strategies are based on greater collaboration among family members and multi-disciplinary professionals, a view of the language learner as a whole person, and recognition of the rights and needs of children to participate in activities with their same-age, normal-learning peers.

Although individual differences are emphasized, general descriptions of normal development nevertheless remain helpful templates for guiding selection of intervention targets, strategies, and contexts when language development is impaired. Part Two therefore provides perspectives from normal development as the dominant but not the only focus. Chapter 7 examines expectations for the early developmental stages, which include infancy through toddlerhood; Chapter 8 addresses the middle developmental stages, which include preschool through early elementary years; and Chapter 9 addresses the later developmental stages, which include middle elementary through later adolescent years. Chapters 7, 8, and 9 are organized with parallel structure addressing three issues: (1) the identification of children needing intervention aimed at that stage (both those children who can "almost but not quite" meet age expectations and those who are older but more severely impaired), (2) commonly used tools and strategies for measuring the needs and abilities at each stage, and (3) methods and targets of intervention for individuals at that stage of development. Chapters 8 and 9 also address the needs of children who are at middle or later stages chronologically, but who remain at earlier stages developmentally. In this way, a balance between consideration of ages and developmental stages is maintained.

Throughout the book, I blend "facts," theories, issues, and clinical experience to help current and future professionals contemplate the relationships between their own organized thoughts (theories) and actions (interventions) regarding language disorders in children. I believe that such a combination is the one most likely to generate positive and productive change in the lives of children with language disor-

ders and their families. That is the ultimate goal of this book.

SPECIAL FEATURES

A few special features have been included to make the text more readable and applicable. Sprinkled throughout are individuals' personal reflections relevant to service provision to children with language disorders. These encourage readers to think about the body of knowledge related to language disorders in children as dynamic, shaped by the people who have studied it. The personal reflections also introduce meaningful statements from workers in related fields—parents, teachers, and children. In addition, I use case examples liberally to integrate theory and basic information with application. Some illustrate a major point and are more fully developed. Others illustrate minor points and are less fully developed.

Finally, I provide pedagogical tools to help readers organize their approach to the text, to raise issues for discussion, and to provide guidance to further resources. These include outlines of main topics and guiding questions at the beginning of chapters. In addition to traditional tables and figures, boxes and appendices summarize key points and present data for organizing assessment and intervention. Appendix A is a bibliography of formal tests (listed by early, middle, and later stages) to augment the discussions of informal assessment techniques highlighted in the chapters. Appendix B summarizes developmental information in the four domains—cognitive underpinnings, receptive language, expressive language, and social interaction and play. It can be used to assist in making placement and programming decisions for children with severe disabilities. Appendix C presents the scoring criteria for Black English Sentence Scoring (Nelson & Hyter, 1990a, 1990b).

Nothing is sacred about reading the chapters of this book in order. Although there is some logic to this order and some cross-referencing of information, alternative approaches are equally appropriate. Readers who are already familiar with aspects of language, speech, and communication may wish to skim Chapter 2. Readers seeking information on a specific developmental stage may start with Chapter 7, 8, or 9. Readers less concerned about public policy may skip Chapter 5 or save it until last.

ACKNOWLEDGMENTS

Completing a long project brings on a flood of feelings. Relief is certainly high among them, as well as a sense of connectedness with the long cast of characters who helped get the project going and nudged it along.

Sometimes editors are only shadowy characters who have little real involvement with a writing project like this, but I never would have started this book if I had not first been approached by Vicki Knight when the publishing company was still Merrill. As Merrill went through several stages of metamorphosis, eventually becoming part of Macmillan, and as Ann Castel took the reins as editor, I never felt abandoned or guilty when I could not make our original deadlines. Instead, I received her steady confidence along with the support of a wonderful cadre of reviewers—Lynn S. Bliss, Wayne State University; Cheryl D. Gunter, Iowa State University; Mareile Koenig, West Chester University; Marilyn A. Nippold, University of Oregon; Kenneth G. Shipley, California State University–Fresno; and Carol Stoel-Gammon, University of Washington— who read outlines and early drafts, wrote words of criticism, praise, and encouragement, and saved me from a few embarrassing mistakes. They have my appreciation, as do copyeditor Luanne Dreyer Elliot and production editor Jonathan Lawrence.

Another part of the cast is the set of colleagues and close friends known to me but too broad a group to name in full. They listened to me gripe and wax enthusiastic; shared their libraries, references, and prepublication copies of their work; took my phone calls at all hours; stimulated my thinking; and made me look at old ideas in new ways. You will recognize some of them from the impact they had on the ideas represented in this book. I have tried to give them scholarly credit, but I also want them to feel my personal appreciation for making this project a lot more fun.

A third set of active participants is the group of graduate students who endured bad photocopies and missing tables and figures to read early versions of the chapters and give me feedback. It was hard for them to accept that I actually wanted them to take the red pencil to their professor's writing, but their comments and questions were important in making the book more relevant as a learning tool. They were the primary audience peeking over my shoulder when I wrote.

It was a crowded shoulder. Charles Van Riper, who still lives down the road, was also there frequently in my mind, reminding me that I was writing about people, for people, including those "in the trenches."

This, then, is the cast who supported the primary characters. The leading roles in this book are held by the individuals with communicative disorders, their families, and the people who work with them directly— those who really are "in the trenches." Because of this, I particularly appreciate the opportunities that practitioner colleagues and graduate student clinicians gave me to share in their real-life experiences while I was writing. They kept my feet on the ground.

For the most part, I have avoided naming names in these lists because there are so many. However, a few individuals took a stagehand role and helped me with the nitty-gritty details of matching citations and references, preparing tables and figures, and working late hours when I needed an extra pair of hands. The graduate assistants who played that role include Janet Sturm, Whitney Gagnon, Sherry Joines, Sally Ricketson, Andrea Behrns, Kim Robinson, Kelly Wenzler and Alison Wilson. Without their intelligent problem solving and ready laughter, I would be a lot less sane.

Finally, my family tolerated a wife and mother who seemed glued to the computer, spread books and papers everywhere, and never was much of a cook anyway. My sister, Theresa Wolf Baumgartner, was a godsend when she visited in the final stages of writing and manuscript preparation (at that point, I decided that a live-in editor would be even better than a live-in maid). I want her to know I appreciate it. To Larry, David, Nicky, and Clayton I give my love and appreciation for letting me get into things like this without too much complaining. Last, but first, there are the others—my parents and grandmothers who came before. This book dedicated to them.

Contents

PART ONE
**Viewing Childhood Language Disorders from
Varied Perspectives   1**

CHAPTER 1
A Framework   5

The Importance of Asking Questions   6

The Question of Purpose   8

The Forest and the Trees Problem (and How to
    Avoid It)   8
    What Is Wrong Within the Person? Defining
        Impairment   8
    What Does the Person Need? Defining
        Disability   10
    What Participation Opportunities Does the
        Person Have? Defining Handicap   12
    Examining Our Mistakes and Learning From
        Them—Factors Contributing to Failure   15

Strategies for Changing Systems   18
    System Theory and Ecological Thinking   18
    Phenomenology—A Philosophical
        Perspective   20
    Collaborative Consultation and Cooperative Goal
        Setting   21
    Ethnographic Methodology   22

Summary   23

CHAPTER 2
Language, Speech, and Communication   25

Multidisciplinary Perspectives   26

The Linkage of Language, Speech, and
    Communication   27
    Language   27
    Speech and Other Modalities   28
    Communication   29

The Nature of Language   33
    Bilingualism and Dialect Differences   33
    The Subcomponents of Language   35
    Assessing Knowledge of the Rule Systems of
        Language   48

Communication as Social Interaction   51
    The Importance of Context   52
    Reasons for Communicating   53
    Playing the Discourse Game by Different
        Rules   53

Summary   54

CHAPTER 3
Language Acquisition Theories   56

Biological Maturation   57
    Cerebral Asymmetries   58
    Brain Weight Changes During Normal
        Development   59
    Neuronal Growth Patterns   60
    Roles of Nature and Nurture in Brain
        Development Revisited   60

Linguistic Rule Induction   61

Behaviorism   62
    Behaviorist Explanations of the Acquisition of
        Phonological Characteristics   63

Behaviorist Explanations of the Acquistion of
    Words   64
Behaviorist Explanations of the Acquistion of
    Sentences   64
Behaviorist Explanations of the Acquistion of
    Varied Functions   64
The Importance of Environmental Factors—
    Issues of Nature and Nurture Revisited   65
Information Processing   65
    Parallel Distributed Processing Models   66
    Explanations for Individual Differences and
        Language Universals Revisited   66
Cognitivism   67
    Thought and Language as Viewed by
        Cognitivists   72
Social Interactionism   72
    Thought and Language—The Chicken and the
        Egg Question Revisited   74
    Social Interaction and Development of the
        Concept of Self   74
    Social Interaction Theory and Later Language
        Development   75
Clinical Implications   75

Summary   77

CHAPTER 4
Causes, Categories, and Contributing
Factors   78

The Elusiveness of Cause   79
    A Definition of Language Disorders   79
    Attributes of Causes, Categories, and
        Contributing Factors   80
    To Categorize or Not to Categorize? That Is the
        Question   82
    Problems With a Developmental Focus   83
    Categorization and Prototype Theory   83
    Problems With a Categorical Focus   83
Categorical Conditions Associated With Language
    Disorders   84
Central Processing Factors   85
    Specific Language Disability   85

Mental Retardation   98
Autism   103
Attention-Deficit Hyperactivity Disorder   110
Acquired Brain Injury   115
Other Central Factors   122
Peripheral Sensory and Motor System
    Factors   123
    Hearing Impairment   123
    Visual Impairment   131
    Physical Impairment and Speech Motor
        Control   134
Environmental and Emotional Factors   139
    Neglect and Abuse   139
    Behavioral and Emotional Development
        Problems   143
Mixed Factors and Changes Over Time   149

Summary   150
    Prevention of Childhood Language
        Disorders   151

CHAPTER 5
Public Policy and Service Delivery   152

Public Policy Influences   153
    Federal Policy   153
    State Policy   162
    Intermediate Policy   162
    Local Policy   163
    Implications of Knowing About Policy and How
        It Is Made   163
Service Delivery   164
    Setting Variables   164
    People Variables   171
    Scheduling Variables   180
Summary   186

CHAPTER 6
Making Assessment and Intervention Work for
Children   187

A Sequence of Questions   188

Theoretical Perspectives Guiding Assessment and
    Intervention Practices   194

    Biological Maturation Theory Influences   194
    Linguistic Rule-Induction Theory
        Influences   196
    Behaviorist Theory Influences   200
    Information Processing Theory Influences   205
    Cognitivist Theory Influences   209
    Social Interaction Theory Influences   211
    Integrating Influences From Six Theoretical
        Perspectives   213
Assessment and Intervention as Integrated
        Processes   214
    Using Team Contributions Effectively
    Using Assessment to Diagnose Disorder   215
    Using Assement to Determine Eligibility for
        Service   219
    Using Assessment to Establish a
        Prognosis   233
    Using Assessment to Outline the Parameters of
        Impairment, Disability, and Handicap   238
    Selecting Goal Areas and Gathering Baseline
        Data   240
    Designing and Implementing an Intervention
        Plan   244
    Monitoring Progress During Intervention   249
    Using Exit Criteria to Decide When to
        Quit   252
    Judging Program Accountability   253
Summary   254

PART TWO
Balancing Ages and Developmental
Stages   255

CHAPTER 7
Early Stages   258

**Children Needing Intervention Aimed at Early-
    Stage Developments   260**

Identifying Infants at Risk for Developmental
        Problems   260

    Risk Factors and Early Identification   260

Child-Find Efforts and Screening   262
Identifying Children With Severe Communicative
        Impairments Who Need Language
        Intervention and Augmentative and Alternative
        Communication Services   263
**Measuring Early-Stage Abilities, Needs, and
    Accomplishments   266**
Contexts for Early Stage Assessment and
        Intervention   266

    Hospital   266
    Home   266
    Infant Center or Clinic   266
    Classroom   267
    A Family Systems Approach to Early-Stage
        Assessment   267
    Models for Assessing Older Children With
        Early-Stage Abilities   268
    Tools and Strategies for Early-Stage
        Assessment   276
    Formal Assessment Tools   276
    Informal Procedures: Blurring the Boundaries
        Between Assessment and
        Intervention   278

**Methods and Targets of Early-Stage
    Intervention   281**

Getting the Basics Together   282

    Organization and Early Sensing of Care and
        Safety   282
    Establishing Mutual Communicative Efficacy
        and Reciprocal "Dialogues"   282
    Early Vocal and Phonological Behavior   284
    Early Feeding Behaviors and Needs   287
    Early Comprehension of Routines and Making
        Sense of Events in the World   290
    Reciprocation, Imitation, and Scaffolding   292
Intentionality and Early Communicative
        Functions   293

    Effects of Context on Early Comments and
        Requests   293
    Ranges of Communicative Functions Expected
        at Different Levels   297
    Aberrant Expression of Communicative
        Intentions by Children With Profound
        Disabilities   297

Limited Expression of Communicative
Functions by Persons With Profound
Disabilities   300

Early Symbols   302

How Children Appear to Learn Early
Words   303
Assessing Early Word Knowledge   304
Word, Referents, and Meanings: Selecting
Symbol Systems   304
Symbol Learning by Individuals With Profound
Impairments   305
Selecting Words to Target in Intervention:
The Meanings and Functions of First
Words   306
Potential Problems With Early Word
Acquisition   308

Encoding Semantic Relations and Combining Two
Words to Do More   310

Specialized Assessment Techniques for Early
Multiword Utterances   310
Targets and Methods of Intervention at the
Two-Word Stage   311

Parental Roles in Helping Children Go Beyond the
Here-and-Now   314

Early Learning About Literacy   316

Building More Complex Ideas Through Play   317

Developments in Decentering, Object
Symbolism, and Social Relations in
Play   318
Targeting Play Skills in Intervention   318

Making Speech More Clear   322

Summary   323

CHAPTER 8
Middle Stages   324

Children Needing Intervention Aimed at
Middle-Stage Developments   327

Identifying Language Disorders in the Middle
Stages   327

Child-Find Efforts and Preschool
Screening   327

Prekindergarten Screening   329
Early Elementary School Referral Criteria   329
Considering the Middle-Stage Needs of
Individuals With Multiple and Severe
Disabilities   331
Summary   333

Measurement of Middle-Stage Abilities, Needs,
and Accomplishments   334

Contexts for Middle-Stage Assessment and
Intervention   334

The Continuing Importance of the Family and
the Child's Primary Culture   334
Increased Interactions With Peers   335
Making the Shift From Home to School in the
Preschool Years and Kindergarten   335
The Elementary School Classroom as a Context
for Language Learning and Use   336

Tools and Strategies for Middle-Stage
Assessment   340

Gathering Background Information for
Contextually Based Assessment
Language Sampling and Other Informal
Assessment Techniques   341
Formal Assessment   358

Methods and Targets of Middle-Stage
Intervention   360

Roles of Adult Partners and Contexts in Language
Intervention   360

Modifying Parent Discourse as Part of
Intervention   360
Modifying Teacher Discourse as Part of
Intervention   362
Enhance the Auditory Language-Learning
Context   363

Developing Skills in Symbolic Play   365

Using Language to Accomplish Expanded
Conversational Purposes   366

Goals Related to Individual Patterns of
Communication   366
Making Requests   366
Being Polite   368
Taking Turns, Managing Topics, and Making
Repairs   368

Pragmatic Functions   370

Producing and Comprehending More Complex
     Content–Form Constructions   371

Producing More Complex Content–Form
     Constructions   371
Comprehending More Complex Content–Form
     Constructions   376
Content, Contexts, and Strategies for
     Content–Form Intervention   378

Continued Phonological Development   379

Acquiring and Recalling Words and
     Concepts   379

Building a Lexicon: Fast Mapping and Other
     Processes   379
Intervention for Word-Finding
     Impairments   381

Participating in Storytelling: Emerging
     Literacy   382

Beginning School   385

The Early Stages of Learning to Read   385
The Early Stages of Learning to Write   387
Other Uses of Language in Classrooms   389

Functional Goals for Older Students at Middle
     Stages   390

Summary   392

CHAPTER 9
Later Stages   393

Children Needing Intervention Aimed at Later
     Stage Developments   397

Identifying Language Disorders in the Later
     Stages   397

Screening   398
Referral   399
Considering the Later Stage Needs of
     Individuals With Multiple and Severe
     Disabilities   400

Measuring Later Stage Needs and
     Abilities   400

Contexts for Later Stage Assessment and
     Intervention   400

Changing Roles of the Family and Continued
     Influence of the Primary Culture   403
Increased Interactions With Peers   404
Influences of Cultural and Language
     Mismatches at School   404
Participating in Nonschool Contexts   406
Transitions to Higher Education, Employment,
     and Other Postschool Activities   406

Tools and Strategies for Later Stage
     Assessment   407

Gathering Background Information for
     Contextually Based Assessment   407
Formal Assessment in the Later Stages
     407
Informal Assessment in Later Stages   408

Summary   433

Methods and Targets of Later Stage
     Intervention   434

Modifying Language Learning Contexts   435

Starting With Respect for Sociocultural
     Backgrounds of Learners   435
Using Mediational Discourse in Curriculum-
     Based Language Intervention   436
Mediated Reading and Miscue Analysis   438
Using Other Strategies to Modify the Language
     Learning Contexts of Classrooms   439

Fostering "Metaskills" and Other Executive
     Strategies   440

The Prevalence of Learning Strategies
     Models   440
The Rationale for Learning Strategies
     Models   440
Using Metapragmatic Strategies to Develop
     School Survival Skills   441
Using Metacognitive Strategies to Improve
     Memory and Higher Order Thinking   443
Using Metacognitive, Metalinguistic, and
     Metatextual Strategies to Focus on Process
     Rather Than Product   466
Summary of Metaskills and How to Teach
     Them   450

Developing Competence in Varied Discourse
     Genres and Events   451

Interacting for Business or Pleasure: The
     Conversational Genre   451
Understanding and Telling Stories: The
     Narrative Genre   458
Getting and Giving Information: The Expository
     Genre   461
Summary   468
Encouraging Later Stage Syntactic–Semantic
     Developments   468

Problems of Later Stage Syntactic
     Development   469
Judging Level of Syntactic Development   469
Potential Targets and Methods for Later Stage
     Syntactic Intervention Programs   469
Developing Abstract and Nonliteral
     Meanings   474

Acquiring a Literate Lexicon   474
Figurative Language   478
Helping Individuals With Severe Disabilities Move
     Into Adulthood   480

Providing Equal Opportunity   480
Facilitating Transitions   484
Fostering Independence   484
Summary   486

APPENDIX A
Annotated Bibliography of Selected Screening
and Assessment Tools Appropriate for
Measuring Three Stages of Language
Development   487

APPENDIX B
Summary and Reference Charts to Use in Making
Service-Delivery and Augmentative and Alternative
Communication Decisions About Children With
Severe Communication Impairments   501

APPENDIX C
Developmental Sentence Scoring and Black
English Sentence Scoring   509

REFERENCES   521

AUTHOR INDEX   571

SUBJECT INDEX   581

PART ONE

Viewing Childhood Language Disorders from Varied Perspectives

Part I lays the foundation for understanding the needs of children with language disorders. The dominant perspective is developmental, in preparation for the second part of the book, which is organized into three chapters covering early, middle, and later stages of language learning. The developmental perspective, however, is only one of several that can be used when working with children with language disorders.

Other perspectives considered in Part I relate to general concerns that extend across developmental ages and stages. Chapter 1 builds a basic framework for working with children with language disorders and their families and teachers. It introduces the importance of asking questions and presents a framework of questions to address the needs of these children. The traditional question about *impairment*, "What is wrong with the way this person processes language?" should be supplemented by questions about *disability*, "What does this person need to do to succeed in this particular context?" and *handicap*, "What opportunities does the person have to participate in desired contexts?" (Beukelman & Mirenda, 1992).

The focus on contextually based need is important for exceeding the limitations of strictly developmental approaches for assessment and treatment. This focus is part of treating these children as members of whole systems, rather than fragmenting them into a collection of separable parts. The "fragmentation fallacy" (Damico, 1988) is one of several potential problems that language specialists should avoid. Others, also suggested by Damico and considered in Chapter 1, are therapist bias, acquiescence, lack of follow-up, and negative effects of bureaucratic policies and procedures.

Strategies for avoiding these mistakes are suggested, using **system theory** as a general framework and tools borrowed from several other disciplines. **Ecological**

thinking, borrowed from biology, is critical for understanding the contextual nature of change and the interactive influences at all levels of environmental and biological systems. **Phenomenology,** borrowed from philosophy, is critical for understanding the relativity of truth and the influence of observational perspectives and tools on how truth is perceived by different observers of the same event or person. **Collaborative consultation** and **cooperative goal setting**, borrowed from educational theorists and group managers, are critical tools for creating change within larger systems. **Ethnographic methodology,** borrowed from anthropologists, is critical for understanding a culture, whether an ethnic group or an elementary school classroom, through the eyes of its participants. These tools provide a framework for considering the information about childhood language disorders in the rest of the book.

Chapter 2 addresses questions about multidisciplinary perspectives regarding language, speech, and communication. The strong linkages of language, speech, and communication are stressed, but evidence of some degree of isolation of each is presented as well. This chapter suggests that professionals should be clear about the relative impairment and retention of speech, language, and communication variables when working with children with language disorders. Chapter 2 reviews basic organizational principles about language rule systems and nonlinguistic and paralinguistic communicative features. (Readers with a strong background in linguistics and communication theory may wish to skim these sections.) The reviews summarize key aspects of systems that children must learn to become competent communicators; later chapters consider evidence about what can go wrong with those systems. Because not all children learn the same language, speech, and communication systems, issues regarding dialect and language differences are also considered here. Summaries of key features follow in the areas of phonology, morphology, syntax, semantics, and pragmatics, plus traditional methods for measuring knowledge of linguistic rule systems. Here, the key distinction is between naturalistic methods that assess **intrinsic knowledge** of linguistic rules, by inferring regularities based on observable evidence such as spontaneous language samples, and controlled methods that assess **metalinguistic knowledge,** by asking individuals to reflect on and to talk about language. Chapter 2 ends with an overview of sociolinguistic contributions related to the importance of context, reasons for communicating, and cultural variation in discourse interactions.

Chapter 3 explores varied developmental perspectives in preparation for considering multiple aspects of assessment and intervention services for children with language disorders. Contributions from six theoretical perspectives are considered: (1) **biological maturation,** (2) **linguistic rule induction,** (3) **behaviorism,** (4) **information processing,** (5) **cognitivism,** and (6) **social interaction.** These six theoretical categories are used again in Chapters 4 and 6 to organize discussions of language disorders, their causes, assessment, and treatment. Readers who have internalized some of the key characteristics of each theoretical perspective from Chapter 3 will find it easier to read those later chapters and the sections on early, middle, and later stage language disorders in Part II.

Chapter 4 explores categorical views of childhood language disorders. This is a touchy area because there are advantages and disadvantages to applying labels to problems. Labels can stereotype children and can seem to reduce the need for individualization. Labels do not always accurately predict an individual child's language abilities and needs, and care must be taken so that labels do not function as blinders. On the other hand, knowledge of labels, and the causative conditions they represent, can open doors to past learning about those conditions and can even reduce the likelihood of repeating previous mistakes. The chapter begins with a discussion of causes, categories, and contributing factors, emphasizing that they are heterogeneous, changeable, layered, multifaceted and interactive, and elusive.

The categorical system used in Chapter 4 is divided into three major sections: (1) central factors, (2) peripheral factors, and (3) environmental–emotional factors. The first grouping includes **specific language disability** (including conditions labeled as learning disabilities and dyslexia), **mental retardation, attention-deficit hyperactive disorder**, and **acquired brain injury**. The second grouping includes **hearing, visual,** and **physical impairments**. The third grouping includes **child neglect and abuse** and **behavioral–emotional impairment**. Mixed factors are also considered. A unique feature of this chapter is the repeated use of the six theoretical perspectives introduced in Chapter 3 to discuss the varied symptoms associated with each causative condition. I suggest that factors associated with biological structures, linguistic rule learning, stimulus–response reinforcement patterns, information processing, cognition, and social interaction are involved to varying degrees in each disorder. Table 4.1 summarizes the relative weights that I assign to the six factors. These might be somewhat controversial. I hope they stimulate readers to think, discuss, and even argue about the assignments I have made. Particularly, I hope that they will stimulate readers to think about the relative fit of varied factors and theories for explaining conditions observed among real people and to examine the theoretical underpinnings of their own assessment and intervention practices with all kinds of children.

Chapter 5 addresses questions about public policy and service delivery. The public policy sections are based on laws and regulations in the United States related to service provision in schools. The service-delivery system is divided into federal, state, intermediate, and local levels. I recognize that readers from other countries and nonschool settings must learn about different public policy systems that apply to them; perhaps the public policy portion of this chapter will provide a framework for doing so, even if it does not apply directly to everyone's needs. The second part of Chapter 5 is a more generic discussion of service-delivery variables and it is divided into three major sections: (1) setting, (2) people, and (3) scheduling. Preferences of children and their parents regarding service-delivery decisions are also considered.

The final chapter in Part I, Chapter 6, overviews factors related to assessment and intervention. It starts with a decision-making flowchart (Figure 6.1) that characterizes the major stages in providing services to children and a sequence of questions asked from the time concern is voiced until the child appears no longer to need special services. After consideration of the sequence of steps for an individual infant, child, or adolescent, the contributions and limitations of the six theoretical perspectives introduced in Chapter 3 are related to assessment and intervention practices. The remainder of the chapter describes procedures to implement assessment and intervention as an integrated process. Assessment topics include using team process and assessment activities to diagnose disorder, to determine eligibility for service, to establish prognosis, and to outline parameters of impairment, disability, and handicap. Intervention topics include selecting goal areas and gathering baseline data, designing and implementing an intervention plan, monitoring progress during intervention, using exit criteria to determine when to quit, and judging program accountability.

Part I sets the stage for Part II, which considers early, middle, and later stage language disorders. The questions and information in Part I are intended to assist readers to develop rich perspectives for looking at developmental needs in Part II. Both parts are designed to encourage an appreciation of the guiding principle of this book: Problems are not just within children—and neither are their solutions.

1

A Framework

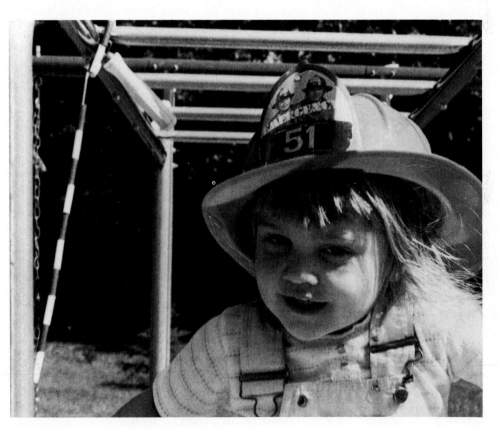

The Importance of
Asking Questions

The Question of
Purpose

The Forest and the
Trees Problem (and
How to Avoid It)

Strategies for
Changing Systems

> ❏   What is wrong (and right) here?
>
> ❏   What does the child need?
>
> ❏   What are the opportunities for participation?

THE IMPORTANCE OF ASKING QUESTIONS

This is a book about childhood language disorders. It is not only an academic description of conditions and effects but is an attempt to influence intervention services for children with language disorders to improve their lives. It is a book about collaborating and, as such, is more about the need to ask good questions than about providing all of the answers.

The importance of asking good questions became clear to me in a new way as I prepared to write this book and encountered Richard Saul Wurman's (1989) text, *Information Anxiety* (see Personal Reflection 1.1). The title of Wurman's book was especially meaningful as I contemplated trying to cover, in a single text, the pertinent information regarding childhood language disorders and related aspects of normal development. I imagined the attempt would be a bit like stuffing an octopus into a box; just when you think you have it contained, another leg pops out. The idea of viewing information management as a process of organizing knowledge in the framework of questions rather than as data banks of facts had considerable appeal.

The ability to ask good questions is a key to the advancement of both science and clinical practice. Background knowledge and the use of highly developed technological skills play relatively minor roles in the scientific process compared to the ability to frame good questions. Background information can be found in books, and research assistants can be hired to gather data, but scientists will never lead the way to truly new discoveries unless they ask insightful questions. The best scientists ask questions of the type that guide others to see the world in a new way.

The same is true of good clinicians and of good teachers. The best diagnosticians are not those who know how to administer standardized tests to perfection but are those who know how to ask the best questions—questions that will lead them to select appropriate procedures, tools, and contexts for assessment, which in turn, will produce additional good questions about what should be done in the intervention process. Good clinicians and teachers can guide themselves and others concerned to view a problem in a new way (referrals generally result when old ways are not working), and they often do it by asking good questions.

Similarly, teachers who are truly effective as educators view their work more as question posing than as information transfer. Recently, a colleague shared with me a cartoon in which two little boys are standing next to a dog. One boy says to the other, "I taught this dog how to whistle." The other boy, staring into the dog's unchanging face, says, "I don't hear him whistling." In the final frame, the first child speaks again, "I said I taught him. I didn't say he learned it."

Effective teachers ask such questions as, "What is important for my students to know in this area? How will I help them learn it? Are they getting it? What parts are still confusing to them? Does it matter? In what contexts does it matter?" Effective teachers view themselves not so much as being in the business of transferring information or "getting through" the curriculum as having the responsibility to help students to become learners (see Personal Reflection 1.2).

As language specialists, our role is also shaped best by the questions we ask. Those questions determine the things we pay attention to, and in many

---

Personal Reflection 1.2   "Teaching is not telling. Being told is not being taught."

David Johnson, Educational Psychologist from the University of Minnesota, speaking at a workshop at Western Michigan University (D. Johnson, 1989). David Johnson and his brother, Roger, have been primary contributors to the development of cooperative learning strategies (e.g., D. W. Johnson & Johnson, 1975).

ways, influence how we work. To a large extent, the work of language intervention involves facilitating others to ask good questions as well.

For example, a major objective of work with language-learning impaired school-age children may be to assist them to comprehend the language of education to facilitate comprehension of the world in the broader sense. During the process, the language specialist starts by asking questions that focus interactions and that direct the student's attention to features of language and to concepts that may not have been apparent to the student before. In this way, the language interventionist builds a scaffold that allows the child or adolescent to obtain access to language and learning events that were previously out of reach. But it cannot stop there. It is important to build the scaffold, but also to take it down, dismantling it carefully, so that the client can function independently without falling flat.

How is that to be done? School-age children become independent when they begin to ask the same sorts of questions that the language specialist has posed. What is needed is a "question transplant." The student needs to start asking such questions as, "What am I supposed to do here? Does this make sense? What does this mean? How does this work? Am I doing this right? Can I do this better? How is this organized? What happens next?" In fact, when I work with school-age language-learning impaired children, one of the things I try to do is to help them use their own "thinking language," which is a form of verbal mediation that I model first for them and then expect them to use to direct their own learning.

This kind of questioning fosters metacognition. *Metacognition* is a conscious awareness of the thinking process (discussed further in Chapter 9). Students must acquire this awareness if they are to acquire *strategies* that will help them direct their own learning processes. The ability to direct one's own attention with questions is clearly important to students who want to compete academically. But what about very young or severely impaired individuals who have difficulty grasping concepts of cognitive self-control or forming linguistically oriented questions? Even then, the words of psycholinguist Frank Smith (1975) (see Personal Reflection 1.3) regarding questions and attention are applicable.

Consider the infant just beginning to make sense of the world. How do babies come to associate sounds with meaning? When a baby begins to pay attention to sounds, such as someone coming in the house through the back door, and to recognize those sounds as possibly having meaning, it is as if the baby is thinking, "What is that? Isn't that something pleasant? Is that my daddy?" Even though, in the early phases of learning, such "questions" are not couched in linguistic terms, the recognition of familiar events and the act of weaving them into organized cognitive perceptions hinges on the natural curiosity of normally developing children. Perhaps this is why the old therapy technique of teaching severely impaired children to "look at me" to be reinforced with some kind of tangible reward was never enough. The mere *appearance* of attention, although it may orient children so that deeper levels of processing have a greater chance of occurring, is not the same as the

Personal Reflection 1.3   "Attention is perhaps best conceptualized as questions being asked by the brain, and our perceptions are what the brain decides must be the answers."

Frank Smith (1975, p. 28).

Box 1.1   The purpose of language intervention

To bring about change in the communicative systems of individuals, and in the important communicative contexts of their lives, that are relevant to their needs for

❑ Social appropriateness, acceptance, and closeness
❑ Formal and informal learning
❑ Gainful occupation (whether paid or unpaid)

---

focused attention that children demonstrate when they want to see or learn or do something. Even with babies, intervention is likely to be most effective if the stage can be set so that their brains will begin to ask questions, to seek regularities in the world and in the language used to represent it, and to communicate.

THE QUESTION OF PURPOSE

Perhaps the most important question language specialists should ask is the question of purpose—"What am I trying to accomplish here?" It should never be far from the language interventionist's mind. Although the ultimate purpose of language intervention may be to facilitate normal functioning, that is not always possible. Some children have such severely impaired biological and neurological systems that they will never support the development of normal language functioning. Given this disparity, can a general statement of purpose be established for language intervention—one that would be appropriate no matter how severe the communicative impairment?

The statement of purpose in Box 1.1 represents such an attempt. It is designed to focus on both change and relevance within the three communicative contexts that are important across the age span—social, educational, and vocational (or avocational). Change is central to the process; if it were not needed, the services of a language interventionist would not have been enlisted. Change should remain a focus of daily efforts and should be measured in systematic ways relevant to a particular person's needs. The questions directing the therapeutic process then shift from "What am I going to do today with this person?" to "What needs to be changed if life is to improve for this person?" The process is also tempered by the question, "What can be changed here?" In addition, it is important to keep in mind the communicative contexts in which change is needed

so that one does not lose sight of the forest for the trees. Clinicians can easily become so absorbed in efforts to "fix" isolated language and speech behaviors that they lose sight of the whole picture. The forest and the trees problem is a classic one in clinical intervention for language disorders.

THE FOREST AND THE TREES PROBLEM (AND HOW TO AVOID IT)

The need to maintain perspective arises partly because language and communicative behaviors can be analyzed into component parts and processes. A traditional approach in language intervention has been to analyze a person's linguistic skills, usually relative to some normative standard, and then to design intervention activities to facilitate the acquisition of missing or delayed skills. Beukelman and Mirenda (1988, 1992) called this assessment approach the *communication processes model* and contrasted it with two other models, a *communication needs model* and a *participation model*. Avoiding the forest and the trees problem requires use of all three of these models to guide processes of language assessment and intervention. Each asks a different critical question that is uniquely related to definitions of impairment, disability, or handicap.

What Is Wrong Within The Person? Defining Impairment

In the communication processes model (Beukelman & Mirenda, 1988), the primary question is "What is wrong *within* the individual?" This model is designed to ask questions about impairment.

Impairment, as defined by the World Health Organization, is "any loss or abnormality of psychological, physiological, or anatomical structure or function" (Wood, 1980, p. 4). Essentially, the questions asked when implementing the communication processes model are, "What is wrong here?" and "Can it be fixed?"

Although it is less often articulated, a related question that should be asked when using a communication processes model to guide clinical practice is, "What is right with this individual?" "What skills and abilities does this person have that can be used to make the intervention work?"

Because the communication processes model is the one most frequently used in providing traditional intervention services, it will be covered in greater detail in later chapters. Here, it is sufficient to describe this approach as one in which an individual's language skills are analyzed, often as relatively separate components within the categories of phonology, morphology, syntax, semantics, and pragmatics (see Chapter 2 for explanation of these rule systems). In most cases, such rule systems are observed by using specially designed tasks presented in carefully controlled contexts, often as components of standardized tests.

The problem with such an approach is that, rather than simply controlling contextual variables, an entirely new context is introduced that is unlike almost any other in which the individual participates. This results in an attempt to define the parameters of a person's language-related difficulties using tasks that alter the essence of those difficulties as they occur in real-life contexts.

Part of the problem seems to stem from an attitude adopted by clinicians from researchers that "universal truths" can only be demonstrated when they occur in all contexts. Therefore, when using traditional models, researchers and clinicians act as if they can conduct their work properly only if they can strip away contextual variability and still demonstrate the phenomenon of interest. In an article called "Meaning in Context: Is There Any Other Kind?," Mishler (1979) pointed out the fallacies of such context-stripping approaches. He noted that in everyday interactions, we humans "rely on context to understand the behavior and speech of others and to ensure that our own behavior is understood, implicitly grounding our interpretations of motives and intentions in context" (p. 2) (see also Personal Reflection 1.4).

Recognizing the importance of context, language specialists may be more likely to see impaired communicative processes not as static, measurable elements, but as the outcomes of interactions between internal systems and external contextual expectations. Children therefore may appear to be relatively more or less impaired depending on the nature of a particular task and the current environmental support. In making the communication processes model more relevant, specialists must abandon the basic assumption that language and communication processes can exist as intrinsic entities with unwavering and quantifiable characteristics.

By making a slight shift, however, the description of the communicative processes approach can be expanded to include the evaluation of the child's processing systems when interacting in certain contexts. The key question of this approach then becomes "What is wrong (and right) with the way this child's communicative processes function in these varied contexts?" If the question is phrased in this way, some of the usual pitfalls of the approach can be avoided, while retaining its value.

One way to avoid the pitfalls of the isolated skills assessment approach is to evaluate language processes within the context of spontaneous communicative interactions. The point of spontaneous sampling is to obtain representative evidence of an individual's language abilities in natural interactions. To evaluate babies, language specialists may collect and analyze videotape samples of interactions with different care givers in different contexts. To evaluate preschoolers, they may collect interactive language samples involving play with an unfamiliar adult, conversation with parents, or play with peers. To evaluate school-age children, they may study social interactions with peers or academic interactions in classrooms.

A modified version of the communication processes model may avoid the problem of splintering language processes artificially and studying them in isolated contexts, but alone, it is not enough. It misses a perspective provided by the communication needs model.

What Does the Person Need? Defining Disability

In the communication needs model, as defined by Beukelman and Mirenda (1988, 1992), the focus shifts from what might be wrong (or right) within the person—in terms of knowledge, skills, and sensory and motor processes—to what the person needs to do to function in important life contexts. This model is designed to ask questions about disability.

Disability is defined within the World Health Organization as reduced ability to meet daily living needs. Disability therefore varies in different contexts and life stages (Frey, 1984; Wood, 1980). For example, a person who has dyslexia and cannot read but who functions normally in other ways may only be disabled in certain societies, such as ours, where literacy is valued highly. (Dyslexia is a neurologically-based language-learning disability that involves severe impairment in learning to read.)

This point was illustrated by the eminent neurologist Norman Geschwind (1984), in an address to the Orton Dyslexia Society shortly before his death. The address was published in a collection of three papers providing personal perspectives on disability. The second paper was written by Thomas Mautner (1984), who holds a doctorate in mechanical engineering. Mautner was relieved to be diagnosed with dyslexia as an adult; it explained some troubling occurrences from his youth. The third paper was written by the parent of a young adult technical-trainee whose dyslexia had been severely disabling during his school-age years but was less so now (Hartwig, 1984).

In his unique contribution, Geschwind (1984) described what it was like to grow up as an otherwise normal person who could read and write and speak multiple languages with ease but who could not carry a tune, discriminate two musical tones, tap to a beat, or learn to dance. The only reason that this *dysmusic* person was not considered disabled, Geschwind commented, was that musical abilities are not as central to success in this society as reading is. This fact made the pain only slightly less poignant when the young Geschwind found himself in social situations where he needed those skills, and no one could understand why he could not learn them as easily as they.

Because disability is defined by the contexts in which an individual needs a particular skill or ability,

disability is amenable to intervention either (1) by modifying the expectations of the context or (2) by providing access to the important activity through compensation. When using compensations, a person can accomplish what needs to be done but only by using tools and strategies that differ from those used by individuals without impairments in the same contexts. For example, a nonspeaking person who needs to communicate orally might use a communication board or computerized augmentative communication device. A person who has a severe spelling problem might write with the aid of an electronic spelling device.

Choices must be made wisely about when to reduce disability by modifying contexts and when to reduce it by providing compensatory devices and techniques. It is fairly easy to engineer special contexts where even individuals with severe impairments can succeed. Before placing individuals in isolated "special" contexts, however, intervention teams increasingly are asking questions about the future as well as the present. In the short term, what skills does this person need to participate in classrooms? In the long term, what skills are needed to lead to independent adulthood? At what price come special classrooms in segregated settings, where children can succeed, if they only appear more disabled when they attempt to meet the greater demands of the "real world"? That is the dilemma faced by the mother whose priorities for her child were illustrated by her frustrated comment, "We'll buy him Velcro!" (see Personal Reflection 1.5).

The dilemma of the mother in Personal Reflection 1.5 indicates that questions about what a child with a language disorder needs should be formed with two grammatical clauses: the first, asking about need, and the second, an *if*-clause, stating the contexts important to the child or likely to become important to the child. For example, teams of individuals, including parents, certainly, and children, if appropriate, might ask questions such as "What does this child need if he is going to become an independent young adult?" or "What does this child need if she is going to function in a regular classroom?" Such questions should be balanced with those that ask, "How can we build contexts supportive enough so that a child is willing to risk new tasks and still prepare the child for less supportive contexts?"

A related dilemma is based on the question whether it is better to label a disability overtly or not.

Personal Reflection 1.5

"We'll buy him Velcro!"

Ann Barnes, mother of a child with cerebral palsy, commenting during an exchange with school district personnel about the Individualized Educational Program (IEP) objectives for her son. The school personnel, following a strictly developmental model, told this mother that her son was not close to being ready to work on reading in his special classroom, because dressing came earlier in the developmental sequence, and he could not yet even zip his pants. The boy's mother surveyed the relative merits of what her son needed to do to compete in school, and decided that pants zipping was less necessary (and perhaps impossible, given his motor impairments) than reading, despite its developmental precedence. As a result, she pronounced that his dressing impairment could be minimized through an adaptive device, but that if he did not learn to read, he would be permanently disabled in an area for which he could not easily compensate. (Courtesy of Barbara Hoskins.)

In Thomas Mautner's (1984) case, it is hard to know. Although he eventually became highly successful in mainstream academia, even earning a doctorate, it was not without a great deal of struggle. As mentioned, Mautner was relieved when, at the age of 32 (he earned his doctorate when he was 38), he was finally identified as dyslexic. The discovery occurred when Mautner's wife learned about dyslexia, and the couple recognized the symptoms in him (see Chapter 4 for a description of the symptoms of dyslexia). Based on Mautner's experience, questions arise: Is it better to provide special services in special contexts or not to pull children out of regular classroom experiences? Would Mautner's struggle have been less if the special nature of his learning disability had been recognized earlier in his life and if he had been given special treatment then?

Such questions, although not directly answerable, are important to ask, especially as regular and special educators in America seek to understand the implications of the Regular Education Initiative (REI) (Will, 1986). The REI is considered further in Chapter 5 as one of several governmental influences on the delivery of special services to people with disabilities. Briefly, the initiative is a commitment to "serve as many children as possible in the regular classroom by encouraging a partnership with regular education" (Will, 1986, p. 20). It is part of a broader move nationally to integrate more people with special needs into contexts where they will interact with persons without disabilities.

When considering the advisability of serving children with language impairments in regular education contexts, it is helpful to consider the histories of individuals such as Mautner (1984), whose disability was based on an impairment that was not identified during his childhood. Although his oral and written language difficulties were not called a disability at the time, it was clearly disabling to Mautner not to have the skills he needed to participate in the important contexts of his life.

As a preschooler, Mautner (1984) was identified as having superior intelligence when he scored in the top 2% of the population. This intelligence seems to have carried Mautner through the early grades, where he earned high marks and apparently met all demands in one way or another (despite weak reading and writing skills that were evident in retained samples of his spontaneous work). Only in a couple of contexts did the disability show clearly, and even then it was not recognized as a disability. For example, in the summer after fifth grade, Mautner refused to read a single page of a book even though that had been the direct assignment from the school principal. He decided he would rather take the punishment his parents threatened than to attempt a task for which he knew he did not have the needed skills. He also decided that he would rather take a failing grade than to try to memorize and recite the Gettysburg Address in front of his seventh-grade English class. Yet Mautner continued to earn high marks in math and other subjects. Not until the context changed dramatically did the disability begin to show clearly.

When Mautner entered eighth grade, his parents decided to place him in private school because of overcrowding in the public school. His entrance tests

Personal Reflection 1.6	"I spent four years in the private school doing the minimum amount of work I could get away with, going to summer school, and excelling in sports. During my high school years, friction between my parents and me increased. There were ugly scenes at grade time, and I was constantly told by teachers, administrators, and my parents that my grades would improve if I would stop being so lazy and begin to apply myself. I graduated with a C minus average (a gift) and was mysteriously accepted by a college. I did not want to go to college, and I certainly did not have the academic background or the maturity. However, my parents insisted that I attend college; there was no other choice. My college experience lasted one semester—I flunked out" (pp. 304–305).
	"Being constantly told, 'You are lazy . . . you don't apply yourself . . . if you would only try harder' creates long-term damaging results. It is very difficult to try hard or to apply yourself when you believe you cannot do the work because nothing will 'sink in.' If you are told these things often enough, eventually you will believe what you hear and give up" (p. 310).
	Thomas S. Mautner (1984), mechanical engineer, talking about what it was like as an adolescent to have dyslexia when everybody knew that he was not doing his work, but nobody knew why.

showed that, although his scores in most areas were above average relative to those of students in the public schools, they were average or below when compared with his private school classmates. Mautner's measured IQ also had dropped from the superior range to average. (Concepts related to intelligence and IQ testing, particularly for people with language disorders, are considered in Chapter 3.) An important point is that, in the contexts of the value system of Mautner's home and of the private school he attended during his high school years, he did not possess the linguistic and reading skills expected of him. His problems may have been relatively subtle in some contexts, but in his life, they were highly significant (see Personal Reflection 1.6).

Although Mautner (1984) reported that he eventually pulled himself "out of the failure mode and into the success mode" (p. 310), he also reported anger, not so much at the dyslexia itself, but from the knowledge that his parents and educators could not recognize the problem, for whatever reason, and thus did not give him the help he needed. Instead, they lectured him, established social restrictions, and required him to attend summer school. Thomas Mautner was clearly disabled without being labeled "disabled." In hindsight, he viewed his condition as having been worse for lack of special recognition of the nature of his difficulties.

No one is immune from the "forest and the trees" problem, but often parents ask more relevant questions than professionals. At least they ask different ones. In his article about living with a son who has severe reading and communication problems, Hartwig (1984) phrased the question that is foremost in the minds of many parents, regardless of type of disability or when it is discovered: "What implications does dyslexia [or any other disorder] have to the future success and well-being of my child?" (p. 314).

Contrast Hartwig's (1984) parental question regarding need with the question that motivates most traditional assessment activities, "What is wrong with this child's processing system?" Which question is more relevant? Perhaps the answer is that each is important for its own purpose and probably both are essential if a child's comprehensive needs are to be met. This suggests the need for including varied perspectives in the intervention planning process (see a later section of this chapter).

What Participation Opportunities Does the Person Have? Defining Handicap

In the third type of assessment model described by Beukelman and Mirenda (1988, 1992), the focus shifts again. In the participation model, the focus shifts to the individuals' opportunities to participate in the important contexts of their lives. This model is designed to ask questions about handicap.

Handicap is defined within the World Health Organization as the social disadvantage that results either from impairment or disability. Its extent depends on impairment, disability, and the attitudes and biases of others in contact with the individual (Frey, 1984; Wood, 1980).

Implementation of the participation model is consistent with the philosophical stance, taken throughout this book, that *problems are not just within children—and neither are the solutions.* Questions should be asked regularly about whether intervention contexts provide sufficient opportunity for children to practice communicative skills and abilities needed for participating in the broader social, educational, and vocational contexts of their lives. A philosophy underlying this approach is that if intervention can be provided in the real world, rather than separate from it, individuals with visible handicaps may be less isolated from the rest of society throughout their lives.

Contributions of the participation model to decision making might be viewed on two levels—conservative as well as radical. Advocates of the conservative version seek to exploit participation opportunities present in the child's current context. Advocates of the more radical version seek out (and even demand) opportunities for children with severe disabilities to be included in contexts with persons who are not disabled.

Many communities are beginning to reinterpret the federal requirement in Public Law 94–142 that all children with disabilities must be educated in the least restrictive environment (LRE) (see Chapter 5 for further discussion of policies). The Education for All

Handicapped Children Act (EHA; PL 94–142) was originally passed in 1975. Reflecting changes in labels and definitions, the act has now been reauthorized as the Individuals with Disabilities Education Act (IDEA). Within the act, the definition of LRE for a particular child continues to be left to interpretation by the Individualized Education Planning Committee formed for that child. In many states and communities, the LRE has traditionally been interpreted to mean that children with severe disabilities should have access to specialized facilities and professionals (e.g., physical therapists, occupational therapists, speech-language pathologists, and special educators).

The result of such an interpretation, however, has too often meant that children with severe disabilities have been educated in isolated classrooms and even in isolated buildings, sometimes necessitating long bus rides from their homes. Advocates for full inclusion of all children with disabilities in the schools and classrooms within their home communities have pointed out that segregated contexts do not provide opportunities for children with or without disabilities to interact with each other (Knoll & Meyer, 1987; Ruben, 1988). As a result, such advocates suggest, long-standing biases and attitudes perpetuate situations that exacerbate the severity of disabilities.

Advocates for change note that individuals with disabilities have the right to be integrated within the mainstream, emphasizing the similarity to civil rights movements of the past (Markus, 1988). When applied to decision making about special services for children, *integration* refers to a process whereby children with special needs interact with normally learning children in an ordinary school structure that represents an educational whole (Flynn, 1990).

Attempts to integrate children with severe disabilities into regular education settings represent a dramatic shift away from a philosophy of "change the child" to "adapt the mainstream." This shift in philosophy was expressed by W. Stainback, Stainback, Courtnage, and Jaben (1985):

> In order to foster change in regular education, special educators need to reduce the current emphasis on classifying, labeling, and offering "special" programs for students who do not fit within the present regular education structure. Instead, they should put more emphasis on joining with regular educators to work for a reorganization of regular education itself so that the needs of a wider range of students can be met within the mainstream of regular education. (p. 148)

Integration for children with language disorders is a goal not only during their school-age years but during preschool years as well. Amendments to the federal act that were passed as PL 99–457 have resulted in services being delivered in many states from the moment of birth and in most states between the ages of 3 and 5 years. In addition, services may be delivered to children "at risk" as well as to those with identified disabilities.

Implementing a participation model of assessment that asks questions about opportunity as well as impairment and need is consistent both with the legislative mandate and with recommended practices for infants and toddlers to be assessed as part of family and cultural systems (Bailey & Wolery, 1989; Greenspan et al., 1987). It is also consistent with intervention activities for modifying care-giver/infant interactions to increase communicative opportunities (Greenspan et al., 1987; Odom & Karnes, 1988; Snow, 1984).

An important function of the current advocacy movement is to shake some old stereotypes about special education contexts for children with special needs. It should lead us away from the strategy of testing and labeling children and then placing them in

---

Personal Reflection 1.9

"For years . . . we have maintained a public policy of protectionism toward people with disabilities. We have created monoliths of isolated care in institutions and in segregated education settings. It is that isolation and segregation that has become the basis of the discrimination faced by many disabled people today. Separate is not equal. It wasn't for blacks; it isn't for the disabled."

Lowell Weicker, former U.S. Senator, making the connection between full inclusion and other civil rights movements explicit when testifying in support of the Americans with Disability Act (quoted by Blackstone, 1989, p. 17).

service-delivery models, classrooms, and even school buildings simply by matching labels. A new flexibility in decision making may benefit many children with language disorders and other disabilities by focusing on their opportunities to participate.

That promise, however, is not a foregone conclusion. If instituted as a blanket policy, this approach has the same potential as any other to overlook the needs of individual children and to reduce the continuum of services available to them. Some parents and professionals also express concerns that if the bandwagon rolls too quickly, and without adequate preparation, existing attitudes and methods may preclude its success. Others worry that the movement may simply represent a swing of the pendulum to former times when the needs of their children for individualized programming were not recognized and they were left to fail in regular classrooms (as Tom Mautner was). For many children with severe disabilities, however, the difference was that, in those days, they were not allowed to go to school.

Examining Our Mistakes and Learning From Them—Factors Contributing to Failure

The forest and the trees problem is based on the premise that holistic needs of language-impaired children will not be met if intervention and education practices become bogged down in piecemeal definitions and activities. It is also possible to lose sight of the trees for the forest. That sometimes happens to administrators of large programs when they become so involved with looking at enrollment figures and program costs that they tend to lose sight of individual children.

Thus far in this chapter, I have suggested that both problems can be avoided by asking questions about desired outcomes and by using differential perspectives to illuminate communication processes, needs, and opportunities. Another strategy for avoiding problems is to look at what happens when things do not work as planned. Learning from mistakes was the courageous approach taken by Jack Damico (1988) in the case study summarized in Box 1.2.

What went wrong in Debbie's case? Damico (1988) identified five factors that contributed to the failure (additional factors are identified relative to the perspectives discussed in this chapter): (1) the fragmentation fallacy, (2) therapist bias, (3) acquiescence, (4) lack of follow-up, and (5) bureaucratic policies and procedures.

The fragmentation fallacy. As described by Damico (1988), the fragmentation fallacy arises out of discrete-point approaches to assessment. Such approaches are related to the communication processes model (Beukelman & Mirenda, 1988, 1992), discussed earlier. They are based on modular models of language proficiency in which the various subcomponents of language (phonology, morphology, syntax, semantics, and pragmatics) are viewed as discrete "modules" that can be evaluated and treated separately. This approach results in fragmentation because it "breaks the elements of language apart and tries to test them separately with little or no attention to the way those elements interact in a larger context of communication" (Damico, 1988, p. 56). Modular views can be contrasted with molar views of language as a system that can be understood only in the contexts of real communicative interactions, not contrived tasks. Although quantifiable, contrived tasks often act to trivialize language in ways that make it lose its essence. The fragmentation fallacy might have been avoided in Debbie's case by asking comprehensive questions about the skills she would need in the social and educational contexts of school, and about opportunities for her to develop and use those skills in the important contexts of her life.

Therapist bias. The problem Damico (1988) identified as therapist bias is tied to theories of cognitive dissonance. According to such theories, therapists internalize a view of their client as a cognitive structure and tend to filter and reinterpret evidence contrary to that view to eliminate dissonance with it. Therapist bias can have two kinds of effects (Nisbett & Wilson, 1977). Based on the halo effect, the therapist sees results of therapy as more positive than they actually are. Based on the Rosenthal effect, the therapist actually introduces subtle, and often unconscious, biasing factors into the collection, analysis, and interpretation of data.

Types and levels of impairment, stages of development, communicative needs, and contextual demands and opportunities all enter into decisions about intervention. Fragmentation and therapist bias are less likely to occur when language and communication skills are observed as whole systems in real-life contexts that shift with the child's age—rather than as isolated sets of behaviors that remain relatively static over time. Language specialists cannot afford to adopt a theoretical stance that any one aspect of lan-

Box 1.2   Damico's example of failed language intervention

Debbie was first seen by Damico in 1976, during her first-grade year, for a language problem that her teacher described as "lack of correct pronouns and the omission of words during conversation" (p. 52). Damico described Debbie as a sociable child of well-educated, involved parents. She made frequent eye contact with the examiner and was curious and readily engaged in the assessment tasks. Her scores on most standardized measures, however, were below her chronological age level. In addition, Debbie's spontaneous language sample included an error rate higher than 40% for some grammatical forms, including pronoun case substitutions (e.g., *her* for *she*), omitted auxiliary verbs (e.g., "The dog running"), and irregular plurals (e.g., *womens* for *women*) and past-tense markers (e.g., *comed* for *came*). Further analysis of the language sample showed 34 instances of "semantic confusion" in which Debbie used excessive generic terms (e.g., *stuff* and *thing*) or misused deictic terms when referring to concepts of space (e.g., *here* versus *there*), time (e.g., *tomorrow* versus *today*), or person (*I* versus *you*).

For the remainder of her first-grade year, Debbie participated in a traditional language-intervention program that was designed to target her grammatical form problems and did not address semantic confusions. At the end of the period, although Debbie's grammatical errors had not disappeared entirely, her error rate involving grammatical forms in spontaneous language sampling had dropped significantly, while her mean length of utterance remained at 5.0. These findings were taken as evidence that she was in a phase of spontaneous carryover. Therefore, and because the teacher requested a reduction in the time Debbie was pulled out of the classroom, a decision was made to dismiss her from therapy. After the first 3 months of the following school year, Debbie transferred to another in-district school.

Damico did not see Debbie again until 1983, when he was asked to evaluate a seventh-grade student who was exhibiting a severe communication disorder. When Debbie entered the evaluation room, Damico did not immediately recognize her: "While she still presented an attractive appearance, she was less friendly and somewhat introverted. Upon identification, however, the significance of the situation was realized. A student dismissed from language management as 'normalized' several years ago still manifested language difficulties. Indeed, she exhibited more severe problems" (p. 54).

Debbie was now reading four grades below grade level and was unable to perform tasks expected of most seventh graders. She claimed to have only three friends (two of whom were in special education programs) and was described by others as being shy, quiet, and having poor social skills. At this point, formal testing showed Debbie to have severe difficulty in recognizing and expressing semantic attributes and in being pragmatically appropriate. Although analysis of grammatical form in her expressive language showed Debbie still to be capable of producing sentences with few grammatical errors that were fairly long and complex (with a mean length of utterance of 8.4 morphemes), Debbie had many problems using pragmatic rules to participate in interactive discourse. Problems included difficulty judging the amount of information to provide to a listener, giving appropriate answers to questions, maintaining conversational topics, and producing an unusual number of linguistic nonfluency and revision errors, both with her peers as well as with the clinician. Based on these findings, Debbie was described as a "severely [language] disordered individual with concomitant academic and social problems" (p. 56).

Note. From "The Lack of Efficacy in Language Therapy: A Case Study" by J. Damico, 1988, *Language, Speech, and Hearing Services in Schools, 19*, pp. 51–66. Copyright 1988 by American Speech-Language-Hearing Association. Adapted by permission.

guage and communicative processing is primary without the risk of missing an individual child's needs at a particular stage of life (see Personal Reflection 1.10).

Acquiescence. By *acquiescence*, Damico (1988) was referring to "the tendency to agree or assent to the impressions or opinions of others without dispute" (p. 59). Professional uncertainty or a desire to build a personal or working relationship with others may contribute to a tendency to acquiesce when making decisions.

The potential danger of acquiescence has some interesting implications for the use of cooperative goal setting and collaborative consultation strategies, described later in this chapter. Because such strategies involve mutual goal setting by teams, the potential for one person to acquiesce to others in the process might seem high. Acquiescence, however, suggests that someone wins and someone loses. Competitiveness is avoided when collaborative techniques of mutual goal setting are used to define what the child needs.

In Debbie's case, for example, perhaps the teacher's request to reduce the frequency of Debbie's pull-out sessions stemmed from her growing concern that Debbie was having increasing difficulty in the classroom. Perhaps a team meeting and some classroom observation could have resulted in a clearer perspective on the specific language and communication skills Debbie needed to develop to be successful in the classroom context. When a teacher, speech–language pathologist, and parent all collaborate in the setting of goals, no one must acquiesce because all have worked together to establish mutually defined goals.

Lack of follow-up. The need for follow-up after children have been "dismissed" from therapy has rarely been discussed in the literature (Damico, 1988). This is perhaps because management strategies for language intervention services have evolved largely out of management strategies for children with speech impairments involving articulation, stuttering, and voice (L. Miller, 1989). Although not invariably, some speech impairments may actually be "corrected." The strategy that seems to have been adopted —by analogy—for children with language disorders is to work with them until their language skills reach normal limits according to some standardized test and then to dismiss them from therapy as corrected. This, essentially, is what Damico (1988) did with Debbie.

Such a strategy can have devastating life effects, however, if the skills measured by assessment tasks are not the same as those required in real-life contexts. In Debbie's case, although she developed sufficient skills to produce well-formed sentences of adequate length, she did not have the skills she needed to meet the communicative demands of real educational and social contexts. Part of the problem may have been due to increased classroom communication expectation and decreasing nonverbal contextual support (N. W. Nelson, 1984), causing Debbie's symptoms of early language disability to shift over time (S. E. Maxwell & Wallach, 1984). Unless follow-up services are provided in the form of classroom observations and interviews, problems that are barely noticeable in some contexts may evolve into highly significant disabilities (see Personal Reflection 1.11).

Another advantage of providing follow-up monitoring is that it liberates the intervention-planning process from the assumption that one must work steadily on a problem using a schedule of regular sessions until the child meets preestablished criteria, at which point a decision is made to stop services. Perhaps the most appropriate intervention services for children and families, in some cases, may be provided in spurts. Such an approach should be possible under current PL 94–142 requirements unless local district rules are overly restrictive. Using flexible scheduling, children and families might receive intensive services for brief periods to foster new skills, strategies, and opportunities, followed by intermittent monitoring and consulting to ensure that appropriate language skills are available and supported in real-life contexts. Such an approach might solve both problems, the overly restrictive environment as well as the lack of follow-up.

Bureaucratic policies and procedures. Damico's (1988) explanation of bureaucratic policies and procedures fits the analogy in which the forest obscures the trees. In the system responsible for meeting Debbie's needs, professionals carried 45 to 90 children on their caseloads; furthermore, children were likely to receive only one kind of special education because of funding formulas. Children were "taken and molded to fit the service plan rather than the reverse" (p. 61). The biggest problem, however, stemmed from a bureaucratic philosophy that children should be provided opportunities and services that were adequate rather than optimal.

Perhaps, if a different set of accountability criteria had been used, problems with Debbie's case could have been averted. The rights of children can be abused without rules to protect them, or they can be abused with the very same set of rules. Writing a rule or establishing a policy to meet children's needs is not easy, but if rules are written and implemented consistent with goals to reduce impairment, meet needs, and increase opportunities, children are more likely to be helped than hurt. The need for transdisciplinary cooperation in goal setting is discussed further in the following section. Professionals are urged to participate in writing rules in Chapter 5.

STRATEGIES FOR CHANGING SYSTEMS

System Theory and Ecological Thinking

Effective programming for infants, children, and adolescents with language disorders is complex. Problems of too narrow a focus may be avoided by viewing language as one aspect of a much larger system. This allows one to view language disorders as behavioral manifestations of subsystems operating both within and beyond the child, not as the outcome of simple cause and effect relationships. Language specialists who seek to reduce language disorders using system theory do so with strategies that include both nonlinear and linear thinking processes.

System theory offers a theoretical framework for conceptualizing complex nonlinear problems. System theory was developed in the 1920s by German biologist Ludwig von Bertalanffy (1968) to avoid mechanistic explanations for biological phenomena. Bertalanffy advocated an "organismic" view of biology "which emphasizes consideration of the organism as a whole or system" (p. 12). Although Bertalanffy's ideas did not meet with immediate acceptance, they eventually merged with similar thinking from other disciplines (e.g., economics, physiology, and physics), articulated as general system theory.

The principles of system theory have been applied therapeutically in a wide variety of work, including disturbed families (Minuchin, 1985), adults with aphasia as a result of stroke (Norlin, 1986), and children with language disorders (L. Miller, 1978; N. W. Nelson, 1986). Six basic principles have been discussed:

1. Any system is an organized whole, and elements within the system are necessarily interdependent (Minuchin, 1985). When describing ecosystems, Capra (1982) commented that "what is preserved in a wilderness area is not individual trees or organisms but the complex web of relationships between them" (pp. 266–267). This principle is also illustrated by Damico's (1988) "fragmentation fallacy" discussion about systems whose properties are lost when one attempts to reduce them to smaller units. It suggests that childhood language disorders can only be understood within a network of complex external and internal relationships.

2. Causative patterns in a system are circular rather than linear (Minuchin, 1985). The principle of complex causality is illustrated by research on the communicative interaction patterns of parents with their language-delayed children. When children have language impairments, parents tend to be more directive, ask more questions, and do more correcting (e.g., Conti-Ramsden & Friel-Patti, 1983; Cross, 1984; Lasky & Klopp, 1982; Leonard, 1987). Given these results, it might be tempting to suggest that the slower language development of such children is caused at least partially by their parents' interaction styles. The causative system theory principle, however, suggests that parents' interaction styles may also be partially attributed to the reduced communicative capabilities of their children (Cross, 1984; Leonard, 1987). Attempts to assign blame for language disorders are counterproductive. Understanding that neither problems nor solutions lie simply within children is not a matter of assigning blame. It involves looking for circular causative patterns so that negative cycles may be broken and replaced by positive ones.

3. Systems have homeostatic features that maintain the stability of their patterns. This principle of homeostasis represents the tendency of biological systems, family systems, and classroom systems to remain stable (Minuchin, 1985). Without it, change would occur randomly, and chaos would result. Yet homeostatic forces tend to maintain systems in maladaptive as well as adaptive states. For example, children who have never raised their hands to speak in class may find it difficult even after they have the basic skills to do so. It just does not "feel" right to them, and no one expects them to talk in class. For such a student, carryover will come only when the homeostatic pattern of the classroom is altered.

4. Evolution and change are inherent in open systems (Minuchin, 1985). The principle of morphogenesis balances the principle of homeostasis. The openness of systems means that they will inevitably change. The question is whether the change be positive or negative. The purpose of language intervention is to influence change within systems to be positive. For example, to change classroom patterns about asking questions, participants may need to agree first that talking when appropriate is a valuable goal. Then, it may be possible to modify the classroom system so that the teacher gives the child more opportunity to participate, the language interventionist helps the child acquire new language skill for participating, and the child commits to risk participation.

5. Complex systems are composed of subsystems (Minuchin, 1985). This fifth principle provides a balance to the first. Although systems are wholes that cannot be reduced without losing some of their essence, they do nevertheless have subsystem components. The ability to analyze complex systems in smaller units allows the language specialist to examine various dimensions of a problem sequentially to

understand how subcomponents work together simultaneously (which is the point of the exercise described in Box 1.3). For example, elements of systems as large as a state or nation may determine the policy for serving a child (see Chapter 5); elements as small as the child's understanding of the relationship between a single sound and symbol are also part of that system. Choosing the size of the units to address is an important part of the decision-making process. Language specialists must learn to shift their focus from whole systems to subsystem components and back again without ever losing sight of the whole. Important subsystems for children with language disorders include, as a minimum, their internal linguistic, psycholinguistic, neurolinguistic, sensorimotor, emotional, and cognitive subsystems; their external family, classroom, peer, ethnic, and other social subsystems; and the physical environments in which they participate.

6. The subsystems within a larger system are separated by boundaries, and interactions across boundaries are governed by implicit rules and patterns (Minuchin, 1985). This final principle about subsystem boundaries also applies to multiple levels of the intervention process. For example, an intervention team will be effective with a teenage mother who feels estranged from the values and methods of the team only if the team acknowledges the existence of the boundaries and works with the mother to design an intervention plan that is ecologically valid. Similarly, a language specialist will be effective consulting with a classroom teacher only if the classroom is acknowledged as the teacher's domain and if they both establish mutual goals to address the child's needs to use language to learn and the teacher's needs to educate the child. A school district will be effective in providing a continuum of services for students only if the boundaries established at state and federal levels allow it to do so.

Patterns are interactive. Systems are whole. Subcomponents, however, can be viewed separately within the context of the whole. Patterns tend to perpetuate themselves. Change is inevitable, however. These are the essential principles of system theory, and they can be used to make a difference in the lives of children with language disorders.

Ecological viewpoints, borrowed from biologists, represent attention to environment systems. They emphasize balance between living beings and their environments and recognize disrupting effects of

Personal Reflection 1.12	"We live today in a globally interconnected world, in which biological, psychological, social, and environmental phenomena are all interdependent. To describe this world appropriately we need an ecological perspective which the Cartesian world does not offer." "Reductionism and holism, analysis and synthesis, are complementary approaches that, used in proper balance, help us obtain a deeper knowledge of life."

Fritjof Capra (1982, pp. 16, 267–268) in his book *The Turning Point*.

aberrations on ecosystems. Because children with language disorders may be more or less disabled depending on context, ecological implications are important. Capra (1982), writing about physical and social systems (not language disorders), described the distinction between rational and ecological approaches as a distinction between linear and nonlinear thinking. Nonlinear (ecological) thinking requires "awareness of the essential interrelatedness and interdependence of all phenomena" (p. 265). Capra noted that "ecosystems sustain themselves in a dynamic balance based on cycles and fluctuations, which are nonlinear processes" (p. 41). These he viewed as conflicting with linear, mechanistic enterprises (see also Personal Reflection 1.12).

Language disorders are associated with unnatural balance. When language disorders interfere with a child's ability to communicate, families, classrooms, and other social systems are disrupted. Maladaptive patterns tend to sustain problems and evolve with them. Homeostatic forces for maintaining the status quo are countered by morphogenic forces of inevitable change. Every person who enters such a system becomes part of it, and this includes the language specialist.

To be effective, language specialists must envision systems holistically (in collaboration with others), while using specialized knowledge to analyze system subparts and modify interactions among them. This requires a sort of inner switching between rational thinking about linear relationships and holistic thinking about interactions. Such skills can be learned (see Box 1.3).

Phenomenology—A Philosophical Perspective

When childhood language disorders disrupt systems, confrontational situations often arise. When this happens, the philosophy of phenomenology may help. **Phenomenology** is the philosophical perspective that phenomena are influenced by the methods used to observe them. It counters the notion that any phenomenon (e.g., a child, a classroom, a school system) has an identifiable, objective essence that can be discovered if all of the contributing variables are stripped away. Rather, the theory holds that any phenomenon contains multiple, equally valid truths, and its essence can only be understood by considering the multiple viewpoints used to observe it (Mishler, 1979). This perspective allows professionals and families to move

---

Box 1.3	Steps for maintaining balanced focus on client needs

1. Focus on one small aspect of a particular language problem.
2. Think about possible immediate causes and effects of the problem and their implications.
3. Shift to a medium level of focus, perhaps thinking about other aspects of the problem and effects within a particular family or a classroom context.
4. Use your cognitive "wide-angle lens" to imagine how the problem might interact with needs the child has (or will have) to communicate in the broader contexts of life and to imagine circumstances in which it might be less of a problem. Try to keep multiple factors all in focus at the same time.
5. Switch back and forth between thinking about a subpart of the problem and the whole system in which the problem appears in various forms.

away from the need to determine what is "right" and "wrong" regarding a particular child's needs.

For example, John was a first-grade student with a severe language-learning disability who had trouble handling the communicative demands of the regular curriculum. John's teacher felt that he should be moved to a self-contained classroom in another building. John's mother felt that John belonged in his home school and that his problems did not warrant moving him. What was the true picture of John's abilities and needs? The contribution of phenomenology to this dilemma was to accept that each participant had a valid perspective of John's problem. In John's case, participants included not only his parents and regular classroom teacher but also the school psychologist, two special education teachers (one who worked with him in the morning and one in the afternoon), his building principal, and the district's special education administrator. The varied perspectives of each of these participants had developed through observation of different aspects of the problem. Each was "true." My students and I also had a perspective that had grown out of our formal tests and informal observations and interviews. To act as effective consultants in this complex system, we had to recognize that the varied perspectives were the natural outcome of the tools and contexts used to observe the problem. We could help the participants expand their views of the problem only if we first accepted their current viewpoints as valid.

Accepting viewpoints as valid does not mean accepting them as unchangeable. If "truth" about a phenomenon is a natural outcome of the attitudes, tools, and contexts used to observe it, then views of phenomena can be altered by helping observers modify their observational approaches. For example, one math teacher was disgusted with a language-impaired child who never asked a question during class but missed all of the questions on a quiz. The teacher wondered why the student did not ask for help if he did not know what to do. As we looked together for clues to the student's understanding in the pattern of errors on the quiz, however, the teacher began to ask different questions. Instead of focusing on the lack of "trying," this teacher began to focus on the lack of knowledge of a particular kind. His view of the "truth" about this boy shifted from one of lack of trying to lack of knowing. The teacher also began to recognize that perhaps the boy did not ask questions because he did not know when he did not understand and would rather fail the test than ask

a stupid question in front of his peers. Based on this modified perspective, the teacher devised a plan to meet with the boy each day to make sure that he understood that day's math lesson. In this case, an "unteachable" boy became "teachable," not because of an inherent change in the child, but because of a shift in the nature of the interaction between the boy and the teacher.

Collaborative Consultation and Cooperative Goal Setting

Because systems function as complex wholes, intervention for language disorders requires the mutual efforts of multiple participants. When a child has a problem, and when people in the child's system identify language as part of the problem, a language disorders specialist may be contacted to act as a direct service provider or consultant.

A variety of service-delivery models may be used in the intervention process (see Chapter 5). Regardless of which is chosen, **collaborative consultation** is a problem-solving strategy that applies across situations, service-delivery settings, and types of disability. Collaborative consultation is

> an interactive process that enables teams of people with diverse expertise to generate creative solutions to mutually defined problems. The outcome is enhanced, altered, and produces solutions that are different from those that the individual team members would produce independently. (Idol, Paolucci-Whitcomb, & Nevin, 1986, p. 1)

The mutual definition of problems mentioned in this description relates directly to the previous discussion about the importance of asking questions. When collaborating participants begin with more questions than answers, they avoid confrontational approaches to problem solving.

Increasingly, I have learned the power of entering problem-solving situations in a collaborative mode. This is what happened when my student and I observed John in his regular and special education classrooms after his mother asked us to consult about his placement needs. When we left the observations, our thank-you notes included the message that the next step would involve joint problem solving. The school staff called the next week to arrange the meeting. At the meeting, all three of John's teachers and his speech–language clinician explained John's interactions with them and the problems they had observed. This focused the group on John's needs for functioning in the varied learning contexts of his school day rather than whether he should be removed from the school. His teachers realized, for example, that John had two spelling lists to learn in a week (one for regular classroom and another for his special education classroom), while his normally developing classmates had only one. Based on such realizations, John's teachers began to coordinate their curricular demands and to design deliberate program interfaces. For example, his speech–language clinician decided to use some regular classroom materials to teach direction following, because his first-grade teacher identified that as a major problem. The catalyst for this problem solving was a set of questions such as, "What must John do in your class? What seems to give him the most trouble?" By formulating mutual questions, the group abandoned confrontational goal setting for mutual goal setting. Rather than arguing over where John should be placed, they began to decide how best to meet his educational needs and eventually decided to keep John where he was.

Another key concept in the definition of collaborative consultation is the emphasis on **diverse expertise**. Individual problems are best understood and solved when approached through multiple perspectives. Collaboration can result in an intervention system that is more than the sum of its parts. That is what is meant by producing creative solutions "that are different from those that the individual team members would produce independently" (Idol et al., 1986, p. 1).

As John's case exemplifies, collaborative consultation works best when it involves **cooperative goal setting**. Cooperative goal setting has been contrasted with two other kinds of goal setting (D. W. Johnson & Johnson, 1975):

1. Competitive goal setting. Competitive goal setting involves "negative interdependence" (D. W. Johnson & Johnson, 1975) among the participants. It is typical of games that have an "I win/You lose" quality. In competitive goal setting, members perceive that they can obtain their goals if, and only if, other members fail to obtain theirs. In John's case, the participants had become locked into a competitive goal-setting mode. John's first-grade teacher wanted him to move out of her classroom, his mother wanted him to stay, and his two special education teachers seemed ambivalent. As mentioned, part of the intervention process for John involved backing away from premature placement goals to focus instead on what he needed to do each day in school.

2. Individualistic goal setting. Individualistic goal setting involves "no interdependence" (D. W. Johnson & Johnson, 1975) among participants. It occurs when actions of one team member are unrelated to those of others. Individualistic goal setting is typical of some multidisciplinary assessment teams when members do not have time or opportunity to interact with each other. Report writing in such cases may be of the variety, "I'll do mine, and you do yours, and we'll staple them together and call it a team report."

3. Cooperative goal setting. Cooperative goal setting involves "positive interdependence" (D. W. Johnson & Johnson, 1975) among participants. It occurs when members of a team perceive that they can obtain their goals if, and only if, other team members also obtain theirs. The essence of using cooperative goal setting to escape from competitive goal-setting contexts is for participants to find a level where they can agree on goals for a particular child and to work from there.

Ethnographic Methodology

For cooperative goal setting to work, participants must start with rich concepts of systems. Techniques may be borrowed from cultural anthropologists for studying children as part of the "cultural systems" of their families, classrooms, and peer groups.

To learn about a culture through the eyes of its participants, anthropologists use ethnographic techniques of informant interview, case history, case study, and participant observation. Using field notes, they map and chart patterns that appear and recur, define events the way participants do, and identify unspoken rules of behavior. When a cultural description is developed, ethnographers validate it by checking it with the participants. In the process, they become participants themselves. They do not judge what occurs as good or bad; they simply describe what is occurring. In the traditional anthropological sense, the process of ethnography is one of

> studying a "whole" culture. The product of an ethnography is a definition of what the culture under study is, what being a member of that culture means, and how the culture under study differs from other cultures. In carrying out an ethnography, the anthropologist generally spends an extended period of time in the field in order to develop a description of the whole culture under study. (Green & Wallat, 1981, p. xii)

To already overextended language specialists, the thought of spending "an extended period of time in the field" is prohibitive; many barely have time to conduct traditional assessment and intervention activities. The process of studying must be streamlined. If intervention were to begin only after all the pertinent information were gathered, it would never begin.

Intervention starts as soon as the language specialist first begins to participate in the child's system (see Personal Reflection 1.13). The techniques of ethnography are useful for obtaining multidimensional perspectives of the system. In the process of information gathering and learning about a problematic situation, the system begins to change.

This smaller version of the holistic process has been described as "microethnography" by Green and Wallat (1981). They defined microethnographies as producing "descriptions of what it means to participate in various social situations that occur within the whole culture" (p. xii). The key to success when using this level of analysis, noted Green and Wallat, is to lay out carefully which part of the culture will be studied and define what size units are "whole." F. Erickson (1977) commented:

> It is in this sense that ethnographic work is "holistic," not because of the size of the social unit, but because the units of analysis are considered analytically as wholes, whether that whole be a community, a school system . . . or the beginning of one lesson in a single classroom. (p. 59)

For the language interventionist, units of analysis are events and contexts that are relevant to the child's needs and opportunities as defined by the important players in the child's life. It is not necessary to define everything relevant to a child's needs; it is only necessary to define something relevant to the child's needs and to begin to work there.

The tools that are used in the ethnographic process are described in Chapter 6. Guided by the questions and theories presented in this chapter, they include such methods as participant interviews, onlooker observation, participant observation, and analysis of artifacts.

SUMMARY

The theme of this chapter has been the need for change and the need for good questions to guide the process of change. Change is needed not only in the language and communication skills of children with disorders but in the systems designed to serve them. Old methods guided by limited theories may not be adequate for meeting the needs of children with language disorders. To those who have a history of serving children with language disorders in traditional ways, the need for change may be seen as either a threat or an opportunity.

Language assessment and intervention services generally are provided by speech–language pathologists and other specialists within the network of educational and health-care organizations. Changing ways of thinking about language disorders in children necessitates changing ways of thinking about such organizations and how they operate. The need for change and innovation is not unique to educational and health-care organizations, however. The same kinds of strategies discussed here for application to problems of children with language disorders have also been discussed for application to problems of business.

Rosabeth Moss Kanter (1983) (see Personal Reflection 1.14) has studied the factors characterizing successful change in American business corporations. Her comments about change echo those about system theory and ecological approaches discussed throughout this chapter. In Kanter's summary of the

Personal Reflection 1.14   *"Stop looking at change as an obstacle to be surmounted and start looking at it as an opportunity to improve."*

Rosabeth Moss Kanter (1983) Professor at Harvard University's Business School, summarizing the message of her book *The Change Masters: Innovation and Entrepreneurship in the American Corporation.*

critical factors associated with successful change, she contrasted segmental and integrative approaches. Kanter explained *segmentalism* as being "concerned with compartmentalizing actions, events, and problems and keeping each piece isolated from the others. Segmentalists see problems as narrowly as possible, independently of their context, independently of their connections to any other problems" (p. 28). Kanter contrasted this with more effective *integrative* approaches:

> Integrative thinking that actively embraces change is more likely in companies whose cultures and structures are also integrative, encouraging the treatment of problems as "wholes," considering the wider implications of actions. Such organizations reduce rancorous conflict and isolation between organizational units; create mechanisms for exchange of information and new ideas across organizational boundaries; ensure that multiple perspectives will be taken into account in decisions; and provide coherence and direction to the whole organization. In these team-oriented cooperative environments, innovation flourishes. (p. 28)

To facilitate the process of change when dealing with childhood language disorders, a philosophical framework has been developed in this chapter based on the central idea that problems are not just within children. Rather, problems arise in interactions between children and contexts when children's skills are inadequate to meet specific contextual demands.

Assessment and intervention should go beyond fixing isolated impairments. The traditional communication processes model should be expanded to include elements of a communication needs model and participation model of communication assessment and intervention as well (Beukelman & Mirenda, 1988).

The "forest and the trees" analogy was used to describe a clinical process that is affected adversely by fragmentation, professional bias, acquiescence, lack of follow-up, and bureaucratic policies and procedures (Damico, 1988). A system theory framework, guided by ecological, phenomenological, and ethnographic theories and methods could be used to avoid such problems. As communities begin to address questions of early intervention, family involvement, and integration of people with disabilities, techniques of collaborative consultation will be essential.

Change in children enhanced by innovations in systems—those are the goals that occupy language interventionists heading into the 21st century. Those goals undergird the remainder of this book as questions are addressed about language and related processing systems, about what children need to do in varied contexts, and about the opportunities provided in collaboration with parents and teachers to encourage growth and development of children's language and communicative skills from infancy through adolescence.

2

Language, Speech, and Communication

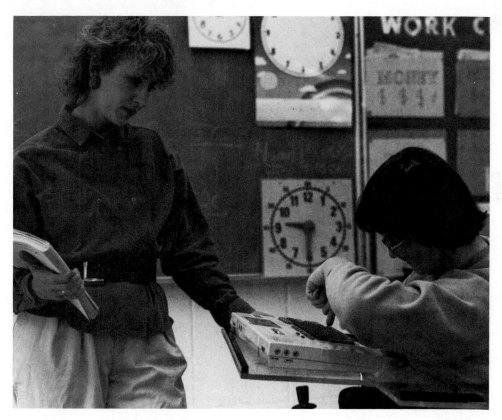

Multidisciplinary
Perspectives

The Linkage of
Language, Speech,
and Communication

The Nature of
Language

Communication as
Social Interaction

❑   What must children learn?
❑   What do they, and others, bring to the task?

Language acquisition is one of the most remarkable processes of human development. How do babies around the world learn most of the rules of their language before they reach their fifth birthday? Is there something unique about human brains that preprograms them for learning language? Why may a severe but specific brain injury early in life cause problems that seem to disappear after a short time; yet why do many children with no detectable brain injuries demonstrate marked difficulty learning the rules of language even after extended help?

MULTIDISCIPLINARY PERSPECTIVES

The preceding questions, and others just as puzzling, have been viewed from the perspectives of scientists from numerous fields as they have studied language, language development, and social communication. Contributions have come from linguists and psycholinguists, neuropsychologists, neurolinguists, and sociolinguists.

It is difficult to understand or to intervene in language disorders unless professionals can grasp what a language learner must learn and the processes normally employed to do so. The discipline devoted to the study of language and its rules is linguistics. *Linguistics* may be defined as the study of unconscious knowledge that underlies the ability of humans to understand and produce utterances in their native languages (Parker, 1986).

The field of linguistics has spawned the subdomain of *psycholinguistics,* which is sometimes defined as the study of language and the mind (Aitchison, 1976). Although the goals of the two disciplines are related, they are contrasted by the relatively greater focus that linguists place on structures and conventions of language compared with the relatively greater focus that psycholinguists place on processes for acquiring and using those structures. The goal of psycholinguists is to study the interrelationships between the structures and processes underlying the ability to speak and understand language. Psycholinguists generally confine themselves to studying processing within individuals. They "are not necessarily interested in language interaction between people. They are trying above all to probe into what is happening within the individual" (p. 11, Aitchison, 1976).

Scientists who probe the contributions of the central nervous system to language processing are called *neuropsychologists* or *neurolinguists.* The fields of neuropsychology and neurolinguistics involve a melding of techniques and concepts from neurology, psychology, and linguistics. They contribute to understanding the physiology of linguistic processing and the unique nature of language and language processing. Like linguists and psycholinguists, neuropsychologists and neurolinguists are interested in language processing as it occurs within individuals.

Important sources of data for neuropsychologists and neurolinguists are studies of individuals with brain damage through trauma, stroke, or other agents such that the site and extent of the lesion can be identified (e.g., Benson, 1967; Benson & Geschwind, 1976; Whitaker & Whitaker, 1981). By studying the variations in processing demonstrated by such individuals, scientists have learned much about the brain and how it contributes to language processing. Some of this information has been useful in remediating problems resulting from acquired brain injuries. Many neuropsychologists assess and intervene with individuals with cognitive processing impairments resulting from brain injury. Neurolinguists also study the effects of brain injuries but focus more specifically on the linguistic aspects of the impairments. Like linguists and psycholinguists, neuropsychologists and neurolinguists traditionally have concentrated on language processing within individuals rather than studying acts of communication in social contexts.

Language, however, is not confined to the brains, ears, and mouths of those who use it but is learned in social interactions. Language is needed to conduct social transactions. Because language is primarily a tool of social communication, it is insufficient to consider language as residing only within individuals. Before babies learn the syntactic rules of their languages, they learn many of the expectations of social interaction within their cultures. The study of the communicative interactions of people in social systems is called *sociolinguistics,* the study of how "children use language in particular social settings" (Cazden, 1972, p. vii).

Cazden (1972) described an early call for "contrastive sociolinguistic" research at a meeting of anthropologists, linguists, psychologists, and sociologists in the autumn of 1965. The first session of the federally funded preschool program, Head Start, had just concluded. Head Start was initiated to address some of the problems associated with school learning in children from families with few financial resources. At the 1965 meeting, a group of distinguished scientists decided that a more productive way to explain school problems was not to look for psycholinguistic problems within children but to look for language differences between home and school. A new set of tools and perspectives was required. The field of sociolinguistics was born to address these and other questions.

Sociolinguists address questions about language use in social contexts. Along with anthropological linguists, they describe language and communication variation within and across cultures. Sociolinguistic interactions provide the warp for the individual strands of psycholinguistic processing that are woven into the fabric of human communication.

THE LINKAGE OF LANGUAGE, SPEECH, AND COMMUNICATION

Because this book is about childhood language disorders, language is the primary system of focus, but this system is intertwined inextricably with related systems of speech and communication. Issues of interconnectedness and separability of language, speech, and communication are critical to assessment and intervention decisions about language disorders in children. Although the three systems overlap and intersect, the fact that it is possible, either in normal or disordered development, for speech and communication to be relatively more advanced or delayed than language leads to some intriguing questions about the brain, behavior, and social contexts.

For example, a college student who is profoundly deaf and communicates primarily through sign language or written language has both language and communication, but not speech. When a child with autism produces speech sounds but combines them in ways that are noncommunicative to most other people, such as in strings of jargon (spoken strings that sound like language but include few or no intelligible words) or as echolalic utterances (repetitions of previously heard phrases that appear to be meaningless or are used in nonconventional ways), that child has speech-like behavior but demonstrates low levels

of language and communication. If this child is to communicate, the child's interaction partners must learn to use special interpretative techniques to understand unconventional messages. A baby who uses squeals and speech sounds to communicate delight at seeing someone has aspects both of speech and of communication but not language. An adolescent with motor impairments who communicates with electronic switches and computerized speech has both language and communication—but does he have speech?

What are language, speech, and communication when examined closely? The following sections examine the interrelatedness, but separability, of these three systems.

Language

Although most normally functioning adults have an intrinsic sense of what language is, language is slippery to define. The definition proposed by the Committee on Language of the American Speech-Language-Hearing Association (Box 2.1) was written to guide public policy regarding language assessment and intervention activities. Its perspective therefore is broad, with a heavy sociolinguistic influence.

Bare-bones definitions of language (e.g., L. Bloom, 1988; Owens, 1992) usually include several key elements. *Language is a socially shared code that uses a conventional system of arbitrary symbols to represent ideas about the world that are meaningful to others who know the same code.* What are the key elements of this definition? Language is a code in the respect that it is not a direct representation of the world, as a drawing or a photograph might be. It is a socially shared code in the respect that, to qualify as a language, a group of people must know the same code and use the same conventions or rules to generate and to understand the symbols of the language. Language uses arbitrary symbols in the respect that words and their components and combinations generally bear no physical resemblance to the concepts they represent (except for some onomatopoetic words, e.g., *buzz* or *click* and some iconic symbols in sign languages, e.g., two hands formed as wings to represent *butterfly*).

The association of arbitrary symbols and abstract meaning is particularly difficult for some children with language disorders. For some children, the problem seems to be confined primarily to attaching meaning to bound morphemes, like plural and possessive

---

Box 2.1   Definition of language proposed by the Committee on Language, American Speech-Language-Hearing Association (1983)

"Language is a complex and dynamic system of conventional symbols that is used in various modes for thought and communication. Contemporary views of human language hold that:

❑ language evolves within specific historical, social and cultural contexts;

❑ language, as rule governed behaviors, is described by at least five parameters—phonologic, morphologic, syntactic, semantic, and pragmatic;

❑ language learning and use are determined by the interaction of biological, cognitive, psychosocial, and environmental factors;

❑ effective use of language for communication requires a broad understanding of human interaction including such associated factors as nonverbal cues, motivation, and sociocultural roles."

Note. From "A Definition of Language" by Committee on Language, American Speech-Language-Hearing Association, 1983, *ASHA, 25*(6), p. 44. Copyright 1983 by ASHA. Reprinted by permission.

---

endings, that are tied closely to the form of language. Rather than arbitrary, such morphemes seem to be expendable. For others, the problem extends to content vocabulary representing things in the world. Children with autism have particular difficulty in acquiring language symbols that represent conventional meanings. These children are more likely to use words and phrases idiosyncratically, as "giant words" for labeling a particular kind of situation (see Box 2.2 for an example).

When used to communicate, language provides a meaningful way of representing ideas about the world to others who speak the same language. Ideas, not things, are encoded into words. Words represent speakers' and listeners' concepts about what words mean. Because speakers and listeners share similar life experiences, they have similar concepts about the world. Because they share words and rules for com-

bining words, they can communicate with each other. Finally, because people share language, they can develop new concepts about the world through language alone.

Speech and Other Modalities

Speech is also made up of arbitrary bits of information that are combined in conventional ways to convey meaning. Speech is one modality through which language can be expressed. As Slobin (1971) pointed out, an important distinction between speech and language is that speech has a corresponding verb form, whereas language does not. People *speak*, but we do not say that they *language*. Speech is behavior and can be recorded with audio or videotape as it is produced. Language is a body of knowledge. It is represented in the brains of people who know that language, but cannot be observed directly. To be as-

---

Box 2.2   An example of unconventional language use

A teacher of autistic children described being present when a student of hers first learned a phrase as a "giant word" label for a particular kind of emotional situation. It started when Robbie, while visiting the home of a classmate, was attracted to play in the cat litter box. The classmate's father, quite upset, yelled, "Get the hell out of there!" Robbie's teacher reported that, thereafter, whenever he was particularly upset, and especially when he was trying to control himself from engaging in a forbidden activity, Robbie repeated the phrase with the original intonation. Such language can be described as delayed echolalia that serves a self-directive function (Prizant & Rydell, 1984), but for Robbie, it also seemed to be a giant word that was evoked by a certain kind of situation much as a proper name goes with a certain person or place.

sessed, language must be observed as behavior produced by users of the language. Speech is one of the most readily available modalities for doing so.

Speech is the oral modality for communication that is used both for speaking and listening. Other modalities include written language and conventionalized systems of gesture, or sign language, which can also be used either expressively or receptively. Speech, however, holds a special place in the development and use of language. Individuals in all cultures learn to speak and understand speech if their auditory, motor, and central nervous systems are intact, and if they receive a minimal amount of exposure to it. On the other hand, written language is generally learned in the context of formal schooling (not invariably, however; the Vai culture in Africa, studied by Scribner and Cole, 1980, provides an interesting exception to this rule by teaching their children to read and write at home, as a part of carrying out the transactions of family business). Not all cultures have developed systems of literacy for communicating through writing.

Language can be learned without speech. Some deaf individuals learn sign language as their first language. When language is learned without speech, however, some other modality must serve as a substitute behavioral system to represent the knowledge system of language, and special circumstances influence the language-learning process. Some studies of deaf children of deaf parents have shown that the acquisition of American Sign Language (ASL) by these children is comparable to the acquisition of spoken English by normal-hearing children (Bellugi & Klima, 1982; Collins-Ahlgren, 1975; Meier, 1991; Newport & Ashbrook, 1977). However, ASL was not developed to be spoken or written; it evolved as an alternative to oral communication for use by deaf individuals. That can be a problem when people who have learned to communicate using ASL attempt to learn to read and write standard English.

Other factors can make it difficult to learn to speak. Individuals who have severe motor control problems but normal cognitive abilities may find it impossible to produce speech, but their lack of speaking ability may

interfere minimally with their reception and comprehension of spoken language. Such people may need to use augmentative and alternative communication (AAC) devices such as computers with synthesized speech to talk and to write. When using AAC devices to write, the individual's expressive language weaknesses may become evident. The written language that nonspeaking individuals produce independently is in many ways remarkable but also often demonstrates predictable limitations, particularly omission of bound morphemes and function words and problems with complex syntactic structures (Kelford-Smith, Thurston, Light, Parnes, & O'Keefe, 1989). Legitimate needs to conserve time and physical effort make it desirable to omit many of these same elements intentionally when users of AAC systems engage in face-to-face communication. It is difficult to determine whether their written language problems are tied directly to such expressive language practices, indirectly to reduced educational opportunity, or to some combination of factors (Koppenhaver, Coleman, Kalman, & Yoder, 1991; Koppenhaver & Yoder, 1988).

Listening, speaking, reading, and writing all are closely intertwined, but their separability must be considered as well, particularly when developmental and acquired disorders of language or speech affect some modalities more than others.

Communication

Communication may be defined as the sharing of needs, experiences, ideas, thoughts, and feelings with other persons (Wood, 1976). It can occur through a variety of modalities. It is possible to communicate without using speech or language. For example, humans use nonlinguistic systems when they communicate messages such as how to move a huge airplane into its bay (with large arm movements and standard gestures). Babies engage in fairly sophisticated communication exchanges with their care givers before they can control their speech-production systems sufficiently to produce intelligible words or their linguistic systems sufficiently to produce or comprehend syntactically formulated utterances (e.g., Bateson, 1971; Bullowa, 1979; Trevarthen, 1974).

Nonverbal communication behaviors can be produced in isolation or in conjunction with messages being transmitted via speech or writing. Two kinds of communicative features that intersect with speech and language processing in unique ways are termed *nonlinguistic* and *paralinguistic*.

Nonlinguistic communication. Nonlinguistic features may communicate information alone or in conjunction with linguistically encoded messages. Examples of nonlinguistic communicative features that researchers have studied are gestures, body posture, facial expression, eye contact, head and body movement, and physical distance or proxemics (Owens, 1992). In Western cultures, the proxemic communication system defines a distance between communicative partners of 12 feet or more (to a visible limit) as public, a distance of 4 to 12 feet as social-consultive, a distance of 18 inches to 4 feet as personal, and a distance of direct contact to 18 inches as intimate (Higginbotham & Yoder, 1982). Box 2.3 summarizes features of nonlinguistic communication that use kinesic communication channels.

Nonlinguistic features are particularly evident when two people engage in face-to-face communication. For example, when given the opportunity, mothers and neonates communicate with intensity during the first few moments after birth. Nonlinguistic features also influence written language communication events. The choice of writing utensil, stationery, text format, and punctuation style (punctuation helps to signal paralinguistic features in written language, discussed

later) all communicate something about the formality of a note or letter. Students with language-learning disabilities risk social disvalue by their peers when they fail to master nonlinguistic rules for communicating via social notes. They also risk making unfavorable impressions on teachers and potential employers when they fail to learn nonlinguistic expectations for formal written communication. Similarly, readers who are insensitive to nonlinguistic context may have difficulty comprehending broader meanings when they read. For example, knowing that an article about human neuroanatomy was written in the 1890s could lead a college student to approach that piece much differently from knowing it was written in the 1990s.

Some forms of nonverbal communication are universal and appear to be part of human genetic makeup. Examples are the smiling faces humans give each other when happy and angry faces when provoked. Other forms of nonspeech behavior communicate different meanings depending on the culture in which they were learned. It can be confusing, for example, for some African-American and Native-American children, who have learned in their home cultures to drop their eyes as a sign of respect while listening to adults, to be reprimanded by their teachers for not looking at them when they talk (Taylor, in press).

Paralinguistic communication. Paralinguistic features are related to speech because they are produced with the vocal tract, but they differ from speech because they are not produced as articulated speech sounds or words. Speech-production elements

---

Box 2.3	Nonlinguistic features of the kinesic communication system (Adapted from Higginbotham & Yoder, 1982)

❏ **Emblems:** Convey meaning, modify associated linguistic message.
   Examples: "yes/no" headshake, hitchhiking gesture, finger pointing, middle finger gesture.
❏ **Illustrators and other body motions:** Modify or clarify linguistic message; indicate level of interpersonal involvement and attention; mark phonemic, syntactic, and semantic boundaries.
   Examples: Gestures, such as those tracing the outlines of a referent; other fine and gross body movements using eyes, fingers, facial expression, head, limbs, or trunk, often in temporal synchrony with speech rhythms.
❏ **Regulators:** Initiate and terminate conversations, regulate turn taking, provide listener and speaker feedback, maintain or direct attention of communicative partner.
   Examples: Head movements, gaze direction and shifts, arm movements, hand tension and gesticulation, postural shifts, facial displays.
❏ **Adaptors:** Indicate psychological anxiety, discomfort, or emotional arousal.
   Examples: Body or object focused movements, such as biting fingernails, picking nose, touching face, cracking knuckles, tapping foot, rotating ring, twirling pencil.

such as vowels, consonants, and syllables are considered to be the segments of a language. Paralinguistic devices, on the other hand, extend across the individual segments of speech that form a message. Hence, they are called *suprasegmental* devices. Rather than resulting in the production of articulated sounds and words, suprasegmental devices are used to modify the more extensive envelopes of the utterances they affect. They provide the melody of speech that is known as its *prosody*. Prosody is sometimes defined as the "residue" that is "left after one has studied the vowel/consonant/syllabic system of sounds" (Crystal, 1979, p. 33). Traditionally, the term has referred primarily to variation in such features as pitch, loudness, speed, and rhythm (including pauses) when speaking. Such features are related to the production of linguistic meaning, but whether they are truly linguistic is subject to debate. To Crystal (1979), such features are linguistic; to others, they are paralinguistic. Box 2.4 contains an outline of types of devices used to produce prosodic variation in linguistic messages. Suprasegmental devices can play multiple roles in influencing message meaning. Box 2.5 outlines common functions of prosodic devices.

Prosodic features seem to function differently in speech directed to persons of different age levels. Fernald (1989) found that the prosodic patterns of

adult speech to infants were more informative as to communicative intent (when judged by a group of adults who heard filtered versions of the speech that removed the linguistic content) than were the prosodic patterns in adult-to-adult speech. This makes sense, given that infants are less likely to understand the linguistic aspects of messages, which is a feature to keep in mind when consulting with care givers of infants at risk for developmental and communicative disorders. Some care givers may need to be shown how to be extra demonstrative with their youngsters. Others may need to tone down their exuberance when their babies are overstimulated. In either case, parents may need to become more sensitive to contexts where different styles are warranted.

At the discourse level, paralinguistic features can be used to convey such indirect shades of emotionally toned meaning as sarcasm, teasing, mocking, or parody. In such cases, the paralinguistic aspects extend beyond single words or sentences to influence an entire piece of coherent discourse (see Personal Reflection 2.2). Anyone who has parented or communicated with junior high school students (or can remember being one) knows that many of them practice such skills as sarcasm and mocking to the point of distraction. When describing first-, third-, and fourth-grade children's arguments in an article titled

---

Box 2.4	Prosodic devices (based on Crystal, 1975, 1979)

1. **Intonation.** The linguistic use of pitch is one of the several prosodic characteristics of speech that is integrated with others to produce a totality that expounds meaning.
2. **Pitch direction and range.** Directional tones may rise, fall, stay level, or do some combination of these things within a given phonological unit such as a syllable. As a system of contrast, tones may also vary in their range. For example, a falling pitch may occur within a relatively high, middle, or low range, and the range itself may be relatively wide or narrow. This results in syllable tone that may be characterized by linguists as high-falling-wide, low-rising-narrow, and so on.
3. **Tone-units.** When features of pitch direction and range are organized into prosodic configurations along with features of rhythm and pause, they are known as *tone units, primary contours,* or *sense groups.* Slant lines are used by linguists to mark off tone-unit boundaries, which generally correspond to grammatical clauses but expound meaning beyond the accompanying linguistic meanings. For example:
   If you want/I'll come along/
4. **Syllable prominence.** Prominent, or *tonic,* syllables are produced primarily using pitch movement, but extra loudness, duration, and pause may also be used to heighten the contrast. Tonic syllables may be indicated with capital letters when spoken utterances are coded for prosodic features. Two contrasting views of syllable prominence are (a) that it acts mainly as a syntactic feature to disambiguate sentences and (b) that it acts mainly as a semantic feature to signal new information in context.

Box 2.5   Functions of prosodic devices (based on Crystal, 1979)

1. **The grammatical function.** Speakers can signal a contrast with prosody that could be coded as morphological or syntactic, such as positive–negative, singular–plural, or statement–question. For example, tag questions might be distinguished as asking–telling by shifting tonality:

   You're còming/àren't you.

   You're còming/áren't you.

2. **The semantic function.** Speakers can indicate the organization of meaning in discourse and can reflect presuppositions about shared information with listeners by using prosodic features to emphasize the relative importance of some elements of meaning and to indicate that others are parenthetical. When prosody is used semantically, it serves the classical role of denotation:

   Sàm /you know, Bónnie's boy/ is marrying the girl from Indepèndence.

3. **The attitudinal function.** When prosody is used attitudinally, it serves the classical role of connotation. In this function, speakers indicate personal emotions such as puzzlement, anger, sarcasm, surprise, or disgust about the subject matter or context of an utterance. It is as yet unclear whether such devices are specific to individual languages or represent universal characteristics of emotional expression.

4. **The psychological function.** Studies have shown that the psychological ability to perform recall, perception, and short-term memory tasks is affected by variation in prosodic features, with words containing tonic features being more easily perceived and recalled.

5. **The social function.** Prosody signals sociolinguistic characteristics of the speaker such as sex, class, and professional status and is an important part of facilitating social interaction in dialogue. Contrast, for example, the role of prosody in differentiating the illocutionary force (basically the speaker's intention) of a speech act such as persuading or commanding when the speaker is boss versus when the speaker is employee.

"You Fruithead," Brenneis and Lein (1977) noted the importance of suprasegmental stylistic conventions in marking a speech event as an argument and enabling the audience to anticipate the structure of ensuing exchanges. They noted that, "Even without hearing the words, most listeners can tell what sort of speech event is occurring by noticing such gross stylistic variables as pitch, volume, and speed" (p. 53) (see Chapter 9 for further discussion of this research).

Personal Reflection 2.2   "If you haven't got the melody, you can't decipher the words."

Sylvia O. Richardson, M.D. (personal communication, September 21, 1989), speech-language pathologist, pediatrician, and former President of the American Speech-Language-Hearing Association and the Orton Dyslexia Society, commenting on the diagnostic significance of aberrant prosody among babies, which Richardson believes indicates a risk for lack of sensitivity to the paralinguistic features of human speech, a negative prognostic indicator for learning language easily.

Richardson relates this to the difficulty she experienced herself when attempting to learn Portugese as an adult in South America. Although she had learned Italian easily (her family was Italian and she had heard it spoken at home) and the two languages had seemed similar on the surface, they had different rhythms. She said: "They were doing the Samba; I was doing the foxtrot."

Prosodic emphasis can also enhance semantic comprehension among listeners. Bean, Folkins, and Cooper (1989) found that listeners could answer multiple-choice questions better when words associated with the correct answers had been emphasized in passages that had been read aloud to the subjects. Leonard (1973) also found that prosodic stress on key words could influence the recall of verbal material.

Paralinguistic features appear at early stages of normal development in expression as well as comprehension. Most toddlers, for example, have mastered the intonation pattern of whining sufficiently to keep it up over an entire grocery shopping trip (at least throughout the checkout line).

The importance of paralinguistic devices to the effective communication of emotional tone and other nonsegmental levels of meaning, even among adults, may be appreciated by observing what happens when messages usually produced orally are written instead. Shapiro and Anderson (1985), for example, recommended that senders of electronic mail label their emotions, opinions, jokes, witicisms, or sarcasm to avoid misinterpretation.

AAC system users sometimes find that the invariant synthetic speech of their communication aids results in similar kinds of miscommunication. It is difficult to program paralinguistic features with such devices. Proficient AAC users and their communicative partners learn to use natural voicing, laughter, and nonlinguistic gestures (impaired though they may be by cerebral palsy and other motor disorders), such as twinkling eyes and extra body movement, to signal when they have made a joke or twisted the literal meaning of their words slightly in some other way. Message interpretation aids can also be programmed linguistically into AAC systems to assist in cuing listeners who might misunderstand, perhaps as a result of absent paralinguistic features, such as "that was a joke."

THE NATURE OF LANGUAGE

Linguists and psycholinguists study the nature of language and the language acquisition process. They are most concerned about what language is and how it is acquired by children and processed by adults. The question of which language system a child might be attempting to learn is also important and relates to issues of dialect difference and bilingualism.

Bilingualism and Dialect Differences

Bilingualism.   Language specialists and language textbooks in the United States often seem to approach issues concerning language disorders in children as if all children were learning standard English. The evolving demographics of North America, however, are not at all consistent with that assumption. It is projected that, by the turn of the century, at least one third of the school-age population in the United States will be either black, Hispanic, Asian, or Native American (Bouvier & Gardner, 1986). In summarizing recent related demographic changes, K. G. Butler (1985) noted that minority groups, including blacks, Hispanics, Asians, and Native Americans, are growing at a much faster rate than whites in the United States. As evidence, she cited that the population as a whole increased 26% from 1960 to 1983, while the black population increased 50% and other minority groups increased 295% during those same 23 years. Currently, the fastest growing minority group is Hispanic, with a 61% increase from 1970 to 1980; an additional estimated 6 million to 8 million Hispanic individuals crossed the border from Mexico without being officially counted during that same time. Meanwhile, the proportion of immigrants from Asia jumped to 34.1% between 1969 and 1979.

Although membership in a minority group provides some hint about cultural and linguistic differences, primary language is by no means isomorphic with cultural heritage (O. Taylor & Payne, 1983). L. Cole (1989) summarized the heterogeneity of linguistic minority populations and commented on the problems that result when trying to use or develop norm-referenced measures for providing speech and language intervention services to members of such populations:

> Linguistic minority populations cannot be categorized into the same four groups as have racial/ethnic minorities. The vast majority of Hispanics in this country are Mexican, Puerto Rican, Cuban, Central American, or South American, each representing varying dialects of Spanish. Asian language populations rank among the five largest linguistic minority groups, including about two million speakers of Chinese, Philippine languages, Japanese, Korean, Vietnamese, Cambodian, and Laotian. About 250 different languages are spoken by American Indians, some of which are spoken by only a few. Others, such as Cherokee, Dinneh, and Teton Sioux are spoken by many thousands. (p. 70)

It is impossible to provide contrastive linguistic information here about all of the rules from the differ-

Personal Reflection 2.3   "My English is terrible. My English to me I understand what I am saying; to other people, they don't understand. I just don't wanna speak; don't know what words to use. My English crashes into Spanish. It mixed together. If I ever try to speak Spanish, Spanish people would say, 'Are you Spanish?' I say, 'Yes.' They say, 'You don't talk like you're Spanish; you don't know how to speak well.' My mother is always telling me I should be ashamed. I don't feel like I'm Spanish; I don't feel like anything. I just feel . . . like a plant."

Carlos, a pseudonym given to a high school student, described by Cleary (1988, p. 62). Carlos was born into a large family in a large city to a Puerto Rican mother, who spoke Spanish, with 11 brothers and sisters, who taught him what he called "street talk," a dialect of English that showed both Spanish language and Black English Vernacular influence.

ent languages that might be first languages for children having trouble acquiring any language. Language interventionists need to bear in mind, however, that legitimate variation is possible even within a language and that such variation should be explained as language difference rather than language disorder.

Dialect differences.   Not all children who acquire language systems other than standard English acquire completely different linguistic systems. Some acquire dialectal variations of English. A *dialect* is defined by linguists as "any aspect of variation which differentiates groups of speakers" (Wolfram, 1979, p. 1). Such variation is systematic and patterned, and it is always governed by regular rules. Everyone who speaks a language speaks a dialect of it. The development and maintenance of dialects is affected by multiple factors, not just linguistic ones. "Dialects develop when speakers of a common language are separated from each other, either by geographical or social distance" (Fasold & Wolfram, 1970, p. 42).

The boundaries that differentiate dialects and languages are not always clear because language evolves in concert with a variety of social and geopolitical influences. Many of the features of the dialect called Black English Vernacular (BEV) can be traced to features of West African languages via Caribbean Creole languages, which developed through processes of pidginization during the years of slave trading (Dillard, 1972; O. Taylor, 1972). As a result, BEV exhibits features not shared by other dialects of English. In fact, Bickerton (1983) noted that "the grammatical structures of creole languages are more similar to one another than they are to the structures of any other

language" (p. 121). Children who come from homes where languages other than English are spoken, but who interact with speakers of a variety of English dialects, also may show mixed influences in the dialects they speak.

Problems related to language dialect occur because of mismatch between the linguistic expectations of the context and the dialect of a person who must communicate in that context (see Personal Reflection 2.3). Some of the problems associated with using a different dialect relate more to the differential prestige with which individuals hold various dialects than to any risk of actual miscommunication. When the rules of a dialect, however, diverge sufficiently from the linguistic rules used in a particular context, communication may be misunderstood in either direction. For example, a teacher who speaks only standard English may have difficulty understanding the communicative attempts of a speaker who uses BEV, just as such a child may not always understand the teacher.

Discriminatory educational practices may be deeply intertwined with language differences. For example, the "ability" tracking that goes on in many of America's schools may actually be based in a profound way on language. Cleary (1988) suggested that social class distinctions are perpetuated by a practice that relegates "basic" writers to "work at the word/exercise level, thus preventing them from becoming fluent in written expression, from getting any joy in the process, or in practicing abstract thought" (p. 63). Cleary also reported that, although it might seem that children whose language was influenced by completely different systems such as Spanish might be at the greatest risk for difficulty, actually "working class English" and BEV were as troublesome to students because the language problems related to them were so subtle, and teachers were more likely to see problems of poor "grammar" and ignorance rather than use of dialect.

Such problems highlight the influence of attitude toward low-prestige dialects. Linguists have been pointing out that all language systems are equally sophisticated and rule based since the late 1960s (Baratz, 1969; Labov, 1966, 1969; O. Taylor, Stroud, Moore, Hurst, & Williams, 1969). U.S. District Court Judge Charles W. Joiner, in the well-known "Ann Arbor case" (*Martin Luther King Junior Elementary School Children et al. v. Ann Arbor School District Board*, 1979), ruled that a school system must appreciate a child's dialect (BEV, in this case) within the context of the community and must use knowledge of dialectal difference in the educational process. Furthermore, the judge ruled, consistent with the requirements of Public Law 94–142, that children must not be found to have language disorders when they are developing normally within their own linguistic communities. However, old attitudes die hard. Smitherman (1985) commented that, even now, "research on language attitudes consistently indicates that teachers believe Black English speaking youngsters are non-verbal and possess limited vocabulary. They are slow learners or ineducable. Their language is unsystematic and needs constant corrections and improvement" (p. 50).

Difficult questions arise for language disorders specialists when they attempt to differentiate language disorder from language difference. Professionals may either "undercompensate" for language difference—and run the risk of identifying children as disabled when they are merely using language skills different from those tapped by most testing methods—or they may "overcompensate" for language difference, and assume that any child from a sociolinguistic community that differs from the mainstream must *not* have a language disorder (S. L. Terrell & Terrell, 1983). Both practices are discriminatory and must be avoided. Strategies for doing so are discussed later in this book (see Chapter 6 in particular; also Chapters 7 to 9).

The Subcomponents of Language

Language intervention specialists need to understand the subcomponents of language so they can conduct language assessment and intervention in culturally and linguistically fair ways. They also need a cohesive model of language and a taxonomy (a categorical system) of its subcomponents so they will not have to rely exclusively on published language tests and intervention programs but will have the flexibility to vary their approaches and expectations in varied contexts. Although formal language tests and intervention programs are useful tools, they often reflect the views typical of a particular point in time, a particular theorist, or a particular linguistic system. They are just tools, not definitions of what needs to be done.

A variety of categorical systems may be used to cut the language pie into manageable slices. Two distinct but compatible taxonomies are used frequently by speech–language pathologists and other language specialists. The traditional set includes the five linguistic categories (1) phonology, (2) morphology, (3) syntax, (4) semantics, and (5) pragmatics. These categories organize this section and are also useful for guiding detailed assessment and intervention activities with children. The other set of categories (L. Bloom & Lahey, 1978; Lahey, 1988) consists of: (1) form, (2) content, and (3) use. Because there are fewer of them, and because the terms are more easily understood by the general public, the categories *form*, *content*, and *use* are particulary helpful when discussing language deficits with teachers and parents.

It is not always clear how different taxonomies of language relate to each other. For example, linguists have described the *structure* of language to include "speech sounds and meanings, and the complex system of grammar, which relates sounds and meanings" (Slobin, 1971, p. vii). According to this definition, the rules for language form include those of semantics as well as of phonology and morphology. Some morphological rules relate more closely to representing language content, whereas others are more closely related to conveying language form. Even the rules of language use are not clearly confined to conventions of pragmatics. How a person chooses to say or interpret a given utterance in a particular context is influenced not only by knowledge of the pragmatic rules of interactive discourse but by syntactic and semantic competence as well.

Not forgetting caveats about overlap and inseparability, it is nevertheless helpful for specialists in language disorders to consider what a child knows about each of the different rule systems of language. Full delineations of the systems of phonology, morphology, syntax, semantics, and pragmatics are still beyond the scope of linguistic explanation (and of this book). Following are brief summaries of some of the major features of these systems and the difficulties they sometimes present to children with language disorders.

Phonology.   *Phonology* is the speech sound system of language. It plays both an early and a significant role in language acquisition. Babies come equipped with sound-detection systems that are sensitive to fine distinctions in the acoustic properties of human speech. In the early days of life, certain aspects of speech and communication seem to be more ready to be put into operation than others.

Probably owing to limitations of the anatomical structure of the human vocal tract and associated brain structures, the possible set of distinctive features that can be used to differentiate classes of speech sounds is limited. In a classic article, linguists Jakobson and Halle (1956) outlined a universal set of binary features (e.g., aspirated–nonaspirated, consonant–vowel, voiced–voiceless, and stop–continuant) that can be combined in unique ways in different languages to set up distinctive classes of sounds called *phonemes*. Linguists define the *phoneme* as a sound class that is the smallest unit that can make a difference in word meaning by its presence or absence.

As babies are exposed repeatedly to the set of features that distinguishes phonemes in their own languages, especially in meaningful and emotionally satisfying contexts, they learn to make sharper perceptual distinctions among those particular acoustic cues (A. M. Liberman, Cooper, Shankweiler, & Studdert-Kennedy, 1967) and to distinguish more sound classes in their own productions (Jakobson, 1968). Eventually, they learn to ignore distinctions that do not distinguish sound classes in their own languages. This kind of first language phonological specialization is what makes it so difficult to learn to speak a second language without accent later in life.

For example, speakers of English do not perceive the /p/ in *pot* and the /p/ in *spot* as representing different sound classes, even though in *pot*, the /p/ is aspirated (i.e., produced with a little puff of air) whereas in *spot*, it is not. For speakers of English, such distinctions are experienced as the phonetic artifacts of coarticulation, not as sound-class (phonemic) differences. That is, they are phonetic differences in the ways that the same phoneme is produced in different articulatory contexts. In English, voiceless stop conso-

nants are aspirated if they occur in the prevocalic position (as in the word, *pit*) but are not aspirated if they follow /s/ in a consonant cluster (as in the word, *spit*). Yet, speakers of English perceive both of these phonetic variations as the same phoneme, /p/. In some other languages, such as Hindi and Thai, whether a stop consonant is aspirated or not at the beginning of a word is a phonemic distinction and not just a phonetic one. That is, the feature of aspiration can make a word like *pit* sound like two different words depending on whether the /p/ is aspirated or not, just as *bit* and *pit* are distinguished by speakers of English because the feature of voicing (voice-onset time) that distinguishes between /b/ and /p/ is phonemic.

Word pairs that are distinguished by a single phoneme are called *minimal pairs*. For example, *bat* is a different word from *at* because of the phoneme /b/. Similarly *pat* is a different word from *bat* because of a single phoneme difference (distinguished by the single distinctive feature of voicing). *Bat* is a different word from *sat*, as well, but in this case the single phonemes that distinguish the meanings of the two words are distinguished from each other by several distinctive features (stop–continuant, bilabial–alveolar, voiced–voiceless) rather than just one. When speech–language pathologists work with children with language disorders who have difficulty discriminating speech sounds, they generally start with sounds that are maximally discriminative and work toward finer and finer distinctions. Recognizing phonological relationships determined by distinctive features can help them do so.

An example of a phonologically based language difference is the different way that the feature of voicing functions in Spanish than in English. Even though both /s/ and /z/ sounds are produced in Spanish, the two sounds are members of the same phoneme class. Native Spanish speakers therefore may have difficulty distinguishing words like *price* and *prize* and *ice* and *eyes* in English. Although this difficulty may seem strange to native speakers of English, native English speakers themselves learn to ignore the voicing distinction between /s/ and /z/ when those two phonemes serve as a single morpheme, such as when they both represent plurality as in *toys* and *trucks*. In both these words, the plural ending is spelled as -*s*, and it is generally experienced as the same sound, even though coarticulation with the voiced vowel leads the sound to be voiced (pronounced /z/) in *toys*, and coarticulation with the voiceless stop consonant leads it to be voiceless (pronounced /s/) in *trucks*.

Similar phonetic distinctions in the spoken productions of the possessive morpheme and in the past-tense morpheme are ignored in the spelling and in the perceived meaning of words like *Jason's* (pronounced /z/) and *Janet's* (pronounced /s/), and in *walked* (pronounced /t/), *used* (pronounced /d/), and *needed* (pronounced /əd/), respectively.

Rules for the phonological system of a language extend beyond the production and perception of individual sounds. They also apply to constraints on the ways sound segments can be combined to form meaningful words in a language. Such rules are sometimes called *phonotactic* rules. Two types of phonotactic rules are distributional rules and sequencing rules. Distributional rules allow some sounds to appear in some positions of words but not others. For example, in English, the sounds ŋ=/ng/ and ʒ=/zh/ can occur at the ends (e.g., *bring* and *beige*) and in the middle of words (e.g., *singing* and *vision*) but not at the beginning (except in words borrowed from other languages). Sequencing rules govern the types of sound combinations than can occur in a particular order. They are often combined with distributional rules so that it is acceptable for certain sequences to occur in some word positions but not others. For example, although in English words do not start with a /ks/ sound combination, they can end with one, as in the word *breaks*.

Of course, idealized adult productions of speech sound sequences do not appear immediately in the developing phonological systems of children. David Stampe (1969) theorized that children's early attempts to reproduce adult models of speech, when their motor abilities are immature, are simplified as a result of application of an innate system of phonological processes children bring with them to the language-learning task. Box 2.6 summarizes phonological processes commonly observed in the speech of preschoolers (with different subsets of processes used by different individuals). Part of Stampe's (1969) theory was that children must learn to suppress these innate simplifying processes as they learn the adult phonological system of their language. Some simplification remains during conversational speech by adults, which is due primarily to constraints on speed and extent of movement of the articulators during rapid speech (Newman, Creaghead, & Secord, 1985), but adults have also learned to vary their articulatory precision with varied contexts in the process of becoming competent communicators. They are likely, for example, to use more careful articulation in formal communicative interactions than in informal ones. Young children, in contrast, are more likely to demonstrate consistency in the application of certain phonological simplification processes at a particular point in their development.

Many, but not all, children with language disorders persist in using phonological simplification processes long after most children have moved past them. Articulatory difficulty is not the only way that children with language disorders may show evidence of having difficulty with the phonological system of language. Internalization of the rules for mapping phonological sequences onto lexical meanings has broad implications not only for early acquistion of oral language but for later acquisition of written language decoding and spelling skills during the school-age years as well.

For example, Lisa, a kindergartener with language-learning disabilities, was asked to retell the story of "Goldilocks and the Three Bears." The word *porridge* apparently was not in Lisa's expressive vocabulary (at least not in a way that she could retrieve it). Thus, when Lisa told the initial episode of the story, she told about how the mother bear had made *soup*, how the family of bears had decided to let it cool, and how Goldilocks had come into the house and had ended up tasting it. The interesting thing about Lisa's phonological rule system was the inconsistency with which she pronounced the word *soup*. At various times in the retelling, she pronounced it as *soup*, *thoup*, *thoot*, and *suit*. Although she did not demonstrate a typical pattern of consistent misarticulation in her speech (such as lisping), Lisa was certainly demonstrating wobbly concepts of the phonological shape of words. If we view this set of productions as being generated based on a rule system for differentiating sound classes, Lisa (at least in the context of the word *soup*) was behaving as if her rule system included /s/ and /th/, both initial voiceless continuant consonants, as members of the same phoneme class. She also seemed to have grouped two other English phonemes as one: the final voiceless stop consonants /t/ and /p/. It was no wonder that this kindergarten child was having such difficulty learning the sound–symbol associations that are an important part of most kindergarten curricula.

But was the problem even bigger? For her, it seemed to be. In another part of the story, after talking about the hot and cold characteristics of the bowls of soup that Goldilocks tasted, Lisa began to

Box 2.6   Phonological simplification processes

Simplification processes are observed in the speech productions of normally developing children but often persist among children with speech–language disorders beyond the ages when they usually disappear normally (based on Ingram, 1976).

Syllable structure processes

    Final consonant deletion (usually eliminated by 3 years)—[bU] for *book*

    Unstressed syllable deletion (usually eliminated by 4 years)—[næ nə] for *banana*

    Cluster reduction, deletion, or substitution (may last beyond 4 years)—[bænki], [ænki], [bwænki] for *blanket*

Assimilatory processes

    Contiguous assimilation between consonants

        Labial assimilation (probably eliminated by 4 years)—[bweɪn] for *train*

        Final consonant devoicing (eliminated by 2 years)—[bɪk] for *big*

    Contiguous assimilation between a consonant and a vowel

        Alveolars become velars when adjacent to a back vowel—[ku] for *two*

        Prevocalic voicing (may last a few months)—[da] for *top*

        Vowel lengthening before a voiced consonant—[ha:] for *hog*

        Vowel nasalization (common)—[fã] for *farm*

    Noncontiguous assimilation between consonants

        Back assimilation—[keɪk] for *take*

        Labial assimilation—[bap] for *stop*

        Nasalization (not common)—[mæ̃məmə] for *grandmother*

    Noncontiguous assimilation between vowels

        Progressive assimilation—[wawa] for *water*

        Regressive assimilation—[bibi] for *baby*

Substitution processes

    Affecting obstruents

        Stopping of fricatives and affricates (may persist over several years)—[ti] for *see*

        Fronting of palatals and velars (most common before 3½ years)—[tæt] for *cat*

    Affecting nasals

        Fronting (occurs with fronting of other velars)—[bin] for *bring*

        Denasalization (not common)—[bæba] for *Grandma*

    Affecting liquids

        Stopping (early in development)—[da] for *rock*

        Gliding (may last for some time)—[wæbɪt] for *rabbit*

        Liquid replacement (may occur late in development)—[særi] for *Sally*

    Affecting glides

        Frication (not common)—[zã] for *yawn*

    Affecting syllabic liquids and nasals

        Vocalization (very common)—[watə] for *water*

    Affecting vowels

        Neutralization—[bəbə] for *baby*

    Deletion

        Can affect any segment (earliest process; must be eliminated before others can occur) tell about the characteristics of the bears' chairs. When she began to talk about the Daddy Bear's chair, Lisa searched overtly for the correct word. "Hard [drawing the word out in a questioning tone] . . . or cold?" she asked herself. And then, with confidence, answered, "I think cold." What happened here? Was Lisa treating the words *hot* and *hard* as if they were homonyms? It seemed that she was. Aside from demonstrating some healthy metacognitive strategies of self-questioning and some healthy metalinguistic strategies of word search using categorical opposites, Lisa seemed to be getting short circuited by her wobbly phonological concepts into confusing word meanings that were not related to clearly distinguishable and stable phonological shapes. We wondered how much this difficulty might be associated with Lisa's other difficulties in learning pronoun case (she consistently substituted *him* for *he* and *her* for *she*), in pronouncing multisyllabic words without *metathesis* (she tended to mix up sound sequences, such as in the word *pasghetti*), and in learning the rules for inflecting verbs (she tended to leave out the auxiliary *"is"* in *"is + Ving"* constructions). Those were problems that represented difficulty in learning some of the other rule systems of language, but they may have been intertwined with the phonological confusions that Lisa demonstrated in her word-production inconsistencies.

What happens when a child learns a word? When a toddler produces a word, how much of the word's essence is tied up in getting enough of the phonological information in the word to match the adult model so that the word is recognizable? What causes the child with the normally developing phonological system to keep improving word pronunciation even after words are recognizable? What causes some language–impaired children to seem to have difficulty doing so? If, because of speech motor control problems, a child has difficulty learning to put phonological rules into practice for producing speech, what happens to the ability to acquire new words and inflectional morphemes? If, because of auditory perceptual problems, a child has difficulty learning to put phonological rules into practice for discriminating speech, what happens to the ability to acquire new words and inflectional morphemes? Can either of these problems occur in isolation or are they always intertwined? In other words, how are phonological rules represented in the brain? Are they tied up with the phonological production system or with the phonological discrimination and word-recognition system? Or are phonological

rules represented as some more abstract entity that is stored separately from modality processing centers? Should speech–language pathologists concentrate on teaching children with articulation and language impairments to say words correctly or merely intelligibly? What happens when a child recognizes a word? What happens when a child retrieves a word to say it as part of a conversation? What happens when a child retrieves a word to spell it in a piece of written language?

These are not easy questions to answer, and in most cases sufficient evidence is not available to allow us to answer them with confidence, but they are good questions to ask. Their answers all seem to involve the internalized representation of speech sounds and speech sound patterns in the brain. Such questions arise again in discussions related to assisting children with language disorders to acquire their first words, to retrieve words in different modalities, and to develop the skills they need to become literate.

Morphology.   Linguists usually define *morphemes* as the smallest meaningful units of language. *Morphology* refers to the study of word formation (Parker, 1986). Whereas phonemes distinguish word meaning, morphemes carry meaning by themselves. However, not all morphemes can stand alone. Some are called *bound morphemes,* and some, *free morphemes.* Bound morphemes are always attached to free morphemes (sometimes called *base morphemes*). Free morphemes can be attached to other morphemes or can stand alone.

Some morphemes have a lexical meaning of their own. They are called *lexical morphemes* (and sometimes, *content words*). Examples are nouns, main verbs, and adjectives. Other morphemes (bound or free) play a grammatical role in that they specify the relationship between one lexical morpheme and another. These are called grammatical morphemes (and sometimes, *function words*). Examples are prepositions, articles, conjunctions, auxiliary verbs, and plural, possessive, and verb endings. It is not always easy to separate lexical morphemes from grammatical ones, and yet the distinction is sometimes important when analyzing language disorders in children. In adults with acquired language disorders, lesions in Broca's area in the frontal lobe (see Figure 2.1) are associated with better retention of content words and severe difficulties in using function words and grammatical morphemes. Lesions in Wernicke's area in the temporal lobe are associated with better retention

FIGURE 2.1
Left hemisphere of an adult brain showing the major lobes and primary sensory and motor cortical areas; the arcuate fasciculus, a subcortical white matter fibrous tract, is shown connecting Wernicke's and Broca's areas in the temporal and frontal lobes.

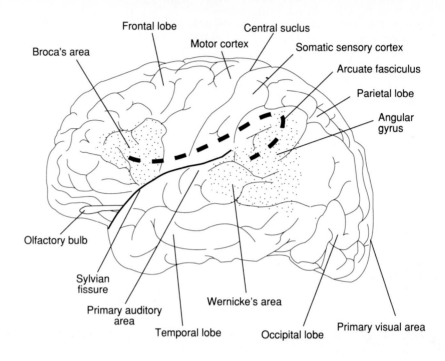

of grammatical morphemes, and content words are either lost or produced as paraphasias (word substitutions that may or may not be real words that are semantically or phonologically related to the target word) (Goodglass & Kaplan, 1983).

Bound morphemes are attached to words as affixes. When they attach to the beginning of words, they are prefixes, and to the ends, they are suffixes. Bound morphemes also can be classified as either *derivational* or *inflectional*. The set of inflectional morphemes is limited, and they are all suffixes that serve a grammatical function in specifying the relationships among words in a particular sentence. Inflectional morphemes are those used to form plurals ("two ti*es*"), possessives ("the tie*'s* pattern"), third person present tense ("he ti*es* his shoes"), past tense ("he ti*ed* his shoes"), past participle ("He has ti*ed* his shoes." Note, the past participle inflectional morpheme is also often *-en* as in dri*ven*), and present participle ("he is ty*ing* his shoes"). Some linguists also include the comparative ("the gaudi*er* tie") and superlative ("the gaudi*est* tie") morphemes on adjectives as inflectional morphemes.

Derivational morphemes are those used to derive new word forms. For example, the related word forms, *event, eventful, eventfully, eventual, eventually, eventuality*, are all constructed using derivational

morphemes. Derivational morphemes may be either prefixes or suffixes, and in many cases they are borrowed from other languages, particularly Latin and Greek. Examples are the Greek prefixes, *hypo-* and *hyper-*, and the Greek suffixes, *-logy* (also Latin), *-ize*, and *-geny*. Other examples are the Latin prefixes, *re-, dis-*, and *de-*, and the Latin suffixes, *-tion*, and *-ate*.

The degree to which languages use morphological inflection to express relationships varies considerably. English uses fewer inflectional morphemes than many languages and relies to a greater degree on word order to convey meaning. The English dialect known as BEV uses numerous inflectional morpheme rules that differ from those of standard English (SE). For example, in several instances, BEV uses an optional zero-morpheme rule (i.e., no bound morpheme is spoken), whereas SE requires a morphological ending to be produced, such as for forming plurals ("She have two marble"), third-person singular verb endings ("He sing the best in our class"), and possessive and copula forms ("That Jason ball"). Language disorders specialists need to carefully consider such language differences when evaluating children's knowledge of morphology.

Syntax. Syntax is the system of rules used in constructing and understanding the form of sentences. Although the two terms are related, *syntax* is not synonymous with *grammar*. Linguists define grammar as the set of rules that will generate all and only the grammatical and meaningful sentences of a language. This suggests that the grammar of a language needs to represent its way of encoding meaning (semantics) by using syntactic rules. As modern linguistic concepts of grammar have evolved, they have been influenced more by the work of Noam Chomsky (1957, 1965, 1981), at Massachusetts Institute of Technology, than by any other person.

In his earlier works, Chomsky (1957, 1965) developed concepts of transformational generative grammar (TGG) as a finite set of rules speakers could use to generate and to understand an infinite number of sentences to represent an infinite number of meanings. TGG comprises two kinds of rules. Phrase structure rules are rewrite rules that define the constituents of simple sentences. For example, Chomsky (1957) provided the following set of rewrite rules that would generate the sentence, "The lightning hit the roof."

i.   Sentence → NP + VP
ii. NP (noun phrase) → Det + N
iii. VP (verb phrase) → Verb + NP
iv. Det (determiner) → the
v.   N (noun) → *lightning, roof,* etc.
vi. V (verb) → *hit, lit,* etc.

Syntactic constituents that are defined in this way can be represented as those coming off from the same node in a tree structure diagram such as the following:

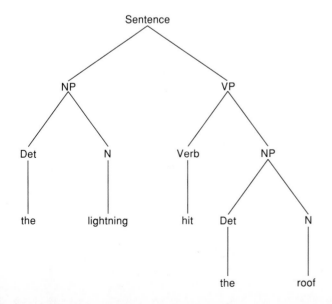

Phrase structure grammar (PSG) works fine for explaining the rules of simple sentences but cannot explain sentences that involve coordination or subordination of ideas, asking questions, stating something in the negative, or forming passives. For instances such as these, Chomsky (1957; J. P. B. Allen & Van Buren, 1971) described a different set of transformational rules. Transformational rules act on the basic constituents of sentences to move them around and to generate more complex sentences. They are needed for transforming the more abstract deep structure of sentences, which are related most closely to their meaning, into the surface structure forms that are actually spoken. They allow active declarative sentences, such as "He eats chili cheese dogs," to be transformed into: (1) negatives: "He doesn't eat chili cheese dogs" (notice that this one requires use of the "dummy do" auxiliary transformation rule), (2) questions: "Does he eat chili cheese dogs?" (the "dummy do" is needed here as well), (3) passives: "The chili cheese dog was eaten by him," and (4) combinations of these: "Didn't he eat the chili cheese dog?" (among a variety of other sentence types).

More recently, Chomsky (1981) revised his ideas of grammar in his government-binding (GB) theory. Never known for being easy to understand (to be differentiated from being eager to understand, in a variation on one of Chomsky's own examples of two sentences with parallel surface structure but different deep structures), Chomsky's newer ideas are as complex as his old ones (see Box 2.7 for an outline of the main points of the theory). They were interpreted for speech–language specialists by Leonard and Loeb (1988). In GB theory, Chomsky's focus shifted slightly from the abstract structure of language to the learnability of language and to constraints on the kinds of hypotheses a human can form about the structure of language, no matter what language that person speaks. According to GB theory, internalized grammar must consist of a universal grammar (UG) that is compatible with the existing and possible grammars of the world, and it must also be possible to develop on the basis of limited evidence.

In GB theory, four levels are posited for UG: (1) Deep structures (D-structures) are characterized by a categorical component and a lexicon, with the rules of the categorical component resembling the rules of phrase structure grammar described in Chomsky's earlier work but with the added possibility of intermediate structures between lexical (verb, noun, determiner) or phrasal (noun phrase, verb phrase)

Box 2.7   The levels posited for universal grammar in Chomsky's (1981) government-binding theory

1. **D-structures** (deep structures) have two components:
   a. A categorical component, in which the rules resemble those of phrase structure grammar described in Chomsky's earlier work (1957, 1965), but with the added possibility of intermediate structures between lexical (verb, noun, determiner) or phrasal (noun phrase, verb phrase) constituents
   b. A lexicon, which specifies both the abstract morphophonological structure of each lexical item as well as its syntactic features
2. **S-structures,** which are similar, but not exactly the same as the surface structures of Chomsky's earlier work, because, although closer to the spoken form than the D-structure, they are still abstract
3. **PF** (phonetic form) rules operate on an additional level that result in an abstract characterization of sound (Leonard & Loeb, 1988, point out that this may be a contribution from Broca's area.)
4. **LF** (logical form) rules operate at the same level as PF rules but provide an abstract characterization of logical interpretation.

Government-binding subtheories, which Chomsky developed to explain grammatical principles and constraints that might allow language to be learned quickly:

1. **Bounding theory** suggests that boundaries imposed by noun phrase nodes and clause/sentence nodes in sentences (explained in text) limit the movement of constituents in transformations.
2. **Government theory** suggests that certain kinds of nodes have privileges for governing other nodes (e.g., prepositions exert governing influences over their accompanying noun phrases).
3. **Case theory** involves the rules by which abstract case (e.g., nominative or objective) is assigned to noun phrase nodes (it makes use of governing principles because some nodes influence others).
4. **Binding theory** concerns the way in which more than one noun phrase can refer to the same entity, including the following:
   a. Reflexive pronouns that refer back to nouns in the same sentence (e.g., John shaved himself) are considered bound in their governing category and are called *anaphor* by Chomsky (however, do not be confused by this; the term, *anaphoric reference* is often used in more general ways to describe the use of one linguistic element (often a pronoun) to refer back to another).
   b. Pronominals that can refer to other entities not included in the same sentence (e.g., "John kissed *her*") are considered free in their governing category.
   c. R-expressions, which are noun phrases that have no antecedents in the same sentence or elsewhere in the current discourse (e.g., "John saw *the zebra*"); considered free.
5. **Θ-theory** concerns the assignment of thematic (hence, *theta*) roles such as agent of action and goal of action. It is closely aligned with case theory, working with it so that both grammatic case (e.g., nominative) and semantic (thematic) case (e.g., agent) can be ascribed to the same node (e.g., *John* in the previous examples).
6. **Control theory** concerns the ways in which the subject of an embedded infinitive phrase may be controlled (in some of the same ways that pronoun reference is) but may be ungoverned (because of the embedding process). "John wondered what to do" implies *John* as subject of the infinitive phrase, but this sentence could be paraphrased "John wondered what one should do."

constituents. (2) The surface structures (S-structures) of GB theory are not exactly like those of Chomsky's earlier work because, although closer to the spoken form than the D-structures, they are still abstract. (3)

Phonetic form (PF) rules operate on an additional level that result in an abstract characterization of sound. Leonard and Loeb (1988) point out that this may be a contribution from Broca's area in the left hemisphere of the brain. (4) Logical form (LF) rules operate at the same level as PF rules but provide an abstract characterization of logical interpretation. In addition, the new GB theory includes numerous subtheories to explain other grammatical principles.

Although GB theory is beginning to influence research questions and design, it has not yet exerted major influence on clinical practice. Chapter 8 presents information regarding more traditional views of the syntax of auxiliary verb constructions and simple and complex sentences that are acquired during the middle stages of language acquisition. Professionals who work with individuals with language disorders at middle and later stages also need to consider the syntactic complexity evident in the curricular contexts in which children and adolescents participate. The demands placed on language comprehension systems when processing complex texts may present problems for children with weak systems even when their productive language appears to be errorless.

Semantics. *Semantics* is the system of rules for relating meaning to words, phrases, sentences, and texts. The sense that is represented semantically, as part of linguistic meaning, can be separated from the kind of sense that varies with a speaker's intentions, which is a part of pragmatic meaning (to be considered in the next section). In this section, in addition to linguistic sense, I discuss linguistic reference. These are the categories suggested by Parker (1986) for outlining the area of semantics. Parker also considers philosophical explanations of linguistic truth as part of semantics, but I have incorporated some aspects of those issues in the other two categories. See Parker or his sources to learn more about the more esoteric philosophical concepts related to linguistic truth.

Linguistic sense. Words do more than represent things. They represent ideas about the essence of things, actions, people, animals, states, qualities, manner, time, number, location, and so forth. One way to attempt to understand semantics is to think about linguistic concepts not as unitary ideas but as clusters of features. Semantic features, like phonological features considered previously, are thought to be binary (either present, +, or absent, −). For example, some of the key distinctive features of the meaning of *nail* are ⟨−animate⟩, ⟨+concrete⟩, ⟨+metallic⟩, ⟨+long⟩, ⟨+pointed⟩, ⟨+head⟩, ⟨+used with hammer⟩, ⟨+fastener of wood⟩. Many more positive features representing the meaning of *nail* can be listed, but

most are probably not important most of the time. You activate them when you need them to perform a particular linguistic task. For example, if you are trying to learn to discriminate between *nail* and *screw*, you might activate the feature ⟨−spiral threads on shaft⟩. What if you do not yet have concepts for *spiral*, *threads*, or *shaft*? You might still be able to attach a feature resembling this to the word in your brain as a nonlinguistic perceptual feature. If you started reading this example with a different meaning for *nail*, thinking of a fingernail instead of a carpenter's nail, you must have activated a different set of semantic features. In this case, you would have included features such as ⟨+animate⟩, ⟨−metallic⟩, ⟨+can be broken⟩, and many others. When you realized that I was describing a different kind of nail, you would have had to shift to a different part of your mental lexicon. Were you thinking about two different words or two different meanings for the same word? When considering how words are acquired, in Chapter 3, I will return to some of these psycholinguistic concepts. The following discussion addresses more of the ways that words might be related to each other in lexicons and language structures.

The following is a list of semantic qualities that characterize the **linguistic sense** of words (based on Parker, 1986, with modifications to include semantic properties of phrases and sentences as well as words):

1. Lexical and syntactic ambiguity. Sometimes called *multiple meaning*, this quality refers to the possibility that a word can have more than one meaning. For example, *nail* can refer to two different objects and can also be used as an action verb, as when one talks about "nailing a doghouse together." *Nail* can also have figurative meanings, as in the idiomatic uses, "She hit the nail on the head," "He got nailed to the wall on that one," or "She really nailed that contract we've been wanting." Multiple meanings may share some of the same semantic features, but different meanings signify that different clusters of semantic features separate them. Context usually disambiguates meanings when necessary.

Phrases and sentences can be ambiguous as well as words. Consider the ambiguity of Chomsky's famous sentence "Flying planes can be dangerous." Another one is "Visiting relatives can be a nuisance." Can you explain the differing meanings of these two sentences?

2. Lexical and syntactic synonymy. *Synonymy* refers to the possibility that more than one word can mean approximately the same thing. For example, *lovely* and *beautiful* are synonyms. Phrases and sentences can be synonymous as well as words.

When two sentences mean the same, we say that one is a *paraphrase* of the other (this concept is related to the concept of syntactic *entailment,* which is considered in the next subsection). As an example of syntactic synonymy, consider the sentence, "Complex machines are made up of several different simple machines" and its paraphrase, "Several different simple machines together make a complex machine." This example is drawn from some curriculum-based language assessment work with a third-grade girl with language-learning problems who could not understand that the two sentences meant the same thing (N. W. Nelson, 1986). For her, they were two entirely different sentences. This lack of flexibility made it quite difficult for her to answer questions that paraphrased material in the text.

Although there are many ways to say the same thing, choices of words and sentences are not arbitrary. Speakers generally choose their words and syntax based on the purposes of the intended communication. This is one of the ways that semantics, syntax, and pragmatics are intertwined.

3. Hyponymy and entailment. "A hyponym is a word whose meaning contains the entire meaning of another word, known as the superordinate" (Parker, 1986, p. 33). For example, *penny* is a hyponym of *coin,* and *coin* is a hyponym of *money.* That is, *penny* includes all of the meaning of *coin,* but *coin* does not include only the meaning of *penny.*

Phrases and sentences can be related in meaning in ways similar to the ways words are related. As noted by Parker (1986), "Just as hyponymy describes an inclusive relation between words, so entailment describes an inclusive relation between sentences" (p. 41). Entailment occurs when one sentence includes the meaning of the other. For example, in the sentences, "Monica has pneumonia," and "Monica is sick," the second sentence is entailed in the first because the second sentence is always true if the first one is, and the first one is never true if the second one is not. The first sentence, however, is not entailed in the second because Monica could be sick with a variety of ailments other than pneumonia. Entailment is related to syntactic synonymy in that if one sentence is a paraphrase of another, each is entailed in the other.

4. Overlap. When two words share some semantic features, but not all, they can be said to overlap. For example, the words *teacher* and *woman* overlap because they contain some of the same features but not all. Not all women are teachers, and not all teachers are women, but both are ⟨+human⟩ and both are ⟨+adult⟩ (usually).

5. Antonymy. When words share all semantic features except one, we say that they are *antonyms.* For example, *long* and *short* both represent degrees of linear dimension, but they differ in the feature of ⟨±degree⟩.

Reference.   Semantic reference is not the same as general sense. Reference differs depending on context, so that the same word may refer to one thing in one utterance and to a different thing in another. For example, in the sentences, "I like your new tie. I have one just like it. I love wearing ties," the first instance of the word *tie* refers to a particular tie around the neck of a friend. When *tie* occurs again in the third sentence, it refers not just to that particular tie, but to the class of things we call ties. Notice that two other references to things called *tie* are made in the middle sentence of this triplet. In that sentence, *one* refers to a tie owned by the speaker, and *it* refers to the tie owned by the listener. Is it any wonder that many children with language disorders get confused about what words refer to during natural communication exchanges?

Semantic qualities that characterize **linguistic reference** include the following (based on Parker, 1986):

1. Referent. The thing referred to is the referent. In the preceding example, three different referents for *tie* appeared: the listener's tie, the speaker's tie of the same kind, and the general class of things called ties.

2. Extension. The third type of referent is considered an extension because it includes all possibilities in the class called *tie.*

3. Prototype. The kind of tie people think of first, as a best example, might be a long skinny piece of folded cloth, worn by men in Western societies with their business suits. A bow tie or string tie is not usually considered a prototype. If you were imagining women in the preceding roles of speaker and listener you may have been thinking in terms of a prototype of a feminine tie, perhaps made of softer silk.

4. Stereotype. When a prototype becomes widely agreed on by many speakers, the list of semantic features that characterize it become a stereotype.

5. Coreference. When two linguistic expressions have the same referent, they are coreferential. For example, the phrases "apple blossom" and "Michigan's state flower" have the same referent but not exactly the same meaning.

6. Anaphora and cataphora. In the tie example, the first instance of the word *tie* and the pronoun *it* both have the same referent. They are coreferential, but they also provide an example of anaphoric reference in that one linguistic element is used to refer to another. Although Parker (1986) did not differentiate anaphoric and cataphoric reference in his listing, other linguists sometimes do, and the concepts are useful to language disorders specialists because so many school-age children with language-learning disabilities have difficulty understanding both kinds of reference when school language becomes complex. Anaphora occurs when a linguistic element (often a pronoun) refers *back* to a term that came before it, as in the example of *tie*, later referred to as *it*. Cataphora, however, is a referential cue for a linguistic element that is due to come up in the next sentence or so. For example, if the speaker in the preceding exchange were to say, "Listen to this. I have two dozen ties at home in my closet," *this* would be an example of cataphoric reference. Teachers often use cataphoric reference in school to mark content for children and to draw their attention to important linguistic information.

7. Deixis. When reference shifts depending on the perspectives of the speaker and listener, the rules of deixis are brought into play for expressing relative concepts of person, place, and time. Deixis of person, for example, involves knowing that the same person can be referred to with the pronouns *me* or *you* depending on who is speaking. Deixis of place in-

volves knowing that the position of a book that stays in the same place may be referred to as *here* when the speaker is standing beside it but *there* when the speaker is some distance away. An example of deixis of time is contained in the phrase, "Today is the tomorrow we talked about yesterday."

Syntactic–semantic relationships (case grammar). A third set of concepts (one not considered by Parker, 1986, in his chapter on semantics) concerns the semantic role assumed by words in a particular sentence. Some issues of ambiguity may be resolved by understanding the rules for relating syntax and semantics in a language. Syntax is formulated by combining words representing such semantic cases as agent, action, patient, and object. An example is the typical English sentence, "Donna made her mother a cake." Even finer distinctions are sometimes made. For example, when Fillmore (1968) proposed case grammar (see Box 2.8) as an alternative to strictly syntactic models, he identified the case served by the *cake* in this sentence as factitive, in that it resulted from the action of the verb. Children may use their understanding of how the world works (e.g., who can do what and how) to develop their semantic concepts and to guide their acquisition of syntactic ones, but these relationships are not fully understood.

Pragmatics. Pragmatic rules differ somewhat from the other four rule systems of language because they relate to ways in which language is *used to communicate* rather than how it is generated. The grammatical rule systems discussed thus far specify how language is pronounced (phonology), how it is formulated (syntax and morphology), and how meaning is represented (semantics and morphology). Now I

Box 2.8	Case grammar rules suggested by Fillmore (1968) to characterize the influence of semantics on syntax	
	Agentive	Perceived instigator of action (usually animate)—"*Mom* made the cake."
	Dative	Animate affected by state or action named by verb—"We gave *her* some."
	Experiencer	Animate who experiences event, action, or mental disposition—"*She* loved it."
	Factitive	Object or being resulting from state of the verb—"Mom made the *cake.*"
	Instrumental	Inanimate object or force which brings about the process of the verb but is not the instigator—"She mixed it with the *beaters.*"
	Locative	Place or spatial orientation of the state, action, or process of the verb—"Some fell on the *floor.*"
	Objective	Animate or inanimate noun whose role in the state or action of the verb depends on the meaning of the verb—"The girl ate *it* anyway."

discuss how each of these rule systems is modified in different communicative contexts depending on contributions from the internalized system of pragmatic knowledge.

Like language itself, pragmatics is rather hard to define. Carol Prutting (1982) quoted Susan Ervin-Tripp, at a discussion during a Child Language Forum at Stanford University in 1978, as saying that "pragmatics is everything we used to throw out when we analyzed language" (p. 123). Levinson (1983) also used a strategy of definition by comparison for pragmatics when he commented that "the most promising definitions are those which equate pragmatics with 'meaning minus semantics' or with a theory of language understanding that takes context into account, in order to complement the contribution that semantics makes to meaning" (p. 32).

To appreciate this emphasis, imagine that someone has just commented on your new hairstyle—something like, "You got your hair cut"—and you are not sure how to interpret it. Whether you say it or not, you will probably think, "What do you mean by that?" Although "You got your hair cut" is a declarative statement, it is more than a simple statement of fact. Your friend certainly did not need to inform you that your hair was cut. It should be obvious to everyone that you were there when it happened. The underlying meaning is probably more like, "I noticed that you got your hair cut." But it is also unlikely that you will interpret the statement as a neutral exposition of your friend's observational powers. Rather, the meaning that probably concerns you the most is the evaluation that is implied in the statement. How you choose to finally interpret the statement and whether you decide to pursue the topic will depend on such complex factors as the cultural backgrounds of you and your conversational partner (in some contexts, you might be offended at such a personal statement, and in others, you might be honored that someone noticed); the tone of voice used in making the statement (was it admiring, shocked, or something else?); the environment in which the exchange occurs (are people watching? did you get a Mohawk?); and many other factors. If you are on the other side of such a potential communicative event, a similar set of factors will determine the language choices you make yourself when possibly introducing the topic.

How can we organize our understanding of the kinds of rules that govern social communicative exchanges? It helps to partition this set of conventions into rules of several different types. In this section on pragmatics, we will use the categories of speech acts, discourse management, and contextual variation.

Speech acts. The concept of speech acts was introduced in 1955 by the British philosopher John L. Austin (1962) when delivering a lecture series at Harvard University (Parker, 1986). Austin's revolutionary idea at the time was that, in uttering sentences, speakers are doing things as well as saying things. That is, they are performing acts with their words. Austin listed six kinds of speech acts that were performed simply by uttering them and called these *performatives.* They were constrained by the conditions that they all had to have a first-person subject and had to be in present tense: "I promise," "I apologize," "I name," "I give and bequeath [in a will]," "I bet," and "I pronounce [you man and wife]."

Others have since extended the concept of speech acts to other kinds of utterances. John Searle was one of Austin's students. In Searle's book *Speech Acts* (1969), based on his doctoral dissertation, he developed the theory that everything speakers say constitutes some sort of speech act (not just Austin's original six performatives). Searle also adapted another key idea of Austin's which, although it may seem to be only linguistic jargon at first, can prove quite useful in providing services to language-impaired children (see Part II). Searle held that every speech act consists of three separate acts: (1) the locutionary act, (2) the illocutionary act, and (3) the perlocutionary act.

The **locutionary act** is the simple utterance of the sentence. In the example we have been considering, the locutionary act is your friend's utterance of "You got your hair cut." Locutionary acts, by virtue of being sentences, are made up of the two parts, a *referring expression*, which is a noun phrase that names the subject of the sentence (in this case, *you*), and a *predicating expression*, which is a verb phrase or predicate adjective that says something about the subject (in this case, "got your hair cut"). But as we considered above, there may be more to the meaning than the simple utterance of the sentence implies.

The **illocutionary act** (Searle, 1976) represents the speaker's intention in uttering the sentence. Sometimes called *illocutionary force*, this act is the one that the speaker intends to perform by producing the utterance. (Numerous categorical systems have been proposed for cataloguing the types of language functions that speakers intend to perform at various stages of development, e.g., Dore, 1975; Halliday, 1975—these are considered later in Chapters 7 and 8). It was the nature of our friend's illocutionary intention that we questioned when we asked about the "true" meaning of the haircut comment. Only the speaker can be sure at the point of utterance whether the meaning underlying the sentence is intended as a compliment, as an "It's about time" comment, or as an "I can't believe you did that!" comment. We may wonder if our friend is using this kind of statement to soften or camouflage an evaluative, exclamatory statement, because we have acquired an understanding of pragmatic rules related to indirect speech acts.

An **indirect speech act** (Searle, 1975) occurs when speakers choose to use one syntactic form on the surface, while their intended meaning is more closely aligned with another. For example, if you say, "I am allergic to shellfish," when invited to a friend's home in New Orleans for dinner, you may appear to be using a simple declarative sentence to state a fact, but the indirect speech act is really a conditional imperative, "Don't serve shellfish (unless you want to see me get sick)." When you arrive, your friend may call to you, "We're out on the balcony." What is the indirect speech act in this case? Of course, it is also possible for a speech act to be direct, such as when a parent says to a teenager, "Go get a haircut," and means it as an imperative.

The speech act may also be either literal or nonliteral. For example, your father may attempt to get you to hurry by saying, "Shake a leg." This act is direct because the locutionary act is formulated as an imperative, and the illocutionary act is intended as an imperative, but it is nonliteral. To comply appropriately, you must understand that the meaning of the idiomatic expression, "Shake a leg," is to hurry up. On the other hand, if you are learning a new dance step, the direction to "Shake a leg" might be intended to be taken literally.

Finally, the third act that is a part of every speech act is the **perlocutionary act**. The perlocutionary act is the effect of the locutionary act on the listener. In the haircut example, the perlocutionary act might be alternatively a sense of being insulted, or of being complimented. One determinant of what communicative partners experience as "smoothness" in communication and being "on the same wavelength" is that the intended message and the received message match at both referential and emotional levels. This is an experience that may escape many children with language disorders. They may recognize that they have irritated their listeners, but not know why.

Discourse management. Different kinds of rules are put into play for managing different kinds of discourse genres. Even before babies can produce locutionary acts, they begin to acquire pragmatic rules for discourse management. The first discourse genre that children experience is conversational. Even before they can carry on a true linguistic conversation, babies engage in what Bateson (1971) called *protoconversations*. Similar to the prototypes that are built before a new automobile is put into full production, protoconversations are the turn-taking exchanges that can be put into practice before full linguistic conversations are possible between infants and their parents.

Among the pragmatic rules that contribute to the orderly management of conversations are the following (Prutting & Kirchner, 1987):

1. **Topic control rules:** for selection, introduction, maintenance, and change
2. **Turn-taking rules:** for initiation, response, repair/revision, pause time, interruption/overlap, feedback to speakers, adjacency, contingency, and quantity/conciseness
3. **Lexical selection rules:** across contexts for specificity/accuracy, cohesion
4. **Stylistic variation:** for varying communicative style depending on listener characteristics
5. **Paralinguistic aspects:** intelligibility, vocal intensity, vocal quality, prosody, fluency
6. **Nonverbal aspects:** physical proximity, physical contacts, body posture, foot/leg and hand/arm movements, gestures, facial expression, and eye gaze

Although conversational interaction is the discourse genre that is most characteristic of early language learning, other genres that become important speech events in the school-age years originate during the preschool years. The presence of varied discourse genres can be illustrated by the fact that young children can answer questions about speech events. If someone walks in while a parent is reading a book to a child and asks, "What are you doing?" a preschool child can answer, "Reading a story." This represents an awareness of the discourse genre of narratives, or story telling. Story telling can be announced, as when adults say, "Let me tell you a story," or when children request, "Grandma, tell me a story," or it can be interwoven with conversations. Think of the times when you have said or heard, "Did I ever tell you about the time that . . ." Such entrees are introductions to the narrative discourse genre.

When someone begins a narrative, everyone else begins to assume the discourse posture of spectator (J. N. Britton, 1979). The speaker begins an organized, somewhat preplanned discourse sequence with a setting and characters, problem, action, outcome, and ending (Applebee, 1978), and everyone else gets ready to listen. This kind of discourse genre differs considerably from conversations, in which both speaker and listener assume the discourse posture of participant (J. N. Britton, 1979). In conversations, participants negotiate the sequence of the discourse within the general rules for conversational interaction outlined previously.

When children grow older, they encounter yet another discourse genre. Expository discourse is typical of academic discourse that explains the hierarchical and parallel organization of concepts in formal education. Lectures and textbooks that are arranged to present factual material in the forms of organized outlines with elaboration are examples of expository texts. Children who understand how different kinds of texts are organized are better able to handle the varied expectations of the curriculum, such as their science books, which are organized as expository texts, and literature books, which are organized as narrative texts.

Contextual variation. The ability to say (and interpret) things differently depending on linguistic and nonlinguistic contextual variables is a key part of knowing the rules of pragmatics. Recall how important contextual variables were in deciding what to say and how to interpret speech acts in the haircut example. The importance of context is one of the primary considerations of sociolinguistics, as discussed in the final section of this chapter.

A major element in contextual sensitivity is being able to make predictions about discourse based on prior experiences with human communication as a medium and with particular communicative partners as individuals. Some of the expectations that play a role in how conversations proceed are based not on overt statements and evidence but on implications that can be inferred from immediate data. Such inferences, which are based on knowledge of context and extend meaning beyond the immediate linguistic statements made, are called *implicature* (Grice, 1975). A part of the predictability of communicative

events is based, in addition, on the four conversational maxims that the philosopher Paul Grice (1975) outlined. These include (1) the *maxim of quantity*, which states that speakers should provide no more or less information than required by the context and the listener's prior knowledge; (2) the *maxim of quality*, which states that speakers' contributions should be truthful and based on sufficient evidence; (3) the *maxim of relation*, which states that speakers' contributions should be relevant to the topic under discussion, and (4) the *maxim of manner*, which states that speakers' contributions should not be vague, ambiguous, or excessively wordy.

Assessing Knowledge of the Rule Systems of Language

This brief overview has outlined the main features of the five rule systems of language that are part of the intrinsic knowledge of normal adult users of a language. Although an important function of language specialists is that of assessing an individual's intrinsic knowledge of language rules (considered further in Chapter 6), that knowledge cannot be measured directly. Intrinsic linguistic knowledge differs from explicit or metalinguistic knowledge in that it can only be inferred by observing the output of a system. A common method used by psycholinguists and by speech–language pathologists for assessing intrinsic knowledge of language rules is to gather samples of oral or written language expression and comprehension using audio- and videotape recordings and to analyze them to see if the person acts as if he or she has been using the expected rule system to generate the observable communicative behaviors. In some cases, the individual may appear to use the rules of a dialect other than standard English but at a level appropriate for his stage of development in that dialect. Such occurrences need to be distinguished from cases of a child showing evidence of using rules typical of a younger speaker or listener (often called *language delay)* or of a person whose intrinsic knowledge of the rules of language is disordered in some other way (often called *language impairment, deviance,* or *disorder*). Evidence regarding distinctions between language delay and language disorder is considered further in Chapter 4.

Some individuals with language disorders may appear to use highly consistent (although limited) rule systems to produce and understand language. Others may not. In either case, it is helpful for language specialists to take the perspective that nothing a person does in participating in language activities is accidental (if not always predictable). Measurements of language comprehension and production always represent multiple factors, including combinations of influences from both within and beyond the individual. These multiple factors work together to result in a particular set of behaviors being observed within a particular context.

This perspective was developed by Kenneth Goodman (1973) in designing strategies for observing knowledge of written language using miscue analysis of "errors" produced by readers when reading aloud. For example, when a child reads the printed sentence, "The baby was cold," as "The baby saw cold," and does not make any effort to self-correct the reading miscue, evidence is available that the child is confusing words that look alike and is not using knowledge of the rules of language syntax or semantics to notice that the resulting sentence is anomalous (this method is discussed in greater detail in Chapter 9).

The perspective that nothing a language user does is accidental is also one taken by developmental psycholinguists when analyzing the childlike "errors" made by preschoolers as they are learning to talk (McNeill, 1966). For example, when a 3-year-old says, "My daddy taked my shoes off and tickled my feets," evidence is available to suggest that the child has rules for adding regular past-tense and plural inflectional endings (the bound morphemes -*ed* and -*s*) but has not yet worked out all of the irregular exceptions to those rules.

Sometimes intrinsic language knowledge is assessed by devising special tasks rather than by gathering spontaneous communication samples. For example, a person's intrinsic knowledge of semantic or syntactic rules might be assessed by asking the individual to judge whether it is acceptable to say particular sentences in certain ways, while manipulating features of the sentences to make some of them anomalous. This type of task differs from one that requires a person to demonstrate explicit knowledge of language rules. Explicit knowledge of language rules is demonstrated, for example, when a person tells what the rule is for forming passive sentences or for forming plurals. The demonstration of explicit knowledge of language rules is something that is practiced as a part of formal education and, occasionally, by language intervention specialists with older children or adults.

Language judgment tasks are not explicit, but they are *metalinguistic*. Metalinguistic tasks require individuals to treat language as an object of focus in its own right, in which it becomes "opaque," rather than the "transparent" tool that it usually is as a medium of communication. Metalinguistic tasks involve conscious focus on language, on using language to talk about language, and on thinking about language on more than one level at once.

Any task that is metalinguistic introduces an extra variable into the process of assessing children's knowledge of linguistic rules. If a child fails to demonstrate knowledge of a language rule when metalinguistic strategies are used, language specialists must consider the possibility that it may be failure to understand the task that prevents the child from demonstrating knowledge rather than lack of intrinsic knowledge of the rule under question. Different kinds of tasks make different levels of metalinguistic demands. A continuum of some sample tasks is shown in Figure 2.2. Notice in this figure that there is no way to gain access directly to a person's language competence or intrinsic knowledge of the rules. (Although at present, there is no way to open up the brain to measure intrinsic knowledge of language rules, Sussman, 1989, in his review of recent research on the auditory–spatial feature-detection mechanisms in the brain cells of barn owls, has suggested that there may be evidence of specific linguistic–type knowledge represented in individual brain cells.)

Noam Chomsky differentiated between nonobservable intrinsic linguistic knowledge and the observable extrinsic evidence of that knowledge as the difference between language competence and language performance. Chomsky (1965, 1968) defined *language competence* as the idealized internalized grammar that allows native speakers of a language to judge sentences as being grammatical, ungrammatical, or ambiguous, and to generate all and only the sentences of the language. He accounted for the observation that native speakers of a language sometimes produce agrammatical sentences or fail to analyze perfectly grammatical ones by saying that these represent errors of *performance*. Performance errors might include such things as lapses of memory or attention and malfunctions of the psychological mechanisms underlying speech.

As Slobin (1971) noted, the difference between linguists and psychologists in regard to language can be characterized somewhat by the primary interests of linguists in the underlying ability that makes it possi-

FIGURE 2.2
Continuum of tasks for using language performance to assess
knowledge of linguistic rules.

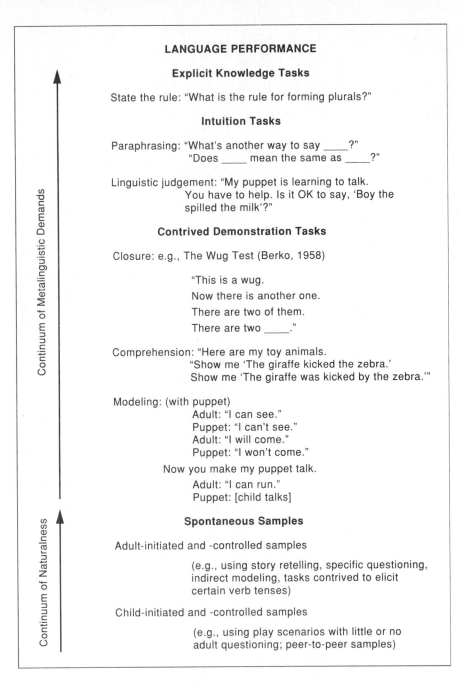

LANGUAGE PERFORMANCE

Explicit Knowledge Tasks

State the rule: "What is the rule for forming plurals?"

Intuition Tasks

Paraphrasing: "What's another way to say _____?"
            "Does _____ mean the same as _____?"

Linguistic judgement: "My puppet is learning to talk.
            You have to help. Is it OK to say, 'Boy the
            spilled the milk'?"

Contrived Demonstration Tasks

Closure: e.g., The Wug Test (Berko, 1958)

            "This is a wug.

            Now there is another one.

            There are two of them.

            There are two _____."

Comprehension: "Here are my toy animals.
            "Show me 'The giraffe kicked the zebra.'
            Show me 'The giraffe was kicked by the zebra.'"

Modeling: (with puppet)
            Adult: "I can see."
            Puppet: "I can't see."
            Adult: "I will come."
            Puppet: "I won't come."
        Now you make my puppet talk.
            Adult: "I can run."
            Puppet: [child talks]

Spontaneous Samples

Adult-initiated and -controlled samples

            (e.g., using story retelling, specific questioning,
            indirect modeling, tasks contrived to elicit
            certain verb tenses)

Child-initiated and -controlled samples

            (e.g., using play scenarios with little or no
            adult questioning; peer-to-peer samples)

Continuum of Metalinguistic Demands

Continuum of Naturalness

ble for people (generally linguists) to identify such things as grammaticality in ideal situations and the additional interests of psychologists in the factors that cause performance to deviate from competence. Psycholinguists are also interested in finding ways to cut through performance irregularities to convince themselves of the "psychological reality" of underlying linguistic rules of varied sorts.

Personal Reflection 2.4   "A child is not a computer that either 'knows' or 'does not know.' A child is a bumpy, blippy, excitable, fatiguable, distractible, active, friendly, mulish, semi-cooperative bundle of biology. Some factors help a moving child pull together coherent address to a problem; others hinder that pulling together and tend to make a child 'not know.'"

Sheldon H. White (1980, p. 43), psychologist at Harvard.

If performance errors are typical of normal speakers in everyday situations (and they are, as evidenced by the sample of classroom discourse shown in Box 2.9), how can language disorders specialists hope to identify children who are not learning and using language normally? The answer to that question often lies in four kinds of judgments that will be considered further in Chapter 6 on assessment and intervention: (1) judgments of degree (children with language disorders may be observed to make more performance errors than their peers in similar contexts); (2) judgments of kind (children with language disorders may be observed to make different kinds of performance errors than their peers in similar contexts); (3) judgments relative to some standard (children with language disorders may be observed to make more and different performance errors than a standardized sample of their peers did in a highly controlled context); and (4) judgments relative to assessment of need and opportunity (children with language disorders may be observed and described as not having all of the language skills they need to take advantage of the opportunities that are, or could be, available to them).

COMMUNICATION AS SOCIAL INTERACTION

Communication does not "happen" within an individual. Communication happens when a listener or a reader understands the language that a speaker or

---

Box 2.9   **Discourse from a regular third-grade classroom (from data gathered by Sturm, 1990)**

Student 1: XXX [three unintelligible syllables] Nintendo (um my) you know my friends and on Mario Brothers went into this elevator, and (it's um) I jumped on it, and (um) my friend thought there were XXX (um) that I was dead, but (um right that um) and other (um) logs caught me. Then I caught up, and (um) . . .
Student 2: What game?
Student 1: Mario Brothers, why?
Student 3: One or two?
Student 1: One, and (um) . . .
....
Teacher: We'll have a quick little review here (where you can. . .) We have talked about learning how to carry [pause] one time (and now today we're gonna see. . .) We may have to carry more than ones in a multiplication problem. So I'll do a quick warmup. I'll put problems up on the chalk board for (ah) people to complete. If everyone gets theirs correct with their partners, then we'll assign the assignment.
Teacher: Quick review: From the ones to the ones, ones to the tens, ones to the hundreds. Three times four. Alisha, do you remember what three times four is?
Student 1: Twelve.
Teacher: Terrific! What number do I put down here?
Student 1: The two.
Teacher Great! Penny, what do I do with the one?
Student 2: Put it on top of the five.
Teacher: OK, in the tens column. (Ah) Renee, three times seven?

a writer has produced (Hoskins, 1990). In other words, it takes two (at least) for language to be communicative. Of course, people can "talk" to themselves either overtly or subliminally (try following a complex set of directions without talking to yourself), but talking to oneself is a different kind of language use. It relates more closely to cognitive processing than to communicative social interaction. Most talking and writing occurs in social contexts that involve not only the influence of immediately present environmental and cultural variables, but the past histories and future expectations of the participants as well.

The term *sociolinguistics* has been used in more than one way. In their book *Child Discourse*, editors Susan Ervin-Tripp and Claudia Mitchell-Kernan (1977) pointed out that the term has been used "both to refer to differences in the linguistic structures of socially defined groups, and to those rules of speech that incorporate contextual features rather than purely linguistic or referential choices" (p. 3). They also noted that the two uses of the term are related. The central themes of the sociolinguistic perspective (as compared with the traditional linguistic perspective) were outlined by Ervin-Tripp and Mitchell-Kernan to include the following five points: (1) Natural conversations, rather than contrived tasks, are used as the data source to learn about the nature of language and communication. (2) Discourse structures, rather than sentences, are treated as the highest level of analysis. (3) Social context, beyond the linguistic structure of sentences, is recognized as influencing how language is interpreted, such as knowing whether to interpret an utterance as a question or a command. (4) Variability is viewed as a systematic component of linguistic rules, including those of phonology and grammar, and it appears to be related not only to linguistic context but also to social features such as sex, age, and setting. (5) Language functions are viewed as diverse, rather than merely representational, in that functions are not mapped directly by any structural features, but are partially related to cultural and developmental expectations (see Box 2.10).

The Importance of Context

The sociolinguistic perspective plays a critical role in decision making for language-disordered children. The questions introduced in Chapter 1 about what language skills a child needs and the opportunities available for communicating in the important contexts of the child's life cannot be addressed without taking a sociolinguistic perspective. The variability inherent in the difficulties many children with language disorders experience can also be understood more readily against a backdrop of understanding that a certain amount of variability represents normal expectations associated with different kinds of speech events. Because contexts vary, and because they play such a role in determining how communication events proceed, the ethnomethodological tools of sociolinguistics become important to language specialists as they conduct language assessment and intervention activities, especially when issues of multicultural expectations are involved.

Box 2.10	Sociolinguistic rules (summarized from Ervin-Tripp & Mitchell-Kernan, 1977)

1. **Alternation rules** involve the selection of alternative events, acts, topics, and linguistic forms from the speaker's repertoire. The choices are based on linguistic and social variables such as the rank and sex of addressees, expected compliance (in the case of requests), and inferred knowledge of the audience.
2. **Co-occurrence rules** govern the stylistic coherence of linguistic features in code switching, such as when a child talks "baby talk."
3. **Sequential rules** provide the structural organization of interaction that are divided between:
   a. **Conversation rules** for entering conversations, leaving conversations, taking turns, getting attention and changing the topic, acknowledging moves, handling digressions, and querying
   b. **Speech event rules** that are genre specific for managing a variety of events that may be more or less tightly structured, such as court trials, classroom lessons, and informal conversations

Reasons for Communicating

The assessment and intervention process should include some focus on factors within the child and within the important contexts of his or her life that maximize reasons for communicating. Whether one is working with an infant in the context of family or a school-age child in the context of the regular or special education classroom, one should determine whether the child has sufficient reasons for communicating and should encourage increased reasons for communicating that are both positive and culturally specific (see Personal Reflection 2.5).

In consulting with others to develop opportunities that encourage children to want to use their language skills, language specialists need to consider that different contexts have different expectations. Although a child's language skills may be reasonably appropriate (or accommodated) in some contexts, other contexts may place demands that are so far outside of the child's abilities and experience that the child cannot hope to participate unless some demands are altered. Part of the intervention process is to work with the people who have the greatest influence over the communication contexts in the child's living and learning environments to help them facilitate the child's opportunities and reasons for communicating.

Playing the Discourse Game by Different Rules

The sociolinguistic perspective encourages practitioners to appreciate the language development of children in ways that are relevant to the children's own cultures. Aquiles Iglesias (1989) noted that an important shift among the research community in speech–language pathology occurred from a time when there was "study after study comparing how the performance of minority children is inferior to that of White children" (p. 75) to a time when cultural sensitivity is more the norm. Personal Reflection 2.6 illustrates a situation when cultural mismatch could have led a clinician astray.

For language specialists charged with the responsibility to provide culturally fair and nonbiased language assessment and intervention services, it may not be possible to start with a full understanding of the differing expectations of communicative interactions in a culture different from their own, but it is always possible to start with an attitude of recognition that some of the rules may be different. Professionals can also seek opportunities to learn about the other culture by using published sources, cultural informants, and participant observation within the culture itself. Ethnographic techniques, including strategies of participant observation and interviewing, can be used by professionals who must be careful to remember that their own cultural backgrounds and expectations will affect the perceptions and behavior of the interview (Westby, 1990). The phenomenological perspective that was introduced in Chapter 1 can also facilitate this process.

One example of cultural sensitivity that can be used to influence the way one conducts ethnographic interviews has been cited by Westby (1990). She commented that *why* questions should be avoided in ethnographic interviews because they have a judgmental tone. They also "presume knowledge of cause–effect relationships, an ordered world, perfect knowledge and rationality" (p. 106). Rather than asking *why* questions, ethnographic interviewers ask participants to describe what they have experienced, how they feel, and what they know. For example, rather than asking parents what they mean when they describe their child as "lazy" or "hyper," parents should be asked to describe what their child does when acting that way. When parents are bilingual, they may also be asked to use the words of their first language to describe their child, so that the interviewer can seek to understand what those terms mean to the parents. If the interviewer does not speak that language and no translator is immediately available, translation should be sought from the taped interview transcript, interpreting cultural as well as literal meanings.

| Personal Reflection 2.6 | *"The researcher's perspective.* One of the boys was particularly intriguing even from the beginning of taping. His language seemed advanced for his age, and he talked frequently. His tapes had more entries per minute than any other child's tapes. From my perspective he was a very bright and very verbal little boy. As time went on I became curious as to why he seemed to talk more than the others. I asked an Inuk teacher for her reactions to this child. |

"The Inuk teacher's perspective. The teacher listened to my description of how much he talked and then said:

> Do you think he might have a learning problem? Some of these children who don't have such high intelligence have trouble stopping themselves. They don't know when to stop talking.

I was amazed by her response. It was as if my perspective had been stood on its head."

Martha Borgmann Crago (1990, p. 80), in an article based on her doctoral thesis at McGill University. Crago used ethnographic techniques to analyze cultural differences in such discourse exchanges as question asking and answering.

SUMMARY

Chapter 2 addressed the question of what children must learn to acquire language normally, viewed from the perspectives of multiple disciplines: linguistics, psycholinguistics, neuropsychology, neurolinguistics, and sociolinguistics. Speech, language, and communication are linked as intertwined but somewhat separable systems. The relatively normal language learning of many individuals with deafness or severe physical disability illustrates this relative separability. The written language-learning deficits these individuals often experience, however, suggest links between language and speech that require further exploration and attention in assessment and intervention. Elements of paralinguistic and nonlinguistic com-munication also may be linked with speech and language in varied ways.

Many factors influence the nature of the language a child learns. Some children are exposed to more than one language (bilingualism) or more than one dialect of English. It is important to recognize the special challenges that face children with language disorders when they are also learning a second language or when they speak a different dialect. It is also critical to separate language disorder from language difference when examining the needs of these children.

All children eventually must develop competence with five different rule systems of language: phonology, morphology, syntax, semantics, and pragmatics. Elements of each rule system were discussed.

| Personal Reflection 2.7 | "Don't put the other fellow in your shoes — wear his. 'Tis true, if 'I were you' I could use the logic that you espouse to solve my problem. But, since I am me, we must find a solution that fits well into the scheme of my mold. We must cloak the solutions of my problems in garments wrinkled by my needs and desires, otherwise, what you are saying to me is not, 'If I were you,' but 'If you were me'; and since I am not, your answers help me little." |

F. Poyadue (1979), a parent of a child with a disability, quoted by Carol Westby (1990, p. 111) in an article entitled "Ethnographic Interviewing: Asking the Right Questions to the Right People in the Right Ways."

When assessing the knowledge of the rule systems of language the specialist must consider how the nature of the task may influence what a child appears to know. For example, tasks that involve metalinguistic awareness add a level of processing demand that may obscure a child's intrinsic knowledge of the rule systems of language.

Finally, the role of communication as social interaction was stressed. Social interaction theory is one of six language acquisition theories discussed in Chapter 3. In Chapter 2, the importance of context, different reasons for communicating, and sociolinguistic variation across cultures were discussed as critical factors when language is learned in a social context.

3

Language Acquisition Theories

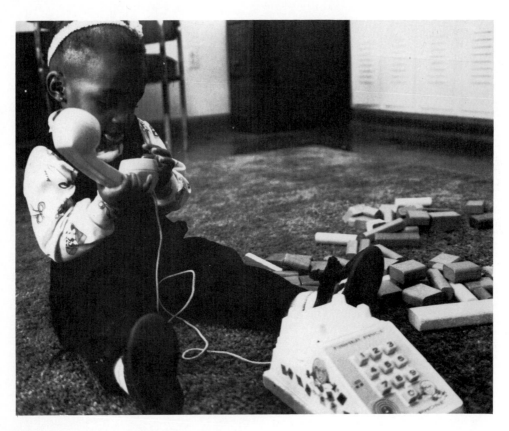

Biological Maturation

Linguistic Rule
Induction

Behaviorism

Information
Processing

Cognitivism

Social Interactionism

❏   How do children learn language when it happens normally?

❏   What are the implications when it does not?

This chapter includes a review of varied explanations of normal language acquisition. This is not a traditional review aimed at identifying which single theory best explains normal language development. Rather, multiple theories are presented, each of which appears to explain some aspects of normal language development. The purpose of the review is to contribute to an understanding of what happens when language development does not proceed normally and to pave the way toward encouraging more normal development.

What are the characteristics of a well-developed theory of language development? Such a theory would have to organize facts from varied sources, generate testable and verifiable hypotheses, explain all aspects of the acquisition process (Bohannon & Warren-Leubecker, 1989), and include all of the necessary and sufficient factors for explaining language acquisition. "A theory of language acquisition must account for the language behavior of children at any point in development as well as the processes responsible for language growth" (p. 168). Bohannon and Warren-Leubecker noted, however, that "none of the extant 'theories' qualifies according to these requirements" (1989, p. 167).

Language development, as considered here, is organized according to theoretical positions of six types: (1) biological maturation, (2) linguistic rule induction, (3) behaviorism, (4) information processing, (5) cognitivism, and (6) social interactionism. Of these, only linguistic rule induction and behaviorism have been proposed as comprehensive theories that attempt to account for both the necessary and sufficient conditions for language learning (some might put the strong form of cognitivism in this category as well). All of the theoretical positions, however, have proponents who advocate more or less extreme views.

Most of the theoretical perspectives discussed in this chapter organize factors that are *necessary* for language acquisition to proceed normally rather than describing factors that are *sufficient* for explaining it. Theories of this type are often considered to be interactionist because they acknowledge the presence of multiple contributions from various sectors (both within and outside the individual). Interactionist positions present organized views of factors essential to the process of language acquisition but do not claim that any single factor can explain the process completely.

BIOLOGICAL MATURATION

Theories that tie normal language acquisition to biological maturation are related to observations of the universality of language acquisition by human beings (Box 3.1). Because a system so complex as language is learned with such rapidity and at such a young age, its learning must be made possible by innate mechanisms. Such theories are called *nativist*. They contrast with *empiricist* theories, which emphasize the role of learning and influences of the environment on language acquisition (e.g., Bohannon & Warren-Leubecker, 1989). Basically, this is the traditional nature versus nurture debate, but with the admission by each side that some (although limited) contribution comes from the other. That is, empiricists do not claim that biological mechanisms are entirely inactive in language learning. Rather, they claim that biological maturation plays a generalist role that is not unique to language.

Box 3.1	Primary assumptions of biological maturation theories of language development

1. Some macrostructures of the brain are more critical than others for language learning (e.g., the left hemisphere, parts of the temporal and frontal lobes, the arcuate fasciculus, and some subcortical structures).
2. Microstructure factors—including brain cell organization, branching and spines on dendrites, myelination of axons, and axodendritic synapses—contribute to language acquisition and other developmental advances (but in ways as yet unknown).
3. Although scientists who study biological maturation of the language system adopt nativist views of language acquisition, they recognize both genetic and environmental factors as influencing human brain development and by consequence, language acquisition.

Conversely, nativists claim that the human brain is specially designed to learn language, but they accept the environment as playing a relatively minor role.

In the statement that "Language is a purely human and non-instinctive method of communicating ideas, emotions, and desires by means of a system of voluntarily produced symbols" (p. 8), anthropological linguist, Edward Sapir (1949) argued for the uniqueness of language as a human feat (suggesting that it was part of the specialized genetic makeup of humans) but emphasized that language was inherently different from the kinds of inborn, "preprogrammed" instincts observed in other animals, for example, instincts leading certain kinds of birds to sing particular kinds of songs.

Linguists who followed Sapir proposed that in some respects the acquisition of language was instinctive to humans. Chomsky (1965) and others (e.g., Lenneberg, 1967; McNeill, 1966) proposed an abstract mechanism, which they called the language acquisition device (LAD), as the innate language component necessary to explain why a developing child can acquire the majority of the rules of language in such a short time and with relatively limited exposure. Chomsky (1976) argued that the growth of language could be viewed as analogous to the development of a bodily organ, noting that no one would regard seriously a proposal that the human organism learns to have arms rather than wings through experience. (Of course, somehow language acquisition theories must account for the fact that children learn a particular language because of their experience.)

Marshall (1979) described the biological unfolding of structures and functions of the LAD as being controlled by a combination of forces, including some extrinsic ones, as well as some intrinsic to the individual. He included (1) genetic programming, including chromosomal contributions to growth, cell division and protein synthesis; (2) multiple principles of embryological growth, specialization, and neural connectivity; and (3) "various properties of the external environment in which the postpartum LAD finds itself" (p. 437).

To explore how normal development of the brain proceeds, this section considers maturational evidence regarding cerebral asymmetry, brain weight, myelination, dendritic elaboration, and cellular organization. Both these sections and the clinical implications section presented later in the chapter look for evidence of specialized brain structures that support the normal development of language as a unique set of skills. These sections also consider the evidence for nature and nurture, and their interactions, in guiding biological maturation.

Cerebral Asymmetries

Evidence of cerebral asymmetry in the developing human brain has implications for theories of language development that rest on biological predisposition. Concepts of equipotentiality and plasticity have been debated ever since Pierre Paul Broca first claimed in 1865 that "although the left hemisphere was 'innately' pre-eminent in language skills, its dominance could be strengthened, modified or reversed by experience or injury during certain critical periods" (cited in Marshall, 1979, p. 446). The traditional wisdom about such periods suggested that:

1. The two cerebral hemispheres are equally capable at birth of supporting the acquisition of language.
2. They remain equipotential in this sense for approximately 2 years.
3. Then, a slow process of specialization begins, with complete lateralization reported to be complete by puberty, or in the opinion of some, by age 5 years.

This traditional view, however, has been contradicted by evidence from several sources. First, rather convincing evidence now indicates that right–left brain asymmetries are present at birth (Galaburda, Corsiglia, Rosen, & Sherman, 1987; Geschwind & Levitsky, 1968; Wada, 1977; Wada, Clark, & Hamm, 1975) and even before—as early as 31 weeks of gestation (Chi, Dooling, & Gilles, 1977). A particularly interesting finding is that the asymmetries are greatest in areas that are known to be critical for normal language functioning in adults. For example, the Sylvian fissure is longer and the planum temporale is larger on the left than on the right in the majority of fetal and newborn brains (see Figure 3.1). The degree of asymmetry, however, seems to grow as brains mature. It is greater in adults than in infants (Wada et al., 1975), suggesting at least some role of maturational factors. As Marshall (1979) put it, "To assert that the left hemisphere is 'innately pre-eminent' as a neurological substrate for language still leaves open the possibility that the young brain is more 'plastic' than the mature brain" (p. 448).

Second, evidence has accumulated that infants as young as 3 months of age, and even as young as 3 weeks, can make highly sophisticated perceptual dis-

FIGURE 3.1
Illustration of left-right brain
asymmetry present in the Sylvian
fissure and planum temporale of
the majority of newborns at birth.
Typical left-right differences are
shown. The posterior margin
(PM) of the planum temporale
slopes back more sharply on the
left than on the right, and the
anterior margin of the sulcus of
Heschl (SH) slopes forward
more sharply on the left.

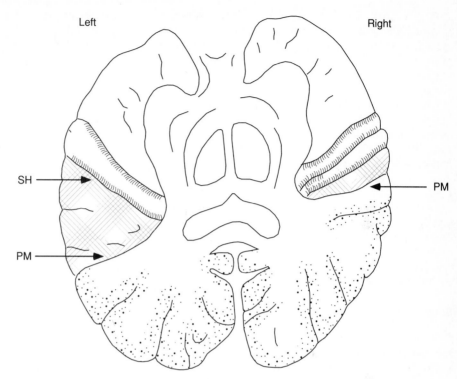

Left

Right

SH

PM

PM

Note. From "Human Brain: Left–Right Asymmetries in Temporal Speech Region" by N. Geschwind and W. Levitsky, 1968, *Science, 161*, pp. 186–187. Copyright 1968 by the AAAS. Reprinted by permission.

criminations in the speech mode and that this processing is lateralized to the left hemisphere. This evidence has been gathered by using dichotic stimulation techniques, which involve presenting two different stimuli to opposite ears with precise simultaneous timing and measuring the relative response strength to each stimulus. Researchers infer that the hemisphere opposite the stimulus that elicits the strongest response is dominant. With infants, the technique usually involves presentation of a repetitive syllable until the infant habituates to it, then shifting the syllable and measuring the response to the change (e.g., from /ba/ to /pa/). Researchers have measured response strength in infants by using a variety of techniques, including electrophysiological measurements (Molfese, Freeman, & Palermo, 1975), and cardiac conditioning (Glanville, Best, & Levenson, 1977). Sucking strength has been measured by using a nonnutritive nipple attached to an electronic recorder (Entus, 1977).

Marshall (1979) has concluded that the evidence of both early structural and functional asymmetry suggests "that cerebral dominance does *not develop*" [italics in original] (p. 447) but is innate. On the other hand, establishing the existence of an innate biological matrix for phoneme perception is not the same as saying that language is lateralized at 3 months (Wada, 1977). Although certain aspects of phoneme perception are innate, a child must learn to recognize such fine details as the particular values of voice onset time (VOT) and the nature of first formant transitions that are distinctive in the child's native language (Simon & Fourcin, 1978) (see Chapter 2 for information on phonemic distinctive features).

Brain Weight Changes During Normal Development

The relationship of function and structure in the developing brain can be addressed in other ways. Brain size and weight changes have been studied with regard to theories of innateness which rely on evidence of orderly structural developments that correlate closely to functional developments.

The human brain increases in size and weight in a series of spurts. The most rapid period of brain growth is in the first 2 years of life, when the brain more than triples its weight (Love & Webb, 1986). The timing of brain weight gains is summarized in Table 3.1.

The analysis of behavioral development and brain weight growth has led to the observation that increments in brain size of mammals are closely associated with the appearance of new behavioral competencies (Epstein, 1974, 1978). In particular, Epstein noted that the first four stages of brain growth coincided with the four main stages of cognitive development outlined by Piaget (1969) (see Box 3.6, later in this chapter). Of course, general increments in brain weight and size, even if they correlate closely to cognitive advances, offer no additional support for theories regarding the presence of an innate LAD, but neither do they provide proof that language acquisition is just like any other component of generalized behavioral or cognitive development.

Neuronal Growth Patterns

Increased brain weight probably represents several kinds of increments in the complexity of the neural network, including increased elongations and branching of axons (long cellular processes that transmit signals away from neuronal cell bodies) and dendrites (shorter cellular process with numerous branches that transmit signals toward neuronal cell bodies) (D. L. Maxwell, 1984). In fact, the two kinds of changes that are the primary parameters of neuronal growth are (1) axonal myelination and (2) dendritic arborization (branching) and synapse formation (axodendritic connections that let the axon of one cell transmit messages to the dendrites of other cells).

TABLE 3.1
Correlations between brain weigth growth and critical stages of cognitive development (Epstein, 1974, 1978)

Age	Percentage of Adult Brain Weight	Epstein's Five Stages
birth	25%	3–10 months
6 months	50%	
12 months	60%	
18 months	75%	2–4 years
5 years	90%	6–8 years
10 years	95%	10–12 years
12 years (puberty)	Full brain weight	14–16+ years

Myelination is the process by which the long axon projections of neurons undergo "anatomical and chemical changes as they are wrapped progressively in several alternating layers of lipids and proteins" (D. L. Maxwell, 1984, p. 45). Myelination is considered to be a prime correlate of speech and language development and one of the more significant indices of brain maturation (Love & Webb, 1986; D. L. Maxwell, 1984). The general blueprint for myelination seems to be that pathways involved in meeting basic physiological needs are myelinated before those that regulate complex mental activity, such as language.

The second kind of evidence about neuronal development is based on observation of *dendritic arborization* (the branches of dendrites resemble tree branches), synaptic connections, and neural organization, including trimming in some areas where neuronal quantity appears to be superfluous. Of interest is the degree to which such developmental changes are preprogrammed and the degree to which they represent a response to the environment.

Animal research has illuminated several interrelationships between brain structures and environmental influences. Evidence suggests that enriched environmental experiences can exert influences on the gradual elaboration of neural elements and the alteration of neural pathways (Goldman-Rakic, 1981; Kandell, 1977). Exposure of rats to an environment enriched with toys and exercise equipment results in increases in the sizes of their cortical and subcortical structures compared with those of sensorially deprived or normally stimulated laboratory rats (Rosenzweig & Bennett, 1976). However, specific connections between dendritic connections and other neuronal variations with maturation and with exposure to environmental influences are yet to be demonstrated in the developing child, particularly in the language area. Nevertheless, "it is a fair guess that modifiable synapses do indeed exist in the central nervous system, and it may well be that environmental influences can lead to hypertrophy, branching and atrophy of these dendritic synapses" (Marshall, 1979, p. 451).

Roles of Nature and Nurture in Brain Development Revisited

The theme of all of this evidence is that it is no longer appropriate to dichotomize nature and nurture in the area of brain maturation. The equipment that a language learner has at birth and before interacts with the things that the learner experiences in complex

Personal Reflection 3.1   "However much experience is necessary for growth, the experience writes on a slate that is plainly predisposed to accept some messages more readily than others, the predispositions reflecting a long evolutionary history."

Jerome S. Bruner (1968, p. 4), Harvard psychologist, delivering a lecture in honor of psychologist Heinz Werner.

ways. Both nature and nurture are part of the same interactive system (review system theory in Chapter 1). Restak (1979) quoted Edward O. Wilson, Professor of Zoology at the Museum of Comparative Zoology at Harvard University, as saying that scientists no longer believe in the tabula rasa (blank slate) theory of child development. "Actually," Wilson said, "only small parts of the brain resemble a *tabula rasa*. The remainder is more like an exposed negative, waiting to be slipped into developer fluid" (personal conversation between E. O. Wilson and R. M. Restak, quoted by Restak, 1979, p. 74).

LINGUISTIC RULE INDUCTION

Linguistic theories of language acquisition have been constructed to describe the essence of the "exposed negative." That is, linguistic theorists propose that the LAD is a biologically based, innate system that needs only to be triggered by evidence in the environment. Thus, theories of biological maturation and theories of linguistic rule induction are not separate theories but are alternate sides of the same coin. The reason for considering them as distinct perspectives is that biological maturation not only is related to confirmation of the linguistic induction theory but may be related to other theories as well.

A major element of linguistic theories of rule induction is that a child learning language is very much like a small linguist working in the field (McNeill, 1970). When presented with a finite number of examples, the child therefore must use the limited and imper-

fect linguistic evidence to induce the general rules of an idealized grammar (see Box 3.2 for a listing of the major assumptions of linguistic rule-induction theorists). Linguistic theorists argue that, because this process is accomplished with such relative ease at a time when children seem unable to use sophisticated inductive reasoning for other purposes, some aspects of the grammar must be preprogrammed. McNeill (1970) held that children come equipped with such innate linguistic universals as concepts of sentences, grammatical classes, and some aspects of phonology. More recently, theorists have tended to emphasize that what is innate is a set of inherent constraints and biases that lead children to treat linguistic evidence from the environment in special ways. For example, linguistic theorists (Slobin, 1979; Wells, 1986) have proposed that children function with a special set of "operating principles." These lead children to do such things as (1) to pay attention to the ends of words (thus allowing children to acquire inflectional morphemes); (2) to recognize that linguistic elements encode relationships between words (thus allowing children to recognize basic differences between classes of words such as *things* and *acts* and ways they relate in sentences); (3) to analyze the utterances they hear into smaller units (thus allowing children to comprehend and construct unique sentences by selecting and rearranging pieces); and (4) to prefer to work with principles of maximum generalizability (thus allowing children to induce the rules but also leading them to produce such "errors" of overgeneralization as *foots* and *goed*).

Personal Reflection 3.2   "There are very deep and restrictive principles that determine the nature of human language and are rooted in the specific character of the human mind."

Noam Chomsky, in his book *Language and Mind* (1968).

Box 3.2   **Primary assumptions of linguistic theories of language acquisition**

1. The end product of language learning is an internalized formal *grammar*, which is a finite set of rules, shared by all of the speakers of a language, that can generate an infinite variety of possible sentences.
2. The majority of the rules of formal grammar are learned very early (before age 5 years), with similar patterns of development observed across languages and cultures, indicating that the environment must play a relatively minor role in the process and, therefore, that human genetics must play a major role.
3. Only indirect links can be observed between the language input the child hears and the language output the child produces; furthermore, direct teaching efforts (e.g., correction) are rarely ever observed.
4. Yet children learn (in ways that cannot be explained by current learning theory and with little or no formal training) to do such things as to understand ambiguous sentences (those with the same surface structure but different deep structures) and to understand and produce paraphrases (those that are different surface structure versions of the same deep structure sentence).

The primary proponent of the linguistic theory of rule induction is Noam Chomsky, from Massachusetts Institute of Technology. As noted in Chapter 2, Chomsky (1957, 1965) originally developed concepts of transformational generative grammar (TGG) that comprised a finite set of rules that speakers could use to generate and to understand an infinite number of sentences to represent an infinite number of meanings. As part of his theory, Chomsky proposed the innate LAD. The actual functioning of the LAD, however, he left largely a mystery. In his more recent work, Chomsky's (1981) focus shifted slightly from the abstract structure of language to the constraints associated with "learnability." He did this by developing government-binding (GB) theory (see Leonard & Loeb, 1988, for an explanation designed for speech–language pathologists, and Box 2.7 for an outline summary of its major features). According to GB theory, internalized grammar must consist of an innate universal grammar (UG), which is compatible with the existing and possible grammars of the world, and it must also be possible to activate the grammar on the basis of limited evidence.

Chomsky is primarily a linguist. Although recently he has focused on language learnability, it has been largely left to other psycholinguists to show how the acquisition process actually takes place. Linguistic induction theorists have not always agreed on the course through which the end product of internalized grammar is acquired. Most have accepted that the child's grammar differs from adult grammar, but psy-

cholinguists have held alternate views regarding its interim states. Some claim that it is always related to adult grammar, developing in stages as a primitive subset of that grammar (Gleitman & Wanner, 1982; Wexler, 1982). Others argue that children go through stages in which their internalized grammar qualitatively differs from that of adults (L. Bloom, 1970; Bowerman, 1982, Pinker, 1987). Wells (1986) noted that, as their grammar develops, children at each stage can deal with evidence of a new level of complexity, which they do in a recursive process that enables them progressively to construct a representation of the language of their community (see Personal Reflection 3.3).

BEHAVIORISM

The general assumptions of behaviorist theories of language development are outlined in Box 3.3. Behaviorists are more interested in explaining the mechanisms of language acquisition than the linguistic system that children learn; they are more interested in function than structure. This contrasts with greater emphasis of linguistic theorists on aspects of structure over function.

The primary proponent of behaviorist theories of language acquisition has been B. F. Skinner (1957). It is interesting that Skinner's book *Verbal Behavior* was published in the same year as Chomsky's (1957) first major book on TGG, *Syntactic Structures*. The polarity of concepts advocated by these two authors in the

Personal Reflection 3.3   "Children learn language because they are predisposed to do so. How they set about the task is largely determined by the way they are: seekers after meaning who try to find the underlying principles that will account for the patterns that they recognize in their experiences."

Gordon Wells (1986, p. 43), British psycholinguist (now at the Ontario Institute for Studies in Education), in his book *The Meaning Makers: Children Learning Language and Using Language to Learn.*

areas of function versus structure, performance versus competence, and nurture versus nature contributed to interesting discussions in the scientific community at the time. It still does (see Personal Reflection 3.4).

The mechanisms proposed for language acquisition in behaviorist theories are the same kinds of stimulus – response–reinforcement mechanisms used in other types of learning. The processes of **classical conditioning** are used to explain aspects of language learning that involve the establishment of associations between arbitrary verbal stimuli and internal responses, such as those needed for establishing word meaning (Staats, 1971). The processes of **operant conditioning** are used to explain aspects of language learning in which selective reinforcement is used to shape key verbal behaviors in a series of successive approximations. As explained by B. F. Skinner (1957), "Any response which vaguely resembles the standard behavior of the community is reinforced. When these begin to appear frequently, a closer approximation is insisted upon. In this manner very complex verbal forms may be reached" (p. 29). Behaviorists also propose that **imitation** plays a major role in language

learning. To explore how these mechanisms are proposed to work, the next section briefly addresses how behaviorists explain the acquisition of such language behaviors as phonological characteristics, words, sentences, and communicative functions.

Behaviorist Explanations of the Acquisition of Phonological Characteristics

The behaviorist mechanism used to explain the acquisition of the phonological system of language is operant conditioning. Elements of modeling and imitation also play a role. Behaviorist theory suggests that parents provide models to demonstrate for their child the important phonological characteristics of their native language. Then they selectively reinforce the child's attempts to imitate those characteristics. As parents reinforce attempts that come closest to those of their native language through attention, soothing, feeding, and handling, the frequency of appearance of desired phonological characteristics is shaped. Meanwhile, phonological characteristics that are not distinctive in the child's native language are ignored, and they eventually become extinguished because of lack of reinforcement.

Box 3.3   **Primary assumptions of behaviorist theories of language development**

1. Language acquisition can be explained by focusing on the observable and measurable aspects of language behavior.
2. Explanations of language acquisition should not rely on mentalistic constructs such as intentions or implicit knowledge of grammatical rules.
3. Rather, language acquisition is related to observable environmental conditions (stimuli) that co-occur with specific verbal behaviors (responses).
4. The term *verbal behavior* is preferred over *language* because the structural aspects of linguistics are irrelevant to the language-learning process; language as a skill does not differ essentially from any other behavior. Language is something people do, not something that they know.
5. The units of focus in the acquisition of verbal behavior should not be words or sentences but "functional units."

Personal Reflection 3.4   "These were the mental and physiological theories I opposed. But I did not oppose them because they appealed to unobservables. Private events had to be taken into account in any successful analysis of human behavior, but they were mediators or by-products, not initiators of behavior."

B. F. Skinner (1983, p. 279), writing in his autobiography, *A Matter of Consequences*.

Behaviorist Explanations of the Acquisition of Words

Principles of both operant and classical conditioning are used to explain the acquisition of words. Of course, when operant shaping principles shape phonological characteristics, they also contribute to the development of words. Phonological productions that sound like words (such as vocal play productions of *mamama* and *dadada)* are responded to with enthusiasm by parents. (I remember trying to reinforce *mama* in my oldest son's early babbling but having to admit that his first true word was a surprise production of *cookie* /kUkU/ instead, showing me where his real priorities lay.)

Behaviorists use classical learning principles to explain how children build associations between words and the things they represent. According to behaviorists, the child has an internal reaction to some thing or event in the environment that the parent labels. For example, the child may have an internal reaction to the environmental stimuli associated with going "bye-bye" (which may have been conditioned earlier). When the parent labels this event, the child begins to associate the conditioned stimulus with the now unconditioned internal response related to going somewhere. In similar ways, other conditioned stimuli (words) are associated with the event, with each other, and with other mediating stimuli. This process is sometimes called *stimulus clustering.* When the child learns to respond "bye-bye" under slightly different stimulus conditions (e.g., when someone else leaves, but the child stays put), the process is called *stimulus generalization.* Stimulus generalization is necessary to explain how children learn that the word *dog* is associated with furry, four-legged creatures that can look widely different from one another.

Behaviorist Explanations of the Acquisition of Sentences

The development of early two-word combinations and later sentences is explained as successive associative learning. Children learn to associate one word with the next in a left-to-right response chain. Meanwhile, they learn to associate the word chain with events in the environment. This is where the idea of functional units comes in. To explain how children can produce and understand unique sentences, behaviorists claim that what children learn is a set of increasingly larger functional units and how to combine them. For example, children might learn to treat prepositional phrases as a functional unit (or grammatical frame). Then, to create or understand novel utterances, they need only insert previously learned lexical items into the slots of the grammatical frame that they have already learned.

Behaviorist Explanations of the Acquisition of Varied Functions

Behaviorists do not rely exclusively on explicit reinforcement from parents to explain the learning that takes place. Reinforcement patterns are more complicated than that. B. F. Skinner (1957) differentiated between several kinds of verbal responses, depending on their effect and other control factors. An *autoclitic* is the type of verbal behavior just described, in which speakers fill slots in grammatical frames (e.g., as subject-verb-object chains). It is a speaker response that is controlled by other verbal behaviors of that speaker. A *mand* is a verbal behavior, such as a demand, command, or request (e.g., "I want to see you") that specifies its reinforcer. In a sense, it is controlled by the reinforcer it specifies. An *echoic* verbal behavior is an imitative one. According to behaviorist theory, this kind of response is important so that a child can be reinforced and thus can develop conditioned responses that can be elicited by environmental stimuli without the intervening model. An *intraverbal behavior* has no one-to-one correspondence to the stimuli that immediately evoke it. It is thought to be stimulated (and controlled) by previously learned associations from within the speaker's own system. For example, social rituals and spontaneous comments in conversational small talk fall into this category. A *tact* is a verbal behavior that relates to elements of the nonlinguistic context that speakers discuss. When speakers learn to name items in their environment, they are learning to treat those items as discriminative stimuli that elicit tact responses.

The Importance of Environmental Factors—Issues of Nature and Nurture Revisited

To summarize, the major difference between linguistic and behaviorist theories is the emphasis of behaviorists on *how* children learn language, with a focus on observable stimuli, reponses, and reinforcers, rather than on *what* they learn. The behaviorists accord more importance to what occurs outside the child than possible brain activity. Behaviorists avoid talking about events that are not directly observable. They do not think it necessary to hypothesize that what children are learning is a set of linguistic rules. They argue instead that discussion of verbal behavior is enough.

INFORMATION PROCESSING

Like behaviorist theories, information processing theories focus more attention on how language is learned than on an abstract set of rules that are assumed to underly language knowledge (see Box 3.4). Johnson-Laird (1983) argued that an adequate theory of language acquisition would be represented by a working model and that the model (often but not always simulated with computer software programs) would "not require any decisions to be made on the basis of intuition or any other such 'magical' ingredient" (p. 6) (see Personal Reflection 3.5).

Linguistic models primarily emphasize language structure; cognitivist models, logical structure; and behaviorist models, language function. In contrast, information processing models propose to relate structure and function. At least in the "competition" information processing model proposed by Bates and MacWhinney (1987), function is primary. It is communicative function that spawns language structures, not abstract grammar, which, according to linguistic theorists, can operate essentially apart from any functional context.

Some of the work of information processing theorists can be traced to publication of Kenneth Craik's book *The Nature of Explanation*, in 1943. Craik proposed that human beings are processors of information, using three distinct reasoning processes to build internal models of external realities: (1) translating some external process into an internal representation in terms of words, numbers, or other symbols; (2) deriving other symbols from those with some sort of inferential process; and (3) retranslating these symbols into actions, or building a correspondence between the new symbols and external events. These are the essential mechanisms used by computers and, according to information processing theorists, by human language processors, as well.

Although human information processing uses biological processing mechanisms, Johnson-Laird (1983) pointed out that "the mind can be studied indepen-

---

Box 3.4	Primary assumptions of information processing theories of language development

1. The human information processing system is a mechanism that encodes stimuli from the environment, operates on interpretations of them, stores the results in memory, and allows retrieval of information previously stored.
2. Language acquisition depends on empiricist principles in that experience with linguistic evidence from the environment causes changes within processing mechanisms.
3. Rather than starting with innate patterns of (probably neural) connections, all original connections are equal; only through experience, some connections become strengthened by repeated activations, whereas others (primitive patterns) are weakened (owing to lack of empirical evidence to activate them) until they disappear.
4. The patterns of information processing that account for language learning are parallel (i.e., occurring on multiple levels at once) rather than serial (as suggested by linguistic models in which deep structures are generated and then transformed, in sequence, into surface structures).
5. The order of acquisition of language forms is cued by the functions (e.g., requesting, identifying location) of the forms. Forms that appear more frequently and that regularly serve the same function (even if they are less frequent) are learned first.

dently from the brain" (p. 9). Johnson-Laird also proposed that human beings can acquire language because of their ability to build internal mental models that are essentially analogous to external linguistic evidence.

Parallel Distributed Processing Models

Information processing theorists attempt to explain what happens internally during the language acquisition process (while avoiding reliance on "magical" elements to do so) by simulating aspects of it with computers that employ parallel (rather than serial) processing. Parallel distributed processing (PDP) models (McClelland, Rumelhart, & PDP Research Group, 1986) consist of networks of multiple level connections that act on information that serves as input to the system. In PDP models, several different encoding nodes can be activated at once. From the encoding nodes, information is sent to a set of parallel pattern associator nodes, where decisions are made based on comparisons to stored criteria for adjusting the relative strength of connections among the association nodes (this is the learning process). These adjustments also influence the activation of output nodes, such that some connective patterns are strengthened and others are weakened.

One example of a PDP system, proposed by Bates and MacWhinney (1987; MacWhinney, 1987), is the competition model. According to this model, when children begin the language-learning process, the only thing that is considered innate is a powerful PDP mechanism. Their systems are subject to no other innate biases or constraints. At first, all phonetic patterns, words, and syntactic forms compete equally to represent any particular meaning or communicative function. As children have repeated experience with language exemplars and experiences in their environment, however, some activation patterns are strengthened (among the nodes in the PDP system) and others are weakened. Over the course of development, the patterns that most closely match the evidence are those that win the competition and are thus used for communication.

David Ingram (1986) offered a comparative analysis between the functionalist theory of language acquisition proposed by Bates and MacWhinney (1979, 1982) and Chomsky's (1957, 1965) nativist views. He contrasted them along three dimensions: (1) **modularity** (whereas Chomsky views language structure as modular, having its own unique formal properties distinct from those in other domains such as cognition and perception, according to Bates and MacWhinney, language is not modular but is under the influence of other cognitive systems); (2) **innateness** (whereas Chomsky views language structure as innate—in the form of the LAD—according to Bates and MacWhinney, language structure is not innate but develops through interaction of several psychological factors that change over time); and (3) **timing** (whereas Chomsky views acquisition of language structures as virtually instantaneous, with properties appearing in their adult state and showing little change over time, according to Bates and MacWhinney, development is gradual and occurs in stages).

Explanations for Individual Differences and Language Universals Revisited

In several key ways, the views of language acquisition proposed by Bates and her colleagues (see also Bates, Bretherton, & Snyder, 1988) are similar to cognitive and social interaction views (discussed later). Information processing views hold a functionalist focus in common with social interaction views. They hold a generalist focus in common with cognitivist views.

The generalist focus is called on to explain individual differences. By avoiding reliance on a unique LAD to explain language acquisition, information processing theory shifts the emphasis from a set of specialized linguistically tuned "operating principles" (proposed by linguistic theory) to a set of generalized cognitive "mechanisms," which can be used to serve the developing child in a variety of ways. Such mechanisms are influenced considerably by the type of input presented to them and by the functions that children attempt to perform. For example, mechanisms are affected by information processing factors related to frequency, perceivability, memory load, and semantic transparency (Bates & MacWhinney, 1987).

Bates et al. (1988) argued that it is possible to accept that children are creative language learners, that they are predisposed to learn language (among other things), and that there is a biological basis for the acquisition process, without accepting that what is biological is necessarily universal or that what is universal is necessarily biological. They pointed to individual differences that have been observed in the normal language acquisition process, both within and across cultures, as evidence of this. By examining this evidence (both their own and that gathered by others), Bates and her colleagues argued against a modular status of language with divisions based on the traditional linguistic categories of phonology, morphology, syntax, semantics, and pragmatics. Instead, they proposed that children learning language divide it up in entirely different ways, by using dissociable mechanisms that cut across traditional linguistic system boundaries.

Based on observation of differential patterns of normal development within and across languages (including Bates's own daughter as she learned Italian while on sabbatical leave with her parents), Bates and her colleagues differentiated mechanisms for rote reproduction of forms from those that children use to segment and analyze the internal structure of forms. They also differentiated mechanisms responsible for comprehension from those responsible for production (comprehension can exceed production by as much as 10 months for some forms). As an explanation for their observations, Bates et al. (1988) proposed the underlying assumption that, "Individual differences in language development can be brought about by the differential strength and/or differential timing of two or more underlying mechanisms responsible for language acquisition and language processing" (p. 7). On the other hand, although the researchers found considerable continuity in language development (i.e., ability to use early language characteristics to predict later developments), they decidedly did not attribute variation in language acquisition patterns to contributions of general intelligence (questioning whether general intelligence exists).

COGNITIVISM

Cognitive theorists are more likely to claim that the sequence and rate of cognitive development determine the sequence and rate of language development. Theorists of all types generally accept that language acquisition has some relationship with general cognitive development, but the essence of cognitive theory (see Box 3.5) is that development can be explained across domains by postulating a general set of cognitive structures and processes, among which language holds no particularly special position.

The classic example of cognitive development theory is the work of Jean Piaget (1896 to 1980), a Swiss scientist who directed the International Bureau of Education in Geneva for much of his life, and whose work has profoundly influenced current understanding of normal cognitive development. Originally, Piaget was a biologist with an early interest in natural history (publishing his first paper at age 10 on an albino sparrow he had observed). Perhaps it was through this interest that Piaget developed his strategies for observing natural phenomena. Piaget applied his

---

Box 3.5	Primary assumptions of cognitivist theories of language development

1. Language is not innate in and of itself, but nonlinguistic, cognitive precursors are.
2. Language is neither innate nor learned but emerges instead as a result of the child's constructivist activity.
3. Language is only one of several symbolizing abilities for representing and manipulating mental concepts about the world, all of which result from cognitive maturation, which is triggered by states of disequilibrium between current cognitive structures and new evidence from the environment.
4. A child's cognitive capacities differ qualitatively as well as quantitatively from those of adults.
5. Yet, a constant across all stages of development is that adaptation processes are used either to assimilate new information into existing schemas, or, if they do not seem to fit, to accommodate the schemas by extending and combining them into new ones that are more complex.

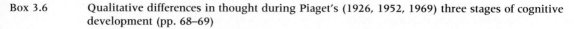

Box 3.6   Qualitative differences in thought during Piaget's (1926, 1952, 1969) three stages of cognitive development (pp. 68–69)

Sensorimotor Stage (birth to 18 months or 2 years): Piaget subdivided the sensorimotor period into six substages, through which children gain increasing control over their environment by learning to differentiate and coordinate schemes (schemata) for acting on it:

❏ Substage i (birth to 1 month). Children rely on reflexive actions but demonstrate the beginnings of adaptive intelligence.
❏ Substage ii (1 to 4 months). Children demonstrate primary circular reactions, in which they demonstrate the ability to repeat a successful cycle of action, such as thumb sucking, for its own sake (with no apparent attempts to use them to an end).
❏ Substage iii (4 to 8 months). Children demonstrate secondary circular reactions, in which they may try out all of their existing schemes in a new situation but will repeat an activity that works especially well with the apparent aim of maintaining the effect (e.g., shaking a toy that rattles). In this substage they can also imitate an action if the behavior is already in their repertoire.
❏ Substage iv (8 to 12 months). Children exhibit coordination of secondary schemas as a means to solving new problems, as, for example, grasping strings and shaking them to dislodge entangled toys. In this substage they also begin to demonstrate the ability to imitate behaviors not in their repertoire, to demonstrate intention to communicate, and to demonstrate concepts of object permanence by looking actively for an object that has disappeared from view.
❏ Substage v (12 to 18 months). Children exhibit tertiary circular reactions in which they actively experiment to achieve new and interesting results, and they can imitate behaviors that differ markedly from those in their repertoire.
❏ Substage vi (18 to 24 months). Children begin the transition to representational thought in which they are able to invent new means through mental combinations and to engage in deferred imitation; they use symbols for representing objects and people not currently present, both in the acquisition of words (e.g., using the word *bird* to represent a thing that flies and sings and has wings and feathers), and in symbolic play (e.g., using a building block to represent anything from a hairbrush to a can of food).

Representational Stage: Children further differentiate and coordinate their representational schemes within two major substages:

Preoperational Thought (18 months or 2 years to 7 years): As in the sensorimotor period, children start with undifferentiated and uncoordinated schemes, but they acquire more mature schemes in a step-by-step fashion:

observational perspective to the task of developing a standardized test of reasoning in 1920 at the Binet Laboratory in Paris (where the first broadly used intelligence test was being developed). As Piaget worked on the standardization task, he was fascinated by the patterns of "errors" that children made on the problems he posed. He noted that the difficulties demonstrated by younger children in attempting to solve the problems were not just quantitative but qualitative. He noted that the approaches taken by children of similar ages were similar and that they appeared to occur as a result of the internalized cognitive structures with which the children approached the task.

Over the ensuing years, Piaget wove his ideas into a theory of cognitive development, which he described as a series of qualitatively different stages (see Box 3.6) in which the child plays an active role in constructing an internal representation of the world.

Piaget's theory extended some ideas proposed earlier by the American psychologist, James Mark Baldwin (for a history of 20th century shifts in theories of children's cognitive development, see Case, 1985). Baldwin was interested in showing how the development of a single human being (ontogeny) recapitulates evolutionary development of the species (phylogeny) by moving through a series of stages,

Box 3.6   continued

- ❏ At first the child's words are undifferentiated (e.g., Piaget's daughter, Jacqueline, used the sound "choo-choo" to indicate a train passing by her window but also to indicate any other vehicle, any other sound from the window, or anything that appeared suddenly).
- ❏ Gradually, words are used in a way that shows a differentiation between the child's actions and internal concepts, such that words can be used to *re-present* events from the past.
- ❏ At about the age of 4½ years, children enter an intuitive period, when they still cannot make comparisons mentally but must build them up one at a time in action. However, in this period children begin a transition to the period of operational thought.
- ❏ Thought still tends to be centered on one attribute at a time; it is also considered to be pre-logical in that it is irreversible (i.e., children at this stage have difficulty imagining that the amount of clay is the same when rolled into a snake as when it was formed in a ball), and it remains egocentric (i.e., they have difficulty considering any perspective other than their own).

Concrete Operations (7 to 11 years).
- ❏ Children develop thinking characterized by conservation, decentration, and reversibility (e.g., now they can perform the conservation task related to judging changes in mass of a ball of clay because they can mentally reverse the rolling action that changed the shape from ball to snake, and they can avoid centering on only the characteristic of shape but can hold mass in mind at the same time).
- ❏ They can now group objects and words into categorical and seriational categories without considering them in individual pairs and without overt action.
- ❏ Preadolescents can demonstrate logical thought but continue to demonstrate some difficulty in moving beyond intuitive explanations for world phenomena.

Formal Operations Stage (more than 11 years):
- ❏ Children begin to be able to form classes and series mentally by internalizing earlier physical actions, or "operations."
- ❏ Development proceeds through a series of subdevelopments (as in prior stages) until children have acquired a set of abstract intercoordinated schemes for understanding laws regulating the behavior of objects in the external world, and they can apply the operations to solving complex problems with several parts.
- ❏ Children demonstrate mental hypothesis testing, abstract and flexible thought, and complex reasoning using language.

which he called *epochs,* on the way to mature cognitive functioning. The epochs Baldwin proposed were those of lower vertebrates (4 to 8 months), higher vertebrates (8 to 12 months), and finally human beings (2 years or more). To account for the sequence of cognitive development, Baldwin postulated two processes, which I will consider briefly here because of their important roles in Piagetian theory. These two processes were *habit formation* (i.e., the development of organized but automatic reactions to environmental stimuli) and *accommodation* (i.e., a process of breaking up old habits to build higher levels of adaptation).

The mechanism that Baldwin proposed for habit formation by infants was that of *circular reactions* (Case, 1985)—adaptive responses that human infants exhibit to stimulation from people and objects in their environment. Perhaps the best way to understand the mechanism of circular reactions is to consider Case's summary of Baldwin's explanation of the way in which orientation toward any form of stimulation becomes habitual, starting with primary circular reactions:

> First, the perceptual system detects some change in the environment, such as the arrival of a face, the sound of a voice, or the chance movement of a small object nearby. In response to this stimulation, the motor

system energizes itself. With the increased energization, there is a spontaneous activation of a global set of movements aimed at orienting toward the stimulation and maximizing its intensity. To the extent that certain of these movements actually do produce a slight orientation, the intensity of the stimulation increases because it is now more directly in the center of the perceptual field. The result is that another burst of energization is triggered, in a cyclical or circular fashion. Finally, the source of the stimulation ends up in the middle of the perceptual field, and the infant achieves a state of maximum energization. (Case, 1985, pp. 9–10)

As an outgrowth of habituation in different areas, Baldwin suggested that the developing infant acquires an internalized blueprint (called a *schema*), for directing action in the future. Baldwin theorized that when such a schema becomes habituated, the infant can use it to process new stimuli of the same type by assimilating them into a preexisting schema. However, because assimilation is insufficient to explain the development of human beings to higher levels of adaptation, Baldwin proposed the additional mechanism of accommodation. As Case described it:

> According to Baldwin, the process of accommodation takes place as follows. First, the infant assimilates a new situation to an already existing schema. Second, it discovers that this assimilation is not successful. At this point it experiences conflict, and activates whatever other schemas or components of schemas seem of possible relevance. Finally, these schemas are coordinated into a higher order schema. The new schema is then applied, and the process of habit formation begins again. (Case, 1985, p. 10)

Piaget (1926, 1952, 1969) used the adaptation processes of assimilation and accommodation to explain the cognitive developments that occur in the stages outlined in Box 3.6. He viewed conduct as intelligent only when behavioral or cogitative means are employed to reach a goal (occurring first with certainty in sensorimotor substage iv), and he felt that intelligence itself takes at least two forms, sensorimotor and semiotic-operational (T. Brown, 1985). Although intelligent, sensorimotor schemes are limited be-

cause they are tied to the immediate perceptual field and take place in step-wise fashion. Mistakes are identified only after they occur (hence, trial-and-error learning). These limitations are overcome as the child develops the capacity for performing mental operations by using symbolic models of a situation, thus allowing potential mistakes to be anticipated and corrected before they occur.

The motivating force behind evolution of thought is, according to Piagetian theory, disequilibrium between what children encounter in the world and what they already have organized in their minds. Piaget (1969, 1970, 1977) defined *behavioral adaptation* (sensorimotor knowledge) as equilibrium between sensation and physical (motor) behavior, whereas he defined *cogitative, or semiotic-operational knowledge,* as equilibrium between meanings (semiotics) and operations. He explained the mechanisms of mental evolution as occurring when information that is somewhat foreign to a scheme is partially assimilated into it. This leads to disequilibrium and to compensations that enlarge the system and result again in an equilibrated structure with its property of reversibility.

In testing Piaget's theory, however, neo-Piagetians have encountered problems that revolve primarily around the two assertions (1) that children's development is controlled by the emergence of general logical structures and (2) that the transition from one stage to the next is produced by a process of equilibration (Case, 1985). Problems with generalized logical structures have arisen because evidence has accumulated that certain tasks, which appear to share the same logical structure, actually may be passed at widely different ages (e.g., conservation of number may be passed at 5 or 6, conservation of liquid volume at 7 or 8, and conservation of weight not until 9 or 10), and some, such as imitation, have been observed to appear much earlier than Piaget originally suggested that they could. In addition, correlations among developmental tasks have been found to be low or insignificant. Finally, it has been difficult to define what is actually meant by the abstract concept of logical structure.

Personal Reflection 3.6   "The idea is an organism, is born, grows, and dies."
Jean Piaget (1977; quoted by T. Brown, 1985, p. vii).

The other problem that has arisen in accepting Piaget's view of cognitive development relates to his assertion that new stage developments must occur entirely through processes of equilibration, another abstract concept. Piaget viewed the young child as a young scientist who constructs ever more powerful theories of the world through the application of logicomathematical tools of gradually increasing power. In this process, the source of change is viewed as coming from within the child and as being impossible to hurry. In fact, Piaget (1964) commented that "Every time we teach a child something, we prevent him from discovering it on his own." However, the assertion that the initiation of change must be prompted by disequilibrium within the child runs into trouble in view of experimental results that have shown that, with training, children who were not even on the verge of acquiring conservation could be brought to complete mastery on conservation tasks (Lefebvre & Pinard, 1972).

In attempting to resolve some of the conflicts between Piaget's theory and empirical evidence, neo-Piagetians have offered modifications of his theory that have moved it in different directions. For example, one of Piaget's students, Juan Pascual-Leone (1969, 1984), modified Piaget's theory to be closer to those of behaviorists and information processing theorists by proposing that schematic activation weight could be determined by the interaction of the four factors: (1) cues from the internalized scheme itself, (2) field effects that might make particular features of stimuli stand out for attention, (3) logical cues regarding structural relationships, and (4) mental power or attention.

The Canadian psychologist Robbie Case (1985) has also called on aspects of information processing theory to modify Piaget's theory. Case proposed that children's mental processes can be divided into two categories: (1) *figurative schemes,* or *state representations,* which represent recurrent patterns of stimulation, and (2) *operative schemes,* or *operations,* which represent ways in which these patterns can be transformed. Case's theory brought in aspects of social interaction theories as well, in that, from very early stages (birth or before), the activation of any scheme would be experienced by the child as having a positive, negative, or neutral affective character. Like Piaget, Case proposed that children are active participants in constructing their knowledge of the world, but Case proposed that development occurs in four

major stages of executive development, each of which involves successive substages moving from unifocal coordination to bifocal coordination to elaborated coordination: (1) a **sensorimotor** stage (birth to 18 months), (2) a **relational** stage (18 months to 5 years), (3) a **dimensional** stage (5 to 11 years), and (4) a **vectorial stage** (11 to 18 years). Case does not view transition from one stage to the next as an evolution of logical structures but as a process of integration that may occur across domains through increasing complexity of several distinct, relatively independent executive control structures (voluntary efforts guided intentionally by the child). The end of one stage is marked when executive control structures are consolidated, and the beginning of the next is marked with their integration. In this way, qualitatively different types of learning occur across stages and across domains within stages (Case designed this theory to address the problem of uneven development and to explain why groups around the world begin formal school in conjunction with the stage shift that occurs around age 5). Case proposed that hierarchical transitions occur as a result of the four general processes of problem solving, exploration, imitation, and mutual regulation (including direct instruction) but that information processing is constrained by the availability of short-term storage space (STSS), which increases at each stage as processes become more efficient.

Other recent theorists have questioned whether the stage Piaget (1926, 1952, 1969) termed *formal thought* is actually reached by all normally functioning adults. Yet others have proposed adding stages of postformal thought (see Kamhi & Lee, 1988, for a review). For example, postformal stages might involve systematic reasoning, as the ability to combine sets of formal operations into higher-order structures or systems, and metasystematic reasoning, as the ability to organize general systems into supersystems. Kamhi and Lee (1988) summarized the evidence regarding later stage thought:

> Although questions have been raised about the universal characteristics of formal operational thought and the age at which youngsters reach this stage, most developmental psychologists would agree that adolescents reason differently than preadolescents. (p. 137)

Kamhi and Lee (1988) also pointed out that several theorists have recognized the importance of contextual variables in determining the appearance of later-stage cognitive competence. For example, Shaffer

(1985) noted that nearly all adults are capable of formal thought, but many exhibit it only on problems that interest them (and fall in their area of expertise). Kamhi and Lee cited the classic illustration of the auto mechanic who troubleshoots an engine problem by reasoning hypothetically but relies on more concrete methods for reasoning about other problems. A message here for clinicians is that they should probe multiple kinds of problem solving when adolescents and adults do not seem to be reasoning at the formal level, and they should not accept that formal thought is impossible just because it is not exhibited on traditional assessment tasks (Kamhi & Lee, 1988; see Chapter 9 for discussion of intervention strategies).

Thought and Language as Viewed by Cognitivists

Because cognitive theorists consider language to be only one of many cognitive acquisitions, they do not accord it any special position. As Owens (1988) noted, "There is no Piagetian model of language development" (p. 135). Implications from cognitive theory have been drawn, however, for understanding processes of normal language acquisition. For example, correlations have been found between the acquisition of linguistic concepts and some other cognitive behaviors, including symbolic play with objects, imitation of gestures and sounds, and aspects of problem solving through tool use. Although the emergence of first words is not as highly correlated with object permanence as might be predicted, the use of "disappearance" words, such as *allgone,* is. In addition, children's first words have been found to appear typically after children first notice that other people may serve as agents (Bates, 1976; Bates, Benigni, Bretherton, Camaioni, & Volterra, 1979; Bates & Snyder, 1985; Corrigan, 1978).

The overriding question, however, for those interested particularly in delayed or disordered language acquisition is whether cognitive development is necessary and sufficient for language development. If cognitive development is viewed as necessary for language development to occur, language intervention services might be denied to children whose language skills are commensurate with their cognitive skills or are above them in some areas. According to such a theoretical stance, language intervention services would be predicted to be ineffective. If cognitive development is viewed as sufficient for language development to occur, language intervention services

might be viewed as superfluous, because cognitive development would then be seen as sufficient cause for further language development to occur, and language intervention alone would be viewed to be of no assistance.

Although such strong forms of the cognitive hypothesis are not common in theoretical discussions, clinical decisions apparently are fairly frequently guided by these assumptions (e.g., when eligibility criteria for intervention services specify that children's language ages must be compared unfavorably with their mental ages). These assumptions are made in the absence of proof that varied kinds of logical structures (linguistic and otherwise) are consistently and irrevocably linked in their developmental progress. In fact, the evidence from patterns of individual development and studies in which cognitive advances have been influenced by instruction suggests otherwise (Case, 1985). Nor has it been demonstrated that cognitive development can be assessed (even using traditional "nonverbal" measures) in a way that is not confounded by children's language abilities (or lack thereof). (Perhaps Gardner's, 1983, tasks for assessing nonlinguistic intelligences, such as his doorknob disassembly and reassembly task, will offer some better ways of doing this in the future.)

Nevertheless, as considered here (and again in the next chapter), general cognitive development certainly appears to play a role in children's language development. The intriguing question that remains is whether language can also play a role in the development of cognition. According to social interaction theorists, it can.

SOCIAL INTERACTIONISM

Theories that focus on social interaction differ from linguistic theories in their emphasis on function over structure (even though they do not deny that some aspects of internalized structure may exist). They also differ in their emphasis on the importance of context. Although social interactionists may accept the concept of implicit knowledge of linguistic rules, the competence–performance dichotomy is relatively unimportant to them (see Personal Reflection 3.7) because the rules of social communication, which are the important rules for them, differ in kind from those of linguistic structure (see Box 3.7). Rather than being static representations, social interactions vary with

Personal Reflection 3.7   "If you concentrate on communicating, everything else will follow."

Roger Brown, Harvard psycholinguist in the Introduction to *Talking to Children,* edited by Catherine Snow and Charles Ferguson (1977, p. 26).

the situations in which they occur. They involve situated uses that are "glued to their contextual backgrounds" (Dore, 1986, p. 7). Dore provided as an example of this, when the meaning of *mine* changes in the context of the preschool playroom where objects are temporarily possessed for play purposes (e.g., *my sponge*) rather than being owned outright as they are at home (e.g., *my room*).

Dore (1986) further contrasted structural (linguistic) and pragmatic approaches:

> Structural and cognitive accounts of language typically assume that development is controlled from within the individual (whether by cognitive processes or substantive constraints) and focus on the construction and elaboration of mental products. But pragmatic approaches should begin by postulating that development proceeds from intersubjectively sustained activity to the child's cognitive-linguistic control and should focus on the emergence of self-awareness and the child's personal powers in social interactions. (p. 5)

Social interaction explanations of language acquisition may be traced back to an earlier definition (C. Morris, 1946) of pragmatics as the system of relationships between symbols and symbol users. It was Bruner's (1968) view that it was possible to isolate a special kind of symbolic communication learning in infancy, which, although it could be distinguished from other kinds of doing learning (as represented by communicative eye-gaze, smiling, and vocalizing patterns), it could also be distinguished from language. (These distinctions differentiate the social interactionism theory from either cognitivist or linguistic views.) Bruner (1968) called the "limited subspecies of symbolic learning involved in social interaction . . . *code learning*" (p. 56). Bruner noted the importance of the parental role in establishing this code, very early in infancy, as one of mutual expectancy. Parents respond to their child's initiative (e.g., crying) by converting some feature of the spontaneous behavior into a signal (in later chapters, I refer to this as the *perlocutionary act*). That is, they expect their child to be communicative. In turn, children learn to expect that behavior they initiate will elicit a response.

In addition, care givers systematically assist children to differentiate between objects using a process Bruner (1974–1975) called *joint reference*. This involves

Box 3.7   **Primary assumptions of social interactionist theories of language development**

1. Language develops, not because of any innate linguistic competence or because of strict reinforcement principles, but because human beings are motivated to interact socially and to develop concepts of self and others.
2. The important elements of development are not abstract linguistic or cognitive structures or concrete verbal behaviors, but rather, they are the phenomena of intentional and symbolic acts of speech, their conversational functions, their consequences for participants, and their context-creating power and context-dependent properties (Dore, 1986).
3. Language acquisition occurs in the context of dyadic, dynamic interactions, which are motivated by the child's drive to develop a concept of self and to interact with others socially (not isolated efforts to construct a grammar, or passive processes controlled by external reinforcers).
4. Parents (and other conversational partners) contribute significantly to the language acquisition process by adjusting their linguistic input to be compatible with the child's developing linguistic and communicative abilities and by supplying a scaffold (i.e., supportive communicative stucture) to allow the child to communicate despite primitive abilities (Bruner, 1978).

elaborate routines whose development begins in early infancy with intensive eye contact between care giver and child, followed by behaviors in which the care giver calls to the child, points, names objects, and comments on them, thus guiding both the content and form of language input. As development continues, care givers modify their speech so that it is comprehensible at the assumed level of the child, but they systematically advance it in complexity (Snow, 1977; Snow & Ferguson, 1977). Teachers have also been shown to modify their linguistic input systematically during the elementary school years, perhaps to match the developing language skills of the majority of their students (Cazden, 1988; Cuda & Nelson, 1976; N. W. Nelson, 1984; Sturm, 1990).

Social interaction theory depends on complex interactions among intrinsic and extrinsic factors to explain human communication learning. The interactionist element in the theory, however, relates to more than just social interactions among people. It also relates to interaction among the various elements proposed as critical by all other theories of language acquisition. We have already considered some ways that social interaction theory is related to cognitivist and linguistic theory. In addition, it has ties to biological maturation theory, as illustrated in the supposition that "There is a vast amount of order built into the human body and its nervous system that serves to shape, constrain, and support organic functioning" (p. 66, Bruner, 1968), and it has ties to information processing theory in the recognition of such factors as motivation and attention.

Perhaps the earliest and strongest proponent for a social interaction theory of language acquisition was the Russian psychologist, Lev Semenovich Vygotsky (1896 to 1934). Although Vygotsky died prematurely of tuberculosis at the age of 38, his ideas about child development and the relationships of thought and language continue to exert a major influence on modern educational practices. In 1962, an English translation of Vygotsky's work *Thought and Language* (originally published in Russian in 1934) was published. Vygotsky argued that early in its development, language is primarily a tool for social interaction. As development progresses, however, language becomes a medium through which children control their own private interactions with the environment by talking aloud during play and verbalizing intended actions. Language eventually becomes a way of structuring actions, directing thought, and creating a concept of self.

Thought and Language—The Chicken and the Egg Question Revisited

In summarizing his views of the relationships between thought and language, Vygotsky (1934-1962) presented the following conclusions, which were based partially on studies of thought and communicative behaviors of chimpanzees and apes (anthropoids): (1) "thought and speech have different genetic roots"; (2) "the two functions develop along different lines and independently of each other"; (3) no clear-cut and constant correlation can be identified between them; (4) "anthropoids display an intellect somewhat like man's *in certain respects*" (such as in elementary tool use) "and a language somewhat like man's *in totally different respects*" (e.g., the pairing of vocalization with affective states, its release function, and the beginning of a social function); and (5) anthropoids do not show the close correspondence between thought and speech that is present in humans, suggesting that (6) "In the phylogeny of thought and speech, a prelinguistic phase in the development of thought and a preintellectual phase in the development of speech are clearly discernible" (p. 41).

Social Interaction and Development of the Concept of Self

Contributions of sociocultural contexts to language learning, according to social interaction theory, do not diminish the significant contributions made by language learners themselves. Cooper and Anderson-Inman (1988) noted that the usual interpretation of socialization is that parents and other adults are the teachers or transmitters of culture and that children (or other new members of the society) are the learners. Cooper and Anderson-Inman added that "This view of socialization is not erroneous, but it is somewhat incomplete. Socialization is actually an interactive process" (p. 225).

Social interaction theories depend in part on an assumption that human beings have an innate motivation to want to communicate. Bruner (1968) noted the early tendencies of newborns to seek out human faces and to respond to them. Fostering of the desire to interact and sustaining the motivation to continue to learn language depend on children's social experiences as they develop concepts of themselves as competent, effective individuals.

To describe the nature of the complex social communicative interactions, Dore (1986) used concepts of feeling-form-function-frame analyses. Dore posited feelings between participants as motivating the particular forms, which are chosen to put into effect various intentional and sequential functions, which are relative to the contextual frames in which they occur. In describing this "house-that-Jack-built" view of the transition to language, Dore emphasized its basis in feelings and the "primacy of relationship" (p. 16).

Dore (1986) relied on the concepts of "personhood" and interpersonal motivation for learning language that were proposed earlier by philosopher John MacMurray (1961). MacMurray emphasized that the development of personhood is neither individual nor social in the usual sense of the terms but relies on a concept of personal order, in which two persons are together in a relationship primarily for the sake of being together. A primary example is an infant–mother pair. As explained by MacMurray, the infant's existence requires informed cooperation and sharing with the mother, to which the infant's contribution is merely (but significantly) the ability to communicate. "His essential natural endowment is the impulse to communicate with another human being" (MacMurray, 1961, p. 51). Dore explained the relationship as one in which a child who may be genetically capable of symbolic behavior nevertheless *learns* to function symbolically because of prior input and consequent confirmation of preliminary attempts at symbol making. As Dore expressed it, "It is the infant's mother who thus endows his behavior with meaning" (1986, p. 17).

Different motivating factors are viewed as being relatively more or less powerful at varied points in the development process and in individual language learners. Snow and Ferguson (1977) related the variability associated with individual differences in language learning to social interaction patterns, noting that the value placed on successful communication is so high that many different routes to the goal are tolerated. Dore (1986) stressed the variation across developmental contexts. In particular, he emphasized that relationship (community) is the primary motivating force behind the transition of the child from communicator to language user during infancy; cohesion between word symbols and their contexts is a major focus of the one-word stage; coherence of function is the primary motivating force underlying nursery school conversations; and social contexts are the overriding factors during the elementary school years.

Social Interaction Theory and Later Language Development

No one disputes that infants, toddlers, and preschool-age children make amazing progress toward mature use of language in just a few years. It is now widely accepted, however, that language development continues across the life span. For example, refinements in the areas of discourse, pragmatics, figurative language, and linguistic ambiguity have been reported throughout the preadolescent and adolescent years (Nippold, 1988c). In cultures where literacy is valued, life span development includes preliteracy learning, which now is recognized as starting during the early years before formal schooling begins (van Kleeck, 1990), and continuing into adulthood, with the acquisition of skills related to advanced vocabulary, interpretation, and rhetoric (N. W. Nelson, 1988). Particularly in the later years, the importance of social context to language learning must be considered. Whereas, for preschool children, spoken communication is the major source of language stimulation, for individuals in the later stages of language acquisition throughout adolescence and adulthood, both spoken and written language provide important stimulation (Nippold, 1988c). For social interaction theorists, language acquisition is more than a process of learning how to communicate. It is a process of learning the tools of one's culture.

CLINICAL IMPLICATIONS

What aspects of these six theoretical approaches can we use to guide us in our decisions as language interventionists? Is this merely a case of six blindmen each describing the elephant as a vastly different creature, depending on the areas of evidence they explored, or are there true differences in essence among these theories that go beyond the avenues of inquiry, observational methods, and data they represent? My own sense is that there is probably some of both.

Perhaps the hallmark of language acquisition research in the 1990s and beyond will be that theorists will attempt to use multifaceted methods to describe the same data, and as a result, language interventionists will have richer tools of observation to focus their own work. Katherine Nelson (1989) and a group of colleagues (the New York Child Language Group) initiated such a practice during the 1980s by analyzing a series of monologues of a 2-year-old child, Emily, alone in her crib at naptime or at night. They grouped these multiple-perspective analyses into the areas of (1) constructing a world, (2) constructing a language, and (3) constructing a self. The ability to see discourse, even that produced for oneself, as having more than one form and purpose is certainly a perspective (indeed, a multiple perspective) that clinicians need to take with them into the intervention setting. The book *Narratives from the Crib* is also important to language interventionists because its "findings go against the conventional wisdom in child-language research, which views the development of language as proceeding from word to phrase to sentence to discourse, each larger unit building on the preceding smaller one" (K. Nelson, 1989, p. 306). For example, in Emily's crib monologues, complex clausal structures appeared before many morphological endings.

What caused language advances of this sort to happen for Emily, and how can some of the conditions that led to their development be duplicated within intervention contexts? That question should accompany each of the theoretical perspectives considered in this chapter. In this case, K. Nelson (1989) identified a key element of the process as one of mutual determinism between concept and linguistic form. She noted, "It is hard to escape the conclusion that Emily has a strong conceptual need to express certain relations, a need that drives her to acquire the relevant linguistic forms and structures" (p. 307).

To some extent, the extreme position of any of the theoretical views considered here can make it incompatible with any of the others, but return to the discussion of system theory introduced in Chapter 1. As clinicians who must deal with the complexities of real

people and problems, we cannot afford the purity of focus that a strictly theoretical orientation requires. System theory allows one to conceive of the language acquisition process as an integrated whole involving contributions from subsystems that may be quite different from one another; some subsystems may appear to be internal to the child, and others external, but all are part of the same open and interactive system.

The clinician–educator needs to understand the assumptions of the varied theoretical positions and the evidence used to support them but cannot afford to become so wedded to one theoretical approach that taking a broader perspective becomes difficult. Rather, aspects of all six of these theoretical positions may be useful in facilitating the language acquisition process when it needs a boost. In the contexts of language assessment and intervention, the best theory may be one that allows the professional to conceive of children as having a genetic heritage, a biological mechanism that predisposes them to make cognitive sense of the world, to interact socially, and to acquire linguistic rules, but that can be molded through interactions with an external environment designed to facilitate their needs. The explanations of behaviorism can be accepted as influencing the directions of development but not without reliance on some contributions from internal cognitive strategies that allow children to process complex data in systematic, parallel ways and to alter their future perceptions, memories, recognitions, and expressions as a result. Children can be viewed as active contributors to their own development, with the degree of their sense of control being influenced by both internal and external factors. The adults and the other

---

Personal Reflection 3.8   " . . . now sleeping time
now not sleeping time
Emmy make it bedtime
not sleeping time."

Emily, a child who, at the age of 23 months, 6 days, was using her crib monologue discourse (this piece is from Gerhardt, 1989, p. 225) in more than one way—to construct her world, to construct her language, and to construct herself (K. Nelson, 1989).

children in their world can be viewed, not just as "accidental tourists" who provide abstract linguistic evidence, but as active interpreters of the child's culture and language through a selective framing of stimuli that occur naturally in the environment and as a mirror through which the child learns to perceive aspects of self and to form concepts of personhood.

SUMMARY

Chapter 3 summarized six different theories of language development: biological maturation, linguistic rule induction, behaviorism, information processing, cognitivism, and social interaction. Some of these theories (particularly linguistic rule induction and behaviorism) attempt more comprehensive explanations than others of the necessary and sufficient conditions for language development. All have some relevance for understanding childhood language disorders. These theories may explain varied aspects of language acquisition, with varied applications to language assessment and intervention as well.

4

Causes, Categories, and Contributing Factors

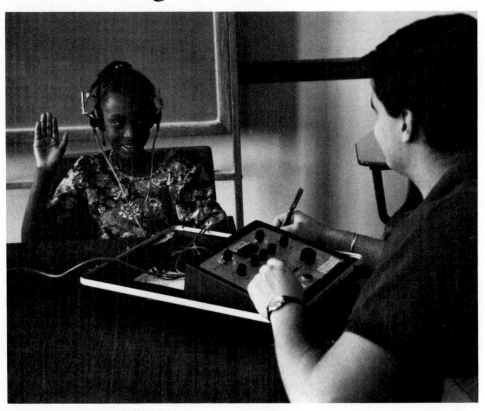

The Elusiveness of
Cause

Categorical Conditions
Associated With
Language Disorders

Central Processing
Factors

Peripheral Sensory
and Motor System
Factors

Environmental and
Emotional Factors

Mixed Factors and
Changes Over Time

❑ What kinds of conditions are associated with difficulty learning language?

In Chapter 3, I asked you to consider theories of normal language acquisition to promote insights regarding factors that might be at work when language development does not proceed normally. This chapter provides a closer look at causes, categories, and contributing factors involved in language-learning difficulty.

In many ways, the topics of Chapters 3 and 4 are integrally related. If certain factors such as biological maturation influence the normal progression of language development, might not disruptions in those same factors cause disorders of language development? If, as proposed at the conclusion of Chapter 3, multiple factors play complex roles in normal language acquisition, might not disruptions in those same factors also play complex causative roles when a language disorder is observed? Furthermore, if causes are seen, not as singular influences that operate at a specific time and then disappear (or possibly remain static), but as vectors that may assume different levels of strength at different times, might not a plan be devised to strengthen the influences of positive contributing factors and to reduce the influences of negative ones? Finally, if causes and contributing factors can be identified that influence language acquisition positively and negatively, won't society have some information that can be used to prevent the occurrence of language disorders (or lessen their effects)? These are questions raised throughout this chapter and addressed throughout the book.

THE ELUSIVENESS OF CAUSE

No one knows what causes children to have language development disorders. Although considerable information has been gathered about the conditions associated with language disorders, clear and predictable causative patterns have not been demonstrated.

Even those factors that appear on the surface to be related to language disorders in fairly direct ways have unclear causative patterns. For example, when children have profound hearing impairments or deafness, they can invariably be expected to have difficulty learning language through speech. Even if they learn sign language, their written language skills are generally affected (review discussion in Chapter 2 about interactions among language, speech, and communication). Yet, two children with highly similar hearing loss profiles may show considerably different language acquisition profiles.

One also might expect that a cause of language disorder can be clearly demonstrated when the disorder follows from a known insult to the brain. Again, causative relationships are not simple. Even when a causative factor such as brain injury resulting from trauma, a cerebrovascular accident, or some other agent is known, long-term effects on language development are difficult to predict. Multiple factors seem to influence the direction and degree of the outcome.

Several reasons explain why causes of language disorders are elusive and why potential causative agents and language disorder symptoms cannot be related in a one-to-one fashion. In this section, causative factors are presented as (1) heterogeneous, (2) changeable, (3) layered, and (4) multifaceted and interactive.

A Definition of Language Disorders

In preparation for considering causes, categories, and contributing factors, a definition of language disorders is useful. As noted in the preface and introduction to this book, I take a broad view of language disorders here. The discussions are not restricted to "specific language impairments" (whether "specific language impairment" is valid as a category is discussed later in this chapter). A definition that comes close to capturing the multiple elements at work when a broad perspective is taken was offered by Bashir (1989):

> Language disorders is a term that represents a heterogeneous group of either developmental or acquired disabilities principally characterized by deficits in comprehension, production, and/or use of language. Language disorders are chronic and may persist across the lifetime of the individual. The symptoms, manifestations, effects, and severity of the problems change over time. The changes occur as a consequence of context, content, and learning tasks. (p. 181)

This definition is a good one because it recognizes the heterogeneity of language disorders, their varied symptoms, and the multiplicity of both developmental and acquired factors that can contribute to them. It acknowledges the chronicity of language disorders but also their changeability. Changeability partially results from developmental shifts and partially from shifts in contributing factors external to the individual (e.g., language contexts, content, and learning tasks) which can influence the appearance of a language disorder.

On the other hand, this definition includes some elements that beg for further definition. What, in fact, *is* a "deficit in comprehension, production, and/or use of language"? That is one of the most difficult questions facing language disorder specialists. It is an integral part of the two more specific questions that practitioners (particularly those working in school settings) face daily: (1) Who should be labeled as language impaired? (2) Who qualifies for what kind of service? In many ways, these two questions underlie and motivate the current discussion of causes, categories, and contributing factors. The discussion is extended further in Chapters 5 and 6 to more specific consideration of assessment and eligibility issues and to the provision of service. Here, it is limited to attributes of causes, categories, and contributing factors.

Attributes of Causes, Categories, and Contributing Factors

Causative factors and categories are heterogeneous.

Different individuals can have different kinds of language disorders for different reasons, which influence programming decisions. For example, when a child has autism, language development concerns may arise that differ from those for a child with Down's syndrome.

Children who exhibit either of these conditions may also exhibit more. Furthermore, they may exhibit associated impairments that might have a more indirect effect on language acquisition than does autism or Down's syndrome. For example, motor impairments can influence children's environmental experiences, as well as their access to speech and handwriting.

In spite of these differences, however, the developmental task facing different children, their parents, and teachers, is basically the same. The broadest elements of the task require all children to learn to communicate and to use language effectively, influenced by others whose job (often unofficial) is to facilitate the process. This partnership is universal. Although cultural differences in communicative interactions and language rules can be found, basic similarities also can be found in the systems to be learned, acquisition strategies, and factors influencing acquisition— across languages, cultures, and language disorders, regardless of cause.

Causative and contributing factors are changeable.

Nevertheless, differences in developmental patterns can be observed both in children developing normally and in those considered to have language impairments. Differences can be seen not only across different children, but also within the same children when they are viewed at different times.

Longitudinal studies have contributed to understanding how interactions of causative agents and contributing factors can change over time for children with language disorders and learning disabilities (Maxwell & Wallach, 1984). A summary of longitudinal studies (Scarborough & Dobrich, 1990) showed that from 28% to 75% of children with language impairments in their preschool years continue to exhibit residual speech and language problems in later childhood, and that 52% to 95% of these children show impairments in reading achievement (Aram, Ekelman, & Nation, 1984; Aram & Nation, 1980; Levi, Capozzi, Fabrizi, & Sechi, 1982; Padgett, 1988; Stark et al., 1984).

An interesting aspect of this quality of changeability is that language disorders may appear to be more or less severe within the same children at different points in their development. Scarborough and Dobrich (1990) reported on conflicting evidence from short-term and long-term studies of changes following early language delay (ELD). Several short-term studies showed that many children with ELD achieve normal levels of language proficiency when they are around 5 or 6 years of age (Bishop & Edmundson, 1987; MacKeith & Rutter, 1972; Morley, 1972; Silva, 1980), but, as noted, longer-term studies have shown residual effects involving oral and written language (Bashir, Wiig, & Abrams, 1987; S. E. Maxwell & Wallach, 1984).

More than one explanation may exist for the apparently conflicting observations that some children seem to recover better than others from ELD. The results may simply represent the heterogeneity present across children. Children with milder delays and those with problems isolated to a single area, such as phonology, may be less likely to exhibit persistent language or reading problems (Bishop & Edmundson, 1987; Hall & Tomblin, 1978; R. R. King, Jones, & Lasky, 1982; Levi et al., 1982). Another possibility, however, is that the same children with ELD who reach apparently normal levels of language skill by about age 5 years may exhibit subsequent oral and/or written language difficulties (Bishop & Edmundson, 1987; Scarborough & Dobrich, 1985, 1990; Stark et al., 1984). Scarborough and Dobrich (1990) termed this second pattern *illusory recovery;* that is, at times of relative plateau (e.g., experienced around age 3 to 5 years for normally developing children, or around age 4 to 6 years for children with language disorders), children with ELD may appear to catch up to those with normally developing skills, but during the next language growth spurt, in conjunction with learning to read, the children who originally exhibited language delay are likely to demonstrate symptoms of language impairment again.

Based on longitudinal studies, two general rules appear to guide the prognosis for the changeable expression of language disorders in children: (1) The greater the severity of earlier impairments, the greater the likelihood that those impairments will be noted across broad areas of language (i.e., that they will be less selective) (Bishop & Edmundson, 1987; Wolfus, Moskovitch, & Kinsbourne, 1980). (2) As children become older, their language impairments tend to become more selective (often involving reading), regardless of the early degree of severity (Aram & Nation, 1975; Scarborough & Dobrich, 1990).

Causative factors are layered. In addition to being heterogeneous and changeable, causative factors are layered. Consider this relationship as being analogous to the multilayered skin of an onion, with the symptoms of language disorder as the outer skin. Peel it away, and a second layer appears, representing the most immediate causes for the symptoms (a level that physicians label *pathogenesis;* Rapin and Allen, 1983). Underneath that layer lies another potential set of causes (in the medical literature, this is considered the true cause), and then another, and another. The final core is never really identified.

To illustrate the complexities of causal relationships, consider a child who has Down's syndrome, which is viewed as a high-risk factor for delayed cognitive and linguistic development and has been fairly thoroughly investigated. What causes it? In 1958, although a chromosomal defect previously had been suspected, a new visualization technique allowed a French geneticist, Lejeune, to demonstrate clearly an extra chromosome in the cells of a child with Down's syndrome (Rynders, 1987) (hence, the current label *trisomy 21;* Jagiello, Fang, Ducayen, & Sung, 1987).

All children with Down's syndrome, however, did not seem to have exactly the same chromosomal defect. Soon, investigators reported that, instead of the extra chromosome, some individuals with Down's syndrome have translocations of chromosomal material (Polani, Briggs, Ford, Clarke, & Berg, 1960) and others have a mosaic condition, in which some cells

in the same individual show the abnormal pattern while others are normal (Clarke, Edwards, & Smallpiece, 1961). Once again, evidence was supplied for the heterogeneity of causative factors.

Research findings like these represent another layer of the onion, but they themselves need explaining. What, in fact, causes the chromosomal aberrations? Two processes hypothesized as functioning within this layer, as the primary causes of disturbance of chromosome behavior, are either nonconjunction or nondisjunction of chromosomes. Jagiello and her colleagues (1987) concluded that now "the bulk of epidemiological and experimental evidence definitely points to nondisjunction or failure of separation of chromosomes as the manifest error in trisomy 21" (p. 24). Yet another causative layer needs to be uncovered to explain the nondisjunction error.

In this case, the research has shown that two apparently different processes are at work, one leading to "maternal age-independent" instances of trisomy 21, which tend to occur at a peak frequency at a maternal age of 28.5 years, and a second, separate process leading to "maternal age-dependent" instances of trisomy 21, which tend to occur at a peak frequency at a maternal age of 43 years (Bond & Chandley, 1983). Some of the 16 or more hypotheses for the cause of nondisjunction in cases of younger mothers (most involving largely "unproven culprits"; Jagiello et al., 1987, p. 27) include x-irradiation, chemical mutagens, viruses, smoking, and alcohol. These are only some of the causative layers that can be peeled away for one specific condition. Every condition associated with language disorders has similar layers of causes when one begins to peel away the surface.

Causative factors are multifaceted and interactive. Peeling the onion, as shown for Down's syndrome, illuminates one set of layers, but there are others. Part of system theory perspective, introduced in Chapter 1, is to consider causative patterns for language disorders to be circular and interactive rather than linear.

Again, using Down's syndrome to illustrate, more specific questions might be asked about how the variations associated with trisomy 21 actually influence brain maturation and language acquisition. As mentioned in Chapter 3, the characteristics of dendritic spines of children with mental retardation related to trisomy conditions differ from those of normally developing children in their sparseness, yielding fewer opportunities for associative synapses with other neurons (Marin-Padilla, 1975). One might hypothesize that these morphological differences may cause some problems exhibited by children with Down's syndrome in forming complex cognitive connections.

Yet, considering the research reviewed in Chapter 3 about influences of reduced and enriched stimulation and experience on brain cell maturation and axonal–dendritic connections, one could hypothesize that neuronal development among such children might be influenced by environmental factors as well. For example, reduced stimulation might interact in particularly negative ways with already weak neurobiological support systems, whereas enriched environmental experiences might facilitate neuronal development in those same systems. What kinds of social interaction variables and other factors might influence the quality of a child's environmental experience and stimulus enrichment?

Again, such factors are multifaceted and interactive. The language development of children with Down's syndrome has a much better prognosis now that physicians no longer routinely recommend that children born with the condition be institutionalized at birth (Rynders, 1987). Today, additional influences on the direction of change in a family with a child who has Down's syndrome can come both from support parents receive for dealing with concerns about causes and the sense of "Why me?" and from support for maximizing long-term outcomes.

Other factors also might influence the quality of stimulation that children with Down's syndrome receive. Audiological factors are particularly significant because of their potential interference with the auditory input crucial for language learning. Pueschel (1987) summarized evidence from several studies that have shown that more than 75% of children with Down's syndrome display some degree of hearing loss. The vast majority of these children demonstrate mild or moderate conductive losses (15 to 40 dB) related to middle ear problems. Here again, the onion analogy regarding layered factors holds. As Pueschel (1987) explained it:

> There are numerous factors that are responsible for increased fluid accumulation in the middle ear with resulting hearing impairment in children with Down syndrome. Insufficient muscle control in the hypopharynx has been described which affects Eustachian tube function and does not allow the pressure in the middle ear to equalize. A blocked Eustachian tube then often

results in negative middle ear pressure, which gives way to secretion of a mucoid fluid from the lining of the middle ear space. If the fluid remains in the middle ear long enough, it may have a permanent effect on hearing. (p. 122)

Miller (1987) summarized the multiple factors that place children at risk for language-learning problems associated with Down's syndrome: (1) potential negative influences of conductive hearing loss; (2) potential negative contributions from deficits in motor coordination, which might adversely affect the synchrony of motor movements within the speech-production system needed for coordinating respiration, phonation, and articulation of the palate, tongue, lips, and jaw; (3) cognitive deficits specific to Down's syndrome, which might result in language-learning problems beyond those typically associated with mental retardation; and (4) social interaction patterns involving decreased expectations for performance, which might result in learned incompetence or reduced opportunity for appropriate experience.

Summary of attributes that make causes elusive.
Why are causes of language disorders so elusive, and why can't potential causative agents be related to language disorder symptoms in a one-to-one fashion? In this section, I suggested several reasons for viewing causative factors as heterogeneous, changeable, layered, multifaceted, and interactive. Although I have drawn illustrations primarily from research about Down's syndrome, similar factors operate in conjunction with other potential causes and categories. In systems as complex as those involved in human development, it is unlikely that simple cause–effect patterns will be found. However, research offers continued hope that more potential factors will be identified that play a role in causing, contributing to, influencing prognosis for, and ultimately, in designing plans for preventing language disorders.

TO CATEGORIZE OR NOT TO CATEGORIZE? THAT IS THE QUESTION

Any categorical approach to childhood language disorders is fraught with difficulty. A primary concern is that causative categories are not predictably related to language attributes. This observation was made by L. Bloom and Lahey (1978) and amplified by Lahey (1988), who make a case for using normal development, rather than diagnostic group membership, to guide language assessment and intervention practices. The rationale for this argument is that the heterogeneity of language skills demonstrated by children within the same diagnostic category and the blurring of language distinctions for children across diagnostic categories lead to validity and reliability problems in using categorical approaches to organize discussions of children's language disorders.

In this book, I consider a child's "membership" in a diagnostic group to be important information relevant to the decision-making process as only one of many factors to be considered, not as the determining factor. Although the overriding organizational framework for this book is developmental, readers are again cautioned that any single perspective can be limiting.

Problems With a Developmental Focus

Some of the problems that can result from a strictly developmental focus were discussed previously. In particular, overreliance on a developmental focus can lead to the prevention of children from participating in communicative opportunities or learning experiences appropriate to their chronological ages because they are not yet considered "ready" for those experiences. As a result, children can be increasingly isolated from their normally developing peers. A related problem is that children's developmental needs may not be uniform across domains of development, and reduced ability in one area may place a "drag" on opportunities in another. This was the reason for the concern expressed by the mother (in Personal Reflection 1.5) who protested that she would buy Velcro when she was told that her son with cerebral palsy was not yet ready to learn to read because he could not yet zip his pants.

Categorization and Prototype Theory

Why use diagnostic categories? People create diagnostic categories for valid reasons. It is a human trait to use categories to organize experience. Each time we talk about a kind of thing or do something, we engage in a category of experience (Lakoff, 1987). Whenever scientists, educators, or health professionals note a particular cluster of characteristics occurring repeatedly, they tend to give that condition a label and then to specify the qualities that define the group. The classic view of categories suggests that "categories are defined solely by the shared essential properties of their members" and that they are ob-

jective representations of real things in the world (Lakoff, 1987, p. 586). This view, however, has been questioned.

Although the classic view that categories are based on shared properties is not entirely wrong, many recent cognitive scientists have suggested that categorization is more complex. Beyond the recognition of shared characteristics, categorization is now thought to involve a kind of subjective processing in which categories are based on prototypes that represent "idealized cognitive models" (Lakoff, 1987, p. 68). This means that potential members of a category may not always be clearly in or out of the category and that some candidates may fit relatively better than others, depending on the closeness of their relationship to the prototype.

As professionals gain experience with persons described with conditions related to language disorders, they begin to form their own idealized cognitive models (prototypes) about such conditions. If you think about your own experience, you may identify some individuals who serve better as "classic" examples of persons with language disorders than others.

Categories and their labels can serve useful functions. When people in remote sites have some commonality of concepts behind a label, they can work together to understand more about the condition it represents; conduct research with subjects who meet criteria for membership in the group; form associations dedicated to understanding the condition and helping others to do so; and design assessment and intervention efforts for other members of the same group. Categories are one tool that people use to avoid having to reinvent the wheel.

Problems With a Categorical Focus

Diagnostic categories can also lead to trouble, such as when *labels*, rather than individual needs, are used to determine the kinds and qualities of services a child from a particular disorder group will receive. Another problem related to categorical labeling is when the label is viewed as being indistinguishable from the individual for whom it is only one of many characteristics. This problem is reduced if care is taken never to use labels as nouns, or even as central identifying attributes. For example, it is better not to refer to a person as an *autistic*, or even as an *autistic person*, but as a *person with autism*. This will help prevent both professionals and persons with disorders from lumping them into categories and inappro-

Personal Reflection 4.1   "I am introducing you to my son, Joshua. Josh is 7 years old. He's diligent to the task, a unique kid, a hard worker and, yes, Josh has Down syndrome. I mention the Down syndrome last because Josh is a person first. Josh is not a 'Down's'; he's not a 'Down syndrome child'; but rather he's an individual who happens to have Down syndrome. He's not a category or a diagnosis. He is a person before he is anything else."

Thomas J. O'Neill (1987, p. xviii), President, National Down Syndrome Congress.

priately limiting their expectations for future growth based on preconceptions about what persons with "condition X" might be able to do in the future. Establishing a prognosis is a responsibility that accompanies clinical intervention, but it should be done with an eye to avoiding stereotyping and to being realistic without limiting an individual's and a family's hopes for the future.

Throughout this discussion of categories, remember that prototypes are being discussed and that space constraints limit the discussion's breadth and depth. The real world does not often offer "textbook examples." It is full of gray areas and overlaps and muddiness. Professionals who realize that categories are inventions for the convenience of thinking and communicating about phenomena will be more likely to maintain the flexibility needed to enter the systems that include people with language disorders, or people at risk for language disorders, and to contribute to those systems in a positive way.

CATEGORICAL CONDITIONS ASSOCIATED WITH LANGUAGE DISORDERS

The outline of categories discussed in this chapter is presented in Box 4.1. For each major diagnostic category, the discussion is further divided into (1) *definitions* (emphasizing associated features of language, speech, and communication) and *subclassifications* and (2) *relationships* of the six contributing factors associated with the theories of language acquisition discussed in Chapter 3: (a) biological factors, (b) linguistic system factors, (c) stimulus–response–reinforcement factors, (d) cognition factors, and (e) social interaction factors.

Using this approach, one can consider how some factors appear to contribute more or less to different conditions. In some cases, a factor may be an essential contributing factor, with known direct involvement in the appearance, course of change, and prognosis

---

Box 4.1   Categorical factors associated with childhood language disorders.

  I. Central factors
      A. Specific language disability
      B. Mental retardation
      C. Autism
      D. Attention-deficit hyperactivity disorder
      E. Acquired brain injury
      F. Others
 II. Peripheral factors
      A. Hearing impairment
      B. Visual impairment
      C. Physical impairment
III. Environmental and emotional factors
      A. Neglect and abuse
      B. Behavioral and emotional development problems
 IV. Mixed factors

of language development and disorders for a particular categorical condition. In other cases, a factor may be recognized as a probable contributing factor, with suspected direct involvement, which may, however, be difficult to prove objectively. Finally, some factors are often found to be involved in the development of language associated with a particular categorical condition, but they may vary widely and are not central to establishing diagnosis or prognosis for the category. The relationships between categories and contributing factors are summarized in Table 4.1.

CENTRAL PROCESSING FACTORS

Specific Language Disability

Definitions, differential diagnosis, and subdivisions. The usual operational definition for identifying children with "specific language impairments" is that they "exhibit significant limitations in language functioning that cannot be attributed to deficits in hearing, oral structure and function, or general intelligence" (Leonard, 1987, p. 1). This definition emphasizes specificity; it assumes that a relatively isolated impairment can affect language development specifically, while leaving general cognitive development and other peripheral sensory and motor functions relatively unscathed.

Although most professionals recognize a condition known by the label *specific language disability* (and by other labels considered later), attempts to establish diagnostic criteria for the category commonly encounter two major problems. These are, first, problems associated with identifying a common set of reliable symptoms that appear repeatedly in different children and, second, problems with isolating language from other cognitive, perceptual, and social functions. The first problem is related to the complexity of language and language processing. Because language is multifaceted, is it possible for children to have specific problems with some areas of language functioning but not others? That question has been addressed by searching for subtypes of children with specific language disability, a topic discussed in a later section (the answer seems to be "yes"). The second problem concerns establishing exclusion criteria in definitions of specific language (or learning) disability.

Because the diagnosis of specific language disability depends on exclusion of other categorical conditions, it becomes problematic to diagnose when children have the essential characteristics of specific language impairment (whatever those are), but mixed either with other problems or with conditions of cultural diversity. Either of these circumstances may make it particularly difficult to identify the problem with standardized measures.

TABLE 4.1

Relationships between categories associated with childhood language disorders and contributing factors to language acquisition

| Contributing Factors | Categorical Conditions | | | | | | | | | |
| | Central | | | | | Peripheral | | | Environmental and Emotional | |
	SLD	MR	Autism	ADHD	BrInj	Hrg	Vis	Phys	Negl/Abuse	Beh/Emot
Biological	b	b	b	b	a	a	a	a	b	c
Linguistic system	a	b	a	c	b	a	c	c	c	c
Stimulus–response–reinforcement	c	b	a	a	b	b	b	b	b	a
Information processing	b	a	a	a	a	a	a	a	b	c
Cognition	b	a	a	c	b	c	c	c	c	c
Social interaction	b	a	a	a	b	b	c	b	a	a

[a] Essential contributing factor with known direct involvement.

[b] Probable contributing factor with suspected direct involvement.

[c] Often a contributing factor, but degree of involvement may vary.

ADHD, attention-deficit hyperactive disorder; Beh/emot, behavioral and/or emotional disorders; BrInj, brain injury; Hrg, hearing impairment; MR, mental retardation; Negl/abuse, neglect and/or abuse; Phys, physical impairment; SLD, specific language disability; Vis, visual impairment.

Diagnostic criteria for specific language (or learning) disability generally include the requirement that children exhibit a discrepancy between reduced scores on at least some language tests and scores on IQ tests that must be normal or near normal (sometimes called *intellectual functioning,* or *potential*). As considered again in later chapters, however, intelligence testing with children with language disorders and related conditions is fraught with difficulty. Often, when intelligence tests are administered to children with disabilities, their performance across tasks is uneven (a condition sometimes called *psychometric scatter*). As Rapin and Allen (1983) have pointed out, in intelligence testing, "The IQ is the summary score derived from performance on a psychological test battery that samples a broad range of behaviors." For children with disabilities, however, "A summary score represents neither their areas of real deficit nor their strengths" (p. 162). Although typically, children with specific language impairments tend to do better on "nonverbal" tests of intelligence than those designed to tap verbal abilities, when a verbal strategy can facilitate problem solving on supposedly nonverbal tests or subtests, children with specific language impairment may also score lower on those tests because of their language deficits.

Professionals are cautioned, therefore, against adopting criteria that are too stringent in hopes of identifying children with "pure language disorder," as some researchers have attempted to do. For example, Stark and Tallal (1981) adopted criteria that children must score at least 85 on the performance scale of an intelligence test (this is a common criterion) and that, if children are age 7 or older, their reading test scores must be within 6 months of their overall language age scores. This criterion might become increasingly problematic as children grow older; it also suggests comparability across tests that may not exist, and it fails to recognize how language symptoms may change over time. For those engaged in clinical or educational practice, Rapin and Allen (1983) commented that it is unusual to see many children with such "pure" syndromes. Instead, they argued that a diagnosis of specific developmental language disorder is justified when children exhibited linguistic skills that "are much more severely deficient than their other cognitive skills and are out of proportion to their IQ" (p. 163).

What to call it?   Perhaps no other categorical condition has been given so many names over the years as *specific language disability*. The reasons for this are also many. First, some of the names reflect theories about underlying causes prevalent at a particular point in the history of concern about the disorder(s). For example, the terms *minimal brain damage, minimal brain dysfunction* (U.S. Department of Health, Education, & Welfare, 1969), and *congenital aphasia* (S. F. Brown, 1959) were prevalent in earlier attempts to describe children who appear to have a specific neurological deficit that makes it difficult for them to learn language. Such diagnoses, however, were based only on "soft signs" (including language development difficulty) in the absence of hard neurological evidence. Gradually, those terms have been replaced by labels such as *learning disability,* which makes fewer assumptions about cause, or by labels such as *developmental language disability* or *developmental language disorder,* which are designed to specify a condition for which no clear cause exists but is apparently congenital.

Second, some terminological differences reflect the varied perspectives of professional disciplines concerned with the diagnosis and remediation of relatively isolated language disorders. For example, whereas physicians might use terms such as *minimal brain dysfunction* and *dyslexia* to describe a child with such problems, speech–language pathologists are more likely to use terms such as *specific language impairment* and *language-learning disability,* and educators may use terms such as *learning disability* and *reading disability*.

Trends in the medical profession, however, are shifting. The *Diagnostic and Statistical Manual of Mental Disorders, Third Edition—Revised* (DSM-III-R), published by the American Psychiatric Association (1987), now uses terms based more on observable symptomatology than on assumptions about cause that cannot be proven. The DSM-III-R refers to a broad category of "specific developmental disorders," which then are further subdivided into "academic skills disorders," including developmental arithmetic disorder, developmental expressive writing disorder, and developmental reading disorder, and a second broad category of "language and speech disorders," which includes developmental articulation disorder, developmental expressive language disorder, and developmental receptive language disorder. In addition, there is a category of "specific developmental disorder not otherwise specified" for disorders in the development of language, speech, academic, and motor skills that do not meet the criteria for a "specific developmental disorder." It includes aphasia with epilepsy acquired in childhood (sometimes known as "Landau syndrome" or "Landau-Kleffner syndrome," discussed in the following section on acquired disorders) and specific developmental difficulties in spelling. Of these subcategories, perhaps only developmental arithmetic disorder does not represent a major contribution from an impaired language processing system (however, as considered later, an intact language system can make major contributions to becoming mathematically competent). The inclusion of subcategories represents the heterogeneity of the conditions related to specific language disability. Such a condition does not look the same in every child for whom it can be diagnosed (Box 4.2 shows a definition of learning disabilities that emphasizes heterogeneity).

Third, some terminological differences reflect evolution of symptoms of language disorders within the same children over time. For example, many children who might be categorized during their preschool years as having early language delay or early language disability may be recategorized during their school-age years as having learning disabilities or language-learning disabilities.

What changes? Do children change or only labels? Recalling the discussions of Chapter 1 regarding contextually based definitions of disability, probably a little of both occurs, set in the context of changes in environmental expectations from the preschool years through adulthood. Out of concern that traditional views of learning disabilities are limited by their restriction to the school-age years, the National Joint Committee on Learning Disabilities (1985) developed

a position paper on "Learning Disabilities and the Preschool Child," in which they noted that learning disabilities must be viewed as problems not only of the school years but also of preschool years and continuing into adult life:

> Indiscriminate premature labeling of the preschool child as learning disabled is not warranted. Normal development is characterized by broad ranges of individual and group differences, as well as by variability in rates and patterns of maturation. During the preschool years, this variability is marked. For some children, marked discrepancies in abilities are temporary and are resolved during the course of development and within the context of experiential interaction. For other children, there is a persistence of marked discrepancies within and among one or more domains of function, necessitating the child's referral for systematic assessment and appropriate intervention. (p. 1)

Fourth, varied terms may reflect the relatedness of a cluster of disorders that may or may not be parts of the same syndrome. In this category are labels such as *specific reading disability* and *dyslexia*, as well as the DSM-III-R categories of developmental expressive writing disorder and developmental reading disorder. Such labels tend to reflect a particular set of symptoms, having to do with the acquisition of written rather than oral language.

Finally, different states, regions, and professional associations tend to adopt different terminology, and their labels evolve over time. Because terminology used to label conditions that society views as handicapping can acquire pejorative connotations, it is particularly likely that such terminology will shift as

---

Box 4.2	Definition of learning disabilities by The National Joint Committee on Learning Disabilities (1991)

> Learning disabilities is a general term that refers to a heterogeneous group of disorders manifested by significant difficulties in the acquisition and use of listening, speaking, reading, writing, reasoning, or mathematical abilities. These disorders are intrinsic to the individual, presumed to be due to central nervous system dysfunction, and may occur across the lifespan. Problems in self-regulatory behaviors, social perception, and social interaction may exist with learning disabilities but do not by themselves constitute a learning disability. Although learning disabilities may occur concomitantly with other handicapping conditions (for example, sensory impairment, mental retardation, serious emotional disturbance) or with extrinsic influences (such as cultural differences, insufficient or inappropriate instruction), they are not the result of those conditions or influences. (National Joint Committee on Learning Disabilities, 1991, p. 19)

perceptions of the disorders shift. This makes it important for parents and professionals to understand the terminology prevalent in a local area or professional group whenever they enter a new setting to be sure that they are communicating clearly about children.

Because of the importance of learning to read in children's lives, and because of the high frequency (noted previously) with which children with oral language impairments experience later difficulty in learning to read (up to 95%), consider terminology related to specific reading disability a bit further. Perhaps no term is more confusing to the general public than *dyslexia*. This term grew out of recognition by a physician, Samuel Orton (1937), that childhood reading disability had some features in common with alexia, or "word blindness." The term *pure word blindness* was first used by the neurologist Dejerine in 1892 (E. Kaplan & Goodglass, 1981) to describe an adult stroke patient who exhibited serious disability in comprehending written material accompanied by a remarkable preservation of writing ability. To contrast with the acquired condition, Orton called the condition involving specific reading disability that he observed in children *developmental alexia*. The term *alexia* then evolved into the term *dyslexia*, partially because the reading disability

is rarely expressed as complete inability to read. Although the general public tends to focus on Orton's explanation of symptoms related to letter reversals and word confusions in the diagnosis of dyslexia, and to think of it as primarily a visual-based problem, Orton's followers in the Orton Dyslexia Society use the terms *dyslexia* and *specific language disability* as interchangeable (see Box 4.3). Kamhi and Catts (1989), in a review of the evidence, also supported the view of dyslexia as a developmental language impairment, with difficulty focused in the area of phonological analysis skills.

Specific language disability: Different or delayed? The validity of a category of specific language disability (or any other of the names by which it has been called) has been probed repeatedly. Some efforts have centered on the question of whether anything is truly "different" about the way children develop language when they fall outside of expected normative patterns in language but not in other areas of development. Are such children qualitatively different in the way they learn language, or are they merely slower in inducing the rules, eventually arriving at a grammar that matches that of the other speakers of their language

---

| Box 4.3 | Characteristics of dyslexia, summarized from Slingerland (1981) |

1. Average or above average intelligence
2. Reversals, transpositions and omissions in reading, spelling, and/or speech
3. Difficulty learning to read, as shown by one or more of the following:
   a. Insertion of small words in reading
   b. Silent reading slow when compared to intelligence
   c. Oral reading hesitant
   d. Poor word recall and decoding skills
   e. Reading comprehension lost during struggle to recognize words
4. Difficulty recalling images for individual letters and letter sequences readily, smoothly, and accurately
5. Features sometimes observed include:
   a. Spelling difficulty
   b. Meager writing vocabulary
   c. Awkward or slow writing
   d. Hesitant in talking, with poor word retrieval
   e. Difficulty expressing self, talking a lot but not getting to the point
   f. Particular difficulty recalling names of acquaintances or places
   g. Poor left-to-right orientation
6. Tends to "run in families," but can occur in isolated cases
7. Language difficulties appear in spite of adequate educational opportunities

(even though it might be slightly less complex)? Such a question seems to be relatively easy to answer. Researchers should merely need to analyze whether the language behaviors observed among children with language disorders are similar to those of younger children or whether they differ. The answers are not so easy.

In earlier studies, some language skills of children with language disorders clearly appeared deviant. For example, Paula Menyuk (1964) used transformational grammar techniques to analyze the language of some children who had been characterized as producing "infantile speech" and showed that their grammatical usage was not simply more infantile than normal nor delayed in time. Menyuk concluded that it is incorrect to say that a 5-year-old child with infantile speech uses the grammar of a normal-speaking child at age 4 or 3 or 2.

Laurence Leonard (1972,1980) also addressed the question "What is deviant language?" In a 1972 article, Leonard reviewed the evidence gathered previously and concluded that any particular structure used by children learning language normally could also be observed in use by children whose language was considered deviant (and vice versa). In answering the question about what might be "deviant," Leonard proposed that "the differences in the use of each syntactic and morphological structure between normal and deviant speakers are probably best described in terms of frequency of usage" (1972, p. 435).

Leonard (1972) also pointed out the clinical dangers in labeling a child's language as *delayed* (thus suggesting the child would be able to "catch up" with other children if only given a little more time) when the evidence suggested that some children do not catch up but plateau in some areas of language learning. They continue to demonstrate a high frequency of early language features, sometimes in combination with such later developing grammatical features as question, negative, and embedding transformations (Menyuk, 1964). Leonard summarized findings showing that children with deviant language, when compared with age-matched peers or peers matched for mean length of utterance (MLU) who are learning language normally, exhibit (1) a lower frequency of indefinite pronouns, main verbs, and secondary verbs; (2) occasional use of some later-developing forms of these types; (3) a lower frequency of transformations involving negation, contraction, auxiliary *be*, and adjectives; and (4) more frequently omitted verb phrases, noun phrases, and articles.

In the 1980 paper, Leonard again pointed out that establishing a case for different (rather than merely delayed) development for children with language disorders might rely not on the observation of unique features in the language of one group or the other but in patterns of frequency of usage. Leonard (1980) tempered his observations of different developmental patterns with the general conclusion that "The phonological, semantic, syntactic, and pragmatic features used by language-disabled children are essentially the same as those used by younger normal children and are not unique to this group of children" (p. 150). Yet Leonard returned as well to mounting evidence that relationships among various linguistic features (phonology, semantics, syntax, and pragmatics) may differ for children with language-learning difficulties.

In a departure from his earlier work, Leonard's (1987, 1991) latest contribution to the study of specific language impairment is to question its existence as an identifiable subgroup. Leonard has reconfirmed that children who appear to have specific language impairments are not simply late in reaching linguistic milestones "but have limitations in their language abilities that are long standing, at least in the absence of intervention" (1987, p. 31). He has also reconfirmed, however, that the characteristics of the language of children with language disorders, when considered singly, do not differ appreciably from those of younger children developing normally. Differences do show up in relationships across areas of language development. Is there such a thing as different language development? The answer is still "yes and no."

The point of Leonard's (1987) article, however, was that, to explain variations in developmental patterns, it is not necessary to use arguments of specific language impairment as if such children belong to a population different from that of normally developing children (see Box 4.4). Leonard reviewed three kinds of evidence (which I will consider further in the following sections regarding contributing factors), all of which have been used to argue for the existence of a special population of children with specific linguistic impairments: (1) differences in the communicative environments of such children, (2) differences in their abilities to perceive rapid acoustic stimuli, and (3) differences in their broader abilities of mental representation.

Leonard (1987) found the evidence noncompelling and argued that little could be gained by considering such children to have a disorder that could be related

Box 4.4   Evidence for different (rather than merely delayed) language acquisition across the rule sys-
                 tems of language for children with specific language impairment based on Leonard's (1980)
                 review of the literature

1. **Phonology**. The most common pattern is for children with language disorders to demonstrate phonological simplification patterns typical of younger children, such as stopping (*pibe*
   for *five*), fronting (*tootie* for *cookie*), and consonant-cluster simplification (*cool* for *school*).
       Although these patterns alone provide more evidence of delay than deviance, co-occur-
   rence patterns differ. Phonological simplification patterns are generally noted in conjunction
   with one- or two-word utterances in normal development. Among children with language
   disorders, they have been observed in conjunction with a wide range of utterance lengths.
   Occasionally, unusual phonological patterns also appear in the speech of children with language disorders (e.g., using a bilabial nasal for liquids and glides), which clearly differ from
   any observed in normal development.

2. **Semantics**. Children with language disorders are slow to acquire their first words, acquire
   additional words more slowly than their peers, and occasionally make lexical errors that are
   similar to the types seen in younger normally developing children. These characteristics seem
   to be more typical of delay than they are of qualitative differences of developmental patterns.

3. **Syntax**. Again, most syntactic differences observed between the language of children with
   language disorders and their same-age peers have been quantitative rather than qualitative.
   When children are matched on the basis of mean length of utterance (MLU) (rather than
   age), the differences are further minimized. Both groups follow similar developmental orders
   in acquiring more complex structures, such as questions (although children with language
   disorders have been observed to use fewer questions even after they can form them). What
   appears to differentiate the groups best is the co-occurrence of later-developing and earlier-
   developing forms in children with specific language disorders. Children with language disorders have also been observed to be delayed in their ability to paraphrase through syntactic
   rearrangement (Leonard, 1980, categorized this as a pragmatic skill).

4. **Pragmatics**. Studies for which children were matched for chronological age again have
   tended to provide more evidence of delay than difference; children with language disorders
   often act more like younger children without disorders. In studies for which children were
   matched for MLU at the one-word level, children with language disorders tended to use
   more nonlinguistic means to communicate about shifting contextual elements. Children with
   longer utterance lengths have not always shown this difference, but they do seem to have
   fewer options for revising their utterances and tailoring them to listener needs. Much of the
   literature on differences in the pragmatic skills of school-age children with language disorders
   came after Leonard's 1980 article. Two of the primary differences noted by Donahue, Pearl,
   and Bryan (1983) for adolescents with learning disabilities were their difficulties in (1) adapting form and content to varied listeners and situations and (2) understanding the rules for
   participating in cooperative conversational turn taking.

to a specific cause. Instead, he commented that "the 'cause' of these children's language limitations is simply the product of the same types of variations in genetic and environmental factors that lead some children to be clumsy, others to be amusical, and still others to have little insight into their feelings" (p. 31).

My view is that Leonard's (1987) focus in this statement on contributions of variable factors to individual differences is consistent with recognizing a category of specific language disability. This is particularly true

in a culture such as ours where oral and written language skills are valued highly and are so important to success. Leonard (1991) himself accepts the current diagnostic terminology. He reported that few changes in clinical practices would be necessitated by acceptance of his hypothesis that many children labeled specifically language impaired are "different solely because they fall at the very low end of the normal distribution in ability" (p. 68). Intervention efforts would be aimed consistently at children's comprehension and use of language rather than at some implied underlying deficit in auditory perception and sequencing skills.

What happens when children are culturally different? Diagnosis of learning disability or specific language disorder becomes particularly problematic when it is inappropriate to use tests standardized on a sociolinguistic population different from that of the individual suspected of having the disability. Historically, because of test bias, children who were culturally or linguistically different were likely to be overidentified as needing special education services (Harber, 1980). Children from different sociolinguistic groups also may be underidentified as having problems, perhaps because language specialists may not be sufficiently comfortable with multicultural assessment to make judgments about whether these children might have language disorders. Terrell and Terrell (1983) frame the question facing clinicians as "How will I know if this child is a normal dialect speaker or if this child's communicative behaviors reflect true language deficiencies?" (p. 3). That critical question is addressed in Chapters 6 and 9.

Subtypes of specific language disability. Although definitions and discussions of specific language disability generally recognize the heterogeneity inherent in the condition, few attempts have been made to differentiate subtypes. This is particularly true in the area of specific oral language impairment. More work has been done in the area of attempting to differentiate subtypes of children who have specific written language problems. In this section, I first consider subtyping efforts made by Aram and Nation (1975), Rapin and Allen (1983), and Fey (1986) in the area of oral language disorders; then, I consider subtyping efforts for differentiating disorders of learning to read.

In one of the first studies of children with developmental language disorders designed to differentiate subtypes based on language symptoms (rather than presumed cause), Aram and Nation (1975) identified six different patterns of deficit among 47 children with developmental language disorders who were between the ages of 3 and 7 years. Using performance on a series of formal language tasks selected to represent the three language dimensions of comprehension, formulation, and repetition (imitation), Aram and Nation divided the children into six subgroups representing (1) better ability to repeat than to comprehend or formulate language; (2) generalized

expressive deficiency involving formulation and repetition; (3) relatively uniform deficiency for all three kinds of language tasks; (4) specific phonological deficiency affecting comprehension, formulation, and repetition; (5) comprehension deficiency with equal or better ability to formulate language or to repeat it; and (6) specific formulation and repetition deficiency.

More recently, Rapin and Allen (1983) compiled longitudinal and cross-sectional evidence (based on such sources as neurological tests, language and cognitive tests, and direct observation) from approximately 100 children who had been referred for a pediatric neurologic consultation with the chief complaint of delayed or deviant speech. From the evidence, the researchers differentiated several developmental language disorder syndromes, grouped into four major subtypes: (1) predominant expressive disorder with three subgroups, (2) verbal auditory agnosia, (3) autism, with two subgroups (considered later in this chapter), and (4) a semantic-pragmatic group with some characteristics in common with autism but lacking the severe affective (interpersonal) deficits of autism.

The most prevalent of the three subgroups of the predominant expressive disorder group described by Rapin and Allen (1983) is the phonologic-syntactic syndrome. It is diagnosed when children are difficult to understand, use few function words, demonstrate limited noun and verb inflection (omitting such endings as plurals and *-ing*), and rarely combine syntactic relations within a single sentence. Although the semantic categories such children use appear to be relatively intact, their abilities vary in all other aspects of language, symbolic, cognitive, and pragmatic functioning. Some, but not all, show additional signs of neurologic dysfunction, particularly oromotor dysfunction. These include signs of mild dysarthria (drooling and a history of difficulty in sucking, chewing, and swallowing) and signs of oromotor apraxia (difficulty in imitating precise movements of the tongue, lips, and jaw).

A second subgroup in the expressive category is *severe expressive syndrome with good comprehension* (Rapin & Allen,1983). These children were completely mute or virtually unintelligible, with productions limited to poorly articulated two-word utterances at most, but with strikingly good language comprehension. The third subgroup in the expressive category is *syntactic-pragmatic syndrome* (Rapin & Allen, 1983). Children in this rare subgroup include those with grossly impaired syntax, severely limited pragmatic use of language, and impaired comprehension. They can name pictures and objects and give and follow simple commands but cannot formulate or respond to *wh-* (e.g, *what, where,* and *who*) questions. This is the only syndrome that Rapin and Allen described in which syntax is affected but phonology was normal or near normal.

The syndrome of verbal auditory agnosia, which Rapin and Allen (1983) described, might be better classified with cases of acquired childhood language disorders in this text. It is comparable to the syndrome of pure word deafness, auditory agnosia, or central deafness in adults, and its cause is thought by some to be related to encephalitic disease processes (others disagree; see Cole et al., 1988) that involve the superior temporal lobes bilaterally. Some children with this rare condition, however, appear to have had it from birth and do not have a history of marked onset; others demonstrate a period of fairly normal vocabulary and language development before the language disorder becomes apparent but with no clear causative incident. A central symptom of this disorder is severe difficulty in interpreting auditory input in the presence of relatively normal peripheral hearing and audiograms. When it appears early, children with verbal auditory agnosia learn language as if they were deaf, being almost totally unable to benefit from auditory input. Thus, they have extreme difficulty acquiring spoken language. Like some children with autism, these children may remain mute, but they can be differentiated from children with autism because of their more normal responses to gestural and facial expressions and tone of voice, their more normal eye contact, and the absence of unusual autistic behaviors, such as insistence on sameness. Academically, children with verbal auditory agnosia often do better in math than in language-intensive course work, and they generally benefit from a total communication approach to language acquisition. Because of their phonological imagery problems, they are likely to have difficulty learning to read as well as to talk.

The final subtype Rapin and Allen (1983) described is *semantic-pragmatic syndrome without autism.* The phrase *without autism* is necessary because this condition demonstrates some similarity to autism because children may demonstrate fluent language that has good phonological and syntactic form but is noncommunicative. Both types of children tend to share a difficulty in the pragmatic skills of considering

the prior knowledge and information needs of their audience and in comprehending language spoken to them. Rather than grasping the full intent of questions, for example, they may focus on single words or short phrases and pursue tangentially related topics of their own. Sometimes this conversational pattern involves overuse of canned phrases that give it a semantically empty "cocktail party" flavor. "Cocktail party conversation" has been described particularly for children who have a history of hydrocephalus, which may impair subcortical white matter while leaving the primary peri-Sylvian cortical language areas relatively intact. However, Rapin and Allen (1983) also describe the occurrence of this syndrome in two brothers for whom a genetically determined developmental (rather than acquired neurological) cause seemed the best explanation.

Children demonstrating semantic-pragmatic syndrome without autism, like those with autism, sometimes may be echolalic (repeating phrases spoken to them in part or exactly, immediately or later), particularly in their younger years, and they may show pronoun confusions. They may also be hyperlexic (precocious in learning to read but often reading without comprehension). They differ from children with autism primarily in their interest and ability in making and maintaining social contacts in spite of difficulties engaging in social conversation. Because teachers do not expect to find children whose verbal expression skills exceed their verbal comprehension abilities, and because school success depends to such a great extent on language comprehension (both written and spoken), these children tend to have great difficulty succeeding in school and may develop behavioral disorders (demonstrating principles of both causative heterogeneity and layering, considered earlier).

A different approach to subtyping children with developmental language disorders was taken by Marc Fey (1986), who devised four categories for grouping preschool-age children based on clinical experience and a theoretical view of conversational interaction (Figure 4.1). By rating children's relative assertiveness and responsiveness, Fey described four groups: (1) Active conversationalists are communicative children high in both assertiveness and responsiveness, although they might have relatively severe impairments of language form (such children might be comparable to those in Rapin and Allen's, 1983, phonologic-syntactic subgroup). (2) Passive conversa-

FIGURE 4.1
Marc Fey's scheme for profiling
children according to their levels of
social conversational participation.

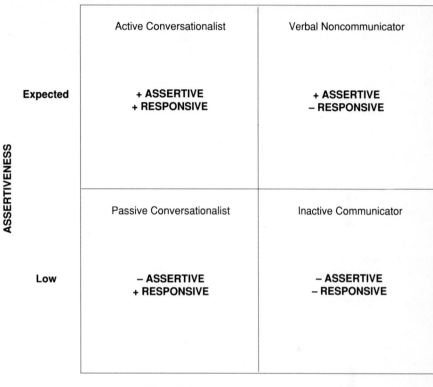

tionalists are low in assertiveness but adequately responsive, rarely adding information to a topic, even though they attempt to answer questions (without a clear parallel in Rapin and Allen's, 1983, system, although children showing severe expressive syndrome with good comprehension might be somewhat similar). (3) Inactive communicators are children low in both assertiveness and responsiveness (perhaps comparable to Rapin and Allen's, 1983, syntactic-pragmatic subgroup). (4) Verbal noncommunicators are children high in assertiveness but low in accommodating the needs of their conversational partners (perhaps comparable to Rapin and Allen's, 1983, subgroup, semantic-pragmatic syndrome without autism).

Readers may notice that my attempts to reconcile categories from two different subtyping systems can illustrate the problems in doing so, as well as poten-

tial benefits. It is a bit like comparing apples and oranges, but it also serves as a reminder that we are ultimately concerned about children, not categories, and they are all individuals.

As noted repeatedly, when children with language disorders enter schools, new sets of concerns arise, and new categories are sometimes devised for grouping children with similarities. Often, the symptom of focus becomes difficulty in learning to read. Some evidence shows that a set of common features is shared by both reading-impaired children without overt language disorders and language-impaired children who also exhibit reading disorders (Kamhi, Catts, Mauer, Apel, & Gentry, 1988). The findings based on multiple measures of phonological, lexical, syntactical, and spatial processing show that children in these two groups perform such tasks similarly to each other and differently from normal learners, suggesting common substrata of difficulties for both kinds of children.

Many attempts to classify subtypes of developmental reading disorders have been made (e.g., see summaries by A. J. Harris, 1983; Satz & Morris, 1981). Some of the subtype classification systems have been based largely on clinical experience. An early example is D. W. Johnson and Myklebust's (1967) division of children with learning disabilities into the two broad subtypes of primarily auditory-based problems (difficulty remembering and sequencing auditory symbols) and primarily visual-based problems (confusion of letters and words that look similar). Others have used sophisticated empirical and statistical analysis procedures.

A. J. Harris (1983) summarized the results of more recent subtyping studies as suggesting that three major subtypes or syndromes occur within the population of developmentally disabled readers: (1) The most common pattern is "general deficiency in language skills (coupled with normal visual and visual-motor skills) and a lower Verbal IQ than Performance IQ" (p. 53). (2) The second pattern involves "difficulty with visual perception and visual-motor tasks, coupled with relatively normal language abilities and a Verbal IQ higher than Performance IQ" (p. 53). (3) The third pattern, which has been called an "unexpected" subtype (Satz & Morris, 1981), is observed among children "whose cognitive abilities fail to show any significant deficits that could account for the reading failure" (A. J. Harris, 1983, p. 53), but whose environmental, economic, cultural, and linguistic conditions often vary widely from the mainstream. In some "disabled reader" populations, this subtype has been observed to account for 70% of the group (Denckla, 1972). A. J. Harris (1983) also identified a fourth subtype observed in some of the more recent studies: those children exhibited normal verbal comprehension and vocabulary but a deficiency in verbal fluency. Harris cautioned that further subtypes may exist, but may not have been illuminated because of the types of reading behavior studied in prior research and because of the tasks used to measure them.

One problem with subtyping studies is that, although recent research on normal reading processes has emphasized the importance of context and syntactic cues in comprehension, studies of reading disability typically have used single-word reading and writing tasks. Many have not even used sentence-comprehension tasks, let alone paragraph or text-comprehension tasks (A. J. Harris, 1983). Therefore, the clinically recognized category of readers who demonstrate a pattern of good word recognition with poor comprehension may have been overlooked in the subtyping studies because of experimental design problems.

Stanovich (1986) used a richer model of written language processing to examine research on individual differences in reading ability. He commented on four classes of cognitive processes often suggested as causes of reading failure: (1) early visual processes, (2) phonological and naming processes, (3) the use of context to facilitate word recognition, and (4) memory and comprehension strategies. Stanovich's analysis of current research strongly supported the conclusion that word-decoding ability, based on phonological abilities, rather than visual processes, accounts for a large proportion of the variance in reading ability at all levels. Stanovich commented that less-skilled readers are not characterized by a general inability to use context to facilitate word recognition. However, problems with comprehension may result from slow and inaccurate decoding of words, which tends to make the context useless.

In a later paper, Stanovich (1988) reiterated evidence supporting the position that the core disability among children with true developmental dyslexia is a phonological decoding deficit. He emphasized that global processes such as "general linguistic awareness, comprehension, strategic functioning, rule learning, active/inactive learning, and generalized metacognitive functioning are the wrong places to look for the key to reading disability" (p. 157). When children do have reading disabilities tied to such overall deficits, their reading problems are described better by a general developmental lag model than by a specific reading disability model. Stanovich did acknowledge evidence in support of a subgroup of dyslexic individuals "who have severe problems in accessing the lexicon on a visual/orthographic basis" (p. 160), but he maintained that the size of this subgroup is extremely small when compared with the subgroup of dyslexic children with phonological difficulties and that one key to fluent reading "appears to be the development of an autonomously functioning module at the word recognition level" (p. 158).

Manis, Szeszulski, Holt, and Graves (1988) reported similar findings regarding 50 children with developmental dyslexia differentiated from 40 normal readers of equivalent reading achievement primarily in phonological skills (spelling-to-sound translation and phonemic analysis). Manis et al., however, also observed limited differences in knowledge of word-specific spellings. The authors identified three major subgroups for the children's phonological processing deficits: (1) specific deficits in the phonological processing of print (53%); (2) deficits in processing both the phonological and orthographic features of printed words (24%); and (3) phonological deficits in oral language (8%). The remaining 16% of the sample had specific deficits in visual or orthographic processing of print or in spelling or did not differ from the control group.

Relationships of contributing factors. *Biological maturation.* Factors of biological maturation are considered probable contributing factors associated with specific language disability in childhood. Generally, some abnormality of central nervous system support for language development is assumed to be present when specific language, learning, and reading disabilities are diagnosed, but the presence of biological factors is difficult to prove. Areas investigated involve brain asymmetry, neuronal development and myelination, and neuronal organization.

Kinsbourne (1981) cautioned against overinterpreting data regarding asymmetry of brain structures. Gone are the days when left-handed children had their left hands tied behind their backs to force them to use their right hands, supposedly to force lateralization to the left hemisphere, which was presumed necessary for normal language and reading development. Now, it is recognized that, although the left hemisphere seems to be structured specially for some aspects of language learning, neither hemisphere is dominant for all functions. Both contribute.

Some intriguing possibilities, however, emerge from brain asymmetry studies for attempting to understand developmental language disorders. For example, Hier and his colleagues (1978) conducted computed tomography (CT) brain scans on 24 children diagnosed with dyslexia and found evidence of a reversed asymmetry in the linguistically important parieto-occipital region among 42%. In those children, the right side was found to be wider than the left. An additional 25% showed symmetrical hemisphere relationships, compared with the expectation that the left planum temporale is larger than the right in 66% of normal brains (Geschwind & Levitsky, 1968). Hynd,

Marshall, and Gonzalez (1991) summarized this and eight other studies using either CT or magnetic resonance imaging (MRI) techniques. They concluded that the studies showed significantly less left–right asymmetry among individuals with severe reading disability or dyslexia but no relationships between brain morphology patterns and handedness.

In a second area of investigation, neuronal development has been implicated. Although immaturity of myelogenesis (delay in myelination) has not yet been conclusively proven to be a cause of speech–language delay, the evidence does point in that direction (Love & Webb, 1986). Other types of disruptive influences on neural organization also have been noted in association with language and learning disabilities. For example, Galaburda and Kemper (1979) conducted an autopsy of the brain of a young person with dyslexia and found evidence of disrupted neural connections in the areas of the brain most responsible for linguistic processing.

More recently, Galaburda (1989) reported on the autopsies of a total of eight brains of individuals with dyslexia. All showed symmetry (rather than the expected asymmetry) in the planum temporale, but in addition, all of the six males and one female showed abnormalities in the organization of neural networks of the perisylvian region, especially in their left hemispheres. Galaburda also noted abnormal cortical cell layering (see Figure 4.2) in some cases and focal evidence of cortical scarring in others. The latter he suspected to be related to injury dated to the end of pregnancy through the end of the 2nd year at the latest.

Linguistic system factors. Linguistic system factors are considered essential contributing factors to specific language disability in childhood. If children learning language do so because they are born with a language acquisition device (LAD) specific to the language acquisition process, they may show isolated impairments that involve only language learning and that spare developmental processes in other areas. This assumption is essential to diagnosis of specific language disability. However, as noted previously, little evidence indicates that the rule-induction process for children with specific language disorders differs qualitatively from that for other children. On the other hand, language group subtyping efforts suggest that individual children

FIGURE 4.2
Arrows point to distorted lamina-
tion of cerebral cortex in the brain
of an individual with dyslexia
(courtesy of Albert M. Galaburda).

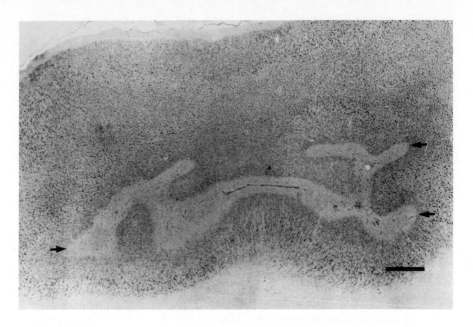

with specific language disabilities may have scattered abilities within varied areas of language phonology, morphology, syntax, semantics, and pragmatics. Phonology, morphology, and syntax seem to
be most frequently involved when children exhibit
specific language disabilities.

Stimulus–response–reinforcement factors. Many specialists in language disorders hypothesize no special
role of stimulus–response–reinforcement patterns for
children with specific language disabilities. These
children, by definition, have intact peripheral sensory
systems. They also tend to respond to social reinforcement in ways similar to those of their normally developing peers. Although some intervention
programs have been designed using carefully programmed behaviorist principles to arrange stimulus–
response–reinforcement patterns to encourage children to notice regularities of linguistic rules that may
have escaped them in natural communicative interactions, many proponents argue (as discussed in later
chapters) that children with specific language disabilities benefit more from approaches that emphasize
communicativeness over language form, even when
the ultimate target is the development of more mature language formulation and syntactic comprehension ability.

Information processing factors. Although it is an
area of controversy, aspects of information processing have been implicated as central to explaining
some of the symptoms of specific language disability,
and are considered probable contributing factors
with suspected direct involvement. In particular, auditory processing of rapid acoustic events has been
shown repeatedly to be more difficult for children
with specific language disability than for their normal
language-learning peers (Tallal & Piercy, 1973, 1975;
Tallal, Stark, Kallman, & Mellits, 1981). As Tallal
and colleagues demonstrated in a series of studies,
children with specific language disability often can
perceive features of nonlinguistic acoustic signals
adequately when they occur in isolation or in slowly
presented sequence but not when they occur in the
rapid sequences more characteristic of the acoustic
patterns of speech.

No one doubts that problems of short-term auditory sequential memory (particularly for rapidly produced stimuli) are associated with developmental
language disorders. The controversy is over whether
they are causally related. Some (e.g., Rees, 1973,
1981) state that these symptoms may represent a
result of disordered language ability, or a concomitant
feature, rather than its cause. When Leonard (1987)
summarized the research regarding "specific lan-

guage impairment" (SLI), he pointed out that "no plausible relation between SLI children's difficulty with rapid auditory processing and their language problems has been established" (p. 21). Whether or not auditory processing should be targeted directly in language intervention plans is also a matter of controversy discussed in later chapters.

Cognition factors. The definition of specific language disability is often based partially on discrepancy between some aspects of language functioning and some aspects of cognitive functioning. Therefore, cognitive factors are probable contributing factors that cannot be viewed as central to the diagnosis except in an exclusionary sense.

The picture is not so clear-cut as the definition implies. Rarely is linguistic processing the only area in which such children experience difficulty. As a general rule, the more that a child's language problems involve language content as well as language form, the more the child will have difficulty with general cognitive processing. Furthermore, for the child with comprehension difficulties, it is particularly difficult to separate comprehension of language from comprehension of the world in general.

The picture is also complicated by a line of research suggesting that some children with specific language impairment demonstrate symbolic deficits in nonlinguistic as well as linguistic areas. Leonard (1987), in reviewing this research, noted the implication "that specific language impairment may not be specific at all" (p. 23). From his summary of the research in symbolic play and mental imagery (often involving mental manipulations of geometric form), Leonard concluded that although some of these children "clearly fall below the performance level of same-age peers on symbolic play and imagery tasks, they appear to perform above the level of younger normal children with comparable language abilities" (p. 29). This is the rationale for considering nonverbal representational ability as a probable contributing factor with suspected direct involvement. Language problems co-occur with weaknesses in other symbolic skills too frequently to be coincidental but with insufficient predictability for cognitive factors to be considered central to the disorder.

Social interaction factors. Social interaction factors are also considered probable contributing factors, and again, the picture is not entirely clear-cut. Although the definition of specific language impairment usually requires that environmental factors be ruled out as the primary cause of delay, several studies reviewed by Lederberg (1980) demonstrated that parents of children with such problems interact with them in slightly different ways, shortening their input and using more assertive and action-oriented speech. When children with specific language impairment have been matched with children at similar language levels, few differences in parental interaction styles have been found. Lederberg's (1980) conclusion in reviewing this research was that "parents of delayed children seem to be as sensitive to their child's abilities as parents of normal [developing] children" (p. 151), and Leonard's (1987) conclusion was the same. Not only do mothers and fathers adapt their speech to the language level of children with specific language impairment, but other adults and children tend to do the same. Again, causative patterns appear to be circular, not linear, and the evidence is certainly insufficient for social interaction factors to be considered a major cause of early specific language disability.

On the other hand, early parent–child relationships are not the only social interaction factors that may contribute to language development. In the school-age years, children must be willing to expend voluntary effort and to risk failure to participate actively in formalized language acquisition activities in school. In attempting to understand the necessary conditions for such motivation, Weiner (1979, 1980) proposed an attribution theory of achievement motivation. The theory suggests that as people experience relative success or failure in life, they search for causes to explain why their efforts are successful or unsuccessful. Four primary causes to which people may attribute their success (or lack thereof) are ability, effort, luck, and task difficulty. The nature of these causes varies in ways that determine subsequent affect, expectancies, and efforts of human beings in the long-term process of development. As Winograd and Niquette (1988) explained it:

> If individuals attribute their failures at some task to bad luck, which is usually classified as an external and unstable factor, then they may not expect to fail in the future. In contrast, if individuals attribute their failures to low ability, which is usually (but not always) classified as an internal and stable factor, then it is more likely that they will expect to fail in the future, and their consequent behavior (i.e., resignation, negative affect,

passivity) will facilitate the realization of this dismal expectation. Subsequent failure will reinforce this attributional pattern, precipitating a cycle of failure, frustration and defeat. (p. 39)

Winograd and Niquette (1988) called on theories of self-concept to understand the learned helplessness they observed among children who have difficulty acquiring later-language skills (especially literacy) in school. Although such factors are unlikely candidates as original causes of specific language disability, they contribute to children's development over time, especially in later childhood and adolescence, and they should not be ignored.

Mismatches between the language system at home and in school may also contribute. Again, it is important to realize that sociolinguistic language differences are not the same as language disorders. When children entering school have a wobbly language system and then encounter a system where the language and communicative interaction rules differ from those at home, they are at a double disadvantage. Professionals must be sensitive to the possible interactions among contributing factors.

Mental Retardation

Definitions, differential diagnosis, and subdivisions.
The definition of mental retardation provided by the American Association on Mental Deficiency (AAMD) has three critical elements. To be considered mentally retarded, a person must demonstrate (1) significantly subaverage general intellectual functioning, (2) concurrent deficits of adaptive behavior, and (3) manifestation of the problem during the developmental period (Grossman, 1983).

The determination of significantly subaverage general intellectual functioning is based on an IQ score of 70 or below (sometimes extended to 75 in educational settings) from an individually administered intelligence test. The phrase *deficits in adaptive behavior* refers to significant lags in general maturation or major limitations in academic learning, personal independence, and social responsibility. In earlier definitions of mental retardation, *developmental period* was defined as birth to 18 years, but in the current version, it extends to conception.

The inclusion of adaptive behavior as a critical feature in the definition and diagnosis of mental retardation is a relatively recent phenomenon. Its inclusion is important for two reasons. First, IQ alone cannot perfectly predict general adaptation. Two individuals with identical IQs may function very differently in society

(Baroff, 1986). Second, IQ tests are known to be biased against individuals from sociocultural communities differing from those of standardization samples (Mercer, 1973). When individuals demonstrate documented limitations of adaptive behavior within their own sociocultural developmental contexts, professionals may be less likely to diagnose them wrongly as mentally retarded than when IQ scores are used alone.

How do psychologists and social workers measure adaptive behavior, and what role might language specialists play? Because adaptive behavior expectations differ with chronological age, settings, and cultural groups, measurement is not an easy process. During infancy and early childhood, identification of adaptive behavior rests on general maturation and the acquisition of basic sensory and motor skills, language, self-help skills, and socialization. During childhood and early adolescence, cognitive and socialization functions replace general maturation as the primary determinants of adaptive behavior. They are measured as school learning, appropriateness of social judgment, and relationships established with peers and adults. In the period of late adolescence and adulthood, adaptive behavior is represented by increasing independence and by the ability to assume varied social roles, for example, as employee, friend, spouse, and parent. Adaptation during this period also includes conforming to community expectations and participating as a citizen (Baroff, 1986). Speech–language pathologists and other language specialists may play key roles in identifying the maturation of speech and language skills and communication functions during each of these developmental periods.

Subtypes among children with mental retardation. Four levels of retardation, mild, moderate, severe, and profound, are recognized by the AAMD (Grossman, 1983), based on the number of standard deviations below the mean on IQ tests (see Table 4.2). The characteristics of mental retardation associated with each of these levels may vary widely among individuals and with time of life (Chinn, Drew, & Logan, 1975).

Mild retardation is associated with delayed development of social and communication skills in the preschool years and with minimal retardation in sensorimotor areas, but the child with mild retardation may not be distinguished from normally developing children before starting school. These children acquire academic skills to approximately the sixth-grade level by their late teens but have difficulty learning

TABLE 4.2
Levels of retardation, corresponding psychometric criteria, and proportions at that level within the population of all retarded persons as identified by the President's Committee on Mental Retardation (1978)

Level of Retardation	Range Based on Standard Deviation	Range Based on Wechsler Scale IQ	Approximate % of All Retarded Persons
Mild	−2 to −3	55–69	89.0
Moderate	−3 to −4	40–54	6.0
Severe	−4 to −5	25–39	3.5
Profound	−5 to −6	0–24	1.5

high school subjects. They need special education, particularly at secondary school levels, and are often labeled *educable mentally retarded* (or *handicapped* or *impaired*), based on state guidelines. As adults, individuals with mild retardation are often capable of social and vocational independence but may need supervision under serious social or economic stress (Chinn et al., 1975).

Moderate retardation is associated with delays in learning to talk and communicate (but eventual ability to do so), with poor social awareness, and with fair motor development in the preschool years. These children typically develop academic skills to approximately the fourth-grade level by their teen years, with special education. In school systems, they are included in the group labeled *educable mentally retarded* (or *handicapped* or *impaired*). As adults, individuals with moderate retardation may be able to work independently at unskilled or semiskilled occupations but often need supervision and guidance under conditions of even mild social or economic stress (Chinn et al., 1975).

Severe retardation is associated with poor motor development, minimal speech development, severely limited communication skills, and difficulty acquiring self-help abilities in the preschool years. During the school-age years, these individuals typically cannot learn functional academic skills, but they may learn to talk or to communicate in other ways, may learn elemental health habits, and generally profit from systematic training efforts. Hence, this subgroup is often called "trainable mentally retarded." As adults, they may be able to contribute partially to self-support under complete supervision. They can also develop self-protection skills to a minimal useful level in a controlled environment (Chinn et al., 1975).

Profound retardation is associated with minimal capacity for functioning in any sensorimotor or communication areas during the preschool years, with continued complete dependence on adults for care. During the school-age years, some motor development may occur, but such individuals continue to need total care and generally do not benefit from training in self-help skills. As adults, some further motor, speech, and communication development may occur, but individuals with profound retardation are incapable of self-maintenance, and they continue to need complete care and supervision (Chinn et al., 1975).

Mental retardation is generally regarded as involving uniform developmental lags across multiple skill areas (only the degree of lag differentiates subgroups), but the group of individuals with mental retardation, even those functioning at the same level, is far more heterogeneous than homogeneous. Anyone who has worked with individuals with mental retardation knows that they are just that—*individuals*. Despite recognized differences, however, it is difficult to find reports in the literature regarding patterns of communicative, speech, and language behaviors that might constitute subtypes within the category of mental retardation.

One distinction often made clinically is whether or not the person with mental retardation is speaking or nonspeaking. Perceptions of subdivisions relating to whether a person is nonspeaking (sometimes called *nonvocal* or *nonverbal*) have evolved over recent years. Whereas in the past, the determination of the potential to talk would have been made before deciding that the individual was a candidate for alternative or augmentative communication (AAC), it is now recognized that AAC strategies and supportive technology (both low-tech and high-tech systems) may be useful at multiple stages and in multiple contexts during the developmental process. No longer does their selection imply that anyone has "given up" on speech development (although professionals should be sensitive to the fact that parents may still perceive the decision in this way).

Another subdivision sometimes made is based on whether a person with mental retardation is capable of symbolic or nonsymbolic communicative functioning (Siegel-Causey & Guess, 1989). To use language, a person must be able to understand that symbols such as words can be used to represent things and concepts. Although not all persons with mental retardation develop symbolic communication, even "children and youth with the most handicapping conditions do indeed communicate; however, this communication is achieved in a variety of ways that are not readily observed or even acknowledged by many attending adults" (Guess, 1989, p. xi). Nonsymbolic modes of communication include such behaviors as facial expressions, gestures, movements, postures, and touch.

At the other end of the continuum, some individuals with mild and moderate levels of retardation may learn to read and write. Again, not much evidence supports the existence of particular patterns of reading and writing disability among mentally retarded children. Yet, the efforts of these children to learn to read and write do not necessarily mirror those of younger normally developing peers, nor are they necessarily commensurate with their oral language abilities. Children with mental retardation may also have difficulty learning to read and write because they are given limited educational opportunities to do so.

Some anecdotal accounts indicate that children with Down's syndrome acquire written language-decoding skills more easily than they acquire global cognitive and comprehension skills. For example, Feuerstein, Rand, and Rynders (1988) presented descriptions of a series of children with Down's syndrome provided by their parents. Jason was a 13½-year-old boy with Down's syndrome whom his mother described as follows:

> In reading, Jason's decoding has always been extraordinarily good—but his comprehension of what he has read still gives him quite a bit of difficulty. He loves playing complicated word games, spelling words backwards, doing crossword puzzles, and performing scenes he has learned from musical shows. But his ability to answer "content questions" has been quite limited. (pp. 125–126)

Tami was a 10-year-old fourth-grade student with Down's syndrome, whom her father described:

> Reading is her worst skill. She has great difficulty in reading a story, and telling us the main idea or episode. She often concentrates on a specific incident which may or may not be essential to the story. On the other hand, given a specific question, she can read several pages to find the answer.
>
> Her writing skills also are poor. She writes (and reads) cursive script, but the letters are still not well formed and not neatly arranged. She has much trouble with creative writing, where she is to make something up. Even her letters to her very dear sisters are stilted and sterile. (p. 124)

Mental retardation: Different or merely delayed? As with specific language disability, some question whether the development of individuals with mental retardation, both cognitive and linguistic, is different or delayed (see Box 4.5).

The evidence for differences in cognitive development, including such functions as attention, discrimination, organization of input material, memory, and transfer (or generalization) has been reviewed by Owens (1989). He concluded that "In general, the mentally retarded population develops cognitively in a manner very similar to the nonretarded but at a slower rate" (p. 243). In a study by Kamhi (1981), retarded and nonretarded individuals matched for mental age performed similarly on most tasks, including those involving haptic (touch) recognition, conservation, classification, number conservation, and linear order. Although the retarded children in the study performed slightly more poorly on tasks involving symbolic skills, on the task involving matching ("mental displacement"), they actually performed significantly better than did their nonretarded mental-age-matched peers.

It is difficult to sort out the evidence for difference versus delay of language development because of the many variables that can influence outcomes of studies. As Owens (1989) pointed out, many early studies of language development of individuals with mental retardation used research designs in which individuals were matched for chronological age. Of course, the results of such studies highlighted the differences in levels of development. More recently, studies have matched subjects on the basis of mental age or language ability, and, as the information summarized in Box 4.5 indicates, more similarities have been found.

Box 4.5   Evidence for different (rather than merely delayed) language acquisition across the rule systems of language for children with mental retardation (summarized from literature review by Owens, 1989)

1. **Phonology**. A higher incidence of articulation disorders is found. Children with retardation demonstrate the application of phonologic simplification processes similar to those used by younger normally developing children, such as reduplication (e.g., /baba/ for *bottle*) and assimilation (e.g., /dɔd/ or /gɔg/ for *dog*).
2. **Morphology**. The same order of development of inflectional morphology (see Chapter 8) has been observed for retarded and nonretarded children. Although no studies are available, one might wonder whether children with mental retardation might have greater difficulty using rules of derivational morphology (e.g., prefixes such as *un-, de-,* and *re-* and suffixes such as *-ly, -tion,* and *-able*) to generate and comprehend derived word forms for which they know the roots.
3. **Syntax**. The order of development of sentence types is similar for retarded and nonretarded children, with a trend to start with simple declaratives, move through negatives, then interrogatives (in the order *what, where, when, why, how*), and later, negative interrogatives. Some differences also appear, however, in that children with mental retardation tend to use shorter, less complex sentences than those used by nonretarded peers matched for mental age. In particular, fewer complex structures such as subject elaborations and relative clauses appear. It has also been suggested that retarded persons have less flexible syntactic structure because they tend to rely on sentence word order (rather than grammatical rules for combining word classes) to formulate and understand sentences. They also tend to rely longer on more primitive syntactic forms.
4. **Semantics**. Word meanings tend to be more concrete and restricted for individuals with mental retardation, who have particular difficulty with nonliteral meanings. Retarded persons also use adjectives and adverbs less frequently than mental age-matched peers do.
5. **Pragmatics**. The pragmatic skills of children with mental retardation vary with their cognitive levels and life experiences (those who reside in institutions show the greatest deficits of communicative use). In the early stages of development, both mentally retarded and normally developing children use imperative and declarative gestures to communicate (imperative gestures enlist help and declarative gestures gain attention). Children with mental retardation, however, use more sophisticated gestures for imperative than for declarative functions. Some pragmatic skills, such as role taking, appear to be more related to social maturity than to cognitive maturity in both mentally retarded and normally developing children. Finally, although persons with mild-to-moderate mental retardation may be as skilled as their mental-age-matched peers at taking the perspective of conversational partners, they are less likely to assume assertive roles in conversation, and this pattern continues to be true of adults with mental retardation of multiple levels, even when speaking to children.

Relationships of contributing factors. *Biological maturation.* Grossman (1983) estimated that biological factors account for only about 25% of the causes of mental retardation; they are considered probable contributing factors to language disorders in children who are mentally retarded. When biological factors do play a role, they are associated with more severe forms of retardation. The identification of mental retardation in individuals for whom socioeconomic variables may play a major role in IQ test performance is highly controversial.

Biologic factors associated with mental retardation can result from vastly different causes. The list includes genetic and chromosomal factors, such as Down's syndrome; infectious processes, such as maternal rubella; toxins and chemical agents, such as fetal alcohol syndrome and lead poisoning; nutrition and metabolic factors, such as phenylketonuria (PKU), gestational disorders, such as hydrocephalus and craniofacial anomalies; complications of pregnancy and delivery, such as extremely low birth weight or prematurity; and gross disorders of the central nervous system, such as tuberous sclerosis and Huntington's disease (Grossman, 1983). The heterogeneity of causative factors easily explains the widely varying symptoms of retardation, yet models of retardation as uniform delays across areas of development tend to persist.

Linguistic system factors.   The summary of the evidence from the studies that Owens (1989) reviewed points to no special causative role for linguistic factors in problems associated with mental retardation. However, they are considered probable contributing factors because linguistic skills are generally affected as a part of mental retardation. Lower levels of linguistic complexity and reduced ability to use abstract symbols may also interact in complex ways with cognitive limitations. Older children with mental retardation, in particular, may have difficulty using verbal mediation to assist in problem solving, but they may benefit from intervention designed to teach them to do so (Feuerstein et al., 1988).

Stimulus–response–reinforcement factors.   Children with mental retardation are thought to benefit less from natural environmental stimulation and reinforcement in the acquisition of language than their normally developing peers, and these are considered probable contributing factors. Retarded children are also more likely to have sensory and motor deficits than other children, which may influence their stimulability and responsiveness (Baroff, 1986; Grossman, 1983). Even in the absence of peripheral sensorimotor impairments, children with mental retardation seem to have difficulty recognizing subtle environmental cues and to need more repetitions of experience before they can internalize concepts based on it. Therefore, behaviorist approaches, which are often recommended for use in intervention with retarded children, are designed to simplify and to highlight discriminative properties of stimuli and to provide tangible reinforcers for targeted behaviors. Structured programs of reward, punishment, and ignoring are also used frequently to modify behaviors of individuals with severe and profound mental retardation (Baroff, 1986). Because inability to generalize is a major problem for persons with retardation, more recent behavior modification approaches tend to emphasize the use of natural contexts and consequences for facilitating the integration and retention of newly acquired behaviors.

Information processing factors.   Information processing theories have been posited to explain why individuals vary in basic cognitive abilities and information factors are considered essential contributing factors in language disorders among children who are mentally retarded. The term *slowness,* which is often used to describe the development of persons with mental retardation, also seems to characterize their processing abilities. Sternberg (1979, 1981) proposed a model with five kinds of functional components of information processing. *Metacomponents* are the executive processes used for planning and decision making, sizing up a situation, considering alternatives, and choosing. *Performance components* are the information processing skills used in solving a problem. *Acquisition components* are the skills used to learn new information by encoding it (usually verbally), transforming raw sensory experience, associating it with other information, and strengthening it through practice and reinforcement. *Retention components* involve short-term memory and the retrieval of information from memory storage. Finally, *transfer components* are involved in generalization, as when a person applies the understanding gained in one context to another.

Persons with mental retardation have significant deficiencies in all of these areas, including problems with planning, encoding, rapid processing, association, retention, and generalization (Baroff, 1986). Furthermore, problems in each of these areas might be expected to affect language and communication development as well as general cognitive development.

Cognition factors.   Obviously, cognitive deficits play an essential role in the diagnosis of mental retardation, but how can theories of intelligence guide the understanding of the cognitive deficits of children with mental retardation? Is intelligence a relatively unitary phenomenon, as Spearman (1923, 1927) suggested when he described the *g* factor as an index of general ability? Can it be differentiated into abilities that are either crystallized (e.g., the capacity to answer questions based on word meanings, general knowledge, and language comprehension), or fluid (e.g., the capacity to reason in nonverbal and visual-spatial contexts), as Cattell (1971) and Horn (1968) suggested? Is it multifactorial in nature, as Guilford (1967) suggested? Is it best represented as a set of gradually unfolding processes for making sense of the world, as Piaget (1970) suggested? Is it a set of information processing abilities, as Sternberg suggested (1979, 1981)?

Or are there multiple, relatively autonomous intelligences, as Gardner (1983) suggested?

Perhaps intelligence is all of these. Any might be shown to be affected in mental retardation (Baroff, 1986). As Sternberg (1981) noted, intelligence has traditionally been described as having the three cognitive components: (1) the ability to learn and to profit from experience and to acquire knowledge in doing so, (2) the ability to reason, and (3) the ability to adapt to changing conditions. Sternberg (1981) also posited a fourth motivational component—the will to succeed. As considered in the next section, motivation is related to social interaction factors and communication as well as to intelligence.

Social interaction factors. Most legal definitions of mental retardation require that diagnostic processes rule out the possibility that a child's reduced IQ results primarily from the influences of economic, social, or cultural factors. Mercer (1973), in particular, has rejected IQ as the sole criterion of retardation, arguing that retardation is a sociological label that refers to particular role expectations and is culture specific. She reserves the classification *retarded* for persons who score below the IQ cutoff of 70 and also fail to meet the adaptive behavior standards of their own culture groups, when pluralistic assessment methods are used (Mercer & Lewis, 1975).

Nevertheless, social interaction factors are thought to be significant in the histories of a substantial number of children with mental retardation and are considered essential contributing factors. Baroff (1986) reviewed the evidence that intelligence can be affected by environmental factors based on studies involving (1) children raised in grossly unfavorable environments (considered later in the section on child neglect and abuse); (2) children reared by retarded parents; (3) children whose biological parents are retarded and whose adoptive parents are of normal intelligence; and (4) studies of identical twins raised in separate homes. General conclusions that can be drawn from all of these studies suggest that "both environmental and genetic factors influence intelligence" (p. 201). Furthermore, Baroff's review showed that intensive modification of the experiences of young children of mothers with low IQs can boost their scores by as much as 10 to 25 points.

The process of socialization is intimately tied to emotional development. Baroff (1986) noted that emotions are commonly generated in social situations. "Ultimately, it is the impulse to *action* created by *emotions* that the child must learn to control in order to achieve social adaptation" (Baroff, 1986, p. 323; italics in the original). Baroff also noted that the emotional responsiveness of young children differs from that of older children and adolescents in normal development, with young children tending to demonstrate intense emotional states of short-lived duration. This may lead children with mental retardation to be judged as overemotional when their levels of emotionality actually may be commensurate with their levels of cognitive development.

Factors related to the development of self-esteem in retarded persons can also influence their further development. Baroff (1986) noted that self-esteem results from the contributions of three factors. First, a need for personal intimacy is experienced by all people, as individuals seek to be accepted, liked, admired, and loved by both parents and peers. Second, a need for success plays a role in motivation, such that, for individuals to learn, "success striving" must outweigh "failure avoiding" (an area in which children with mental retardation seem to be at particular risk). Third is the need for autonomy, as expressed in needs for self-determination, choice, and maximum independence. The dependence of people with mental retardation has been well documented, but this does not mean that it is safe to conclude that they are dependent by choice. All such factors seem to interact with their ability to learn, including their ability to learn to communicate.

Autism

Definitions, differential diagnosis, and subdivisions. A variety of definitions have been offered since Kanner first described the syndrome of autism in 1943. Kanner listed the characteristic features as (1) extreme autistic aloneness, (2) language abnormalities, (3) obsessive desire for the maintenance of sameness, (4) good cognitive potential, (5) normal physical development, and (6) highly intelligent, obsessive, and cold parents (see the following section on social interaction factors for an updated view of the role of parents of children who have autism).

A more recent definition, proposed by the Autism Society of American (see Ritvo & Freeman, 1978), includes the following characteristics:

Box 4.6   Diagnostic criteria for autistic disorder in DSM-III-R

At least eight of the following sixteen items are present, these to include at least two items from A, one from B, and one from C.

Note: Consider a criterion to be met *only* if the behavior is abnormal for the person's developmental level.

A. Qualitative impairment in reciprocal social interaction as manifested by the following: (The examples within parentheses are arranged so that the first mentioned are more likely to apply to younger or more handicapped, and the later ones, to older or less handicapped, persons with this disorder.)
   1. Marked lack of awareness of the existence or feelings of others (e.g., treats a person as if he or she were a piece of furniture; does not notice another person's distress; apparently has no concept of the need of others for privacy)
   2. No or abnormal seeking of comfort at times of distress (e.g., does not come for comfort even when ill, hurt, or tired; seeks comfort in a stereotyped way, e.g., says "cheese, cheese, cheese" whenever hurt)
   3. No or impaired imitation (e.g., does not wave bye-bye; does not copy mother's domestic activities; mechanical imitation of others' actions out of context)
   4. No or abnormal social play (e.g., does not actively participate in simple games; prefers solitary play activities; involves other children in play only as "mechanical aids")
   5. Gross impairment in ability to make peer friendships (e.g., no interest in making peer friendships; despite interest in making friends, demonstrates lack of understanding of conventions of social interaction, for example, reads phone book to uninterested peer)
B. Qualitative impairment in verbal and nonverbal communication, and in imaginative activity, as manifested by the following:
   (The numbered items are arranged so that those first listed are more likely to apply to younger or more handicapped, and the later ones, to older or less handicapped, persons with this disorder.)
   1. No mode of communication, such as communicative babbling, facial expression, gesture, mime, or spoken language
   2. Markedly abnormal nonverbal communication, as in the use of eye-to-eye gaze, facial expression, body posture, or gestures to initiate or modulate social interaction (e.g., does not anticipate being held, stiffens when held, does not look at the person or smile when making a social approach, does not greet parents or visitors, has a fixed stare in social situations)

1. Age of onset before 30 months.
2. Disturbances of developmental rates and sequences in the areas of motor, social-adaptive, and cognitive skills.
3. Disturbances of responses to sensory stimuli. This includes hyper- or hyporeactivity in audition, vision, tactile stimulation, motor, smell, and taste. Self-stimulatory behavior is also included.
4. Disturbances of speech, language, cognition, and nonverbal communication, including mutism, echolalia, and failure to use abstract terms.
5. Disturbances of the capacity to appropriately relate to people, events, and objects, including lack of

social behavior, affection, and appropriate play. Interruption of the idiosyncratic or perseverative use of objects will upset the child.

The definition of autism proposed by the American Psychiatric Association (1987) in the DSM-III-R places it as a subdivision of the more general diagnostic classification *pervasive developmental disorder*. In some service-delivery systems, this label may be preferred for children with autism. Many parents, however, have worked hard to have autism treated as a separate disorder in state and federal regulations and to have it removed from status as an emotional disorder or even

Box 4.6   continued

      3. Absence of imaginative activity, such as playacting of adult roles, fantasy characters, or animals; lack of interest in stories about imaginary events

      4. Marked abnormalities in the production of speech, including volume, pitch, stress, rate, rhythm, and intonation (e.g., monotonous tone, questionlike melody, or high pitch)

      5. Marked abnormalities in the form or content of speech, including stereotyped and repetitive use of speech (e.g., immediate echolalia or mechanical repetition of television commercial); use of "you" when "I" is meant (e.g., using "You want cookie?" to mean "I want a cookie"); idiosyncratic use of words or phrases (e.g., "Go on green riding" to mean "I want to go on the swing"); or frequent irrelevant remarks (e.g., starts talking about train schedules during a conversation about sports)

      6. Marked impairment in the ability to initiate or sustain a conversation with others, despite adequate speech (e.g., indulging in lengthy monologues on one subject regardless of interjections from others)

 C. Markedly restricted repertoire of activities and interests, as manifested by the following:

      1. Stereotyped body movements, e.g., hand-flicking or -twisting, spinning, head-banging, complex whole-body movements

      2. Persistent preoccupation with parts of objects (e.g., sniffing or smelling objects, repetitive feeling of texture of materials, spinning wheels of toy cars) or attachment to unusual objects (e.g., insists on carrying around a piece of string)

      3. Marked distress over changes in trivial aspects of environment, e.g., when a vase is moved from usual position

      4. Unreasonable insistence on following routines in precise detail, e.g., insisting that exactly the same route always be followed when shopping

      5. Markedly restricted range of interests and a preoccupation with one narrow interest, e.g., interested only in lining up objects, in amassing facts about meteorology, or in pretending to be a fantasy character

 D. Onset during infancy or childhood.

Specify if childhood onset (after 36 months of age).

Note. From American Psychiatric Association: *Diagnostic and Statistical Manual of Mental Disorders, Third Edition, Revised* (pp. 38–39). Washington, DC: American Psychiatric Association, 1987. Reprinted by permission.

as a physical or health impairment. They may prefer to have it maintained as a distinctive label.

In the past, the labels *childhood psychosis* and *childhood schizophrenia* have also been used interchangeably with *autism* (sometimes called *early infantile autism*). Those conditions are now thought to be distinct. In DSM-III-R, *childhood schizophrenia* is no longer considered a valid diagnostic category. Those who have attempted to differentiate autism from childhood schizophrenia in the past have pointed out that, in comparison, autism is characterized by early onset (before 3 years of age), less common family history of mental illness, normal or above-average

motor development, lower IQ, good physical health, no periods of remission and relapse, failure to develop complex language and social skills, and absence of delusions or hallucinations (all of which can be contrasted in childhood schizophrenia) (Schreibman, 1988).

The DSM-III-R criteria for diagnosing autism appear in Box 4.6. Because symptoms of "qualitative impairment in verbal and nonverbal communication" are noted as one of the three major sets of diagnostic criteria, language and communication specialists often play an important role in the transdisciplinary diagnosis of the disorder.

Subtypes among children with autism. Although autism is recognized as a disorder with a great deal of heterogeneity, subtype categories have not been clearly differentiated. One suggestion was that, for the purpose of research, the population of individuals with autism might be categorized into three main groups: (1) individuals with the classic symptoms of Kanner's (1943) syndrome, (2) those who have childhood schizophrenia with autistic features, and (3) those who have autism with neurological impairment (Coleman, 1976).

A more broadly accepted clinical and educational subdivision is based on the accompanying degree of cognitive impairment shown by individuals with autism. Approximately 60% of children with autism have measured IQs below 50; 20% have IQs between 50 and 70; and 20% have IQs of 70 or above (Schreibman, 1988). These subtypes combine the critical diagnostic features of autism with features of the accompanying level of retardation. The labels *low, middle,* and *high functioning* are often used in conjunction with these subdivisions.

Wing (1983) suggested a third approach recommending classification of individuals with autism based on their social problems. She designated the three groups as (1) *aloof,* associated with severe impairments of verbal and nonverbal communication, aggression, destructiveness, and self-injury; (2) *passive,* associated with the ability to imitate but lack of understanding of social contacts and meanings and being easiest to integrate into social units; and (3) *active but odd,* associated with production of lengthy monologues and repetitive questioning and significant social difficulties because of their demands for social attention but inability to interact appropriately.

The subclassifications described by Rapin and Allen (1983) for autism, mentioned earlier in this chapter, differentiate between autistic children on the basis of whether they are primarily echolalic or mute. Autistic children who are mute generally have a poorer overall prognosis (including for the development of language) than do children who are echolalic (DeMyer et al., 1973).

Rapin and Allen (1983) described children with autism and echolalia as having variable phonology (more likely than not to be defective); faulty prosody resulting in wooden, nonmusical, robot-like speech; variable morphology (with particular difficulty developing normal pronoun reference); variable word retrieval (with particular difficulty in the absence of visual referents); variable nonverbal intelligence; impaired comprehension and semantic processing of connected discourse (as seen both in the echolalia and hyperlexia that tends to be evident in those with higher levels of measured intelligence); and impaired pragmatic skills (with limited ability to initiate and to participate in conversational discourse even after they become verbal).

Autism: Different or delayed? There is not much debate that children with autism develop in ways that are not only delayed but qualitatively different compared with normally developing children. Qualitative differences in social interaction and communication are central to the diagnosis of autism in the DSM-III-R criteria (see Box 4.7 for an additional summary of language development characteristics).

Within the area of language development, however, is there any evidence that children with autism follow patterns similar to those of normally developing children? Swisher and Demetras (1985) reviewed the evidence.

In the area of syntax, when children with autism are matched for nonverbal mental age with children who are mentally retarded, have specific language

| Personal Reflection 4.2 | I'm as good at a two way conversation as a pile of gramophone records
Or a parrot that is talking from a cage.
Some lasses seem in a rage when they talk to me
I don't seem to hold the keys to their thought processes. (p. 7)

David Miedzianik, a person with autism who lives in Scholes, Rotherham, England, writing about his loneliness in a poem.
    Note. From "I Hope Some Lass Will Want Me After Reading All This" by D. Miedzianik, 1990, *The Advocate* (newsletter of the Autism Society of America), *22* (1), p 7. Copyright 1990 by D. Miedzianik. Reprinted by permission. |

Box 4.7   Summary of characteristics of the development of language, speech, and communication by children with autism (based on reviews by Fay & Schuler, 1980; Schopler & Mesibov, 1985; Schreibman, 1988)

1. Failure to acquire language may be the first signal to parents that something is wrong.
2. Some may initially acquire such words as *mama* and *dada* but then suddenly (between 18 and 30 months) lose the acquired words and fail to progress further linguistically.
3. Approximately 50% never develop functional speech.
4. Those who speak use language qualitatively different from normally developing children and other children with language disorders, as demonstrated by the following:
   a. Echolalia, which may be produced beyond the period when it might appear normally. Echolalia may serve a variety of functions for individuals with autism, and it may be immediate or delayed (based on timing); communicative or noncommunicative (based on its apparent pragmatic function); or exact or mitigated (based on whether it is altered in any way to be more contextually appropriate). Echolalia may appear in the communicative development of other children with language disorders, particularly those with mental retardation.
   b. Pronominal reversals, with the child often referring to self with the pronouns, *you, he/she,* or the child's proper name.
   c. Noncommunicative and self-stimulatory speech, using the same sounds, words, or phrases repeatedly but without apparent attempts to communicate. (However, as professionals look more carefully at behaviors previously thought to be noncommunicative, their possible communicative value may become more apparent.)
   d. Dysprosodic, as characterized by unusual or inappropriate pitch, rhythm, inflection, intonation, pace, and/or articulation.
   e. Confusion of form, function, and context, as, for example, when a child with autism uses question forms to express desires (e.g., "Do you want to go outside?") or make declarative statements (e.g., "Is Joe scared of lightning?").
   f. Impaired ability to produce and understand nonlinguistic communicative behaviors, such as those involving eye gaze, gestures, proximity, and body contact.
5. Some higher functioning and older children with autism demonstrate language problems more similar to those of some other children with language disorders or to normally developing children at earlier stages.
   a. They are likely to have severe impairments of comprehension.
   b. They tend to form rigid semantic concepts and have particular difficulty with abstract words and concepts, including expressing their own emotions or imagination.
   c. They produce and comprehend language with almost total literalness, and they have particular difficulty understanding idioms, analogies, and metaphors (even though their own language may be characterized as metaphoric at times, in that phrases may bear only an indirect relationship to the things and ideas they represent).
   d. They may have great difficulty talking about anything outside of the immediate environment or events, having difficulty discussing past or future, and appearing stuck in the here-and-now.
6. They may be hyperlexic (reading early, but with limited comprehension).
7. Their writing may show evidence of free association of thought, with individual words appearing to have some connections based on the child's own experiences but with lack of semantic, syntactic, or thematic connectedness.

impairments, or are normally developing, the language-form abilities of children with autism are consistently lower than those of normally developing children but as advanced as those of children with mental retardation or specific language impairment. Swisher and Demetras (1985) interpreted these results as evidence that children with autism construct sentences with superficial form, not fully supported by an understanding of their deep structure or generative principles.

Studies of morphology have again shown that children with autism have skills that are delayed with respect to normally developing controls. However, they were not delayed with respect to children with either mental retardation or specific language impairment, who were matched on nonverbal IQ measures (Swisher & Demetras, 1985).

In the area of semantics, surprisingly little research evidence is available to support the common contention that children with autism do not always use meaningful speech. Studies of word and sentence recall have shown children with autism to be impaired in their ability to use semantic cues to aid recall, but in the absence of further evidence, Swisher and Demetras (1985) suggested that the semantic problems of children with autism might be viewed as evidence of language delay rather than difference. They also suggested, however, that "It appears that autistic children can remember words better than they can connect them to a cognitive base" (p. 159).

In the area of pragmatics, evidence indicates that children with autism use language in ways that are not only delayed with respect to normally developing peers but also deviant. In particular, they tend to have difficulty in making appropriate matches between the content and form of the language they use and the contexts in which it is produced (Swisher & Demetras, 1985). This mismatch across domains of language (in the presence of patterns of delay within domains), Swisher and Demetras concluded, best characterizes the uniqueness of language development among children with autism (similar to conclusions drawn earlier by Leonard, 1972, 1980, for children with specific language disabilities).

Prizant (1983) also addressed the question of whether children with autism acquire language in a unique way. He reviewed modes of gestalt (holistic) versus analytic processing with reference to the communicative symptoms of autism. The literature shows that normally developing children are distributed on a continuum, with most children either being analytic or showing both analytic and gestalt characteristics (Peters, 1977). The analytic mode of processing is evident when single words serve as basic language units that can be combined as grammatical constituents using linguistic rules, when early language acquisition involves movement from two- to three-word phrases, and when growth in language production is flexible, creative, and generative. The gestalt mode of processing is evident when multiword utterances appear early and function as single units, when a child's syntactic development appears more sophisticated than it actually is, and when growth in language development involves segmentation and recombinations of unanalyzed chunks, with eventual movement into an analytic mode.

Prizant (1983) suggested that children with autism might function in two different modes during varied points in their development. For some, earlier language development demonstrates a high frequency of echolalia. As this pattern is gradually replaced by more spontaneous, analytic language, children produce some utterances in a gestalt mode, while at the same time, producing other utterances in the analytic mode. This pattern may be confusing to observers because the analytic utterances may appear to be more similar to language produced by younger children (shorter in length and sometimes "telegraphic"), but as Prizant points out, they actually represent a positive sign of growth. They represent the child's emerging ability to generate unique sentences using the building blocks of language as separable units that can be combined in flexible ways, rather than reusing the same inflexible word chunks over and over as unanalyzed wholes.

Relationships of contributing factors.   Theories of the cause of autism have changed dramatically over the years since the condition was first described by Kanner (1943), who attributed its cause to the lack of interaction with cold and unresponsive parents. Although many possibilities for explaining the social, cognitive, linguistic, and neurological symptoms associated with autism have been explored, the exact mechanism by which it operates is still not understood.

Biological maturation.   Numerous attempts have been made over the years to relate the cause of autism to biological factors, but these largely remain probable contributing factors with suspected involvement. Factors investigated have included those associated with pregnancy and birth, genetics, neurology, and biochemistry. Some positive evidence of biological differences among children with autism has been found in all of these categories (Schreibman, 1988).

For example, prenatal histories of children with autism show an increased incidence of early complications but no particularly uniform patterns of influence. Family histories show increased incidence of speech delay (in approximately 25% of one sample) and of close family members with autism (between 2% and 6% have siblings with autism). Some evidence has also been found that autism is associated with "fragile-X" syndrome (in which a weakness or "break" appears in the structure of the X sex chromosome) (Schreibman, 1988).

Investigations of neurochemical factors have focused on neurotransmitters. Unusually high levels of serotonin (a neurotransmitter) have been found in the blood of children with autism at an age when it has begun to diminish in their normally developing peers. Another neurochemical possibility is that children with autism have an abundance of opioid peptides (brain chemicals generated naturally in normal development with the pleasure rush that comes from being cuddled and comforted). It is hypothesized that the preexistence of these chemicals in the brains of children with autism may make them less prone to seek affection and comfort. Treatment with an opioid-blocking agent has been shown to reduce such abnormal behaviors as self-stimulation, echolalia, and a tendency to shut out stimulation by covering eyes and ears (Schreibman, 1988).

Neurological factors have long been suspected to play a role in the cause of autism. Neurological pathology is often inferred from the appearance of such neurological "soft signs" as hypotonia (low muscle tone), poor coordination, and toe walking. Such symptoms are reported in 40% to 100% of children with autism. Abnormal patterns of brain activity have also been identified in 65% of children with autism (as compared with only 39% of children with mental retardation) (DeMyer, 1975).

Structural abnormalities have also been sought in the brains of individuals with autism, for the most part, with limited success. However, Courchesne (1988) used MRI to examine the brains of persons with autism and found an area of the cerebellum that was significantly smaller than expected. This new area of investigation may not be significant for all individuals with autism, but the early evidence suggests that for some, abnormal brain development may have occurred at the end of the first trimester or during the second trimester. For others, abnormality may begin in the first or second year of life. Although the mechanism for cerebellar involvement is not fully understood, the cerebellum regulates incoming sensations, and its cellular irregularities may account for

the sensory deficits so characteristic of autism, including insensitivity to pain or oversensitivity to sounds and textures (Schreibman, 1988). Rapin and Allen (1983) pointed out that the pattern of strengths and deficits of children with autism leads to suspicion of "multifocal brain dysfunction rather than the impairment of a single system, even one with widespread projections" (p. 174).

Linguistic system factors. Competing theories have been proposed regarding the relative roles of linguistic and communication impairments in autism, but these factors are generally considered essential contributing factors. Language deficit is agreed to be a central diagnostic feature of autism; it is always present. The question is whether linguistic impairment is central to the disorder or whether autism is primarily a disorder of cognitive development. Some theorists have suggested that language deficits are pivotal in autism, playing a major role in social interaction problems and other problems associated with autism (e.g., Churchill, 1972; Hermelin & O'Connor, 1970; Rutter, 1965). However, this would not explain the differences noted among children with autism and children with specific language disorder, particularly in the manner in which they approach social interactions.

Stimulus–response–reinforcement factors. The symptoms of autism have prompted the development of theories that children with the disorder may be over- or under-stimulated. Earlier, investigators speculated that such symptoms might be related to an impairment of the reticular-activating system in the brain stem (Rimland, 1964), but, as noted, the findings of several investigators have now pointed in the direction of cerebellar abnormalities (Schreibman, 1988).

For some time, behaviorist methods have served as the cornerstone of many intervention programs for children with autism (Lovaas, Schaeffer, & Simmons, 1965). In recent reports, Lovaas (1987) has even claimed, based on the results of a carefully designed experimental study, that behavior modification therapy can result in apparently normal intellectual and educational functioning in some children with autism when it is provided early (before the age of 3 years) and with intensity (for at least 40 hours/week). Stimulus–response–reinforcement factors are considered essential contributing factors to autism.

Information processing factors. The "islets of excellence" that are sometimes observed in children and adults with autism (e.g., the movie character Rain man's unusual ability to memorize playing cards and his interest in the telephone directory) appear to represent specific information processing skills that are out of balance with the person's other cognitive and linguistic abilities. Without referring specifically to autism, Bruner (1968) cautioned of the dangers of premature overspecificity:

> Human infancy appears to be a guarantor against the achievement of precocities of development, a period in which very general rules of skill, or perceptual organization, and of interaction are learned in preparation for later, species-specific forms of human achievement in action, perception, and communication. In this sense, infancy can be conceived almost as a shield against premature specialization. (p. 9)

In spite of some unusual skills involving short-term memory, children with autism have difficulty integrating information from multiple levels of processing. Hermelin and O'Connor (1967) compared the recall skills of 12 children with autism and 12 children with mental retardation matched for receptive vocabulary and immediate memory span for digits. They found that children with autism had better recall skills than children with mental retardation, but they were less able to use meaning and sentence structure to aid recall. They also tended not to correct anomalous word order (as retarded and normally functioning individuals do), but to repeat agrammatical sentences verbatim. Various aspects of the information processing mechanism appear to function relatively independently of one another in children with autism, rather than to assist each other as they do in normal language processing.

Cognition factors.   Cognitive factors are clearly implicated in the development of children with autism, even among the relatively small proportion (around 20%) who score near normal on IQ tests, and are considered essential contributing factors to language disorders in children with autism. Rutter (1983) has argued that children with autism have a general cognitive deficit that cannot be explained as secondary to their severe problems in social relationships. On the other hand, not all children with autism demonstrate the same degree of cognitive impairment; those who do often show wide scattering in different areas of ability, and many children with significant mental retardation do not show symptoms of autism. Therefore, the two conditions must be relatively independent.

Nevertheless, the degree of cognitive impairment is one of the best predictors of eventual outcome in autism (Schreibman, 1988).

Social-interaction factors.   Qualitative disturbance of social interaction is listed first in the DSM-III-R definition of autism and is an essential contributing factor. Although social disturbance continues to be viewed as central to the diagnosis of autism, few specialists now use pschodynamic theories to explain its primary cause.

This has not always been the case. Kanner's (1943) original description of the parents of children with autism as cold and aloof led to a proliferation of theories about the roles of family environment in causing the disorder during the 1940s to 1960s. The most famous of the parent-causation hypotheses was proposed by Bruno Bettelheim (1967) in a book called *The Empty Fortress.* For many years, psychogenic hypotheses formed the basis for unstructured psychodynamic therapeutic interventions. However, such theories have never been supported with any but anecdotal evidence. In fact, as much evidence indicates that the behavior of children with autism causes their parents to act the way they do as vice versa. Current reviews suggest that "the overwhelming evidence indicates that autism is a neurological rather than a psychogenic disability, and that unstructured, play therapy approaches are quite inappropriate" (Schopler & Mesibov, 1986, p. 4). Most theorists now agree that, as opposed to causing their children's difficulties, the parents of children with autism often play significant positive roles in intervention programs.

Current researchers also recognize that when they reach adolescence, many children with autism show an increased interest in and awareness of others. Their problems appear to be "a lack of social skills rather than a lack of social interest" (Schopler & Mesibov, 1986, p. 5).

Attention-Deficit Hyperactivity Disorder

Definitions, differential diagnosis, and subdivisions. The newest diagnostic category to be considered for its possible relationship to childhood language disorders, although its relationship is unclear, is attention-deficit hyperactivity disorder (ADHD or ADD). In the DSM-III-R (American Psychiatric Association, 1987), ADHD is categorized as a disruptive behavior disorder (see Box 4.8 for a list of symptoms). The current label follows an earlier change in the 1980 edition of DSM-III, in which the terms *hyperkinesis* and *minimal brain*

Box 4.8   Diagnostic criteria for attention-deficit hyperactivity disorder

Note: Consider a criterion met only if the behavior is considerably more frequent than that of most people of the same mental age.

A. A disturbance of at least 6 months during which at least eight of the following are present:
  1. Often fidgets with hands or feet or squirms in seats (in adolescents, may be limited to subjective feelings of restlessness)
  2. Has difficulty remaining seated when required to do so
  3. Is easily distracted by extraneous stimuli
  4. Has difficulty awaiting turn in games or group situations
  5. Often blurts out answers to questions before they have been completed
  6. Has difficulty following through on instructions from others (not due to oppositional behavior or failure of comprehension), e.g., fails to finish chores
  7. Has difficulty sustaining attention in tasks or play activities
  8. Often shifts from one uncompleted activity to anothers
  9. Has difficulty playing quietly
  10. Often talks excessively
  11. Often interrupts or intrudes on others, e.g., butts into other children's games
  12. Often does not seem to listen to what is being said to him or her
  13. Often loses things necessary for tasks or activities at school or at home (e.g., toys, pencils, books, assignments)
  14. Often engages in physically dangerous activities without considering possible consequences (not for the purpose of thrill-seeking), e.g., runs into street without looking

Note: The above items are listed in descending order of discriminating power based on data from a national field trial of DSM-III-R criteria for disruptive behavior disorders.

B. Onset before the age of seven.

C. Does not meet the criteria for a Pervasive Developmental Disorder.

Note. From American Psychiatric Association: *Diagnostic and Statistical Manual of Mental Disorders, Third Edition, Revised* (pp. 52–53). Washington, DC: American Psychiatric Association, 1987. Reprinted by permission.

---

dysfunction were both replaced with the terminology *attention-deficit disorder with hyperactivity* (American Psychiatric Association, 1980). Now, in turn, that terminology has been replaced with the ADHD label.

ADHD is a behavioral syndrome marked by inattention, impulsivity, and hyperactivity that tends to occur as much as nine times more frequently in boys than in girls (Sattler, 1988). The associated "overactivity" typically is first observed by parents and preschool teachers in early childhood. Hyperactivity is difficult to define objectively, particularly for preschool children, who exhibit wide ranges of activity levels normally (Campbell, 1985), and its identification is often controversial, being based primarily on observational evidence.

When children with ADHD reach school age and have difficulty meeting the demands of the classroom, academic underachievement becomes common. At this point, psychologists often look for a profile on the Wechsler Intelligence Scale for Children—Revised (WISC-R; Wechsler, 1974) in which children with ADHD earn scaled scores of 10 to 13 on most subtests but only achieve scores of 6 or 7 on the cluster of four subtests that demand the most selective attention: digit span, arithmetic, coding, and mazes (Newhoff, 1986). Parents and classroom teachers also contribute to the diagnosis by rating children's behavior with such instruments as Conners' Scales (Conners, 1969).

Because many classroom demands are conveyed through linguistic and nonlinguistic communication, it is important for language specialists to participate in the multidisciplinary diagnostic process for children with ADHD. Newhoff (1986, 1990) advocates involvement of speech–language pathologists in identifying the problem and in sorting out its relationship to possible language-learning disabilities whenever children are experiencing academic, social interaction, or psychiatric difficulties. Among adolescents, the risk for increased psychiatric difficulty among children with ADHD is great (Sattler, 1988), and speech–language pathologists should probe for significant signs of previously unrecognized ADHD, along with hidden language-learning disabilities, when they consult regarding the interrelated social, communicative, learning, and self-esteem problems these young people often have.

Although communicative behavior plays a role in the diagnosis of ADHD, it cannot be considered to be central to identification of the disorder. As noted, this category is relatively new, having been differentiated from earlier classifications in which minimal brain dysfunction, hyperactivity, and learning disabilities were considered to be part of a common syndrome, and much of the previous research on those disorders is complicated by confounding of the various factors involved. Currently, the diagnosis of ADHD is considered distinct from the diagnosis of learning disabilities, and the frequency of co-occurrence of the two conditions is a matter of debate. Research efforts are complicated by the newness of the differential diagnosis and the fact that professionals have not yet agreed on exact objective criteria for diagnosing either condition. In most states, ADHD is not currently viewed as an educational diagnosis that justifies special education. However, when children with ADHD exhibit symptoms of learning disabilities or behavioral disorders, they may be placed in programs for children with those disorders (sometimes termed emotional disorders or impairments), or they may receive services under Section 504 of the Rehabilitation Act (see Chapter 5).

One fairly well-controlled study (Rutter, Tizard, & Whitmore, 1970) was designed to look for intercorrelations among psychiatric, learning, and neurological disorders among all of the children of a similar age on the Isle of Wight (an island off the coast of England). Rutter and his colleagues found that children who had "overt behavior disorders" (such as ADD, hyperactivity, or oppositional disorders) had very high rates of learning problems, especially reading disorders. In fact, among children with reading disorders, 25% also had one of these overt psychiatric behavioral disorders.

In another study (Cantwell, Baker, & Mattison, 1979), 600 children who were assessed in a commu-

nity speech clinic were offered free psychiatric evaluations as part of the diagnostic process. Two thirds were boys and 60% were less than 6 years old. The researchers found that 50.3% of the group with communication impairments had diagnosable psychiatric disorders (compared with an estimated 10% of the general population) and that the most commonly diagnosed psychiatric problem was an "overt behavior disorder" (ADD, oppositional disorder, or conduct disorder), which was diagnosed in 26% of the 600 children with communicative disorders.

Evidence for the existence of subtypes. In the DSM-III-R, only ADHD is defined, but an additional category of undifferentiated attention-deficit disorder is included with the following description:

> This is a residual category for disturbances in which the predominant feature is the persistence of developmentally inappropriate and marked inattention that is not a symptom of another disorder, such as Mental Retardation or Attention-deficit Hyperactivity Disorder, or of a disorganized and chaotic environment. Some of the disturbances that in DSM III would have been categorized as Attention-deficit Disorder without Hyperactivity would be included in this category. Research is necessary to determine if this is a valid diagnostic category and, if so, how it should be defined. (American Psychiatric Association, 1987, §314.00)

Relationships of contributing factors. *Biological maturation.* It is inferred that biological factors underlie conditions of ADHD because children with the disorder often respond favorably to treatment with psychostimulant medication. These are considered probable contributing factors to language disorders in children with ADHD. However, neither the exact mechanism for the symptoms of ADHD nor the effect of medication is as yet fully understood. Based on studies of regional cerebral blood flow, the disorder is thought to be related to disruptions in transmission and metabolism along subcortical pathways that connect the midbrain to the prefrontal cortex. These areas play a role in directing attention, self-regulation, and planning (Bass, 1988). One hypothesis for the paradoxical finding that psychostimulants such as methylphenidate (Ritalin) appear to assist children with hyperactivity to control and direct their attention in desirable ways is that the hyperactivity exhibited by children with ADHD is secondary to attentional impairments and that psychostimulants are effective because they stimulate neurotransmitters that enable children to concentrate longer (Zametkin & Rapoport, 1987).

The use of psychostimulants to treat ADHD remains somewhat controversial. Although little evidence suggests that long-term learning or academic achievement are improved (Gittelman-Klein & Klein, 1976; E. Rie & Rie, 1977; H. Rie, Rie, & Stewart, 1976), research has consistently shown that psychostimulants can result in improved parent and teacher ratings of behavior and in enhancing performance on some laboratory measures (Abikoff & Gittelman, 1985; Gittelman-Klein et al., 1976; Rapport, Stoner, DuPaul, Birmingham, & Tucker, 1985). For children who can benefit, psychostimulants seem to normalize their biological systems so that they can participate in other kinds of interactions with less difficulty.

Linguistic system factors. No evidence indicates that children with ADHD have linguistic deficits specific to the syndrome. On the other hand, as noted in the study by Cantwell, Baker, and Mattison (1979), children diagnosed as having language and communicative impairments are at increased risk of also meeting criteria for having ADHD. The study by Rutter, Tizard, et al. (1970) also supports the risk for interrelatedness of ADHD and written language disorders. Linguistic system factors are often found in children with ADHD, but the degree of involvement may vary.

Some evidence regarding the role of linguistic factors in the attention difficulties experienced by children with ADHD is also available from the literature on selective auditory attention. Studies of selective auditory attention typically involve having children perform some auditory task, such as repeating words or pointing to pictures that match words they hear over headphones, while being exposed to an auditory distractor simultaneously over the headphones. Research has shown that when meaningful linguistic distractors are used (e.g., someone reading a story) children with hyperactivity and learning disabilities have much more difficulty relative to their non-attention-impaired peers, than when nonlinguistic distractors (e.g., white noise) are used (Cherry & Kruger, 1983; Lasky & Tobin, 1973). It is difficult to interpret the results of these studies, however, because of earlier tendencies for diagnoses of hyperactivity and learning disabilities to be confounded. Professionals also must be careful not to assume that the controlled conditions of laboratory testing using headphones provide an accurate measurement of children's distractability in natural settings (Dalebout, Nelson, Hletko, & Frentheway, 1991).

Stimulus–response–reinforcement factors. An inherent part of the diagnosis of ADHD is an observation that children with the condition respond differently to stimuli in their environment than do other children of a similar developmental level (with the diagnosis complicated by a lack of clear standards for making these kinds of comparisons). Stimulus–response–reinforcement factors are considered essential contributing factors to childhood language disorders in ADHD. Behavioral analysis is an important part of both assessment and intervention.

Most professionals currently recommend combined behavior and pharmaceutical treatment, although it remains controversial. Kendall and Braswell (1985) have described cognitive-behavioral therapy for "impulsive" children as an approach in which "The client and therapist work together to think through and behaviorally practice solutions to personal, academic, and interpersonal problems with a consideration of the affect involved" (p. 1). Whether or not behaviorist learning principles, in addition to biological influences, can explain the problem of ADHD, behavioral management practices, including positive reinforcement, clearly must be part of the solution. If such practices are not instituted consistently and deliberately, these children tend to elicit primarily punitive responses from the adults and other children around them, and they run increasing risks of depression and delinquency as they become older.

Information processing factors. Information processing factors are considered essential contributing factors for childhood language disorders in ADHD. Levine (1987) noted that individuals of all ages daily confront more data than they can possibly interpret, store, and apply. As a result, selection is necessary and involves a combination of both selective attention and selective intention. As children mature, they gradually become better able to concentrate on important information and to ignore irrelevant stimuli while they become better at selecting rewarding ways to spend their time and rejecting less worthwhile options. Levine said that children with ADHD are predisposed to poor selectivity, concentrating on inappropriate stimuli, and participating in purposeless activities.

Vail (1987) noted that, to focus attention, children need a combination of arousal, a filter, language, and appropriate work. Attention is awakened through arousal, but then it must be focused with a filtering process that keeps out both external and internal distractions. According to Vail, language is also an essential element, enabling children to organize thought and to focus their attention. Language assists them to break down a task into manageable pieces, anticipate cause and effect, and categorize and sort ideas according to their relative importance. She noted that "Some children who appear to have trouble paying attention actually lack the language to structure their work" (p. 141).

Another element in determining how well children can attend, in Vail's (1987) view, is a "need for appropriate work," which conveys the message that problems are not just within children. Before a child is diagnosed with ADHD, it is important that those in the child's environment experiment to see whether the child may be demonstrating the symptoms of ADHD because the schoolwork is too difficult for the child's level of ability. Vail cautioned, "Sometimes the label *attentional deficit* is applied to a student who is merely in over his head" (p. 141).

Cognition factors. To be diagnosed as having ADHD, a child must demonstrate symptoms atypical of children of the same "mental age." This mental age referencing is consistent with a co-occurring diagnosis of mental retardation, as long as the attention deficit appears to exceed attentional immaturity that might be typical of children of a similar developmental level (of course, few standards are available to make this assess-

ment, except for observational ones). Children with ADHD may function at all levels of cognitive ability, although cognition is often at least subtly affected in these children. Children with other kinds of central processing deficits are at particular risk for attention deficits.

As Frank Smith (1975) pointed out, the attention demanded for processing a certain kind of stimulus is relative to the degree of uncertainty about its meaning. It is safe to ignore potentially distracting stimuli, such as an airplane flying overhead, when you understand what the sound represents. Because much of that understanding comes through language, children with language and cognitive deficits may have to work harder than other children to make sense of their world and to ignore information that is not central at the moment.

In the broadest sense, the attentional deficit and information processing problems associated with ADHD might be considered to represent problems of cognition for all children who have the disorder. Although the ability of some children with ADHD to earn IQs in the gifted range (Vail, 1987) suggests relative independence from general intelligence factors, the cognitive approach to learning taken by children with ADHD seems to differ from that of children without the disorder. Children with ADHD are nonreflective in their cognitive style and tend to make decisions too quickly and on the basis of relatively inadequate thought processes. As Cantwell and Baker (1985) noted, the impulsivity that is one of the core symptoms of ADHD "is not only a behavioral impulsivity but also a *cognitive* impulsivity" (p. 49).

Social interaction factors. As noted in Box 4.8, social interaction factors are central to diagnosis of the condition and are considered essential contributing factors to language disorders in children with ADHD. Difficulty in playing, taking turns, participating in conversation, and following the rules of formal conversation without interrupting are all characteristic of children with ADHD. Problems in these areas may lead some children with ADHD to be identified in the preschool years. Others are not identified until they experience difficulty in more structured social settings where rigid rules of interaction are observed, such as in the elementary school classroom. During adolescence, difficulties with social behavior and interpersonal relationships may become primary (Sattler, 1988).

During the preschool years, social interaction difficulties associated with ADHD influence the relationships of young children with their parents. Parents tend to become particularly frustrated when these children appear not to "listen" to parental requests and often fail to comply with behavioral expectations. In such instances, it is difficult to sort out factors of inattention, lack of comprehension, and impulsivity within the child, from methods of behavioral management and control used by the parents and from distractions and other environmental influences. Parents of children with ADHD often doubt their abilities to control their own children and may experiment with alternate behavioral and communicative strategies as they attempt to cope and to "get through" to their children.

The role of psychostimulant medication in this complicated open system of preschoolers and their parents is still somewhat fuzzy. In one study, however, Barkley (1988) found that preschool children decreased their off-task and noncompliant behavior, and significantly increased their compliant behavior to their mothers' directives when the children received appropriately high doses of methylphenidate.

Speech–language pathologists and audiologists may help to sort out whether noncompliance among preschoolers stems from auditory-linguistic factors as well as from pragmatic and behavioral factors. Specialists in language and communication can help youngsters with ADHD during school-age years and early employment to understand the social systems of schools, to use inner communication to direct their own study habits, and to communicate better in interactions with peers and adults.

Acquired Brain Injury

Definitions, differential diagnosis, and subdivisions. Children with acquired brain injury constitute such a heterogeneous group that to consider them to be members of one category is probably misleading. They also differ in some important ways from children with developmental language disorders, making the condition worthy of a separate category. In the past, many texts on childhood language disorders did not include children with acquired brain injury in their discussions, but professionals who work with children of all ages do find them in their practices.

The developing human brain is quite remarkable. It is complex enough to support the development of an impressive array of integrated sensory, motor, linguistic, cognitive, and social skills; yet it is fragile enough to be set back by a bump on the head, the bursting of a strategically placed blood vessel, or the invasion of a microscopic agent. It is also resilient enough to make an amazing recovery when a significant amount of tissue is irreparably damaged or even when an entire hemisphere is removed. One of the great mysteries of childhood language disorders is how a brain that appears normal, even with modern neuroimaging techniques, can lead a child with specific language impairment of unknown origin to have as much or more difficulty in acquiring language (at least some aspects of it) than does the brain of a child who has a frank lesion in an area known to be critical for language processing in adults.

A language disorder associated with a focal-acquired lesion of the brain is termed *aphasia*. This term and its various subclassifications are applied primarily to language disorders associated with brain lesions caused by cerebrovascular accidents (CVAs; strokes caused by blockage or hemorrhage) in adults. When professionals have noted the similarities of symptoms of specific language impairment in developing children to the symptoms of acquired aphasia in adults, they have sometimes used the label *congenital aphasia* to represent developmental language disorders (Eisenson, 1968, 1972). The use of that term, however, can lead to confusion and, currently, is rarely applied to children with congenital problems, except perhaps when a specific language disability is unusually severe.

When brain injury occurs after gestation and birth, it is considered to be acquired. Depending on the cause, timing, extent, and location of the injury, the symptoms and prognosis for continued development by a particular child may vary widely. It is impossible to outline a common set of symptoms, yet, some expectations vary with the cause: (1) focal acquired lesions, (2) diffuse lesions associated with traumatic brain injury, (3) acquired childhood aphasia secondary to convulsive disorder, and (4) other kinds of brain injury or encephalopathy, such as those following injury by infectious agents or treatment for childhood cancer. These are not subtypes in the same sense as the subtypes considered here in other categories, but they do represent subdivisions within the category of acquired brain injury in children.

Focal acquired brain injury in children. Several studies have shown that children who acquire focal (specific and localized) lesions of the left hemisphere during early childhood show generally good recovery and development of language (Aram & Ekelman, 1987; Aram, Ekelman, & Whitaker, 1986, 1987; Hecaen, 1976, 1983). Close examination of results, however, also shows some significant effects on language development and learning ability.

Although we tend to think of CVAs as occurring primarily in older adults, they can occur at any age. Children with congenital heart disorders are particularly at risk because embolic material may break loose and clog the middle cerebral artery, cutting off blood supply to the critical language areas of the brain. Children also may have congenital arteriovenous malformations, clusters of malformed and misconnected arteries and veins that are particularly susceptible to hemorrhaging (another form of CVA).

Dorothy Aram and her research group at Case Western Reserve University and Rainbow Babies and Children's Hospital in Cleveland, Ohio, have done much of the carefully controlled recent research on the linguistic and cognitive sequelae of unilateral brain lesions in children. Aram (1988) reviewed the results of several of her own and others' studies regarding effects of unilateral brain lesions on language development (summarized in Box 4.9).

Traumatic brain injury in children. The language development picture for children with diffuse brain injury that is due to trauma (from falls, vehicular or bicycle accidents, or child abuse) is more mixed than that for children with unilateral lesions. The traditional

wisdom is that the earlier brain injury occurs in child development, the more complete the expected recovery. More recent interpretations of the evidence, however, suggest that age is only one factor in determining recovery (Ewing-Cobbs, Fletcher, & Levin, 1985). Although spontaneous recovery following brain injury is striking, a significant proportion of children exhibit persistent deficits of cognitive and linguistic processing (Satz & Bullard-Bates, 1981).

A summary of studies of long-term deficits in children following traumatic brain injury (TBI) (Ewing-Cobbs, et al., 1985) shows more pervasive cognitive and behavioral sequelae than previously recognized. These include general intellectual, language, memory, and psychosocial deficits, all of which can be expected to interfere both with communication and with academic functioning. Accumulating evidence suggests that younger children may exhibit more severe and long-lasting cognitive sequelae following TBI than either older adolescents or adults (Levin, Ewing-Cobbs, & Benton, 1984).

Levin and Eisenberg (1979) evaluated the language deficits of 64 children with closed head injury within 6 months of injury. Their findings showed linguistic deficits in 31%. The most common symptom was dysnomia, both for objects presented visually (13% of the sample) or to the left hand for tactual identification (12%). Auditory comprehension was impaired in 11% and verbal repetition in only 4%.

In a more recent study, Ewing-Cobbs and co-workers (1985) studied children and adolescents with moderate-to-severe closed head injury, defined by the presence of neurologic deficit, CT scan findings, coma persisting for at least 15 minutes, or a combination of these findings. Their results showed that after post-traumatic amnesia (PTA) was resolved, these injuries were associated with continued deficits in confrontation naming, object description, verbal fluency, and writing to dictation. Not only did younger children fare no better than adolescents in terms of outcome, they actually were more impaired than adolescents on measures of written language functioning.

Some studies of written language processing by children with TBI have been difficult to interpret because their results are based on reading and writing assessments involving single words only. Other complicating factors arise because populations at risk for head injury exhibit characteristics of lower intelligence, social disadvantage, inadequate or interrupted schooling, and interfering behavioral or physical difficulties.

Box 4.9   Features of language and cognition observed following unilateral brain injury in children (based on Aram, 1988)

1. **Cognition**. Results from IQ tests are conflicting (probably because subject groups in many studies have been confounded with children with seizure disorders who have possibly been on medication). In children free from ongoing seizures, IQ scores may be expected to be well within normal limits, but tests may not be sensitive enough to predict persistent language or learning difficulties. The most common finding is distractibility, regardless of lesion site.

2. **Syntactic comprehension**. Studies have demonstrated at least subtle syntactic comprehension deficits following left hemisphere lesions but not right hemsiphere lesions. More research is needed to assess comprehension of connected discourse and syntactic structures that are more complex than those assessed by token tests. The contributions of more primary cognitive abilities such as memory and attention also need to be teased out.

3. **Syntactic production**. In children, the most frequent early observation after acquired brain injury, even when the right hemisphere is affected, is mutism, followed by telegraphic production during the recovery process. Although the expressive syntax deficits of these children appear to lessen considerably with continued development, when tasks become more demanding, evidence of long-standing deficits can be found.

4. **Lexical and semantic aspects**. In rapid-naming tasks, children with left-hemisphere lesions tend to be significantly slower in response time and to make more errors when given rhyming cues than matched control subjects. On the other hand, children with right-hemisphere lesions respond as rapidly or even more quickly than control subjects but produce more errors (suggesting a speed–accuracy trade-off).

5. **Written language development and academic success**. Although the oral language deficits of children with acquired unilateral brain lesions are generally subtle, with few children remaining clinically aphasic, children with both left- and right-hemisphere lesions typically exhibit academic difficulties in school. The reading abilities of children with focal left-hemisphere lesions may vary widely. Although most perform comparably to carefully selected controls on reading tests, a select subgroup (with a variety of lesion sites, including subcortical ones) exhibits severe reading disorders. Efforts to identify commonalities among this subgroup of children have been largely unsuccessful, except to note the presence of concomitant language and/or memory problems in the presence of generally intact nonverbal conceptual skills (Aram, Ekelman, & Gillespie, 1989). Children with both right- and left-hemisphere brain lesions are likely to show residual deficits of brain injury on attention, impulse inhibition, memory, reasoning, and perceptual speed, all of which may affect school functioning (Aram & Ekelman, 1988).

Such characteristics, which are associated with educational and social difficulties in general, make it difficult to identify which elements are due to predisposing factors and which are specific to the brain injury itself (N. W. Nelson & Schwentor, 1990). For example, when Shaffer, Bijur, Chadwick, and Rutter (1980) investigated 88 school-age children who sustained closed head injuries producing depressed skull fractures, they found that 55% had reading ages 1 or more years below their chronological ages, and 33% were 2 or more years behind. However, the authors found it difficult to sort out the effects of the head injury from the confounding predisposing variables.

To reduce some of the problems stemming from earlier retrospective studies, Chadwick, Rutter, Brown, Shaffer, and Traub (1981) conducted a prospective follow-up study of children injured between the ages of 5 and 14 years. They concluded that 25 of those who experienced PTA for more than 3 weeks (defined as the "severe head injury" group) showed reading difficulties attributable to the head injury. Of these children, seven were reported by their teachers either to be experiencing difficulties with their schoolwork or were placed in special schools. These authors pointed out the need to consider the real-life effects of time pressures and contextual demands when evaluating children and adolescents with head injury. They noted that such individuals may be able to complete tasks under optimal, temporally controlled circumstances of psychometric testing but not in other settings.

Are there recognized subtypes of children following TBI? Rather than attempting to identify subtypes of children with brain injury based on specific symptom complexes, rehabilitation teams tend to focus on identifying stages of recovery, because different sets of concerns arise during different points in the recovery process. Thus, the same child may be considered to be a member of different subgroups longitudinally. In addition, subdivisions may be helpful, depending on whether brain injury (and possibly, spinal cord injury) has affected motor functioning, including speech production, eating, and swallowing, as well as cognitive and communicative functioning.

In the early recovery period (sometimes called the acute phase), the primary goal is to increase the responsiveness of a child who may be emerging from coma. Rosen and Gerring (1986) marked the early period from the point of injury to the end of PTA when "patients are consistently oriented to place, date, and time and are able to store long term memories" (p. 25). During the early phase, treatment is aimed at sensory and sensorimotor stimulation to increase arousal and adaptive responses to the environment (Szekeres, Ylvisaker, & Holland, 1985). The middle recovery period involves efforts to channel recovery for confused patients by focusing on cognitive retraining and structured environmental compensations. The late recovery period involves goals for increased independence, withdrawal of environmental supports, the development of functional integrative skills in more natural settings, and development of strategies to compensate for residual impairments (Szekeres et al., 1985). Rosen and Gerring (1986) described long-term recovery as a process that occurs over a period of months to years and that is continually influenced by concomitant processes of development.

Acquired aphasia secondary to convulsive disorder. Another type of language disorder that may be acquired in childhood is acquired aphasia secondary to a convulsive disorder, which is usually of idiopathic (unknown) origin. Normal development, varying in length (see Miller, Campbell, Chapman, & Weismer, 1984, for a review), is followed by either sudden or gradual onset of dramatic language problems (L. S. Jordan, 1980).

The condition was first described by Landau and Kleffner (1957) and is sometimes known as the *Landau syndrome* or *Landau-Kleffner syndrome*. It should be suspected whenever a child loses previously acquired language, before, during, or after seizures (Cooper & Ferry, 1978). It also may be referred to as Worster-Drought (1971) syndrome.

This syndrome is characterized by the presence of electrographic epileptic discharges (whether or not overt seizures are evident), generally accompanied by severe language comprehension deficits, at least initially. Its prognosis is variable. Some children show dramatic recovery after a brief period of impairment, others show fluctuations of ability, and still others show severe, long-lasting language deficits (Mantovani & Landau 1980). The degree of recovery appears to be weakly correlated to improvement of electrographic abnormalities and medical control of seizures.

Encephalitis has been suggested as a causative agent for this syndrome, but a variety of agents likely play a role (Cole et al., 1988). One girl I saw when I was a consultant for Berrien County Intermediate School District first demonstrated comprehension problems when she began to have seizures in third grade. She then retained the ability to read aloud and to talk but began to have difficulty understanding what she read or the teacher's instructions (she was also very embarrassed by her seizures, which often included vomiting). This girl was later found to have a temporal lobe tumor.

The language symptoms associated with Landau syndrome differ from those usually occurring in acquired aphasia (in which expressive symptoms tend to predominate, often in the form of early mutism) (Aram, 1988; Rapin, Mattis, Rowan, & Golden, 1977). In contrast, the most frequent report for children with acquired aphasia secondary to onset of a convulsive disorder is loss of comprehension, sometimes so profoundly that it may be mistaken for deafness. The problem is better described as *central auditory agnosia:* Hearing is intact but the ability to interpret meaning is lost because of damage to auditory reception and association areas in the brain. The loss of expressive speech usually represents an insidious accompaniment to the loss of ability to process receptive oral language. Depending on the age of onset and other factors, reading and writing may be relatively spared. Word-finding difficulties and paraphasic (word-substitution) errors are also common when children acquire the disorder past early childhood.

When symptoms of auditory agnosia are marked, sign language may offer a functional alternative communication mode for these children. In my experience, the condition is more difficult to diagnose in younger children because they have less history of normal development to contrast with the period of impairment, and the children themselves are less aware of their changed status. They also have acquired fewer words in their expressive vocabularies to contrast with the receptive language deficits, and they tend to show a more uniform language deficit across areas.

In cases of suddenly acquired aphasia, one of the most important early services that communication specialists can provide—aside from contributing to the assessment process and assisting families to understand this scary thing that is happening to them—is to ensure that some form of communication is immediately available. Often, this involves encouraging families and educators to take advantage of all modes of communication (particularly low-technology techniques, e.g., gestures, pictures, and written communication materials, if appropriate). This role is critical in reducing frightening feelings of isolation these children are likely to experience with sudden onset.

Encephalopathy secondary to infection or irradiation. Some children exhibit signs of brain injury resulting from agents that are less direct than CVA or trauma and that disrupt the normal biological maturation process over time, rather than precipitously. The direct effects of brain tumors and the aftereffects of encephalitis or cancer treatments fall into this category.

The symptoms may vary widely, again based on factors such as timing, extent, and location of involvement of cortical and subcortical tissue. They also vary qualitatively from those of children with more purely developmental disabilities. Children with acquired brain injuries of any type tend to retain some function and to have information processing and cognitive deficits of varying severity. For acquired brain injury, the risks for either over- or underexpectation, and for knowing how to intervene, are great.

For example, I saw a child, Sarah, who acquired severe language and cognitive disabilities as an after-effect of treatment for acute lymphocytic leukemia (ALL). She developed normally, if not precociously, up to the age of 3, when the ALL was identified. She was then treated with a combination of brain irradiation and chemotherapy (methotrexate in the spine), and, within

a couple of years, the leukemia was basically "cured." Sarah's parents, however, faced a new set of worries 2 years later when she began to lose some of the developmental skills that she had already acquired, and the worries became major concerns as the condition worsened and her seizures became uncontrollable.

The most confusing part of the picture for those who worked with Sarah at school was her scattering of abilities. Because her syntactic construction skills were more intact than her comprehension abilities and because she retained some of her earlier learned vocabulary in her self-initiated speech, people tended not to identify language processing as a major component of the problem. They focused more on the perceptual and apraxia deficits that made it difficult for her to perceive shapes or to dress herself (early developmental skills). Her psychometric level of functioning was placed at the level of trainable mental retardation. Sarah's language comprehension was also severely impaired. An effect of this and her reaction to it was the appearance of refusing to cooperate in most standard assessment and teaching tasks (which are often the "I say and you do," or "I ask and you answer" variety). When she did verbalize in these contexts, it was usually with off-task or echolalic remarks. Yet, when allowed more control of the topic, Sarah participated much more "normally" in conversation and play. Sarah's school district had a great deal of difficulty knowing how to provide appropriate services to meet Sarah's unique needs. She did not "fit" in any of the usual programs designed for children with developmental disabilities. This problem is common for children with acquired brain damage, especially when its effects are severe, as they were in Sarah's case.

Relationships of contributing factors. *Biological maturation.* Biological factors obviously play a central role when a known brain injury or abnormality is associated with a child's language disorder and are classified as essential contributing factors. As mentioned, the cause, timing, extent, and location of lesion(s) all seem to influence the symptoms and prognosis for a particular child. In general, better prognosis now appears to be associated with lesions that are caused by CVAs, that have an early onset, that involve a small area of tissue, and that do not involve subcortical structures. However, the exact relationship of these factors can vary widely in individual circumstances.

Some studies have shown that children who sustain brain injuries before age 2 years may actually be at greater risk for having later difficulty learning to read than those who have already begun (Aram & Ekelman, 1988; Ewing-Cobbs et al., 1985). This leads researchers to suspect that, contrary to the traditional wisdom that earlier lesions are associated with better prognosis because of the assumed superior plasticity of younger brains, periods of normal development before injury actually may give the child certain advantages in recovery.

Relatively speaking, the prognosis for children who acquire focal (specific and localized) lesions of the left hemisphere during childhood to develop language is amazingly good (Aram & Ekelman, 1987; Aram et al., 1986, 1987; Hecaen, 1976, 1983). This leads us to wonder what brain mechanisms are responsible for recovery. When a child experiences a unilateral lesion in the left hemisphere, does subsequent language development shift primarily to right-hemisphere control or does the left hemisphere itself reorganize?

New techniques for studying brain activity may help to answer this question. They involve identifying which hemisphere is doing the most work for a particular kind of task by measuring the tiny evoked electrical potentials (with surface electrodes placed on the skull over the right or left hemisphere), stimulated by presentation of a clear, abrupt "probe" (either an auditory click or visual strobe flash). Measurements are taken both in a control condition, when individuals are instructed to pay close attention to the stimuli when they occur in isolation, and then in an experimental condition, when the person gives primary attention to performing some other kind of task. When the brain is busy with another task while the stimulus probe is presented, the evoked potential to the brief stimulus is reduced (attenuated) relative to the control condition. When tested in this way, children who have recovered significantly from unilateral left-hemisphere lesions show patterns of performance that are more like those of control children and normal adults; they show predominantly left-hemisphere engagement (measured as greater evoked response attenuation) during language tasks and predominantly right-hemisphere engagement during visuospatial tasks. This suggests that, for children with unilateral lesions acquired early, the pattern of recovery and further development involves intra- rather than interhemispheric functional reorganization (Papanicolaou, DiScenna, Gillespie, & Aram, 1990).

The influence of TBI on the biological systems of the brain differs from that of relatively focal, unilateral injuries. The primary mechanism producing brain injury following trauma is the diffuse neuronal damage that occurs at the time of impact with both coup (direct hit) and contrecoup (rebound of the brain inside the skull) forces, accompanied by shearing and stretching of neurons and injury to white matter. Because of the bony prominences inside the skull, certain areas, such as the anterior tips of the temporal lobes and the orbital regions of the frontal lobes, are particularly susceptible to injury (Pang, 1985).

The mechanisms of damage in cases of acquired brain injury following treatment for cancer and insidious effects of disease differ from those of either CVA or traumatic origin. In some children with Landau syndrome, the "damage" may only be inferred from aberrant findings on electroencephalograms (EEGs). In cases like Sarah's, the effects of the irradiation treatment may show up clearly on MRI scans some time after treatment (see Figure 4.3). Childhood cancer survivors may demonstrate mild neuropsychological late effects of brain irradiation without apparent white matter effects on MRI scans (Kramer, Norman, Grant-Zawadzki, Albin, & Moore, 1988). A summary of results of research reports on children with ALL who have been treated with brain irradiation and chemotherapy shows (1) general lowering of functioning, with the effect most pronounced for nonlanguage skills; (2) encephalopathy (brain damage), intelligence deficits, and/or neuropsychological deficits occurring within months or years following cranial radiation and chemotherapy (Hutter, 1986; McCalla, 1985); (3) children receiving irradiation before 5 years of age being more likely to experience cognitive difficulty (Copeland et al., 1985); and (4) children treated with chemotherapy alone showing no global or specific neuropsychological impairment (Tamaroff et al., 1982).

Because the role of biological maturation factors is so critical to the group of children with acquired brain injuries, it is essential that language specialists be vigilant in recognizing any symptoms of childhood language disorder that may involve sudden onset or worsening of a preexisting condition. Immediate medical referral and treatment may reduce the long-term effects. It is not a time for "wait and see."

Linguistic system factors. Throughout these discussions of the varied causative agents of acquired brain injury, I have emphasized individual variability. In some

FIGURE 4.3
A magnetic resonance image of
the brain of an 8-year-old child
who had undergone irradiation
and chemotherapy (spinal cord
injection of methotrexate) from
age 3 to about 5 years. The neu-
roradiologist noted that this image
looked more like the brain of an
elderly adult with dementia than
that of an 8-year-old. The scan
shows signs of pathology in the
form of white matter hyperintensity
off the posterior aspect of the lat-
eral ventricles (spaces filled with
cerebrospinal fluid), which are
enlarged. These changes indicate
reduced white matter, which with
its myelin sheath coverings provides the major means of connecting various centers and
association areas of the brain.

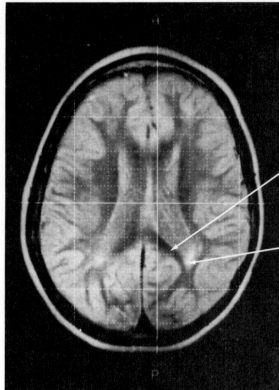

Anterior

Right

Enlarged
ventricle

Left

Abnormal
white
matter

Posterior

cases, such as those involving left-hemisphere lesions
or Landau syndrome, the language processing deficit
may appear to be primary. Yet the liguistic processing
deficits of such children may actually be secondary to
deficits of auditory information processing related to
auditory agnosia (remember, however, that the separation of linguistic and auditory processing may be artificial). In other children, such as those with TBI,
specifically linguistic impairments may appear to be
secondary to more general cognitive and social interaction deficits. In all cases, a comprehensive approach
to assessment and intervention is needed; linguistic
system factors are considered probable contributing
factors.

Stimulus–response–reinforcement factors.   When biological injury is clear, professionals are unlikely to
assume behavioral explanations for symptoms, but, in

"real life," behavioral manifestations often accompany
a dramatic life event such as acquired brain injury, and
they cannot be ignored. They are considered probable
contributing factors to language disorders in these
children. In addition to the variable direct effects of the
brain injury on receiving stimuli from the environment
and on modes of response, parents and teachers generally find themselves dealing with a very different
child after the injury. Children and parents may both
be confused, frightened, and angered by changes in
cognitive, linguistic, and sensorimotor processing.
Particularly following traumatic brain injury, changes in
personality, the ability to concentrate, and compliance
with parental and teacher expectations may be viewed
primarily as problems of behavior.

Of course, in the most general sense, all observable effects of inner processes are manifested as
behavior. Behaviorist principles may, in fact, be quite

useful in providing consistency in environmental organization, stimulation, and reinforcement during the rehabilitation process for children with acquired brain injuries. However, all forms of intervention are best applied within a system theory context in which the child's behavior is seen as emanating from complex interactions among intrinsic and extrinsic forces, including memories of a different past. A hefty dose of understanding and unconditional acceptance mixed with consistent behavioral expectations is also helpful when children undergo dramatic life changes. In particular, language specialists may be able to assist parents and teachers in understanding how the child's lack of compliance with behavioral expectations and learning tasks may be related to shifts in attention and shifts in linguistic and auditory processing capabilities rather than "misbehavior." Specialists thus may help to set realistically revised behavioral standards and to adjust them over time.

Information processing factors. Information processing is invariably affected when the brain is injured and is considered an essential contributing factor to language disorders in these children. Regardless of the injury's cause, problems of attention, concentration, and memory tend to interfere with further development and learning, particularly in natural contexts where many potential distractions are often present. Because these factors are less likely to show up under the controlled conditions of individualized assessment, naturalistic observation is critical to understanding their full impact on recovery and further development.

Cognitive factors. The services needed by children with acquired brain injury extend beyond the area of linguistics and communication. The term *cognitive rehabilitation therapy* is commonly used when children have TBIs requiring intervention (Ylvisaker, 1985) and represents the comprehensive scope of impaired abilities and the extent of rehabilitative needs. Cognition factors are considered probable contributing factors to language disorders in brain-injured children.

At least since the end of the 19th century, neurologists and other rehabilitation specialists have been debating whether the changes that accompany brain injury are best characterized as general diminutions of functioning or as specific deficits. As in other areas of sustained debate, there may be elements of truth in both positions. Kurt Goldstein (1948), who was considered to be a member of the "cognitivist school," noted that brain injury almost invariably involves im-

pairment of the abstract attitude and problems of what he called categorical behavior. Even when they achieve relatively high levels of functioning, many children and adolescents with brain injury have continued difficulty grasping later developing meanings, such as those involved in abstract figurative language and humor. Perhaps the most consistent characteristic of children with acquired brain injury is their wide variability as they continue to mature. (N. W. Nelson & Schwentor, 1990; Rosen & Gerring, 1986, Ylvisaker, 1985).

Social interaction factors. The effect of an acquired brain injury on a child's social interactions and the effects of the child's social interactions following brain injury on subsequent recovery form a complicated picture of interactive cause and effect. Regardless of causative agent, the family likely will have had an emotionally, physically, and economically trying experience. Depending on the length of hospital stay during the acute phase, and the presence of physical and sensory symptoms necessitating long-term rehabilitation, children will have been more or less isolated from their peers and their normal experiences.

In some cases, children may be so impaired following injury that it is unrealistic to expect them to be able to compete in the social and educational contexts where they functioned well before the injury. School placement then becomes one of the most difficult decisions facing transdisciplinary teams, complicated by the fact that such teams must span from hospital to education settings and that most special educators are not accustomed to working in rehabilitation. In discussing educational reintegration following head trauma, Rosen and Gerring (1986) observed the paradoxical situation that "School is the most appropriate place for children to gain reassurance that achievement is possible again, even while being confronted with enormous new difficulties in thinking, remembering, speaking, reading or concentrating" (p. xii). Language specialists may be able to facilitate this process in ways that accentuate the positive and reduce the negative factors involved.

Other Central Factors

The conditions considered thus far are not the only ones that might be found when children have difficulty learning language. Any influence that disrupts central nervous system development can disrupt language, speech, and communication development.

Language specialists need to know about other specific conditions such as Tourette's syndrome, fragile-X syndrome, and other complexes of symptoms that may influence communicative development. Sources for information specific to communication disorders associated with these and other syndromes are Sparks (1984) and S. E. Gerber (1990).

PERIPHERAL SENSORY AND MOTOR SYSTEM FACTORS

Hearing Impairment

Definitions, differential diagnosis, and subdivisions. Of impairments involving hearing, vision, and motor functioning, hearing loss is by far the most certain to be associated with difficulties in language acquisition. The term *hearing impairment* refers to all degrees of hearing loss, ranging from mild impairments, which may result in only subtle effects on language acquisition, to profound hearing loss.

Subtypes of hearing impairment. Within the category of hearing impairment, a traditional subdivision is between *hard-of-hearing* and *deafness*. Two types of criteria are used to make this distinction: (1) the effect of the hearing loss on the ability to process linguistic information and (2) audiometric results (Northern & Downs, 1984).

An audiometric criterion for determining deafness is hearing loss in the better ear of 70-dB or greater hearing level (HL). (HL is the average of pure-tone thresholds at 500, 1,000, and 2,000 Hz, the "speech frequencies"). An audiometric criterion for determining hard-of-hearing is hearing loss in the better ear in the range of 35 to 69-dB HL (Northern & Downs, 1984). M. Ross (1977) argued that, with modern amplification methods, the physiological borderline for determining deafness should be even higher, at 95 to 100-dB HL. Boothroyd (1982) also pointed out that proper amplification can move children from one classification to another, making the audiometric distinction between deafness and hard-of-hearing questionable. Cochlear implants and tactile aids (Roeser, 1988) have also been used to help some children who previously would have been categorized as "deaf" to be aware of sounds and to use them as information, although, even using these aids, they may not be able to discriminate speech without visual help.

Perhaps the more useful criterion is that based on the ability to process linguistic information. Using this criterion, hard-of-hearing children are those who can develop basic communication skills through the auditory channel, whereas deaf children are those whose hearing impairments are so severe that it is impossible to process linguistic information through hearing alone, with or without amplification (Northern & Downs, 1984; Ross, 1982). To these two basic subdivisions, Ross (1982) added a third gray-area group of children who "can utilize their hearing, derive much benefit from it, and may even employ it as a primary channel in certain restricted circumstances, when they have no other choice, such as talking on the telephone on a specific topic" (p. 4). For general communication, however, this group depends primarily on vision to gather information about communicative input.

Categorization of children as either deaf or hard-of-hearing is problematic in another way. The application of the label *deaf* may be a self-fulfilling prophecy (Ross & Calvert, 1973), making a child who has some residual hearing "deaf" by limiting the child's opportunities for language acquisition and influencing the child's self-image as a person who can hear. When parents, teachers, and relatives think of a child as deaf (although that child may have some usable residual hearing), they tend to treat the child as one who cannot hear at all. Ross and Calvert (1973) pointed out that the adults then tend to adopt attitudes that there is little point in speaking to the child, that the child will never speak but will communicate only through an alternate form of communication; that the child will always need special classes for education; that hearing aids will be of little use; and that the child cannot be expected to succeed at intellectual, social, or vocational activities. When children internalize such messages, they may become functionally deaf although their hearing is not completely lost.

A different kind of subdivision is sometimes based on whether the hearing loss occurred prelingually or postlingually. Longitudinal research shows that, as we might expect, children who lose their hearing after they have acquired some language show superior continued development of speech and language compared with those who lose their hearing prelinguistically (Levitt, McGarr, & Geffner, 1988).

Whether a hearing loss is unilateral or bilateral can also make a difference. Although bilateral losses are, of course, most devastating, and traditionally, the hearing loss of a child's better ear is used as the best estimator of auditory functioning, unilateral hearing losses are by no means innocuous (Northern & Downs, 1984). For example, Bess (1982) found that unilateral hearing loss had a significant effect on the linguistic, educational, and auditory perceptual development of children.

An additional subtype of children with hearing impairment. Beyond the basic subdivision of hearing impairment into categories of *deafness* and *hard-of-hearing*, a separate important subtype is made up of children with mild, conductive hearing impairments associated with otitis media with effusion (OME). This condition may be associated with hearing losses of less than 25 dB but with air–bone gaps of 15 dB or more. Therefore, rather than using a cutoff of 25-dB HL to determine normal hearing, Northern and Downs (1984) suggested that hearing thresholds of 20, 15, or even 10 dB in the speech frequencies might be significant enough to be handicapping during the critical language-learning years for some children.

Although not all studies have shown OME to have markedly adverse developmental effects (Brooks, 1986; Fischler, Todd, & Feldman, 1985; Roberts et al., 1986), many studies have demonstrated OME to exert long-term negative effects on language and learning, particularly when the condition occurs in the first 6 to 12 months of life and when episodes are more frequent (J. Klein, Chase, Teele, Menyuk, & Rosner, 1988; Silva, Kirkland, Simpson, Stewart, & Williams, 1982; Zinkus & Gottlieb, 1980). Adverse effects have also been reported for children in a wide variety of ethnic, socioeconomic, and racial groups. For example, G. K. Kaplan (1973) found significant gaps in school achievement between a group of Eskimo children in Alaska whose first documented episode of OME occurred before age 2 and a control group who showed no history of OME. Disturbingly, they also found that the educational gaps tended to widen over the age range from the 7 to 10 years when children were followed. In a longitudinal study in the Boston area, J. Klein et al. (1988) found a significant correlation between time spent with OME and significantly lowered speech and language test scores. They also found that the correlations were strongest for children in highest socioeconomic brackets.

What mechanisms might account for significant negative effects on language and learning from slight losses that were formerly thought to be insignificant? Investigators (e.g., Dobie & Berlin, 1979; M. W. Skinner, 1978) have outlined several sources of potential confusion, including confusion about (1) speech-sound constancy, because of fluctuating acoustic information; (2) acoustic parameters, especially for rapid speech; (3) segmentation of linguistic boundaries, such as for plurals and tenses; (4) prosodic intonation and stress patterns that convey subtle

emotional meanings; and (5) word characteristics, making it difficult to acquire new vocabulary. Significant correlations are also found between second-grade teachers' ratings of classroom attention and task orientation and the number of days of OME before 3 years of age (Roberts et al., 1989).

Hearing impairment: Different or delayed? What are the influences of hearing loss on the acquisition of oral and written language? Is language development of these children different, or merely delayed? As previously noted, it is probably misleading to attempt to summarize characteristics of language difficulty associated with a particular categorical condition from research studies. Patterns of development for individual children, of course, are not all alike. The summary in Box 4.10 should therefore be used with that caveat in mind. It summarizes features identified in a range of studies conducted with hearing impaired children with varied types and degree of loss, as well as at different points along an age-level continuum.

For the most part, the characteristics in Box 4.10 are not unique to children with hearing impairments, or even to children with language disorders. Most also can be observed in normal-hearing children at some points of their development. Like the language of children with specific language impairment, the language of children with hearing impairment may be better categorized as being delayed than different, especially when considering any one system.

That was the tentative conclusion reached by Quigley, Power, and Steinkamp (1977) when they summarized research on syntactic development by 450 deaf students (ranging in age from 10 to 19 years, with 50 subjects in each age group), in comparison with 60 normal-hearing control children (20 each in 8-, 9-, and 10-year old groups). Their results showed that syntactic structures develop similarly in deaf and hearing children but at a greatly retarded rate among deaf children.

In addition, Wilbur (1977) found commonalities in the strategies used by both deaf and hearing children in the language acquisition process, noting that both groups seem to approach the language-learning task by searching for generalities. Similar conclusions have resulted from studies of phonological processing. Evidence of relatively stable, rule-based phonological development has been found both for children with mild-to-moderate hearing losses (Oller, Jensen, & Lafayette, 1978; West & Weber, 1973) and with pro-

Box 4.10   A summary of language development characteristics of hearing impaired children

1. **Phonology.** The phonological systems of deaf children may be so affected that intelligibility is impaired, even with familiar listeners. Phonological simplification processes used by other children with hearing impairments vary with degree of loss and generally are similar to those used by younger, normal-hearing children. They differ more in frequency than in kind. Consonant deletions are numerous, particularly in final position. The most notable differences from normal development involve impaired productions of vowels (with a tendency toward neutralization) and suprasegmental features. Problems with suprasegmental features interact with speech planning and production constraints, such as (a) reduced speech rate, which may reflect extension of consonants and vowels, slow articulatory transitions, and frequent pauses; (b) lack of coordination of breathing patterns with syntactic phrasing; (c) inappropriate use of duration to distinguish stressed and unstressed syllables. Voice and resonation qualities may also be distorted (C. Dunn & Newton, 1986).

2. **Syntax and morphology.** Developmental order of syntactic types is similar to that for normal-hearing children. Negation, conjunction, and question formation are less difficult. Relativization, complementation, the verb system and pronominalization are most difficult. Developmental progression is dramatically delayed for most hearing impaired children, particularly those who are deaf. In some cases, deaf children may produce syntactic structures never used by normal-hearing individuals. These seem to be combinations of English grammar and attempted approximations of English grammar (Quigley, Smith & Wilbur, 1974). Unstressed, final inflectional morphemes (such as plurals and verb endings) and some parts of speech (such as adverbs, prepositions, quantifiers, and indefinite pronouns) tend to be produced with less frequency. Delays in the acquisition of morphological and syntactic rules are noted in both receptive and expressive language, oral and written.

3. **Semantics.** Hearing impaired children encode a wide range of semantic notions using both verbal and nonverbal means from a very young age, although they tend to talk about location more frequently than normal-hearing children do (Curtiss, Prutting, & Lowell, 1979). Vocabulary production and comprehension problems include difficulty understanding and using concept words, figurative meanings of words and phrases, and multiple-meaning words. Comprehension problems also extend to connected discourse in both oral and written modalities, and they persist as children advance in age (Moeller, Osberger, & Eccarius, 1986; Robbins, 1986).

4. **Pragmatics.** Toddlers with hearing impairment employ a wide range of methods, both verbal and nonverbal (including invented gestures) to communicate their pragmatic intentions, and this ability to communicate tends to exceed their ability to encode semantic concepts linguistically (Curtiss et al., 1979). In conversational interaction, preschool deaf children may show a narrow range of complexity when they act as initiators and may be less likely to respond to partners' initiations, particularly when utterances are in the form of comments (McKirdy & Blank, 1982). Older children with hearing impairments show continued difficulty in using pragmatic rules for entering and engaging in conversations. In the rapid-moving and shifting discourse of regular classroom settings, children with hearing impairments may be particularly disadvantaged (Roeser & Downs, 1988; Wiess, 1986).

found congenital deafness (Dodd, 1976). For some sounds that were particularly difficult to lip-read, however, the deaf children in Dodd's study used different phonological processes when lip-reading than when reading aloud. For example, when reading aloud, they made fewer errors involving the /k, g/ phonemes than when lip-reading.

Whereas some have interpreted the evidence as suggesting that the order of development and strategies used are basically the same for hearing impaired and normal-hearing children, others have interpreted the evidence as suggesting that the language of deaf children differs in quality as well as quantity. Particularly, the rigidity of language used by deaf children has been cited, as well as its susceptibility to being molded by a particular language-teaching curriculum (Russell, Quigley, & Power, 1976; Simmons, 1962). To some extent, conclusions reached depend on whether comparisons are made only within systems of language or across them. As noted in the preceding section on mild hearing losses associated with OME, features of language that carry less meaning, are less visible, and are produced with less prosodic stress in natural communication tend to be more difficult to acquire than more salient features when hearing is impaired.

Written language problems of children with hearing impairments.   Written language is difficult for hearing impaired children to master. Geers and Moog (1989) reviewed the association between prelingual hearing loss and reading deficiency, which "has been abundantly documented, beginning as early as 1916" (p. 69).

Demographic studies of reading performance by hearing impaired children show that a plateau occurs at about the third-grade reading level (Schildroth & Karchmer, 1986). Most hearing impaired children reach the plateau by 15 years of age and remain there at least through age 18 (Geers & Moog, 1989). Myklebust (1964) also concluded, based on studies of read, written, and spoken language, that the syntax of deaf children of around age 17 was approximately equal to that of 7-year-old normal-hearing children. Not only that, the deaf children in Myklebust's research tended to persist in a kind of formula writing and depended on written language prompts until the age of 15 years, whereas normal-hearing children had abandoned them by age 9.

Because most studies of reading development among hearing impaired children used cross-sectional data, Geers and Moog (1989) argued that they may not adequately represent longitudinal growth for individual students. Demographic studies also are likely to miss more academically competitive students because they tend to be mainstreamed at earlier ages and may not be represented in subject groups. Therefore, Geers and Moog (1989) cautioned that "the low scores reported for older hearing impaired students may result from an increasing proportion of students with additional and more severely handicapping characteristics who remain in special education settings" (pp. 69-70). Degree of hearing loss is not necessarily the best predictor of educational success, however, because even minimal hearing loss may

place students at risk for language and learning problems involving a number of psychoeducational variables (J. M. Davis, Elfenbein, Schum, & Bentler, 1986).

Geers and Moog (1989) studied 100 profoundly hearing impaired 16- and 17-year-olds enrolled in oral and mainstream high school programs and tested reading, writing, and spoken language abilities extensively. Tasks included those designed to measure both analytic "bottom-up" skills (e.g., phonics, vocabulary, and syntax) and synthetic "top-down" skills (e.g., paragraph comprehension, cloze completion, and narrative retellings). Both kinds of skills were, to the degree possible, evaluated at word, sentence, and text levels. In a multiple-regression analysis, Geers and Moog found three factors that contributed significantly to overall literacy: spoken language, hearing, and early intervention. Three other factors that were found not to contribute significantly to literacy were sign language, socioeconomic status, and mainstreaming. Test results also showed that this special subset of orally educated profoundly hearing impaired youngsters achieved reading skills commensurate with those of their normal-hearing peers (much above those traditionally reported for hearing impaired students). The authors concluded that their reading achievement was possible because they had at least average nonverbal intellectual ability, good use of residual hearing, early amplification, auditory stimulation, and oral educational management, "and—above all—oral English language ability, including vocabulary, syntax, and discourse skills" (p. 84).

Relationships of contributing factors.   *Biological maturation.*   Disorders of hearing have a biological basis that must be clarified as part of the diagnostic process and that is an essential contributing factor in childhood language disorders in these children. The importance of the biological mechanism is described by Bess and McConnell (1981):

> Despite the marvelous intricacy of the inner ear with its thousands of hair cells and nerve fibers providing sensitivity to both frequency and intensity of auditory vibrations, there is only a finite number of such hair cells and nerve endings; if enough of them are destroyed by disease, trauma, or toxicity, or if simply absent by reason of maldevelopment, the individual may have total incapacity for any useful auditory functioning. (p. 120)

Comprehensive assessment, conducted as early as possible by both audiologists and physicians, is a critical element in ensuring that children have as much capacity for useful auditory functioning as possible. Although some states now mandate neonatal screening, particularly for high-risk infants, not all do. Early amplification is also essential. The intricate auditory pathways from the inner ear to the brain are most likely to mature and to assume their usual role in providing linguistic stimulation to key areas of the central nervous system if they can carry acoustic information from the earliest days of life, long before infants can be expected to talk or to understand language. The value of early identification and provision of amplification has been confirmed repeatedly, and their importance cannot be overstated in helping to ensure that children have the best possible biological mechanisms (augmented by hearing aids whenever necessary) for supporting normal language acquisition.

Sensorineural hearing losses may be mixed with conductive losses across the severity spectrum (Northern & Downs, 1984; see Table 4.3). Ongoing audiological and medical monitoring are critical to intervention whenever hearing loss is suspected, even if it is mild and intermittent.

Linguistic system factors. Ample evidence from the auditory–oral language-learning difficulties of people who are deaf from an early age indicates that hearing is critical to normal acquisition of spoken language (Geers & Moog, 1989) and therefore is classified as an essential contributing factor to language disorders in deaf children. However, the evidence is equally striking that people who are deaf, if given sufficient opportunity and if no other handicapping conditions are present, have no difficulty acquiring a fully developed system of sign language (Quigley & Paul, 1984).

An interesting middle ground is occupied by children who basically have had to create their own "language" of natural gestures. This was reported by Goldin-Meadow and Feldman (1977), who studied a group of six deaf children ranging in age from 17 to 49 months. The children's parents had decided not to expose them to manual sign but to concentrate on providing oral education (however, the authors neither described the oral education methods nor commented on the provision of amplification). Nevertheless, at the time of the study, the children had not learned to produce spontaneously generated oral language. The researchers videotaped the children interacting informally at home with their mothers and toys and other objects. Then they analyzed the nat-

urally occurring gestures the children used to augment their communicative needs. The gestures not only were representational, they were produced in phrasal sequences. One child gestured about a shovel, first, establishing the topic by pointing to a picture of one (a nominative meaning), then pointing downstairs where a shovel was stored (a locative meaning), and also producing a digging motion in the air with two fists (a predicative meaning), before finally pointing downstairs again. The authors interpreted such examples as supporting the existence of an innate language processing system.

However, others (e.g., I. M. Schlesinger, 1981) have pointed out that a cognitive level, in which concepts and relations are built on basic understanding of the world, is separate from a semantic level, in which cognitive relations are related to linguistic meaning. Chomsky (1980) also suggested that the semantic component of language may be more closely related to a cognitive/conceptual module; whereas the syntactic component of language is more closely related to the linguistic module.

Although the central meanings of language might be so firmly embedded in human potential that they can be generated spontaneously without exposure to models, a closer look at the spoken or written language produced by most hearing impaired children (even those with some hearing) shows that certain linguistic elements are more difficult to master than others with impaired hearing. As discussed previously, these tend to be the unstressed elements, such as morphological endings and grammatical function words. Such elements are more difficult to hear and also carry less meaning. Thus, syntax and morphology, two central aspects of linguistic functioning, are almost invariably affected by hearing loss, perhaps even by the relatively mild losses associated with persistent OME (although this last contention is still controversial). Not only syntactical systems but lexical and referential systems also can suffer when hearing is impaired. Literal meanings do not appear to be as difficult for hearing impaired children to master as figurative meanings are. This makes sense, of course, if one considers that figurative meanings are learned almost exclusively through language. For example, normal-hearing children have opportunities to be exposed daily to hundreds of idiomatic expressions (e.g., "Don't bug me, I'm talking on the phone"; think here of the more literal meanings of *bug* and *on*) just in the process of hearing or overhearing language used in natural

TABLE 4.3
Hearing handicap as a function of average hearing threshold level of the better ear

Average Threshold Level at 500–2000 Hz (ANSI)*	Description	Common Causes	What Can Be Heard without Amplification	Degrees of Handicap (if not treated in 1st year of life)	Probable Needs
0–15 dB	Normal range		All speech sounds	None	None
16–25 dB	Slight hearing loss	Serous otitis, perforation, monomeric membrane, sensorineural loss, tympanosclerosis	Vowel sounds heard clearly, may miss unvoiced consonant sounds	Possible mild or transitory auditory dysfunction Difficulty in perceiving some speech sounds	Consideration of need for hearing aid Lip reading Auditory training Speech therapy Preferential seating Appropriate surgery
26–40 dB	Mild	Serous otitis, perforation, tympanosclerosis, monomeric membrane, sensorineural loss	Hears only some speech sounds; the louder voiced sounds	Auditory learning dysfunction Mild language retardation Mild speech problems Inattention	Hearing aid Lip reading Auditory training Speech therapy Appropriate surgery
41–65 dB	Moderate hearing loss	Chronic otitis, middle ear anomaly, sensorineural loss	Misses most speech sounds at normal conversational level	Speech problems Language retardation Learning dysfunction Inattention	All of the above, plus consideration of special classroom situation
66–95 dB	Severe hearing loss	Sensorineural loss or mixed loss due to sensorineural loss plus middle ear disease	Hears no speech or sound of normal conversations	Severe speech problems Language retardation Learning dysfunction Inattention	All of the above; probable assignment to special classes
96+ dB	Profound hearing loss	Sensorineural loss or mixed	Hears no speech or other sounds	Severe speech problems Language retardation Learning dysfunction Inattention	All of the above; probable assignment to special classes

*ANSI = American National Standards Institute.

Note. From *Hearing in Children* (3rd ed., p. 89) by J. L. Northern and M. P. Downs, 1984, Baltimore, Md: Williams & Wilkins. Copyright 1984 by Williams & Wilkins. Reprinted by permission.

contexts that are not intended for directly teaching language.

Stimulus–response–reinforcement factors. Sensory impairment can directly affect the ability to receive adequate stimulation to learn language and to be reinforced for using it appropriately and naturally. Therefore, stimulus–response–reinforcement factors are considered probable contributing factors to childhood language disorders in hearing impaired children. Behavioral theory has implications for understanding the influence of hearing loss on other aspects of development. As in other categories of disability, the behavioral patterns that result from disruption of normal stimulus–response–reinforcement options may be deeply intertwined with social interaction considerations, and to separate them for purposes of these discussions is somewhat artificial.

For example, the discovery that a child has a serious hearing impairment can affect the quality of early interactions of parents with their infant, and the specialized stimulation and reinforcement needs of both should be recognized in early intervention efforts. Ling (1984b) described ways in which hearing impairment may reduce the quality of parent–child interaction in complex cycles of causative interaction. He noted that the lack of response to auditory stimulation on the part of the child may reduce the frequency of social behaviors such as looking, laughing, vocalizing, and smiling, which tend to be reinforcing to parents and serve to maintain the frequency of social interactions. The result of the child's reduced responsiveness may be reduced responsiveness from the mother, particularly if she has had any difficulty in accepting the hearing impairment; she may convey elements of rejection without realizing it. Intervention can help to reduce the likelihood that maladaptive cycles will result.

Consider also the effects on parents' behavior management options with their older children when the ability to reason with spoken language is severely curtailed by hearing loss. Noting the problems that parents with normal hearing often experience in becoming fluent in sign language, and recognizing the natural needs of all parents for behavior-management methods, Moeller (1989, October) used behavior management as a context for teaching hearing parents to learn to use more elaborate signed language communications with their children. For example, rather than communicating, "Stop that!," Moeller urged the parents in her training sessions to sign and say, "It is not polite to stare." Rather than saying, "Leave the cat

alone," parents practiced communicating something like, "He likes gentle touching." In essence, Moeller was teaching parents to use more elaborate linguistic stimuli as models for their children's language development, while at the same time using behavior-management strategies that encouraged rational self-control in their children.

Information processing factors. When a child's hearing is sufficiently impaired to interfere with normal language acquisition, reduction of information from the primary linguistic input source affects the entire processing system. Information processing factors therefore are essential contributing factors to language disorders in these children. Auditorily, children have to learn to make more out of less information if hearing is to become a useful avenue for them. The fitting of appropriate amplification as early as possible is a critical feature in maximizing this auditory potential (Bess, Freeman, & Sinclair, 1981).

Questions of information processing are deeply embedded within the long-standing debates about how best to help children to acquire language and learning skills. Essentially, two major types of intervention approaches have been advocated for use with hearing impaired children: (1) oral–aural options, and (2) total communication options (Ling, 1984a).

Those who advocate oral–aural options argue that "spoken language has emerged as the universal means of basic communication not by chance, but because the central nervous system and physiological nature of mankind render it the most efficient means of human communication" (Ling, 1984a, p. 9). To be maximally independent as adults, advocates argue, hearing impaired children must be educated using oral–aural approaches. As a special subcategory of oral communication options, unisensory programs are implemented without formal training of lipreading and do not actively encourage use of the visual modality. Pollack's (1984) "acoupedic" approach is an oral–aural unisensory program in which intervention focuses primarily on the use of audition for language acquisition.

Total communication options are based on the philosophy that all visual–manual and/or auditory roles in communication are complementary and that encouragement of all avenues of communication is a part of full acceptance of the child as hearing impaired, setting the stage for development of a healthy self-concept. Other key elements of this philosophy are that use of a multisensory approach can increase the child's learning potential and can provide an early form of communication, which provides a base for further language development (Ling, 1984b).

Written language acquisition is a goal of both oral–aural and total communication approaches. The obvious difficulties hearing impaired children experience in receiving auditory information might make written language seem to be a preferred input modality. However, there is nothing magical about the written form (Ling & Ling, 1978). The finding that many students with hearing impairments read no higher than the third-grade level by the end of high school provides additional support for the contention that reading is basically an auditory-linguistic skill and not visual.

Cognition factors. Cognitive abilities for hearing impaired children, as measured by performance IQ scores, may appear across the same range as those of normally hearing children. However, they may be distributed somewhat differently. For example, J. M. Davis, Elfenbein, Schum, and Bentler (1986) had to eliminate 4 (out of 45) potential subjects in a study of students with mild-to-moderate hearing impairments and no other exceptionalities because their performance IQs were greater than 130. At the other end of the spectrum, however, evidence suggests that multiple handicaps, including cognitive ones, are more likely to occur among children who are deaf than among children with milder forms of hearing loss. Levitt et al. (1988) found multiple handicaps among 33% of the deaf populations they studied, whereas Shepard, Davis, Gorga, and Stelmachowicz (1981) found them among only 13% of a public school population with milder hearing impairments.

What can the experiences of children with hearing impairments contribute to discussions about the relationships of language and cognition? A primary effect of hearing impairment is to limit auditory-linguistic input as a source of information for forming concepts about the world. By studying the effects on cognitive development, researchers might be able to gain added insight into the question of whether language is necessary for the development of the full range of cognitive abilities.

Myklebust (1964) argued that loss of sensation could impede both the development of language and the development of cognition. He based his argument on a hierarchy of processing that proceeded from lower to higher levels: sensation, perception, imagery, symbolization, and conceptualization. The loss of auditory sensation, Myklebust hypothesized, would result in an organismic shift, in which the loss of auditory sensation (and greater reliance on visual sensation) would impair auditory-linguistic symbolization, and that limitation would, in turn, impair the ability of people with hearing impairments to think abstractly.

Others disagreed with Myklebust's theory and designed studies showing few differences between the cognitive abilities of deaf and normal-hearing individuals (Furth, 1966; Vernon, 1969). For example, based on a study measuring performance on a set of Piagetian tasks, Furth concluded that deaf children's ideas about the world develop in the same sequence as those of children with normal hearing, and with only slight delay (particularly in stages of concrete and formal operations). Furth reasoned that problems demonstrated by children with hearing impairment on IQ tests represented results of communicative difficulties rather than low intelligence.

Others have suggested that the language limitations associated with hearing impairment do interfere with later stages of cognitive development, particularly for performing cognitive activities in which mental manipulation of linguistic symbols is critical (Quigley & Paul, 1984; H. S. Schlesinger & Meadow, 1972). When J. M. Davis et al. (1986) measured a variety of language, intellectual, social, and academic skills, they found that performance IQ was not a good predictor of overall educational success by hearing impaired children (although it was correlated significantly to both reasoning and math scores). The best predictor of concurrent academic achievement in that study was a verbal IQ score, followed by vocabulary scores earned on the Peabody Picture Vocabulary Test—Revised (PPVT-R) (L. M. Dunn & Dunn, 1981).

Somewhat different results were found in a study of 6- to 10-year-old children who were learning a system of signed English language, however, (Watson, Sullivan, Moeller, & Jensen, 1982). In this case, nonverbal intelligence and visual memory skills were found to be the best predictors of language performance. In fact, the average correlation of .45 between nonverbal IQ and language scores for the hearing impaired children in this study was only slightly lower than the .50 correlation reported for intelligence and measure of school achievement for normal-hearing children (Matarazzo, 1972). Watson et al. concluded that nonverbal intelligence is a factor in helping children acquire language (particularly a visually based system such as signed English). Studies like this contribute to growing evidence that language and cognition are closely related but not totally interdependent.

Social interaction factors. Social interaction factors are considered probable contributing factors in childhood language disorders among hearing impaired children. When hearing loss is identified, the cyclical patterns of social interaction between parents and babies are disrupted (see previous discussion of stimulus–response–reinforcement). Moses (1985) described the social aspects of parental discovery that their child has a significant hearing loss as a grieving process, which parents tend to repeat working through each time the child reaches a new milestone.

Although hearing loss is generally recognized as affecting the social interactions of children with their parents, peers, and important others, the degree of loss is not a particularly good predictor of problems in the psychosocial realm. This was one of the conclusions of the study by J. M. Davis et al. (1986) in which they assessed 45 children in a variety of areas who ranged in age from 5 to 18 years and had mild-to-moderate hearing losses. Although degree of hearing loss was not a good predictor of psychosocial difficulty, data from personality inventories administered to these youngsters did suggest that they were more likely than their normal hearing peers to show certain social interaction and self-concept problems, including aggressive tendencies and a tendency to express more physical complaints. In addition, parent observations indicated that a higher than average proportion of the hearing impaired children demonstrated significant behavior difficulties, especially school problems involving isolation and adjustment to school (see Personal Reflection 4.4)

Visual Impairment

Definitions, differential diagnosis, and subdivisions.
Loss of vision does not have the same devastating effect on language acquisition as loss of hearing. Because language is learned primarily through auditory–vocal modalities, vision is less critical than hearing to language acquisition. Vision, of course, plays a vital role in learning to read in the usual way, but the relative ease with which blind children learn braille when they have no concomitant cognitive impairments supports the contention that reading is far more a linguistic-communicative act than it is a visual act. Adaptive technology, such as talking computers and print-scanning devices, can transform printed or computer text into spoken output so that blind children can have more independent access for using language in varied modalities.

This is not to say that vision in unimportant to the process of normal language acquisition and social communicative development. The earliest form of communication between neonates and their mothers is visual. In fact, advocates of natural childbirth emphasize the importance of allowing new mothers to gaze into the eyes of their newborns as part of the bonding process. Furthermore, as considered later in the sections on child abuse and neglect, disruptions of normal patterns of gaze and eye contact tend to accompany maladaptive child-rearing patterns, perhaps in interactive patterns of cyclical cause and effect (see Personal Reflection 4.5).

If vision is so important, what is the effect of visual loss on the language acquisition process? Erin (1990) refuted the "myth of compensatory ability" (p. 181), which suggests that blind or visually impaired children must have exceptional abilities in audition and language production as automatic compensations for their losses of vision. Erin's own research results were consistent with others' in confirming risks for delay in language use in specific areas among children with visual impairments (Fraiberg, 1977, 1979; Kekelis & Anderson, 1984; Mills, 1983; D. H. Warren, 1984).

Both age of onset and degree of loss may influence the effect of visual impairment on language acquisition. Complete congenital blindness is more likely to influence language acquisition significantly than is partial blindness. Erin (1990) compared the language characteristics of four children who were blind (light

---

| Personal Reflection 4.4 | "I don't have very many friends. Oh, people say, 'Hi, Kris, Hi Kris,' but only 'Hi Kris,' never anything—you know—go out for lunch or go out on dates or anything like that. The only friends I almost have are my teachers and my counselors." |

Kris, an adolescent with hearing impairment interviewed by J. M. Davis et al. (1986) during their study of the effects of mild-to-moderate hearing impairments on language, educational, and psychosocial behavior in children.

Personal Reflection 4.5   "Sometimes when we have professional visitors at the project to look at films or videotapes, I steal glances at their faces when the child is seen on the screen. With sighted children it is always interesting to see the resonance of mood on the viewer's face. We smile when the baby on the film smiles; we are sober when the baby is distressed. We laugh sympathetically when the baby looks indignant at the examiner's sneakiness. We frown in concentration as the baby frowns when the toy disappears. When he drops a toy, we look below the movie screen to help him find it.

But the blind baby on the screen does not elicit these spontaneous moods in the visitor. Typically, the visitor's face remains solemn. This is partly a reaction to blindness itself. But it is also something else. There is a large vocabulary of expressive behavior that one does not see in a blind baby at all. The absence of differentiated signs on the baby's face is mirrored in the face of the observer."

Selma Fraiberg (1979. p. 151), University of Michigan Medical School, writing about some of the sociolinguistic side effects when infants are unable to see.

perception or less), four who had low vision (legally blind but able to respond to a flashlight at 15 feet), and four who were sighted (none with other disabling conditions). She found contrasts in several areas (syntactic complexity, pronoun usage, and language functions) between the two groups of visually impaired children and the sighted children. The differences were more prominent, however, in the samples of the blind children than the low-vision children.

Other minor vision problems identified during elementary school years are not insignificant, especially because they may influence written language acquisition and the processing of academic language in school. On the other hand, when recognized, minor losses in visual acuity can be easily compensated by the fitting of glasses. Such problems have never been associated with general delays in language acquisition.

When a child has total or near-total blindness from the earliest stages of development, three kinds of interrelated influences tend to show up in the areas of language and communication. First, a major avenue through which the child learns about the world, forms semantic concepts, and acquires lexical knowledge is lost (Dunlea, 1989). Katherine Nelson (1985) has pointed out that since the time of Augustine, the classic description of word learning has been that of a tutor pointing to objects while uttering their names. Although K. Nelson (1985) notes that referential–perceptual theories are not the only way, nor the most complete way, to explain the acquisition of first-word meanings, evidence has shown that children learn many new words

in this way, including from photographs or other pictorial forms (Ninio, 1983; Ninio & Bruner, 1978).

Second, certain language abilities seem to be more sensitive than others to acquisition without sight. Pronoun use has been shown to be especially difficult for blind children to master (Erin, 1990; Fay, 1973; Fraiberg, 1977; House & House, 1989; Keeler, 1958). Many children with visual impairments are observed to refer to themselves by name or as "you," and, more rarely, to call others "I" or "me." Erin (1990) also found reductions in mean length of utterance and variety of sentence types. Visually impaired children also talked less about past and future events and used language less to initiate imaginative play.

The third area in which children without sight are at risk is in the area of pragmatics. Many of the nonverbal cues for turn taking and other aspects of conversational interaction are unavailable to children who have low vision. Limited opportunities to learn about language and communication through play and other natural interactions also may influence language learning negatively. For example, Erin (1990) hypothesized that the high frequency of questions and imperatives observed among the visually impaired children she studied could be explained by their awareness that others have more access to information from the environment. This could increase their tendency to use language to gather information and to confirm impressions about physical factors in the environment.

Relationships of contributing factors. *Biological maturation.* The loss of peripheral vision represents a frank physiological difference between children who can see and those who cannot. Biological impairment is thus a key aspect of the disability. The effects on communicative development for children who are blind are often complicated by other physiological conditions, including deafness, which may be directly related to a genetic syndrome that causes the blindness and other problems or which may be indirectly related through another common cause. An example of direct relationship is Usher syndrome, which is the most common cause of deaf-blindness. It involves profound congenital deafness accompanied by progressive blindness resulting from retinitis pigmentosa (S. E. Gerber, 1990). An example of an indirect relationship is through the effects of maternal rubella, which commonly results in a combination of hearing loss, mental retardation, and ocular defects. Juvenile diabetes can also lead to diabetic retinopathy, the leading cause of blindness in the United States (S. E. Gerber, 1990). Whatever the cause of the blindness, professionals should always question whether other aspects of the biological apparatus, critical to language and other development, also might be involved.

Linguistic system factors. In blind children, linguistic system factors are often found in association with childhood language disorders, but the degree of involvement may vary. Hypotheses for explaining the problems exhibited by blind children in making the *I–you* distinction vary from psychodynamic to psycholinguistic ones. The similarities noted to the difficulties of autistic children led Charney (1980) to propose that pronoun reversals can be directly explained by cognitive or linguistic deficits taking two forms: (1) Either reversals are a direct by-product of echolalia (attributed to linguistic deficits), or (2) reversals and echolalia are both caused by a common cognitive deficit. Schiff-Myers (1983) lent support to the linguistic-base hypothesis when she analyzed the pronoun reversals produced by her own normally developing daughter when the child was between 21 and 25 months old. Those analyses showed that the pronoun-reversal pattern was related to (1) a tendency to imitate utterances of others (possibly similar to the gestalt language acquisition style discussed earlier in the section on autism); (2) early production of *you* as a productive linguistic form; and (3) a tendency to use a pronoun rather than a noun for self-reference. Other attempts to explain pronoun reversal have ranged from hypotheses about blind children's need for an extended learning

period to master self-representation (Erin, 1990), to more specific sensory input problems in matching the spoken *I* or *you* with the person addressed when that person cannot be seen (D. H. Warren, 1984).

Stimulus–response–reinforcement factors. Obviously, blindness does limit a major source of stimulus input, and stimulus–response–reinforcement factors are probable contributing factors to language disorders in visually impaired children. Blindness influences the child's choice and monitoring of response modes. Although no one has suggested the use of behaviorist methods of selective reinforcement to treat the visual problem for which there is a clear biological cause, behaviorist methods of analysis may promote understanding and prevention of maladaptive communicative patterns that may be more likely to arise in children without sight. For example, children who cannot see should not be reinforced for interrupting others during conversation, just as other children are not. They may, however, need to be guided to become more sensitive to auditory cues that signal an opportunity to enter a conversation, and their conversational partners may need to be guided jointly in setting appropriate standards for these kinds of pragmatic skills at varied points of development.

Information processing factors. House and House (1989) noted that loss of vision represents the loss of the sensory organ most uniquely adapted for synthesis of all perceptions and the data of self. Variations from normal information processing are clearly essential contributing factors affecting general development in individuals with visual impairment, and they necessitate the use of compensatory techniques, particularly for reading and writing. However, the relationships of information processing, as influenced by blindness, to the acquisition of language, have not been extensively studied. When vision and hearing are both lost, the effects on the acquisition of communication are clearly devastating.

Cognition factors. Children who have blindness and no other impairments may show the normal variation in general cognitive ability. Because of causative patterns, however, cognitive deficits may play a role for a greater proportion of visually impaired children than for the general population.

Social interaction factors. Social interaction factors are often associated with childhood language disorders among blind persons, but their degree of involvement may vary. For example, difficulty in constructing an image of self and others in the absence of vision has been hypothesized as one explanation of the delay in the acquisition of *I* as a concept and as a stable pronominal form. For blind children to understand that they must refer to themselves as *I* and to others as *you*, they must clearly differentiate between themselves and others. This is more difficult without sight (Fraiberg, 1977).

Communicative partners' environmental adaptations to the visual deficit may also influence such symptoms as the delay in pronoun acquisition. For example, House and House (1989) studied children who were multiply handicapped and blind, had an MLU of 1.0 to 1.8, and lived in a residential setting. The researchers observed that many staff members addressed the blind children with their proper names in all activities and used the pronouns *I* and *you* infrequently. Perhaps variation in opportunity to learn pronominal reference plays a significant role in its developmental delay for some blind children.

Fraiberg (1979) noted that modifications in social interactions are to be expected when infants are without sight. She commented that, "What we miss in the blind baby, apart from the eyes that do not see, is the vocabulary of signs and signals that provides the most elementary and vital sense of discourse long before words have meaning" (p. 152). The usual milestones of human attachment, however, may be observed among blind infants during the first 2 years of life, who are like their sighted peers in preferences for their mothers, differential smiling and vocalization, manual tactile seeking, embracing, and spontaneous gestures of affection and comfort seeking. From 7 to 15 months of age, blind toddlers, like sighted ones, begin to avoid and manifest stress reactions to strangers and reject them as interaction partners. During the 2nd year, blind children's anxiety at separation and comfort at reunion provide evidence that the blind baby values the mother as an indispensable human partner.

Physical Impairment and Speech Motor Control

Definitions, differential diagnosis, and subdivisions. An estimated 1,225,000 children in the United States alone do not learn to speak or are severely speech impaired as a result of neurological, physical, or psychological disabilities (D. Yoder, 1980). For many of these children, physical impairment co-

occurs with other risk factors, such as cognitive impairment or sensory loss, conditions that may themselves interfere with normal language acquisition. In cases of mixed causes, it is difficult to differentiate the influence of the motor impairment from other factors. Some children, however, exhibit a severe physical impairment, such as cerebral palsy, which greatly impedes their ability to learn to speak but leaves their cognitive and linguistic systems relatively intact. What kinds of variations in language acquisition can be expected for such children?

Returning to the discussions about the relative separability of language, speech, and communication from Chapter 2, apparently children can have normal potential for learning language in the presence of severe deficits of motor functioning that prevent them from acquiring intelligible speech. Limited information is available about the developmental process in such cases, however. In the past, the language development of children with severe motor impairments was rarely studied in detail because the current usual modes of investigation, spontaneous language sampling and analysis, were not available. Widespread provision of augmentative and alternative communication (AAC) avenues is still a relatively recent phenomenon. Even now, when AAC techniques are more likely to be encouraged during early language acquisition stages, the language expression of nonspeaking children, at least before the development of literacy, is heavily constrained by the vocabulary and phrases that someone else has included on their communication boards or programmed into their vocal output communication devices.

It is difficult to obtain a true picture of what nonspeaking children can do with language. The usual assessment techniques simply do not work, particularly for assessment of language expression, but also for assessment of language-input comprehension. Language comprehension skills may tend to be overestimated (Roth & Cassatt-James, 1989). Efforts have been made to study the pragmatic interaction problems that also often accompany the nonspeaking child's efforts to learn to communicate, such as passivity in conversation, but methodological problems abound in the research, and more investigation is needed in all areas of language acquisition with these children (Calculator, 1988; Light, 1988; Sutton, 1989).

Evidence for subtypes related to physical impairment. One question that still needs to be addressed is whether there are recognizable subtypes among children who have difficulty learning to speak as a result of physical impairments. Certainly, physical impairment can differ in degree and kind, based on such factors as varied cause and time of onset. It is beyond the scope of this chapter to consider all of the factors that can lead children to have difficulty acquiring motor control of the speech mechanism (e.g., cerebral palsy comprises several subtypes, and acquired brain injuries can result in others) or to have structural defects of the oral mechanism (e.g., burns and oral-facial anomalies). It is important, however, to differentiate the kinds of oral-motor impairment associated with symptoms of dysarthria from those associated with symptoms of oral-motor and speech apraxia.

There is precedent for considering these subdivisions when relating types of oral-motor impairment and language disorders. As discussed earlier in this chapter, a subgroup of the phonologic-syntactic syndrome described by Rapin and Allen (1983) was one in which an expressive disorder seems to predominate, accompanied by additional signs of neurologic oromotor dysfunction, including signs of mild dysarthria (demonstrated by drooling and a history of difficulty in sucking, chewing, and swallowing) or signs or oral-motor apraxia (demonstrated by difficulty in imitating precise movements of the tongue, lips, and jaw).

The subcategory of *developmental apraxia of speech* (J. C. Rosenbek & Wertz, 1972; Yoss & Darley, 1974) is controversial. It has also been called *childhood verbal apraxia* (Chappel, 1973) and *developmental verbal dyspraxia* (Crary, 1984). The controversy revolves around whether children with specific, severe expressive speech and language delay constitute a legitimate category based on deficits in motor planing that affect primarily the operation of the speech mechanism, or whether the observed delays in speech production capability are more representative of central problems in the phonological conceptualization of sound classes and combinations.

The primary characteristics used in diagnosing children with developmental verbal apraxia are outlined in Box 4.11. It is noteworthy that these characteristics describe speech behavior and generally fail to identify any symptoms of expressive language, except to note its significant delay relative to superior receptive language abilities. In actual practice, many children with signs of oral-motor and speech apraxia also appear to have specific language delays of probable central origin.

Without referring to developmental verbal apraxia (or even testing for it directly), Rescorla and Manzella (1990) reported on a group of 20 toddlers with normal cognitive ability and good receptive language at age 2

Box 4.11   The most common features in developmental apraxia of speech (based on summaries from J. C. Rosenbeck & Wertz, 1972, and Yoss & Darley, 1974)

1. **Neurological findings** of dyspraxia may be generalized, possibly including difficulty in fine motor coordination, gait, and alternating motion rates of the tongue and extremities. The condition may occur in isolation or in combination with aphasia and/or dysarthria. Oral nonverbal apraxia, often, but not always, accompanies apraxia of speech.

2. **Speech development** is delayed or deviant, with receptive abilities markedly superior to expressive ones.

3. **Repetition (imitation) tasks** may result in two- and three-feature articulation errors (e.g., /p/ for /m/ is an error in nasality, voicing and continuancy). Groping trial-and-error behaviors may appear in the form of sound prolongations, repetitions, or silent posturing, preceding or interrupting the imitative utterances. Single-word productions on articulation tests may be surprisingly good, however, considering the unintelligibility of connected speech.

4. **Spontaneous speech** includes a predominance of omission errors but also evidence of other immature phonological processes (and phonetic distortions). Misarticulations include vowels as well as consonants. Errors vary with the complexity of articulatory adjustment, with more frequent errors on fricatives, affricatives, and consonant clusters, and on longer words. Metathetic errors (transpositions of sounds and syllables) and phonetic transition problems are frequent.

5. **Rate and prosody** are affected in spontaneous speaking and on diadochokinetic tasks (e.g., "puhtuhkuh"). Words and syllables are produced with slowed rate, even stress, and even spacing, perhaps in compensation for the problem.

years, whom they followed until the age of 3. They identified this group of children as having specific expressive language delay (SELD). When they compared the group with 10 matched toddlers, the children with SELD continued to be significantly delayed with respect to MLU, use of obligatory morphemes, and grammatical development relative to the comparison children. Because the phonological and oral-motor skills were not reported, it is difficult to know whether any or all of these children might exhibit signs of verbal apraxia.

Written language processing by physically impaired individuals. When individuals with physical impairments become literate, it is somewhat easier to assess their spontaneous expressive language abilities by asking them to write, particularly if they have sufficient motor control to operate a typewriter or computer keyboard (perhaps with scanning or Morse code adaptation). Of course, if they have difficulty learning to read and write, we are back to the problem of knowing whether their difficulties are related to a basic language deficit, a lack of experience (because of their motor impairments) in using formalized written language, a more isolated reading and/or writing disorder, or some other factor(s).

Some researchers have attempted to investigate the relationships of written language acquisition to frank neurological deficits. It is not always clear, however, whether motor deficits or other neurological signs have led to inclusion in the subject groups studied. Seidel, Chadwick, and Rutter (1975) found a higher incidence of reading problems in children who had experienced perinatal brain injury than in the normally developing population. Mattis, French, and Rapin (1975) studied reading disorder subtypes by comparing the abilities of children with diagnosed neurological impairments with and without reading disabilities with those of dyslexic children (without overt neurological disorder) on several tasks. They found no difference in the types of reading disability among neurologically impaired and dyslexic children, and they also found neurologically impaired children who were good readers and showed no signs of dyslexia.

Mattis (1978) noted that many symptoms frequently associated with dyslexia (e.g., dyscoordination, dysarthria, and deficits in drawing and in puzzle and block construction) could be observed in neurologically impaired children who were good readers. If such is the case, Mattis hypothesized, then these underlying skills could not be essential to the reading process. Apparently, input–output modes used in reading and writing can vary without interfering with the central aspect of the written language processing—that is, the representation of meaning. It is recognition of the meaningfulness of orthography that is the essence of written language processing, not the manner in which stimuli and products are received or produced. It is only necessary that individuals have at least one mode of input and output available, not that they necessarily must be able to read or write in the most conventional ways (e.g., braille and AAC users).

Dorman (1987) found results that contrasted somewhat with those of Mattis (1978) regarding individuals with diagnosed neurological impairments. Dorman studied neurologically impaired students with cerebral palsy ($n = 23$), spina bifida ($n = 9$), neuromuscular impairments ($n = 16$), and head injury ($n = 2$) and divided them almost equally into reading disabled and non-reading disabled subgroups. Dorman did find that more neurologically impaired reading disabled than non-reading disabled students could be classified into the three subtypes identified by Mattis (anomic language disorder, articulatory-graphomotor dyscoordination, and visual-spatial-perceptual disorder). Dorman found that 19 of the 23 students with cerebral palsy had symptoms of visual-spatial-perceptual disorder, whether or not they had reading impairments as well. When neurologically impaired individuals with visual-spatial-perceptual disorder did have reading problems, they were likely also to evidence signs of anomic language disorder. The fact that persons with anomic language disorders almost always exhibited reading difficulty (whereas those with isolated visual-spatial-perceptual disorders did not) supports the contention that language skills play a more central role in written language processing than do visual-spatial-perceptual skills.

A problem for clinicians who might wish to draw on Dorman's (1987) data is that Dorman did not specify whether any of the subjects with cerebral palsy could be classified as nonspeaking. It might be assumed that they were not, because nonspeaking children would have difficulty responding to the read-aloud tasks used in Dorman's study. Many questions remain about the influence of inability to produce spoken language on written language processing. In children with specific dyslexia, phonological processing skills seem to be important (Stanovich, 1986, 1988). Therefore, one might assume that inability to speak might influence the processes of learning to read and write, and that, in such cases, the phonological decoding and encoding difficulties might be expected to show up as problems in learning to read and spell.

Not much research is available, however, on the written language processing abilities of nonspeaking individuals (Kelford-Smith, Thurston, Light, Parnes & O'Keefe, 1989; Koppenhaver & Yoder, 1988). Koppenhaver and Yoder summarized existing research on literacy-learning characteristics of AAC users as showing (1) delays and difficulty in learning to read and write; (2) positive relationships between number of decoding strategies and reading achievement; (3) uneven profiles of strengths and weaknesses, with some persistent difficulties even among literate individuals and adults; and (4) reports of beneficial effects from auditory feedback during instructional activities.

One study (Kelford-Smith et al., 1989) sheds some light on the acquisition of written language by individuals with severe physical impairments. Six AAC users with cerebral palsy in Toronto were given formal instruction in reading and computerized access to independent writing relatively late in childhood (at about age 10 years for all but one subject). All of the individuals were in their late adolescence to young adulthood at the time of the study. The researchers gathered and analyzed all written language output that the individuals produced using their home computers over 4 weeks. All six of the individuals had functional writing skills at the time of the study, indicating that they had made the transition from Blissymbols (a graphic symbol system) to traditional orthography "despite decreased access to normal speech upon which written language is thought to be mapped, despite the use of telegraphic output in their face-to-face interactions, and despite the fact that they were all provided with access to microcomputer systems and introduced to literacy programs relatively late in their academic careers" (p. 122). In addition to functional written language skills, however, the six individuals also demonstrated (to varying degrees) limitations in the use of morphological endings, functors, auxiliaries, and complex sentence formulation. The authors speculated that these characteristics may have been due to language-based problems among some of the subjects, performance limitations, or monitoring and editing limitations.

Relationships of contributing factors. *Biological maturation.* Physical impairment can be congenital or acquired, mild or severe, but it always involves a diagnosed impairment of the biological mechanism. The question germane to this discussion is, how much does the impact of the physical disability influence the acquisition of language? Although physical impairment is classified here as being peripheral to the language acquisition process, it almost always (except in the cases of degenerative muscular diseases or peripheral structural malformations) involves abnormalities in the central nervous system. Yet, when central nervous system impairment is marked enough to produce symptoms of motor difficulty in learning to talk, it is difficult to determine to what degree the motor-speech symptoms may be isolated from other aspects of linguistic-cognitive development or to what degree the agent that caused the central nervous system dysfunction in the motor system may have affected other systems as well.

Linguistic system factors. Case study and research reports of individuals who are nonspeaking but appear to have basically normal language suggest that linguistic system factors are only indirectly related to physical impairments that impede the development of speech. It is easier to make this statement with confidence, however, for the subgroup of physically impaired individuals who have neuromotor impairments that result in impaired motor control for chewing and swallowing and dysarthric speech (as caused by cerebral palsy) than it is for those children who have symptoms of oral-motor and speech apraxia. For children with developmental verbal apraxia, morphological development difficulties and other symptoms of specific language impairment are often integral factors.

Stimulus–response–reinforcement factors. Because stimulus–response modes are clearly influenced by physical impairment, behaviorist explanations are rarely invoked to explain any of the learning difficulties related to the biological involvement per se. However, physical impairment can result in changes in the environmental opportunities and natural reinforcers available to individuals who are nonspeaking or who have limited ability to express themselves orally. Such factors need to be considered when designing intervention programs, and are considered probable contributing factors for language disorders in children with physical impairments.

When employing techniques of selective reinforcement, professionals also need to be vigilant, lest they find themselves reinforcing, or failing to reinforce, communicativeness under the guise of modifying the response mode behavior of a child who is physically impaired. For example, Beukelman (1987) commented on the confusing consequences that are sometimes provided to young AAC users when response modes, rather than message communication, are used as criteria for providing natural reinforcement for attempts to communicate (see Personal Reflection 4.6).

Information processing factors. By definition, individuals with severe physical impairments have limitations of output modes in their information processing systems, and, thus, information processing factors are essential contributing factors to language disorders in these children. In addition, Dorman's (1987) research showed that the majority of individuals with cerebral palsy have symptoms of visuospatial-perceptual disorder, which may or may not be associated with difficulties in learning to read. The problems inherent in investigating how these difficulties influence inner processing have already been discussed. Future research, it is hoped, will add to understanding in this area.

Cognition factors. The cognitive skills of individuals with physical impairments affecting speech, language, and communication can vary across the spectrum from severely retarded to gifted. However, individuals with congenital problems involving the central nervous system are at greater risk for having multiple impairments, including mental retardation (Baroff, 1986).

Social interaction factors. Cycles of balanced interactions between care givers and infants are reported to be critical to normal development (see related discussion in the section on neglect and abuse). When children are born with physical impairments, it may be particularly difficult for them to send and receive reciprocal signals with care givers regarding their receptiveness to stimulation. For example, Brazelton (1982) reported on the work of Kathryn Barnard, who found that new mothers were at first repelled by the disturbing movements of their motor-impaired children. However, when the mothers watched therapists synchronize their movements with those of their physically impaired infants, the mother could see that their babies picked up the information and showed positive responsiveness. Subsequently, the mothers were able to imitate the therapist and become more synchronous with their infants for the first time.

Variations in social interaction patterns continue to play a role in language acquisition and communication for developing physically impaired individuals and are considered probable contributing factors to language disorders in these children. Light (1988) reviewed the interaction research conducted with individuals who use AAC systems. She noted, particularly, the variation across AAC users and their parents, reflecting such factors as participants' unique abilities, constraints, personalities, and experiences. Within many dyads, conversational interaction patterns have been found to be asymmetrical, with speaking partners dominating the exchanges. However, interactions are dynamic and transactional with both partners influencing each other. Light summarized the research as

---

Personal Reflection 4.6

"Recently, a language-delayed child with whom I was working vocalized and then pointed to an object in my presence. Quite confident that I understood what she wanted, I reached for the object in question, only to be stopped by her teacher who instructed both of us that she could 'point to what she wants on her communication board.' A few moments later, I was visiting with a preschool child who made a request by pointing to a pictographic symbol and was told that she needed to 'use her voice and ask for it first.' At least one result of both interactions was considerable frustration on the part of both myself and the children. The tendency to assume such narrow, 'either/or,' approaches toward communication options for children is perhaps particularly unfortunate in that it deviates so markedly from the way in which nondisabled children acquire the ability to communicate."

David R. Beukelman (1987, p. 95), University of Nebraska-Lincoln, writing about the choices made for children with communicative disorders in situations where most individuals have the opportunity to make choices for themselves.

showing that "interactions may be influenced by subject variables, by partner variables, by contextual variables, by variables in AAC systems employed, and/or by variables in experience and training" (p. 75). As in other areas, the social interaction picture is complex but rich for mining in the intervention process.

ENVIRONMENTAL AND EMOTIONAL FACTORS

Neglect and Abuse

Definitions, differential diagnosis, and subdivisions. The terms *neglect* and *abuse* refer not so much to a clinical category as to a set of environmental conditions that may affect the development of infants, toddlers, and children in profound ways. Sparks (1989) pointed out that definitions of abuse and neglect differ, depending on whether they have been written for legal, medical, or social purposes. After reviewing the inadequacy of legal definitions, which tend to focus on deliberate intent of the abuser, rather than effect on the child, Sparks suggested the following five subdivisions:

1. Physical abuse: (a) shaking, beating, or burning that results in bodily injury or death; (b) physical acts that result in lasting or permanent neurological damage.
2. Sexual abuse: (a) nonphysical—indecent exposure, verbal attack of a sexual nature; (b) physical—genital-oral stimulation, fondling, sexual intercourse.
3. Emotional abuse: (a) excessive yelling, belittling, teasing–verbal attack; (b) overt rejection of the child.
4. Physical neglect: (a) abandonment with no arrangement made for care; (b) inadequate supervision for long periods, disregard for potential hazards in the home; (c) failure to provide adequate nutrition, clothing, personal hygiene; (d) failure to seek needed or recommended medical care.
5. Emotional neglect: (a) failure to provide warmth, attention, affection, normal living experience; (b) refusal of treatment or services recommended by social or educational personnel. (Sparks, 1989, p. 124)

Of these categories, emotional neglect and abuse is probably most difficult to identify because individual incidents are so common. Child maltreatment occurs on a continuum. Not all occurrences are so severe that they are obvious or justify legal intervention. Yet, professionals cannot afford to ignore the possibility that emotional neglect can influence children's development, particularly because the occurrence of emotional neglect is associated with failure-to-thrive in infancy (Sparks, 1989). Physicians diagnose this condition when a child's weight falls below the third percentile on standard growth charts without known organic cause (Barbero, 1982). Clinical criteria used to diagnose failure-to-thrive syndrome are presented in Box 4.12.

It is difficult to obtain accurate prevalence information on conditions related to neglect, but Barbero (1982) reported that 5% of pediatric admissions in his hospital met the criterion of being below the third percentile in weight and that a significant number of these met all five of the diagnostic criteria summarized in Box 4.12. A report of the U.S. Department of Health and Human Services (1981) also estimated that more than 300,000 children are abused annually, and at least twice as many are neglected. Others have

---

Box 4.12	Clinical criteria used to diagnose failure-to-thrive syndrome

1. Weight below the third percentile with subsequent weight gain in the presence of normal nurturing.
2. No evidence of systemic disease or abnormality on physical examination and laboratory investigation which explained growth failure.
3. Developmental retardation with subsequent acceleration of development following appropriate stimulation and feeding.
4. Clinical signs of deprivation which decrease in a more nurturing environment.
5. Presence of significant environmental psychosocial disruption.

Note. From "Failure-to-Thrive" by G. Barbero in *Maternal Attachment and Mothering Disorders (Pediatric Round Table: 1)* (p. 3) edited by M. H. Klaus, T. Leger, and M. A. Trause, 1982, Skillman, NJ: Johnson & Johnson Baby Products Company. ©1982 by Johnson & Johnson Baby Products Company.

pointed out that, although abuse and neglect conditions co-occur about 50% of the time (Garbarino & Crouter, 1978), they are not interchangeable (Deutsch, 1983).

The relevant question for language specialists out of all of these discouraging statistics is whether conditions of abuse and neglect have any negative effects on the development of language. The picture is cloudy because many factors confound studies associating maltreatment of children with language development (L. Fox, Long, & Langlois, 1988; McCauley & Swisher, 1987; Sparks, 1989). Confounding variables include socioeconomic status, general cognitive delays, predisposition to language delay related to prematurity or poor prenatal care, the tendency of children at risk for communication problems to be more difficult to parent to start with, and lack of clarity in identification of varying degrees of abuse and neglect as separate or co-occurring conditions.

Several studies, however, have produced results suggesting a significant connection between maltreatment of children and developmental delay, particularly when the maltreatment extends beyond the 1st year of life (R. E. Allen & Wasserman, 1985; Egeland & Sroufe, 1981). It has also been suggested that patterns of abuse and neglect tend to have differing effects on different children (Augustinos, 1987). Beyond individual differences, however, the research can be summarized as showing children who have been physically abused to be more noncompliant and aggressive, whereas children who have been both abused and physically neglected to experience more problems at school, including problems of academic performance and problems of adjustment (Lamphear, 1985).

Studies specifically of language development have shown significant correlations between maltreatment and language delay, although cause–effect relationships have been difficult to prove. For example, in an early study, L. Bloom (1975) found that children with a "high certainty" of having been physically abused (but who were also described as frequently neglected) showed significantly lower expressive language scores than did a group of "low-certainty" abused children. Bloom also found a significant relationship between expressive language scores and socioeconomic status for both experimental and conrol groups, however, and suggested that was perhaps the stronger relationship. Blager and Martin (1976) and Blager (1979) also reported finding symptoms of

delayed speech and language development among almost all of the abused preschoolers they evaluated at the National Center for Child Abuse in Denver. By school-age level, however, the children's abilities to produce well-formed language seemed to have matured, but the older children (who were no longer being abused and were in psychotherapy) continued to have difficulty in using communication skills appropriately. These studies have received considerable criticism for their lack of control groups and for inadequate description of experimental procedures (McCauley & Swisher, 1987). More recent and better controlled studies have provided additional evidence that conditions of abuse and neglect, but particularly severe neglect, are associated with language-learning difficulties (R. E. Allen & Oliver, 1982; L. Fox, Long, & Langlois, 1988).

A few cases of neglect have been reported in the literature that are so severe that children have been almost totally isolated from the opportunity to communicate with other people (Curtiss, 1977; K. Davis, 1947). In such instances, both cognitive and linguistic development are impaired, and the prognosis for language development is limited even when stimulation is normalized and language intervention is provided (Curtiss, 1977; Gleitman & Gleitman, 1981). In one case, a child was discovered who was not totally isolated but had been cared for by her deaf-mute mother (K. Davis, 1947). Despite the lack of spoken language in her environment up to the age of 6, she apparently was subsequently able to attain a normal IQ later and adequate language functions (U. Kirk, 1983).

Causative layering and other complexities. Babies who exhibit failure-to-thrive often have parents who are themselves at risk. Several identified factors may play a role in disturbances of maternal attachment (Barbero, 1982) including (1) factors in the mother's past, such as childhood loss of a parent or death of prior children; (2) pregnancy events, such as protracted emotional or physical illness, or loss of key family figures; (3) perinatal events, such as birth complications, acute illness in either mother or infant, prematurity, congenital defects, diseases, and iatrogenic or institutional disruptions; and (4) current life events, such as marital strains, mental or physical illness, alcoholism or drugs, and financial crises.

Another major risk factor is adolescent pregnancy. Osofsky (1990) noted that the proportion of teen births occurring outside of marriage has risen for both blacks and whites since 1960 from 15% to 61%.

Causative layering factors associated with teenage pregnancy are poverty, membership in large or single-parent families, and having a teenage mother or poorly educated parents.

Relationships of contributing factors. *Biological maturation.* Biological maturational factors are considered probable contributing factors to language disorders in neglected and abused children. Under normal environmental conditions of interactions with persons, objects, and events, a child's nervous system becomes progressively elaborated and coordinated (U. Kirk, 1983). However, negative environmental conditions, such as malnutrition, may affect brain growth and cellular development. Restak (1979) summarized evidence from the brains of children who died of malnutrition and noted both reduced numbers of brain cells and decreased whole brain size when malnutrition occurred within the first 2 years of life.

The vestibular system also seems to be crucial to the timing of additional brain development. It is controlled largely within the brain stem and is responsible for transmitting impulses important in coordinating other functions. Vestibular dysfunction has been postulated as playing a role in dyslexia, autism, childhood schizophrenia, and human violence. Its development may be particularly susceptible to influence by environmental events. Some evidence suggests that premature infants given periodic vestibular stimulation by being placed on gently oscillating water beds gain weight faster, develop vision and hearing earlier, and demonstrate regular sleep cycles at a younger age, with a dramatic reduction in sleep apnea (Korner cited by Restak, 1979).

Linguistic system factors. The linguistic system may be at risk under conditions of severe and continuing physical or emotional neglect or abuse, but the degree of risk is unclear, particularly when other contributing factors, such as socioeconomic status, are controlled, and it is also not clear whether the linguistic system is specifically at risk relative to other areas of cognitive and social–emotional development. In Blager and Martin's (1976) report, as abused and neglected children reached school age, specific linguistic abilities were found to be age appropriate. In the broader areas of communication and language use, children experienced ongoing difficulties. However, in Curtiss's (1977) report of "Genie," who spent her first few years in almost total isolation, specifically linguistic behaviors, such as syntax and morphology appeared to be relatively more impaired and more resistant to intervention than did lexical knowledge and general cognitive abilities.

Stimulus–response–reinforcement factors. For normal patterns of communicative interaction to develop, infants need to be exposed to linguistic stimulation (U. Kirk, 1983) and to be reinforced for attempts to gain care-giver attention (Brazelton, 1982). Later in life, children need to continue to receive appropriate attention and social rewards for their attempts to communicate and to advance developmentally in other ways. Therefore, stimulus–response–reinforcement factors are considered probable contributing factors to language disorders in neglected and abused children.

Parents also need to receive reinforcement from their infants. The well-known pediatrician and child development specialist, T. Berry Brazelton (quoted by Fraiberg, 1982), has commented that mothers of failure-to-thrive and abused children say that "This baby affected me differently from the beginning" (p. 13).

The power of the reciprocal stimulus–response–reinforcement relationship between mothers and infants has been demonstrated in experiments (Brazelton, 1982) where mothers first were asked to engage their 3-week-old infants in normal face-to-face interactions. Then, they were instructed to maintain their facial expression without change for 3 minutes. The infants then made a brief attempt at interaction. When their expectations for response were not fulfilled, the infants made several brief, but urgent, attempts to elicit a response, followed by waiting periods. When the attempts failed to be reinforced, infants typically withdrew and seemed to expect no further response. Emphasizing the strength of the effect, Jerome Bruner (1968) noted from his research that "Failure to obtain reciprocation produces an active avoidance—indeed the child will struggle bodily to look away" (p. 57).

Although such response patterns can be quickly reversed when created experimentally for brief periods, with prolonged child neglect, the withdrawal is seen as extreme wariness and aversion. Even in such cases, however, responsiveness to care givers can be increased following interventions that may last around 2 weeks, and such increments are associated with normalized weight gain (Brazelton, 1982).

These are only some of the insights that a mixture of behavioral and social interaction theory can offer for understanding the effects of child abuse and neglect. Some instance of physical or emotional abuse may, in fact, be escalations from misguided behavioral approaches that young parents have acquired from their own parents. That is, in attempting to punish unacceptable behaviors, including communication behaviors, parents may inadvertently punish the normal risk taking and exploration that accompany development in protected and accepting environments. Certainly, a transdisciplinary approach to family intervention in such cases should include social services that help parents acquire more functional behavior management skills. Language specialists can help parents to develop realistic expectations for communicative development and encourage it.

Information processing factors. Information processing factors are considered probable contributing factors to language disorders in abused and neglected children. In normally developing infants, a cyclical curve of infants' attention allows them to modulate the amount of stimulation that they receive to avoid being overstimulated. Brazelton (1982) described this process as one in which:

> all parts of the infant's body move in cyclical patterns, outward toward the person (attention) then back towards his body (nonattention). This ebb and flow of attention occurs several times per minute. Without such an economical homeostatic model, he might be overwhelmed by the many cues flowing from another human in a short period of time. (pp. 49–50)

When care givers are not sensitive to infants' needs to modulate their sensory stimulation, the infants' capacity for prolonged attention may be overloaded. By 6 weeks of age, these infants may exhibit an abnormal pattern of prolonged nonattention followed by brief periods of attention rather than the more normal balanced rhythmic cycle of attention and nonattention (Brazelton, 1982). In one study of videotaped mother–child interactions (Hyman, Parr, & Browne, 1979), mothers who had abused their children tended to respond to fewer of their infants's initiatives, and abusive mothers of boys tended to initiate so often that their sons could not respond effectively. Problems of "reciprocity" are also common when teenage mothers interact with their infants (Osofsky, 1990).

Cognition factors. The picture for general cognitive delay associated with child abuse and neglect is no clearer than that for specific linguistic delay. Studies are confounded with socioeconomic status variables that are generally associated with inability to score as high on intelligence tests and with the possibility that general cognitive delays may be precursors of incidents of abuse and neglect.

Studies have shown that when abuse extends beyond 1 year of age, toddlers who have been abused are less likely to score in the normal range than are abused babies under the age of 1 year (R. E. Allen & Wasserman, 1985). Egeland and Sroufe (1981) identified a similar pattern of declining abilities in a group of abused children they studied longitudinally.

Social interaction factors. The essence of child abuse and neglect is a set of negative environmental interaction factors. Such factors are always involved and are essential contributing factors to language disorders in these children. The social conditions associated with risks to child development from abuse and/or neglect are complex. Although a review of the literature shows that child abuse and neglect occur more frequently in urban families where low income and poor education play a role, parents who abuse and neglect their children can be found in all socioeconomic levels (L. Fox, Long, & Langlois, 1988).

Individual parent–child interactions offer perhaps the greatest opportunity for fostering change. For example, the research discussed earlier on reciprocal stimulus–response–reinforcement patterns falls in this category, particularly when positive as well as negative factors are investigated. Osofsky (1990) observed that teenage mothers interacting with their dependent infants in the 1st year of life were likely to encourage their infants to be independent before they were ready by expecting them to hold their own bottles, to sit up early, or to scoot after toys. They also tended to use teasing behaviors toward their infants. On the more positive side, however, many infants and their teenage mothers demonstrated considerable resiliency under remarkably difficult conditions. Infant factors that seemed to contribute positively were intelligence, positive temperamental characteristics, and the ability to cooperate and nurture oneself to some extent. Maternal factors that seemed to contribute positively were emotional availability and responsivity, even if they were variable, as they often are among teenage mothers.

Among mother–child pairs where abuse has been identified, reciprocity problems are commonly identified as characterizing the interactions (Dietrich, Starr, & Kaplan, 1980; Hyman, Parr, & Browne, 1979; Wasserman, Green, & Allen, 1983). In particular, mothers who have abused their children are less likely to engage in active interactions, such as patting, kissing, or nuzzling, or to produce "baby talk" with their infants than control mothers are. Some attempts have been made to rule out the possibility that maternal interaction style might be a result, rather than a cause, of a less communicative baby. Based on their research, Wasserman et al. (1983) suggested that abnormal maternal interaction may influence problems that children already have and thus may contribute to the maintenance of a maladaptive interaction style, but is probably not simply a response to the problems that the child brings to the interaction.

Although infant–parent interactions seem to be particularly critical during the earliest stages of communicative development, social interaction influences do not stop at infancy. In describing the communicative styles of older children who had been abused or neglected, Blager (1979) reported that they ranged from aggressive and hostile to precociously adaptive and noted that, "Regardless of the amount of talking they did, they avoided any real contact through conversation . . . keeping themselves behind a barrage of words" (p. 991).

Behavioral and Emotional Development Problems

Definitions, differential diagnosis, and subdivisions. The environmental role is less clear with problems of behavioral and emotional development than with direct evidence of maltreatment. Increasingly, as investigators appreciate the intricacies of brain–behavior relationships, behavioral or emotional

abnormalities are seen almost universally to involve some central processing component (Andreasen, 1984). Indeed, as discussed earlier in this chapter, autism is no longer categorized as a "psychotic" disorder but is considered to have a likely basis in central nervous system dysfunction. In this chapter, ADHD has also been categorized as a problem of central functioning more than as a psychiatric disorder, despite its classification with that group in DSM-III-R (American Psychological Association, 1987).

What is a "psychiatric disorder"? One way to answer this question would be simply to use the subdivisions of the DSM-III-R to define the domain. As Prizant and his associates (1990) pointed out, however, because of overlap with other developmental disorders (including those specifically involving speech and language), such an approach creates confusion related to differential diagnosis of communication disorders and psychiatric disorders. Perhaps better for our purposes is a working definition provided by Baker and Cantwell (1987a) of psychiatric disorder as "a disorder of behavior, emotions or relationships that is sufficiently severe and/or sufficiently prolonged, to cause disturbance in the child or disruption of his immediate environment" (p. 193).

Baker and Cantwell (1987a) also differentiated two major subgroupings of psychiatric disorder, behavior disorders and emotional disorders, on the basis of their varied behavioral symptoms. Behavior disorders include such conditions as ADHD, oppositional disorder, and conduct disorder, all of which involve overactivity and aggression, which may disturb the environment and people nearby. Emotional disorders include disorders such as anxiety disorders, phobias, and forms of depression (including dysthymic disorder), all of which are associated with internalized and/or somatic symptoms that do not directly disrupt the environment.

The most crucial question for language specialists is again, of course, whether psychiatric disorders are predictably related to speech and language disorders. Perhaps the most predictable finding is that they are related. The two diagnoses occur together with an alarming frequency that tends to increase as children with language disorders increase in age.

Typically, epidemiological studies have examined children referred to a center specializing in diagnosis of one type of problem for co-occurrence of the other. For example, in a study of children referred to a child psychiatry inpatient facility, Gualtieri, Koriath, Van Bourgondien, and Saleeby (1983) found that 50% of the 40 children had moderate-to-severe language disorders. Prizant et al. (1990) reported that 67% of the children referred to a psychiatric inpatient facility in their Rhode Island hospital failed a speech and language screening on admission.

In other studies, children were examined for psychiatric disorders when they were originally referred to community or hospital-based clinics for speech and language diagnosis. Similar proportions of co-occurrence were found. In the largest study of this type, Baker and Cantwell (1982) found that 44% of 291 children, originally referred for speech and language problems (between the ages of almost 2 years and almost 16 years), had some psychiatric disorder as defined by the DSM-III-R. When they followed up this same group a few years later, Baker and Cantwell (1987b) found that the prevalence rate for psychiatric disorders among the original sample of children with speech and language disorders had jumped from 44% to 60%.

Subgroup analysis from the original study (Baker & Cantwell, 1982) also yielded some interesting differences in prevalence of psychiatric disorders based on whether children had pure language disorders (i.e., involving language expression, comprehension, or processing, but with normal speech), pure speech disorders, or mixed speech and language disorders. Among these three subgroups, those with "pure" language disorders were at greatest risk for also having diagnosable psychiatric problems (95% showed evidence of psychiatric problems). Those with "pure"

speech disorders were at lowest risk (29%), and those with mixed speech and language problems fell in the middle (45%). These groups, however, also differed in mean chronological age, and this may have played a role in the varied prevalence rates. The pure language disorders subgroup had a mean age of 9.3 years ($SD = 3.4$) at time of referral; the pure speech disorders subgroup, 6.0 years ($SD = 2.6$); and the speech and language disorders mixed subgroup, 4.9 years ($SD = 2.3$). One implication of these results is that children with language disorders not involving speech production are less likely to be identified until they are older and, at least at that point in their lives, are more likely to have psychiatric difficulties in addition to their language problems.

Any of these studies might be said to be confounded by the fact that they involved only children whose problems were severe enough to warrant referral. Beitchman, Nair, Clegg, and Patel (1986), in Canada, used a different design in an epidemiological study of 1,655 five-year-old kindergarten children, from the general population. They identified 11% of the children as having speech and language disorders; of these, 48.7% also had a psychiatric disorder.

All of these studies placed the rate for co-occurrence of speech and language and psychiatric disorders somewhere between 40% and 67%. When considering the data, however, it is important to remember that the diagnoses included a wide range of types and severity of psychiatric disorders. Also, the diagnosis of ADD, categorized separately in this chapter, was included within the category of psychiatric disorder for these studies. In the Beitchman et al. (1986) study, emotional disturbance and ADD (diagnosed using DSM-III, APA, 1980, criteria) were far more prevalent in the kindergarten children diagnosed as having speech and language impairments than in those who were not. Of these, ADD was diagnosed in 30.4% of the speech and language impaired group but only in 4.5% of the control group; emotional disturbance was diagnosed in 12.8% of the speech and language-impaired group but only 1.5% of the control group. On the other hand, conduct disorder was diagnosed with similar frequency in both groups (5.5% of the speech and language-impaired group and 6.0% of the conrol group).

One subgroup of children with psychiatric disorder has a problem of communication as its central symptom. Elective mutism is a type of psychiatric disorder

> **Box 4.13**   **Symptoms of elective mutism (based on a summary by Norman, 1983, who reviewed studies by Kolvin & Fundudis, 1981, and Rosenberg & Linblad, 1978)**
>
> 1. Behavioral constriction in the presence of strangers.
> 2. Verbal fluency documented when at home with parents or siblings (although a history of speech problems or late talking has been reported for as high as 50% of the group).
> 3. No evidence of reduction of key symptoms for at least 1 year.
> 4. Personality characteristics may include extreme shyness, timidity, withdrawal, anxiety and fear, and/or willfulness and a manipulative need to control.
> 5. History often shows at least one extremely shy parent.
> 6. History often shows bed wetting and bed soiling.
> 7. No history of disordered thought, bizarre speech patterns, or eating or sleeping disturbance.

in which a child capable of talking refuses to do so, except perhaps to a small group of intimates. Its symptoms are summarized in Box 4.13. A large proportion of children who are electively mute (as many as 80%) have demonstrated long-standing personality deviations before insidious, rather than abrupt, onset of the mutism (Kolvin & Fundudis, 1981; Wolff & Barlow, 1979). Higher instances of elective mutism have also been reported in cases of child abuse (Hayden, 1980), including sexual abuse.

What is cause and what is effect? An important question regarding the relationship between psychiatric disorders and speech and language disorders is whether the relationship is causal. Prizant et al. (1990) summarized four hypotheses about the relationship: (1) Psychiatric disorders lead to communication disorders; (2) communication disorders lead to psychiatric disorders; (3) a third, underlying factor leads to both psychiatric and communication disorders; and (4) transactional factors between children and their environments lead to mutual influence within a longitudinal, developmental framework. Evidence for each of these hypotheses is considered within the following discussions of the six contributing factors based on theories of normal language acquisition.

Relationships of contributing factors. *Biological maturation*. Factors related to biological maturation are often found in children with behavioral and emotional development problems. The level of involvement of these factors may vary, however. As noted, recent research has implicated the central nervous system in many disorders that were previously thought to be strictly psychiatric or behavioral (Andreasen, 1984). It

is, therefore, possible that the third hypothesis of causality (Prizant et al., 1990), which states that a common factor might underly symptoms both of psychiatric and communication disorders, will be supported by the identification of similar central nervous system dysfunction in both types of problems.

Baker and Cantwell (1987a) considered this possibility, along with a variety of other factors, which might underlie both disorders. They found that although factors such as brain damage, intellectual retardation, and marked hearing loss could each be identified in a small percentage of their sample, these did not account for the differences between the psychiatrically well and the psychiatrically ill groups who had speech and language disorders.

As new evidence about possible central nervous system involvement in disorders such as ADHD (see preceding discussion) accumulates, the third hypothesis may receive additional support, especially because ADHD has been shown in several studies to be the most common disorder to co-occur with speech and language impairment. The need for further investigation of a possible underlying central nervous system link is also suggested by Baker and Cantwell's (1982) results showing the highest co-occurrence for problems of "pure language disorders" and psychiatric disorders. Perhaps a common brain mechanism will be identified that is associated with both kinds of problems.

In his work on brain chemistry as a determinant of temperament, Jerome Kagan (1989) raised another possible explanation of biological factors in both psychiatric and communication disorders. Kagan said that the more than 150 different chemicals in our brains (e.g., the neurotransmitters norepinephrine, serotonin, and acetylcholine; peptides; endorphins and opioids; hormones), have the potential to be combined into thousands of different "broths." Although the brain is basically the same in all cases, and the broths do not vary randomly, temperamental differences are caused by the variations in the "broths" in which the brain sits and which determine the firing patterns of its varied parts.

Two of the most dramatic temperamental types Kagan (1989) studied can be recognized for their extremes. One is a group (approximately 10% to 20% of the population) of outgoing, sociable individuals, who, Kagan reported, if raised in middle-class families are generally socialized to be leaders but, if raised in neighborhoods at risk for crime, more likely may become delinquents. As infants, these are the babies who appear to be relaxed and smiling when shown a mobile or played taped speech. They have a high threshold before they experience fear and anxiety, and they are willing to take risks. In the extreme, these are the children who may later show symptoms of conduct disorder. A completely different temperament is evidenced by the approximately 10% of all children who are born with tendencies to be shy (of these, Kagan said that most will overcome the problem through environmental shaping by the time they are 8 years old). These are the infants who become easily aroused by stimulation and who respond with high tension and crying when shown a mobile or played a tape (which Kagan speculated may be due to high arousal in the limbic lobe). Children with this temperament are unlikely to take social risks. This is the group that may be more at risk for such conditions as anxiety disorders and elective mutism.

Linguistic system factors.   The second hypothesis outlined by Prizant et al. (1990) is that disorders of the linguistic system may cause psychiatric disorders. This position has been argued by Baltaxe and Simmons (1988), who noted that speech and language development is a unique feature of being human and that disorders involving such critical processes can therefore be expected to have a negative impact on the developing person. The role of linguistic factors in psychiatric disorders, however, is thought to be an uncertain contributing factor.

Incidents of elective mutism have also been cited as evidence that impairments of the linguistic system may lead to the development of psychiatric disorders (Prizant et al., 1990). In one study, Wilkins (1985)

found that one third of a group of 24 children with elective mutism had histories of delayed development of speech, whereas none of the matched controls had this history.

Expressive language disorders may make it difficult for some children and adolescents to express fully their ideas, feelings, fears, and needs, and eventually this lack of communication might result in the kinds of problems that justify referral to psychiatric facilities (Gualtieri et al., 1983). Prizant et al., (1990) concurred that such a description fits many children and adolescents:

> These children may appear to be immature and restless, and may develop impulsive and aggressive behaviors. Other children who present with language-processing deficits may misinterpret messages and are unable to request further information or clarification, resulting in confusion and frustration. Consequently, they may demonstrate externalizing behaviors (e.g., destroying materials, physical confrontation with peers and adults), internalizing behaviors (e.g., withdrawing from interactions, self-abusive behaviors), or both. (p. 183)

Although both experimental and clinical evidence suggest that some children and adolescents are at increased risk for psychiatric disorders based on the problems resulting from their communication impairments, if the relationship were purely causal, the proportion of communicatively impaired children with psychiatric disorders should be even higher. A related question from the other side of this coin might be, What proportion of children with early speech and language delay grow up to be psychologically healthy adults?

Although no one (to my knowledge) has yet attempted to answer that question directly, a study is underway at the University of Iowa (Tomblin, Freese, & Records, 1990) to look at outcomes following developmental language disorder in terms of language and cognitive skills, social skills, and quality of life variables. Tomblin's group gathered follow-up data on 22 adults (mean age 21.17; *SD* 2.69) with clear histories of developmental language disorder and compared them with a carefully matched group (with similar ages, nonverbal intelligence scores, and socioeconomic status) of 22 young adults with normal verbal and nonverbal skills. The Iowa data showed that, although language impairment continued to be evident across most language measures, the indices of life satisfaction and general affect did not differ significantly for the two groups.

This suggests that at least some individuals with language and speech disorders must be able to navigate through the years of childhood and adolescence with their self-esteem fairly well intact, at least when compared with other individuals of similar nonverbal cognitive ability. For both groups, scores on the Wechsler Adult Intelligence Scale—Revised (WAIS-R; Wechsler, 1981), performance subtest IQs averaged between 90 and 95 (Tomblin et al., 1990). An important clinical question might be "How can professionals differentiate between communicatively impaired individuals who are at risk for psychiatric disorder and those who are not?" Building self-esteem and confidence as communicators may be one of the most important outcomes to target in all intervention programs, regardless of apparent risk. Perhaps clinicians should also learn to be more aware of danger signs, taking particular note, for example, when children have receptive and expressive language disorders not involving speech production difficulties.

Stimulus–response–reinforcement factors. Stimulus–response–reinforcement factors play a critical role in the language problems associated with emotional and behavioral disorders. When "behavior disorders" become so severe as to disrupt the environment, behavioral theories are often invoked to explain why children and adolescents behave the way they do and to design strategies for modifying their behaviors. Problems that sometimes occur with this approach revolve around the fact that human behavior and motivation are so complex that consequences that would be reinforcing or punishing for most children may assume twisted meanings for children with emotional or behavioral disturbances. For example, such youngsters may appear to seek out situations or punishing consequences that most children would avoid, perhaps because they have internalized parental and teacher messages that they are "bad" (L. Fox et al., 1988). Communication specialists, psychologists, and social workers then need to work together to analyze the highly complex sets of variables that may influence a particular behavioral system. Parents and teachers may need consultative help for planning strategies to help these children communicate about their problems and to escape from the boxes in which they find themselves.

The subgroup of children with psychiatric disorders most likely to come to the attention of speech–language specialists is the electively mute group. As noted, a variety of explanations have been offered when children who can talk, do not. No general explanation seems to work for all cases. Individual assessment is critical because knowledge of contributing factors helps to determine which intervention approaches might work best. For example, when a child who is mute has been abused, a pediatric psychotherapeutic approach is warranted (along with legal and social service system action). In most cases, however, because elective mutism is particularly disruptive to a child's ability to participate in school, transdisciplinary teams design behaviorally oriented programs for implementation in the educational setting, perhaps in conjunction with other kinds of approaches implemented elsewhere.

A strictly behaviorist approach to intervention for elective mutism might involve strategies of (1) describing the overt symptomatology without necessarily dealing with the past, (2) reciprocal inhibition, (3) desensitization, (4) shaping, (5) successive approximations, (6) reinforcement, and (7) fading. Such an approach, however, because of its superficiality, may overlook key aspects of the problem. A more holistic approach that uses behaviorist strategies is advocated (Marx & Hillix, 1979; Norman, 1983). For example, a combined approach was implemented by Norman with a 5-year old girl who was electively mute and in a special-needs kindergarten class. Norman employed shaping through provision of natural and secondary reinforcement contingencies, at first when the girl spoke to her sister in the protected environment of the speech room at school, then through successive approximation and desensitization procedures in a variety of rooms, with a variety of people. Later in the program, the child's initial attempts to speak in the presence of her teacher involved mouthing words or whispering. Although Norman noted that the child was always reinforced with natural consequences for talking, comments such as "Good talking!" were avoided. The focus was kept on good communication, not speech production.

In this and other approaches, it is important to avoid techniques that seek to force the child to talk, or to withhold natural reinforcers until the child does. Power struggles that tend to result from application of these kinds of behavioral techniques are, in most cases, doomed to failure (Friedman, 1980). Although elective mutism tends to be frustrating to the adults in a child's environment, it helps to remember that a child who chooses not to speak may in fact be a child who, in the circumstances of the moment, cannot speak. It is not a matter of simple choice or of finding the right reinforcer. Rather, it is a matter of using selective behaviorist principles carefully but within the context of a supportive environment in which the child can feel safe to talk and to participate.

Information processing factors. Information processing factors are often associated with language disorders in children with behavioral and emotional disorders, but the degree of involvement may vary. When ADHD is considered to be a member of the general category of psychiatric disorders, information processing is, by definition, implicated in symptoms of distractibility and self-regulation that children with the disorder demonstrate. Prizant et al. (1990) speculated that ADHD could lead to communication disorders (as stated in the first hypothesis regarding causal relationships) by interfering with the child's ability to sustain attention when language is presented auditorily.

Milder (or more indirect) interference with normal information processing may result from other psychiatric disorders, especially when children are at risk for language acquisition difficulty. It is difficult to concentrate on learning language and using language to learn when basic psychiatric needs such as freedom from anxiety and feeling OK about oneself have not been met. Anyone who can recall times of severe emotional upset can probably appreciate the effect that such a state can have on such information processing abilities as selective attention, comprehension, memory, recall, and production. Add to this picture a child with weak language skills who is trying to process information within such a demanding communicative context as a classroom (Cazden, 1988; N. W. Nelson, 1984), and it is easy to understand why children whose minds are filled with emotional stress might have difficulty.

Cognition factors. A deficit in cognitive development was one of the variables that Baker and Cantwell (1987a) included when they analyzed their data for common factors associated with both psychiatric and communicative disorders. Just as other factors (including brain damage and marked hearing loss) were not enough to account for the differences between the psychiatrically well and the psychiatrically ill groups with speech and language disorders, neither were cognitive impairments.

On the other hand, cognitive impairment should not be ignored as a possible risk factor. The characteristics of mild, moderate, severe, and profound mental retardation, which were summarized earlier in this chapter, include increased difficulty in coping with environmental stress independently as mental retardation becomes more severe. However, no evidence indicates that all individuals with cognitive impairment experience psychiatric distress any more than evidence indicates that all persons with psychiatric distress are cognitively impaired.

Even individuals who are cognitively gifted may experience distortion of their world views and self views in the midst of psychiatric problems. When such individuals are children, their developing attempts to make sense of the world could be jeopardized. Prizant et al. (1990) also suggested that the following question remains unanswered: "Are mild cognitive deficits, weakness, or disorganization—which often co-occur with language disorders—part and parcel of an emotional disorder or behavioral disorder as well?" (p. 190).

Social interaction factors. By definition, psychiatric disorders involve disruptions of social interactions, although types of psychiatric disorders differ in their influences on environmental interactions. Social interaction factors are essential contributing factors to language disorders in children with emotional and behavioral disorders. Psychiatric disorders considered behavioral are defined as overt enough to disturb the environment and people nearby, whereas those that are considered emotional involve internalized symptoms that do not directly disrupt the environment (Baker & Cantwell, 1987a). Environmental factors may cause, or at least aggravate, symptoms associated with psychiatric disorders.

The first hypothesis Prizant et al. (1990) reviewed regarding causal relationships suggests that psychiatric disorders can lead to communication disorders. Evidence showing that communication disorders are more likely to precede psychiatric disorders than vice versa (Baker & Cantwell, 1987b) argues against this position.

This is not to suggest that, for individual children, psychiatric disorders may not contribute to language disorders, just as communicative disorders may contribute to behavioral or emotional disorders. Such a pattern of mutual influence was proposed in the fourth hypothesis discussed by Prizant et al. (1990) and is consistent with the system theory view of language disorders advocated throughout this book.

Certainly, a child's behavior, whether overaggressive and acting out or anxious and withdrawn, influences the child's communicative interactions and social transactions. Adults communicate differently with different children, in patterns that begin in infancy and continue throughout life. A role of the communicative specialist is to help normalize communicative interactions and to contribute toward aiming the system on a new course. Communication specialists and mental health workers may be most effective when they work together for assessment and intervention with young people who find themselves in psychiatric trouble.

For example, Dr. Barbara Hoskins (a specialist in speech–language pathology and learning disabilities in private practice) evaluated the language and learning abilities of a teenage boy who had tried to take his own life (personal communication, March 19, 1991). Hoskins gathered a variety of kinds of data in evaluating this boy: formal test data documenting his language and learning disabilities as well as interview and observational data. The boy went to school every day, but did nothing—no assignments, no homework, no tests. He had simply given up on himself but was still interested enough in meeting his parents' expectations to attend school. As the boy shared this information in an interview with Hoskins, he must have expected more lectures, more fix-it plans, more adult judgments. What he got instead was a person who took his perspective and tried to see the situation through his eyes. She really listened to him and then said something like, "How awful that must have been for you! I am amazed that you stayed in that situation so long. I am not sure what we are going to do, but one thing is for certain. We cannot let you go back into a situation like that one. We will put our heads together and figure out how to make some changes. Are you willing to work with me on this one?" He agreed.

MIXED FACTORS AND CHANGES OVER TIME

Separate discussions of separate categories imply that problems of various types occur in isolation from one another, but of course, problems can co-occur in all kinds of combinations. When they do, they bring characteristics of the separate problems but with outcomes that may appear different because of complex interactions. Part of the diagnostic process is to identify the possible involvement of multiple disabilities when individual children have problems.

Although practitioners recognize the frequency with which varied categories of impairment overlap, federal counts, and most state counts, of handicapped children are not set up to recognize such "duplication." Children can only be counted in one category for funding purposes. Because official agencies do not make "duplicate counts," the number of children and adolescents who have speech and language impairments in conjunction with other disabling conditions is difficult to determine. It is interesting to note, however, the changes across the four age levels in patterns of occurrence of the four types of conditions *learning disabilities; speech and language impairments* (called *speech impairments* in the original wording of PL 94–142); *mental retardation;* and *emotional disturbance* (shown in Figure 4.4, which is based on data from the Tenth Annual Report to Congress on the Implementation of The Education of the Handicapped Act, covering the 1986 to 1987 school year, M. M. Gerber & Levine-Donnerstein, 1989). Rather than speech and language problems disappearing, as Figure 4.4 might imply, it is more likely that they become one more component of a complex problem.

It is also important to recognize other factors that influence interpretations of the data. For example, one reason for the apparent increase in proportions of students with mental retardation in the 18 to 21 year-old "postsecondary" category is that most students with normal learning abilities graduate by around the age of 18, so this category naturally includes a higher proportion of students with mental retardation. Another factor influencing data proportions relates to students' dropping out of school before graduation. M. M. Gerber and Levine-Donnerstein (1989) reported that the proportion of the general population leaving school over the age of 16 in that same time period was less that 16%. It was less than 22% for black, Hispanic, and low-socioeconomic status young men. In contrast, the proportions of teenagers with disabilities dropping out during that same time period was 29%. This group included 59% of the students

FIGURE 4.4

Proportions of students with learning disabilities (LD), speech impairments, mental retardation (MR), and emotional disturbance (ED), identified within four age groups.

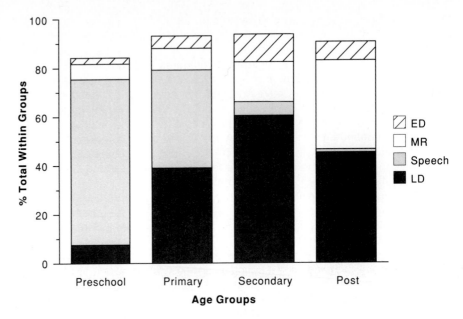

Note. From "Educating All Children: Ten Years Later" by M. M. Gerber and D. Levine-Donnerstein, 1989, *Exceptional Children, 56*, p. 19. Copyright 1989 by The Council for Exceptional Children. Reprinted by permission.

over the age of 16 with speech impairments and almost 60% of those with emotional impairments. In contrast, only 7% of children with multiple disabilities and only 9% of students with both deafness and blindness dropped out.

SUMMARY

In this chapter, I encouraged the viewpoint that not all factors that influence the course of development in children with language disorders need necessarily to be viewed as causes of the disorder. I considered how causes of childhood language disorders may be heterogeneous, layered, multifaceted, and interactive. I also looked at a set of categorical conditions that are often associated with language disorders but are not necessarily related in a linear causative sense. Finally, I used the same six categories of theories of normal language acquisition discussed in Chapter 3 to organize discussion of factors that may contribute to the appearance of language disorders in individual children and their modification over time: biological, linguistic, behavioral, information processing, cognition, and social interaction. One way of looking at theories of normal language acquisition is to think of them as

attempts to identify causes of normal development. Taking this viewpoint a step further, isn't the purpose of language intervention with children to cause language development to proceed more normally?

Discussions of causative factors may be fruitful, but one must also consider ways in which they may be dangerous. In particular, when parents and professionals become stuck in identifying causes that may no longer be active, they may be tempted to do so as a way of assigning blame. The statement that "Problems are not just within children, and neither are the solutions" is not intended to focus attention on determining what factors are at fault when a language-based problem is observed. Rather, it is aimed at helping those wishing to remediate the problem to look at interactions among factors internal and external to the child when designing an intervention plan. The idea is to devise a plan that can facilitate positive developmental factors, while lessening the effects of negative factors. The goals in understanding the causes of a child's difficulty in acquiring language are to reduce the child's problems with language development throughout childhood and adolescence and to reduce the probability that other children will have similar problems.

Prevention of Childhood Language Disorders

Theoreticians generally divide prevention into three types, based on the stage each attempts to address: (1) *primary prevention,* encouraging conditions to prevent problems before they start; (2) *secondary prevention,* early identification and intervention to foster conditions that will minimize long-term handicaps; and (3) *tertiary prevention,* remediating current problems and limiting further ones after they have appeared (S. E. Gerber, 1990).

Primary prevention activities attempt to ensure that children begin life with and develop with the best biological mechanisms possible. These activities include genetic counseling, avoidance of alcohol or drug consumption by mothers during pregnancy, and avoidance of other teratogens throughout life. Teratogens are environmental agents that can cause structural or functional abnormalities in a developing embryo or fetus. Examples are infectious diseases, alcohol and drugs consumed by the mother, and lead in paint chips or gasoline to which the child is exposed (S. E. Gerber, 1990). S. E. Gerber (1990) has noted that the Association for Retarded Citizens—United States believes that "50 percent of mental retardation *could be prevented*" (p. xiii).

Some potential causes and contributing factors are more preventable than others. For example, a child's existing genetic and chromosomal makeup is not modifiable by current techniques. Whether it should be in the future is one of the more difficult ethical questions currently facing genetic engineers and society. Parents of a child whose language impairment is related to genetic factors should certainly have access to genetic counseling as they contemplate having additional children.

Relatively "new" problems stemming from substance abuse should be more preventable, but their underlying causes are also complex and not easily removed. Fetal alcohol syndrome, prenatal drug exposure, and congenital human immunodeficiency virus (HIV, the virus that causes acquired immune deficiency syndrome—AIDS) all are associated with developmental disabilities. They occur in epidemic proportions in some settings, particularly in urban centers and Native American reservations. Prevention efforts to limit causative factors like these require comprehensive social service approaches. Solutions will not be easy.

Secondary prevention, with its methods based in early identification and treatment, is the ultimate focus of Chapter 7. Its topics of expectations, assessment, and intervention for infants and toddlers are clearly related to identifying risk factors and reducing their impact early. Secondary prevention is also an element in the treatment plans of older children and adolescents (see Chapters 8 and 9). It is always important to keep positive developmental targets in focus, but comprehensive assessment and intervention also require that professionals be aware of possible pitfalls and dangers awaiting youngsters who have difficulty communicating (e.g., self- and other-imposed limits on social and academic interactions, which may influence long-term outcomes) to help youngsters navigate around them at any developmental stage.

Tertiary prevention is a part of any attempt to intervene in a system where a problem clearly exists; it occurs each time we become a part of a system to assist in moving the process of change in a positive direction, no matter what the age of the child. It forms the primary motivation for this book.

5

Public Policy and Service Delivery

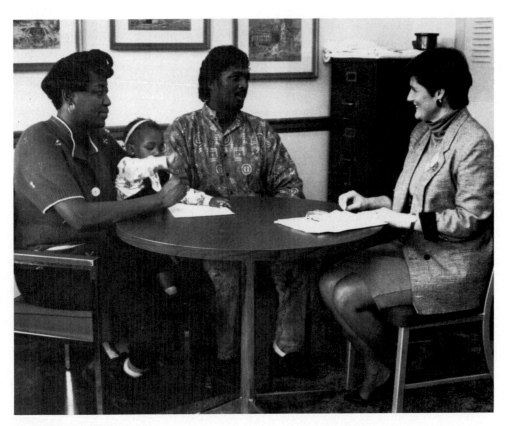

Public Policy Influences
Service Delivery

❏   How, where, for how long, and by whom should services be delivered?

The systems perspective discussed in Chapter 1 can be used to guide decisions for providing services for children with language disorders. Children function within broader systems by participating in multiple contexts that affect them and that they affect in turn, in the recursive causative patterns typical of systems. Problems are not only within children. They occur when the language and communication demands of situations exceed children's language and communication abilities.

Although systems function as wholes and cannot be subdivided without losing some of their essence, they are nevertheless composed of subsystems. Subsystems that exert major influences on service provision to children with language disorders operate on the levels of (1) **public policy**, including influences from federal, state, intermediate, and local levels, and (2) **service-delivery contexts**, including influences related to settings, people, and scheduling. Those two levels provide the organizational structure for this chapter.

PUBLIC POLICY INFLUENCES

For service provision to children with language disorders, even such preliminary steps as how professionals approach children and families are constrained by public policy. Therefore, this chapter begins with a consideration of public policy influences as they occur at federal, state, intermediate, and local levels.

Federal Policy

Federal policy in the United States is guided by laws passed by Congress. Other federal influences are based on court interpretations and on position papers, newsletters, and research priorities issued by federal agencies. Such influences are considered in this section.

Section 504 of the Rehabilitation Act of 1973. Section 504 of the Rehabilitation Act of 1973 (as amended with the Rehabilitation, Comprehensive Services and Developmental Disabilities Amendments of 1978) is significant because it prohibits recipients of federal assistance from discriminating against persons on the basis of their handicaps. This piece of civil rights legislation set the stage for passage of the Education for All Handicapped Children Act in 1975.

The passage of section 504 meant that, for the first time, children could not be excluded because of a handicap from attending schools that receive federal assistance. According to the wording of the law, "No qualified handicapped person shall, on the basis of handicap, be excluded from participation in, be denied the benefits of, or otherwise be subjected to discrimination under any program or activity conducted by the agency" (28 CFR 39.130(a)).

Public Law 94–142: The Education for All Handicapped Children Act of 1975 (Part B). The Education for All Handicapped Children Act was passed by the U.S. Congress in 1975. Often referred to as Public Law (PL) 94–142 (now known as the Individuals with Disabilities Education Act, IDEA, Part B), it is the most far-reaching piece of legislation affecting the education of children with handicaps ever passed in the United States. PL 94–142 guarantees the rights of all children in this country to a **free appropriate public education (FAPE)** in the **least restrictive environment (LRE)** (see discussion of LRE in Chapter 1). These rights are actualized by using an **Individualized Education Plan (IEP)**. The rules and regulations for implementing PL 94–142 were published in the *Federal Register* on August 23, 1977. Their initial implementation was required in 1979.

The regulations for PL 94–142 include requirements for multiple stages of service delivery to children with handicaps. The process starts with a mandate to states to design a child-find process to identify all children of school-age (in many states defined as ages 3 through 18) who might need special services. Other policies address procedures regarding parent notification, comprehensive multidisciplinary evaluation, IEP meetings, IEP content, and periodic reevaluation. Requirements for each of these activities are outlined briefly in the following discussion.

Parent notification.   Signed, informed, parental consent is required at two points under PL 94–142: (1) before a preplacement evaluation and (2) before initial placement in a program providing special education and related services. When obtaining parental consent, school districts must provide information about parental and child rights under both PL 94–142 and the Family Rights and Privacy Act. Those rights include parents' rights to review their children's records and to give permission before records are sent outside the district. When parents are notified, they must also be given descriptions of proposed activities in a way that they can understand.

It is not easy to present so much technical information understandably and concisely and without overwhelming parents. This is true regardless of parents' backgrounds, but it is especially difficult when parents' cultural and linguistic backgrounds differ from those of school officials. To meet requirements for informing parents, districts often develop multiple-copy forms, with preprinted explanations and places for parents to sign and to check off indicating that they have been properly informed. Forms like these are designed to meet the letter of the law and to pass the inspection of state and federal officials who periodically audit districts. Districts must take care, however, that check marks in boxes do not become more important than the actual interactions with parents that lead up to them. When this happens, something has gone wrong. Documentation should be used to represent important processes that have taken place; it should not become those processes.

Evaluators often have the first opportunity to develop relationships with parents. Whoever fills the role of first interpreting the special education process to parents should use culturally sensitive techniques in the interactions. The ethnographic strategy of attempting to view the experience through the eyes of the participants can assist. A face-to-face meeting is generally best for explaining the evaluation process, but if that is impossible, a telephone contact is better than a written one. The ultimate question underlying this phase of the interaction should be,

"Does this parent understand what is about to happen here, and the due process rights that go along with it, in his or her own terms?"

That question should be accompanied by one about potential effects of the notification process on the family system. If you accept the premise, developed in Chapter 1, that intervention begins when the first contact with the family is made (see Personal Reflection 1.13 by Dr. Sylvia Richardson), you also ask yourself at this point, "How is this event influencing this system, and how can I enhance the chances that the influence will be positive?"

Comprehensive multidisciplinary evaluation and determination of handicap.   The comprehensive multidisciplinary evaluation has two basic purposes: (1) to determine whether the child is eligible to receive special education services (see Chapter 4 for a discussion of the terminology differences for children in different categories who might need language intervention services) and (2) to identify specific intervention needs to be included in the first IEP.

Before a child is determined to be handicapped, "a full and individual evaluation of the child's educational needs must be conducted" (§121a.531) using more than one procedure, and those procedures must be "validated for the specific purpose for which they are used" (§121a.532(a)(2)). In addition, they must be selected and administered in ways that are not "racially or culturally discriminatory" (§121a.530(b)).

Concepts of bias in evaluation and eligibility determination may seem to be confined to issues of race and culture. However, an additional requirement of

---

Personal Reflection 5.1

"Since the enactment of Public Law (PL) 94–142, the Education for All Handicapped Children Act of 1975, it has been federally mandated that all test materials and procedures used for the evaluation of handicapped children be selected and administered in such a manner that they are not racially or culturally discriminatory. If this stipulation were enforced today to its fullest intent, most school systems in the United States would be in violation of the law. Eight years after PL 94–142 promised to be the salvation for all handicapped children, little has been done to improve tests and other evaluation procedures for handicapped children, especially those with communicative handicaps, to make the tests linguistically and culturally valid."

Orlando T. Taylor, Ph.D., and *Kay T. Payne, Ph.D.* (1983, p. 8), both of Howard University in Washington, D.C., writing in an article entitled "Culturally Valid Testing: A Proactive Approach."

PL 94–142 (one that is often ignored) pertains to issues of bias in which one type of impairment influences decisions made about another. This regulation has implications for making difficult decisions about children who have both cognitive impairments and language impairments. The regulation states that tests must be selected, administered, and interpreted so that:

> when a test is administered to a child with impaired sensory, manual, or speaking skills, the test results accurately reflect the child's aptitude or achievement level or whatever other factors the test purports to measure rather than reflecting the person's impaired sensory, manual, or speaking skills (except where those skills are the factors which the test purports to measure). (§121a.532(c))

This requirement has important implications when systems have rules using mental age (MA) as a reference point for determining eligibility. Consider a child with a language disorder given an intelligence test. The test requires the child to rely partially on defective language comprehension and production skills (even tests labeled "nonverbal" can rely heavily on language comprehension skills and the ability to use linguistic strategies for problem solving). The child's MA is computed for this test; the age score reflects the child's levels of language development and cognitive development. If this child resides within a school system that requires a discrepancy to be shown between language age and MA (sometimes called MA referencing) to qualify for language intervention services, the compounded test results may make it impossible for her to qualify, even though she has serious unmet needs. For such a child, the psychologist and speech–language pathologist should collaborate to look at multiple measures, including tests and subtests that tap areas of intelligence other than those guided by linguistic processing, as well as evidence of intelligence that might show up in less academic tasks. Such strategies can help the diagnostic team for this particular child tease out the relative influences of linguistic and general cognitive deficits.

To guard against a child being labeled as having one kind of handicap when another is primary (e.g., when a child with an unrecognized hearing impairment is labeled mentally retarded), PL 94–142 requires that a child must be "assessed in all areas related to the suspected disability, including, where appropriate, health, vision, hearing, social and emo-

tional status, general intelligence, academic performance, communicative status, and motor abilities" (§121a.532(f)). Because speech, language, and hearing impairments so often accompany other handicapping conditions, consideration of those areas is especially important when children are evaluated for other possible handicapping conditions.

Not all speech- and language-impaired children, however, receive complete psychological evaluations. In 1977, the following comment appeared:

> Comment. Children who have a speech impairment as their primary handicap may not need a complete battery of assessments (e.g., psychological, physical, or adaptive behavior). However, a qualified speech–language pathologist would (1) evaluate each speech impaired child using procedures that are appropriate for the diagnosis and appraisal of speech and language disorders, and (2) where necessary, make referrals for additional assessments needed to make an appropriate placement decision. (§121a.532)

For children with language and speech impairments, referrals for additional assessments are almost always necessary. Recall the discussion of interrelationships among speech, language, and communication in Chapter 2 and discussions of causes, categories, and contributing factors in Chapter 4. If a child has an impairment involving language as well as speech, then aspects of learning other than those that are obviously part of oral communication most likely are also affected. Learning to read and write and to benefit fully from oral and written language instruction in the classroom all require intact language systems. Children whose language skills do not match the increasingly sophisticated language processing demands of school are at serious risk for failing to learn and for developing accompanying self-esteem problems. Most children with language disorders need to be evaluated by a team of individuals who bring diverse expertise to the process and who can work together with the family and child to decide how to best serve the child's needs.

The use of assessment results to decide which children qualify to receive special services is one of the most difficult problems facing language specialists working in schools. Specific rules and criteria for determining eligibility for special services in school systems are usually established at state and local levels, not at federal levels. The rules and regulations for PL 94–142 provide only a circular definition of "handicapped":

§121a.5 Handicapped children

  (a) As used in this part, the term "handicapped children" means those children evaluated in accordance with §§121a.530–121a.534 as being mentally retarded, hard of hearing, deaf, speech impaired, visually handicapped, seriously emotionally disturbed, orthopedically impaired, other health impaired, deaf-blind, multi-handicapped, or as having specific learning disabilities, who because of those impairments need special education and related services.

You may recall the discussion from Chapter 1 about distinctions among definitions of impairment, disability, and handicap used by the World Health Organization. Remember that, in those definitions, the term *impairment* is reserved for the "loss or abnormality of psychological, physiological, or anatomical structure or function" (P. Wood, 1980, p. 4). The term *disability* is applied to the reduced ability to meet daily living needs, a condition that varies under different contexts and in varied stages of life (Frey, 1984; P. Wood, 1980). And the term *handicap* refers to the social disadvantage that results either from impairment or disability, a condition that varies depending on impairment, disability and the *attitudes and biases of others* in contact with the individual (Frey, 1984; P. Wood, 1980).

The regulations for PL 94–142 do not make exactly the same distinctions but do include the elements of need in determining disability and context in determining handicap. The following comment is pertinent in clarifying these distinctions:

  Comment. In Part B of the Act, the term "disability" is used interchangeably with "handicapping condition." For consistency in this regulation, a child with a "disability" means a child with one of the impairments listed in the definition of "handicapped children" in §121a.5, if the child needs special education because of the impairment. In essence, there is a continuum of impairments. When an impairment is of such a nature that the child needs special education, it is referred to as a disability in these regulations, and the child is a "handicapped" child. (§121a.124)

IEP meetings.   An important vehicle of PL 94–142 is the IEP, which is the document outlining the services to be delivered to a child. IEPs are developed at meetings so that decisions regarding the selection of a program for an individual child are not made unilaterally. After the first meeting, IEP meetings are also held at least annually (more often, if parents or school personnel request), to review and update the child's program. Individuals who must be present at the IEP meeting include the following:

1. A representative of the public agency, other than the child's teacher, who is qualified to provide or supervise the provision of special education.
2. The child's teacher.
3. One or both of the child's parents, subject to §121a.345.
4. The child, where appropriate.
5. Other individuals at the discretion of the parent or agency. (§121a.343(a))

The category of *other individuals* who might attend IEP meetings includes those who may be invited either by the school or district or the parents. At the first IEP meeting, it is specifically required that someone be present who can explain the evaluation results to the parents.

The requirements of PL 94–142 §121a.345 (mentioned in item 3) state that the parents must be notified of the meeting early enough that they will have an opportunity to attend, the meeting must be scheduled at a mutually agreed on time and place, and the parents must be encouraged to participate in other ways if neither parent can attend the meeting. Districts may hold an IEP meeting without parents, but only if the school district shows that it has made concerted, repeated attempts to involve the parents in the process and has been unable to convince them to participate. Other required procedures include keeping records of phone calls and copies of correspondence. The district must ensure that parents are fully informed about the purpose of the meeting and who will be there.

What are the real-life effects of these requirements? When you are involved in this process, it is important to remember that the familiar routine for the professionals in the IEP meeting may seem completely strange and threatening to the parents. When I was involved in many IEP meetings, I tried to interact with parents individually before the formal meetings whenever possible so that we could talk about what would happen at the meeting and the kinds of options that would be discussed. When they work well, IEP meetings offer the opportunity for cooperative goal setting (review goal-setting options from Chapter 1) and collaboration. When they do not work well, IEP meetings can be confrontational arenas of competitive goal setting at its worst.

Consider again the definition of collaborative consultation discussed in Chapter 1. It describes IEP meetings that work well, functioning as

> an interactive process that enables teams of people with diverse expertise to generate creative solutions to mutually defined problems. The outcome is enhanced, altered, and produces solutions that are different from those that the individual team members would produce independently. (Idol, Paolucci-Whitcomb, & Nevin, 1986, p. 1)

IEP content. The components that must be included in a child's IEP (the acronym IEP refers to both *programs* and *plans* in the regulations for PL 94–142) are clearly specified:

> The individual education program for each child must include:
> (a) A statement of the child's level of education performance;
> (b) A statement of annual goals, including short-term instructional objectives;
> (c) A statement of the specific special education and related services to be provided to the child, and the extent to which the child will be able to participate in regular education programs;
> (d) The projected dates for initiation of services and the anticipated duration of the services; and
> (e) Appropriate objective criteria and evaluation procedures and schedules for determining, on at least an annual basis, whether the short-term instructional objectives are being achieved. (§121a.346)

These requirements contribute to good professional practice in all settings. As legal requirements, however, they tend to generate preprinted paperwork monsters, with just a few blank spaces left to "individualize." Professionals and parents must try to keep IEPs concise, clear, and individualized and use them to work for children. It can be done, if the original purpose of IEP is kept forefront in mind, and if questions of the child's needs and opportunities, as well as impairments and abilities, are used to guide the deliberations that result in the written IEP (return to the discussion of Chapter 1).

Periodic reevaluation. A final requirement of PL 94–142 is that children must receive a comprehensive reevaluation, meeting all of the requirements of the preplacement evaluation, at least once every 3 years. Parents must then be notified that a formal evaluation is occurring that may affect the educational placement decisions regarding their child. At this point, parents do not have to give their written permission, but they must be formally informed. At the conclusion of the evaluation, the parents are invited to a meeting where the results are discussed. This meeting can be scheduled to coincide with the regularly scheduled IEP annual review.

PL 99–372: The Handicapped Children's Protection Act of 1986. In 1986, the U.S. Congress passed two new laws that further influence the provision of services outlined in PL 94–142: PL 99–372 and PL 99–457. These laws do not supplant PL 94–142 but augment it.

In the original Education for All Handicapped Children Act (PL 94–142), due process provisions ensure enforcement of the rights of all children to a free appropriate public education. These procedural safeguards grant parents the opportunity to examine all relevant records concerning their child, to obtain an independent evaluation if they disagree with the school district's evaluation, to receive prior notice if the school district proposes to initiate a change in the educational program, and to participate in team placement decisions. If a dispute arises regarding any of these rights, or if the parents and school district have a dispute over the child's education, either party may request an impartial due process hearing before a hearing officer, where parents can be accompanied and advised by legal counsel.

The impartial officer who holds the hearing decides the outcome. Although this decision is considered final, either the parents or the school may appeal to the state department of education for review. If the "administrative remedies" of the state do not result in satisfaction, either party may initiate a lawsuit in federal or state court. These steps are summarized in Figure 5.1.

The result of litigation in federal courts sometimes has been "relief" awarded to the families of handicapped children. The relief has been of three types: (1) **Injunctive relief** has been awarded when courts compel school officials to provide the education the court deems appropriate. (2) **Tuition reimbursement relief** has been awarded when the courts compel school officials to pay the costs of educating children in alternative placements chosen unilaterally

FIGURE 5.1

A due process ladder for parents concerned about educational services being provided for their children. Note that a due process hearing is not requested unless the parent reaches level 8 without satisfaction, and then only if the parent is seriously dissatisfied.

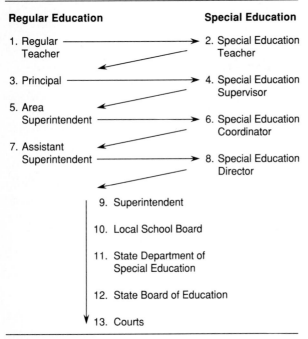

Regular Education	Special Education
1. Regular Teacher	2. Special Education Teacher
3. Principal	4. Special Education Supervisor
5. Area Superintendent	6. Special Education Coordinator
7. Assistant Superintendent	8. Special Education Director

9. Superintendent

10. Local School Board

11. State Department of Special Education

12. State Board of Education

13. Courts

Note. Figure from *After the Tears: Parents Talk About Raising a Child With a Disability* by R. Simons, copyright © 1987, 1985 by The Children's Museum of Denver, Inc., reprinted by permission of Harcourt Brace Jovanovich, Inc.

by parents. (3) **Attorney's fees** have been awarded on a case-by-case basis.

The Handicapped Children's Protection Act was passed by Congress to clarify its intent regarding relief. The law followed a U.S. Supreme Court decision in *Smith v. Robinson* (1984), which held that attorney's fees were not available to parents prevailing in special education lawsuits (Yell & Espin, 1990). The primary effect of PL 99–372 is to establish clearly the authority of courts to award reasonable attorney's fees to the parents or guardians of handicapped children if they prevail in a decision (retroactive to *Smith v. Robinson*, 1984), and to clarify the effect of the Education for All Handicapped Children Act on other laws. The Handicapped Children's Protection Act is considered important because a major factor in the success of PL 94–142 in making free appropriate pub-

lic education truly available to all children is the opportunity for parents to use the due process provisions of the act to resolve disputes between parents and schools (Yell & Espin, 1990).

PL 99–457: The Education of Handicapped Act Amendments of 1986 (Part H). The Education of Handicapped Amendments were passed in 1986. Although they were amendments to the Education for All Handicapped Children Act, they surpass the original act in several important ways, and they "fundamentally alter public policies for children with handicaps or developmental delays—and for their families" (Krauss, 1990, p. 388). PL 99–457 extends the requirement for provision of special education services to children from the ages of 3 to 5 years (by 1990), which is optional in PL 94–142. In addition, Part H of the law (sometimes the label *Part H* alone is used to refer to the new program; *Part B* may be used to refer to the original program requirements of PL 94–142) establishes a discretionary program to assist states to develop and implement a system of early intervention services for handicapped infants, toddlers, and their families.

The involvement of families in Part H represents three shifts in emphasis: (1) It involves the use of **Individualized Family Service Plans (IFSPs)** to redefine the service unit as being the family, rather than the child alone. (2) It requires explicit decisions to be made about the family's service needs. (3) It mandates family representation on the decision-making team. These three modifications represent a dramatic shift in public policy for young handicapped children and their families (Krauss, 1990).

Another distinction is in the way that the law is handled at the level of states. Whereas implementation of PL 94–142 is clearly the responsibility of each state's public education agency, the implementation of PL 99–457 is assigned to different designated lead agencies in the states by their governors. Governors in all 50 states have now affirmed their state's intention to implement the new law. In 21 states or territories, education agencies have been designated as lead agencies. In the others, health agencies or agencies devoted to welfare, human resources, or developmental disabilities have been designated. This is because PL 99–457 is intended to involve a "statewide system of coordinated, comprehensive, multidisciplinary, interagency programs providing appropriate early intervention services to all handicapped infants, toddlers, and their families" (§676.(a)), which does not supplant old ones. Fiscal resources should be coordinated to provide services at no cost to families "except where Federal or State law provides for a system of payments by families, including a schedule of sliding fees" (§672.(2)(B)).

Evaluation and eligibility. The definition of *handicapped infants and toddlers* in PL 99–457 follows:

(1) The term "handicapped infants and toddlers" means individuals from birth to age 2, inclusive, who need early intervention because they—
(a) are experiencing developmental delays, as measured by appropriate diagnostic instruments and procedures in one or more of the following areas: Cognitive development, physical development, language and speech development, psychosocial development, or self-help skills, or
(b) have a diagnosed physical or mental condition which has a high probability of resulting in developmental delay.
Such term may also include, at a State's discretion, individuals from birth to age 2, inclusive, who are at risk of having substantial developmental delays if early intervention services are not provided. (§672.(1))

Issues related to evaluation of infants and toddlers are considered in Chapter 7. Two important policy contributions, however, that need to be considered here for their potential influence on the development of services to children in various states over the next few years are (1) the assignment to states of the responsibility to write more specific definitions and (2) the possibility that states may, at their discretion, choose to serve children at risk for handicap as well as those with identified handicaps. These opportunities will likely result in variations in implementation of the law at the state level.

Individualized Family Service Plan. One requirement of the law that will remain consistent across states, however, is that an IFSP must be written. The IFSP is similar to the IEP but has several important distinctions. In PL 99–457, IFSPs are described as follows:

CONTENT OF PLAN—The individualized family service plan shall be in writing and contain—
(1) a statement of the infant's or toddler's present levels of physical development, cognitive development, language and speech development, psycho-social development, and self-help skills, based on acceptable objective criteria,

(2) a statement of the family's strengths and needs relating to enhancing the development of the family's handicapped infant or toddler,
(3) a statement of the major outcomes expected to be achieved for the infant or toddler and the family, and the criteria, procedures, and timelines used to determine the degree to which progress toward achieving the outcomes are being made and whether modifications or revisions of the outcomes or services are necessary,
(4) a statement of specific early intervention services necessary to meet the unique needs of the infant or toddler and the family, including the frequency, intensity, and the method of delivering services,
(5) the projected dates for initiation of services and the anticipated duration of such services,
(6) the name of the case manager from the profession most immediately relevant to the infant's and toddler's or family's needs who will be responsible for the implementation of the plan and coordination with other agencies and persons, and
(7) the steps to be taken supporting the transition of the handicapped toddler to services provided under Part B [the original PL 94–142] to the extent such services are considered appropriate. (1986, §677.(d))

The idea that an IFSP should be individualized is not new, but the requirement that it involve families to the degree that it does, is new. IFSPs also must be revised at least twice per year, compared with once for IEPs. Families not only must be included as active members of multidisciplinary teams, but they must also be described in the IFSP. Their strengths and needs relative to the infant or toddler with the handicap must be written down, and a case manager must be assigned.

This strategy is fraught with complex implications. Although it is too early to report on broad experience implementing the law, it is possible to imagine a scenario in which a team of specialists, using a traditional assessment model, might approach a family, study it, analyze it, and list the family's strengths and needs. Then, the family might be invited to a meeting where their "strengths and needs" are presented and discussed and where they are presented with a list of recommendations.

Imagine yourself as the parent of a recently born infant with problems. How would you feel if someone decided to intervene this way? Add the consideration that you have had only a few months to become accustomed to the idea that your imagined perfect child has problems. You are likely still to be going through the stages of guilt, anger, and mourning that

---

Personal Reflection 5.2   "I've heard this period called 'nothingness' and that's exactly how you feel. You can't move, can't think, can't do anything but feel—leaden like a rock. There's *nothing* there—but that disability."

Parent of a handicapped child speaking about the early stages of adjustment, quoted by Robin Simons (1987, p. 6), in the book *After the Tears*.

In the book, Simons introduces the task facing parents with these words: "In parenting a child with a disability you face a major choice. You can believe that your child's condition is a death blow to everything you've dreamed and worked toward until now. Or you can decide that you will continue to lead the life you'd planned—and incorporate your child into it. Parents who choose the latter course find that they do a tremendous amount of growing." (Preface written by Simons, 1987.)

---

are part of that process. (See the book *After the Tears*, Simons, 1987, for an explanation of some of these effects; also see Luterman, 1979, for an explanation of how parental stages of adjustment can recur at multiple points in a child's life.) Now someone comes in to analyze your family to tell you how to fix things. To a mind that has already been dealing with issues of guilt, the most rational conclusion might be that, "Yes, I really must be the cause of my child's problems."

Now imagine a different scenario: Two caring professionals begin to get to know your family at times that are arranged jointly. You are asked to show the professionals things that you have learned about your baby. Together, you explore contexts in which your child functions differently—such as places and positions for feeding and playing, food textures, times of the day, toys, pets, and people—that seem to bring out different skills, abilities, and reactions from your baby. Gradually, joint concepts evolve so that it becomes clear that problems that may have seemed to be an inherent part of the baby actually vary with the surroundings and that the baby brings more than just problems to interactions. You become increasingly comfortable in asking the professionals questions and learning about your baby's disability, but you appreciate that the professionals always seem to respect your role as the expert on your own baby. By the time you schedule the first IFSP meeting, you are ready to sit down together and talk about the current situation and about your hopes and expectations for the next few years. You work together to create a mutually defined statement of strengths, problems, and needs that recognize the ecology of your own family. You

are a legitimate member of the team. In which situation would you rather participate?

The qualified service provider requirements of PL 99–457. Another part of PL 99–457 related to service delivery to children with language disorders requires all professionals providing service to meet the highest standards in their state. Therefore, if a state has licensure or requires a master's degree in language, speech, and hearing to work as a speech–language pathologist in any setting, all providers of speech–language intervention services to handicapped infants, toddlers, children, and their families must meet this standard.

PL 101–476: The Individuals with Disabilities Education Act of 1990 (IDEA). On October 30, 1990, President George Bush signed into law the Education of the Handicapped Amendments of 1990, changing the name of the Education for All Handicapped Children Act to Individuals with Disabilities Education Act (IDEA) and adding the numbers PL 101–476 to the list of laws aimed at protecting the rights of all children in the United States to a free appropriate public education. Consistent with international clarification of terminology (see World Health Organization definitions of *impairment*, *disability*, and *handicap* earlier in this chapter and in Chapter 1), the 1990 amendments did more than add provisions to the law when they reauthorized it. They also changed the name of the law and specified that whenever the word *handicap* appeared in the original wording, it should be replaced with the term *disability*.

New categories of disability. Among other changes (including increased emphasis on providing materials and training for parents, providing programs for children exposed prenatally to maternal substance abuse, meeting the needs of ethnically and culturally diverse children with disabilities, and targeting the elimination of illiteracy among individuals with disabilities), the reauthorization expanded the general definition of children with disabilities to include children with autism and traumatic brain injury as separate categories. During hearings preceding the final drafting of the act, considerable controversy was raised over whether attention-deficit disorder (ADD) should also be added as a separate category or subcategory. After much debate, it was decided not to include ADD as a new category at that time but to publish a Notice of Inquiry to gather additional data and viewpoints.

Transition plans. The other major change brought about by the amendments of PL 101–476 with significance for children and adolescents with language and communication disorders involves requirements regarding transition services, defined as follows:

> Transition services means a coordinated set of activities for a student, designed with an outcome-oriented process, which promotes movement from school to post-school activities including postsecondary education, vocational training, integrated employment (including supported employment), continuing and adult education, adult services, independent living or community participation.
>
> The coordinated set of activities shall be based upon the individual student's needs, taking into account the student's preferences and interests, and shall include instruction, community experiences, the development of employment and other postschool adult living objectives, and, when appropriate, acquisition of daily living skills and functional vocational evaluation. (§1401a.19)

The description of what must be included in IEPs is:

> a statement of the needed transition services for students beginning no later than age sixteen and annually thereafter (and when determined appropriate for the individual, beginning at age fourteen or younger), including, when appropriate, a statement of the interagency responsibilities or linkages (or both) before the student leaves the school setting.
>
> In the case where a participating agency, other than the educational agency, fails to provide agreed upon services, the educational agency shall reconvene the IEP team to identify alternative strategies to meet the transition objectives. (§1401a.20)

Transition services may seem to be primarily the responsibility of vocational education specialists, but speech–language pathologists and other language-learning specialists also should be involved in trans-disciplinary efforts to plan and implement transition. Language and communication skills contribute to success, whether a person's transition plan is aimed primarily toward higher education or employment. Language assessment activities, for example, might include observation of functional communication demands and expectations of targeted contexts. Then intervention goals and activities should be coordinated with transition plan outlines to help prepare students to meet those functional communication requirements.

Other federal-level influences. *Outcomes of case law.* Laws present opportunities for varying interpretations. When litigation is used to interpret law, the implications of the outcomes of individual cases for service delivery can extend beyond the individual case. For example, in a recent case in New Hampshire, a U.S. District Judge ruled that 13-year-old Timothy W., who was quadriplegic and severely handicapped, was ineligible for education services because he could not "benefit" from special education. The case (*Timothy W. v. Rochester School District*, 1989) was appealed, and three federal judges overturned the earlier ruling and reaffirmed the intention of PL 94–142 that regardless of severity of impairment, no child is too impaired to benefit from special education. This finding is now known informally as the "no exclusion" ruling.

Practicing professionals can best remain current on case law outcomes by participating in professional associations and state and federal information networks. These groups often monitor and publish summaries of important case results in newsletters and computer bulletin board networks.

The Regular Education Initiative. A prime example of a policy influence not based on law but on a position paper issued by a federal agency is the Regular Education Initiative (REI). It is based on a paper by Madeline Will, Undersecretary in the U.S. Office of Special Education and Rehabilitative Services in 1986, called *"Educating Students with Learning Problems: A Shared Responsibility."* The essence of the REI is its proposal to "serve as many children as possible in the regular classroom by encouraging a partnership with regular education" (Will, 1986, p. 20). As originally conceived, it apparently was aimed primarily at mildly handicapped students, such as students with educable mental retardation or learning disabilities (most of whom have language disorders). These children, especially those with learning disabilities, were pulled out of regular education and served in special education in record numbers in 1986.

The discussion of the REI is in full force in the 1990s. Thus far, the debate has been largely in the special education community. This is curious, considering the broad implications of the REI for regular education (W. E. Davis, 1989). Recently, however, the REI has begun to draw more attention from regular educators. W. E. Davis outlined the arguments of both proponents and opponents of the REI and suggested possible interpretations for why individuals in each group might feel the way they do. He suggested that the debate needed to be moved into the forum of regular education and local policymakers.

Responding to this invitation, Byrnes (1990), a school administrator in Sudbury, Massachusetts, noted the advantages of the REI for students who had potential to keep up with the regular curriculum but expressed concerns about its appropriateness for students with more severe cognitive and behavioral control problems. Her suggestions were to "keep all options open" and to "keep opening the debate" (Byrnes, 1990, p. 348). In responding to Byrnes's comments, W. E. Davis (1990) urged participants in the debate not to see it as an either/or proposition— that is, either to keep the current special education system in place as it is currently implemented or to abandon old methods entirely and move all handicapped students into regular education settings. Both Byrnes (1990) and W. E. Davis (1990) urged a broadening of respect for diversity.

Full-integration initiatives. Byrnes's (1990) comments illustrate the overlap between the discussion of the REI, as the original position paper was written, and discussions regarding integration of all handicapped students in schools with children who are developing and learning normally. Federal policy influences on processes designed to integrate handicapped students or to include them with their normally developing peers are even less formally articulated than the REI position. The idea of community integration is not so much an official policy as it is a philosophy, and yet it promises to exert a significant influence over service provision to many children with language disorders and other handicaps.

Several ideas related to full integration of handicapped students were published in an article called "Community Integration: The Next Step" (Office of Special Education and Rehabilitation Services, 1989):

> Over the last several years the Office of Special Education and Rehabilitation Services (OSERS) has made a major commitment to the goal of fostering greater integration of students with disabilities into the community. This commitment is based on the premise that isolation makes it harder for students with disabilities to develop appropriate interpersonal skills. The lack of such skills often creates obstacles to proper adjustment. Without the experience of living and working in community settings, it becomes more difficult for students with disabilities to succeed in the "real world" after they leave school. (p.1)

Interpretations of the full integration initiative (sometimes called *inclusive education*) and REI in the future will depend on policy decisions made at state, intermediate, and local levels. Those levels are considered next.

State Policy

State education agencies bear the responsibility for implementing the IDEA, which includes Part B (PL 94–142) of the Education for All Handicapped Children Act, in all 50 states, and they have been named as lead agencies for implementing Part H (PL 99–457) in 21 states. As specified in those laws, states have advisory committees. They also employ staff to oversee the implementation of laws. Beyond these similarities, wide differences in public policy may exist among states.

State policies generally influence service provision to children with language disorders beyond federal policies. For example, states often have guidelines for evaluating children and finding them eligible for service. They also have certification or licensure standards outlining the professional preparation needed to provide specialized services to these children. Because states are involved in funding special services, states' formulae and procedures also are likely to exert policy influences. Because states differ widely in their policies, however, readers must seek sources within their own states to understand the policies that affect children with language disorders there.

Intermediate Policy

Different states have different labels for the intermediate-level education agency. For example, Michigan has Intermediate School Districts; Pennsylvania has Intermediate Units; Texas, Independent School Districts; Iowa, Area Education Agencies; New York, Boards of Cooperative Educational Services (BOCES); California, cooperatives or consortiums. Not all states have policy-making bodies at this level, and not all agencies at the intermediate level perform the same functions. However, intermediate-level agencies can exert significant influence on making, implementing, and monitoring the implementation of policy. As PL 99–457 is implemented, a whole new set of intermediate-level agencies, including third-party payers, may become involved in making policies regarding service delivery for infants and toddlers and their families.

One contribution of many intermediate-level agencies has been to provide centralized services for children with "low-incidence" conditions such as moderate-to-severe retardation, autism, and multiple physical and mental impairments. These conditions are considered relatively rare and are not likely to show up frequently in any one local school district (unless it is in a large city; then city-wide school districts tend to take on many intermediate-level functions). Professionals in local districts therefore may be less familiar with the handicapping conditions and their treatment. Local districts (at least small ones) also may not employ the kinds of specialized service providers (e.g., occupational therapists and physical therapists, educators of the hearing impaired, audiologists, and augmentative communication specialists) who can provide the services that such children might need. As a result, sometimes officially, sometimes simply by tradition, children are bused throughout an entire intermediate or "cooperative" district to a central location where "appropriate" services can be provided and where they are isolated from normally developing children in their own communities. The question that local planners and families are beginning to ask is whether services provided in isolation are truly more appropriate than those that might be provided at the local level. (See, however, the following section on service-delivery scheduling, especially Figure 5.2, for an example of some of the difficulties faced by rural districts with few resources when they attempt to serve children with limited help from specialists.)

Some of the changes that will evolve at the intermediate policy level in the 1990s may be a shift away from the model of bringing children to centralized programs to using consultants with specialized expertise who go to the students to provide new and different services. These specialists may continue to be employed at the intermediate level but may function more as consultants. They might collaborate with regular and special education teachers and speech–language specialists in local districts rather than providing direct service themselves.

On the other hand, some children may benefit fully from educational experiences only when they are provided in specialized contexts (with control of variables such as room acoustics and group sizes) and by teachers who have specialized expertise in meeting their learning needs and encouraging them to develop more mature skills. Furthermore, as the sections on people variables later in this chapter attest, merely placing children side by side does not ensure that they will interact. As new opportunities are explored and as new questions are asked, the events are certain to be interesting. It is hoped that the outcome will be decisions that are beneficial for children.

Local Policy

Local policy may be articulated in official documents, or it may be implemented as a part of long-standing traditions. It is, of course, impossible to outline here all of the kinds of local policy decisions that might affect provision of services to children with language disorders. In general, local policies influence factors such as which school buildings house special programs or classrooms and which rooms are used for what kinds of services.

Because public policy established at local levels can vary widely, parents and service providers have more opportunity to influence it there than at any other level. For example, parents may serve on parent advisory councils, work with others in special interest groups, and run for positions on local school boards. Parents can also work cooperatively with their local school officials, both special and regular educators (building principals are perhaps the single most important individuals to have on one's side when working at the local level) to design programs that will accomplish mutually defined goals that are good for children.

Implications of Knowing About Policy and How It Is Made

Because public policy can profoundly influence service provision to children, families, and teachers, part of being an effective language interventionist involves knowing how to participate in the process of establishing public policy. Doing so involves several strategies.

The first and most important strategy is to understand current policies and their sources. Knowledge is power when it comes to making public policy. If someone tells you that you cannot do something that you think would be good for a child with a language disorder because of policy, first try to understand thoroughly the current policy that prohibits the activity. What is the actual wording of the rule? Where is it printed? Who made the rule? To answer these questions, you may ask your supervisor (in a nonthreatening manner) for a copy of the document that established the rule, or you may go to agencies at the other levels to obtain copies of important policy documents from them.

Once you believe that you understand the current policy, you can look for flexibility within it. Maybe the policy itself does not prohibit the activity, but overinterpretation does. This is where your collaborative negotiating skills are needed. Again, go to your immediate supervisor, but first be sure that your plan represents a collaborative effort with others involved in the problem-solving activity. If the problem involves a child in school, the building principal is an essential participant, in addition, of course, to the child's parents. At this meeting, present an organized plan to show how the desired activity is good for the child, is consistent with the current IEP or IFSP (if there is one), can be conducted so as not to violate written policy, and represents the results of collaborative planning efforts.

If current policy clearly prohibits the activity you wish to employ, you have several choices. First, you can seek to understand the rationale for the original policy and may, in the process, give up your idea. Second, you can decide that your idea, although inconsistent with prior established policy, is an innovative one, worth pursuing and good for children. In such cases, you may obtain special approval to implement your plan as an experimental or model program. Most states have provisions for these kinds of activities and may even have special sources of funding, as long as you can satisfy the appropriate groups that your idea is worthwhile and of benefit to children. Third, you can work to change the official policy.

If you elect the third choice, you will need to know not only what the current policy is, but how it was established and how it can be changed. Then you will have to set about moving through those channels. This may be a long and frustrating course, and it generally requires association with others (e.g., regional or state speech-language-hearing associations and other advocacy groups), but if the potential benefits

to children with language disorders are great enough, the effort will be worth it (see O'Brien & O'Leary, 1988, for a description of a case in which they chose this course). Individuals can make a difference in public policy. It just takes patience, persistence, understanding the political process, and watching for the right place and time.

SERVICE DELIVERY

Although it is important to understand policy and how it is generated, the crucial decisions that influence children are those that are made for them as individuals. These decisions are of two broad types. One concerns daily activities of individual assessment and intervention. That kind of decision is considered in Chapter 6 as well as in Chapters 7 to 9. Another kind of decision involves the broader selection of settings and people and the timing of events involved in those activities.

Variables related to settings, people, and scheduling are combined to design service-delivery models. In this section, I discuss variables in those three areas separately to highlight their individual contributions to the acquisition and generalization of language by children with language disorders (see Table 5.1, later in this chapter, for service-delivery models and caseload sizes recommended by the ASHA Committee on Language, Speech, and Hearing Services in Schools, 1984).

As in other cases, choices should be guided by good questions. An important question underlying the selection of service-delivery variables is "How can we use intervention settings, people, and schedules to maximize the opportunities for this child to acquire the language abilities the child needs for participating in important life contexts?"

Setting Variables

When selecting service-delivery settings for individual children, it is helpful to start by considering the contexts where children would spend most of their time if they were developing normally. Such contexts serve as a baseline for determining least restrictive environments.

Infants and toddlers spend most of their time at home and in day-care settings. At age 3 years, some enter preschool. Preschoolers also accompany their parents more often to the grocery store and on other errands, and they may play with other children in the park or neighborhood. By the time they are 5 or 6 years old, they enter school, and, unless they drop out, they spend most of their days, for 9 or 10 months out of the year, in regular education classrooms until they are age 18. Increasingly, during these years, they try to spend more time with their peers and less with their parents. When they are 16 years old, they might get a job, they probably begin to drive, and they attempt to pursue actively the independent lives for which they have been lobbying since their years of preadolescence. Yet, in functional families, part of the pushing seems to involve making sure that adults are there to push against. There is safety and security in a consistent family context and in feeling successful at school.

Children who need assistance because of language disorders have probably experienced some degree of failure in communicating in one or more of these contexts. If the natural contexts of the child's life have limitations for meeting the child's needs and opportunities for language growth and communicative participation, parents and service providers may attempt to modify the contexts, making them more conducive to meeting needs and providing opportunities. In some cases, however, either instead of a natural context, or in addition to it, specialized contexts are required to meet children's individualized language learning needs. Special contexts may also be used to provide communicative opportunities that cannot be met within the child's natural contexts. If, in such cases, intervention teams (including parents) move carefully and deliberately through the decision-making process, children will not be removed from the natural contexts of their lives unless removal appears to meet their needs. Furthermore, once a child has been placed in a special learning context, steps should be taken to monitor the child's function-ing to ensure that the child's needs continue to be met and that intervention efforts act to increase the child's ability to function in the least restrictive environment and not to decrease it. Monitoring should also be provided after children are returned to regular contexts (remember the problems that occurred as a result of lack of follow-up in Damico's 1988 case study, discussed in Chapter 1).

Language intervention setting options. Options for intervention settings include home, preschool, regular classrooms, special education classrooms, small clinic-like rooms (called "pullout rooms" here), and various work and social settings. Traditionally, language specialists have used pullout rooms most frequently as contexts for providing language intervention services.

Pullout rooms. The practice of using pullout rooms to provide language intervention services has been prevalent for many reasons. Services to children with language disorders tend to have evolved out of services to children with speech impairments in schools and clinics (L. Miller, 1989), and those services traditionally have been provided in special rooms, either one-on-one or to children in small groups. The advantages of this setting relate to the control the language specialist can exert over communicative contexts. Ironically, so do its disadvantages.

Consider first the advantages. On the basis of practicality and cost, more children can be seen in a week if the children come to the specialist than if the specialist goes to the children. On a more philosophical basis, it can be argued that if children could learn language normally without specialized intervention, they would have done so already, and they never would have been referred for special attention. In

---

Personal Reflection 5.3   "Decisions about where handicapped students should be instructed have received more attention, undergone more modifications, and generated even more controversy than have decisions about how or what these students are taught. Handicapped students' educational journey has come nearly full circle. Their odyssey, which began in general education classrooms, took them first to special schools, from there to full-time special classes, and on to resource rooms with part-time placement in regular classrooms, and now they appear to be headed in the direction of full-time placement in general education classrooms."

Joseph R. Jenkins and *Amy Heinen* (1989, p. 516).

such cases, pullout rooms allow professionals to exert control over the many variables that influence whether or not a child can perform specific tasks such as speaking in sentences, taking conversational turns, and using new words meaningfully. For example, in small pullout rooms, auditory and visual distractions can be controlled and contexts can be structured so that children have more turns to talk, more guidance, and more positive reinforcement for attempting to use new language skills than they do in more natural settings. Pullout rooms also allow older children with difficulties to practice new skills in environments that reduce the stress of trying to look good in front of their peers and to avoid being embarrassed by needing special help.

A major advantage of pullout settings is that they permit intentioned adults to design special contexts allowing children to experience success and to acquire new skills and knowledge in small increments using organized formats. Such contexts are particularly important when evidence indicates that the children are unable to acquire such skills and knowledge in less controlled and less systematically organized contexts. In pullout rooms, children may have more time to talk with an adult who is working to facilitate that skill and checking to ensure that the children really understand.

A major danger of such settings, however, is that, in redefining the child's world, adults may create a world so different from the child's natural world that, at best, newly learned skills do not transfer to the regular contexts of the child's life, or, at worst, the child is increasingly isolated from those contexts. Another disadvantage is that it is difficult to provide rich opportunities for developing language content and to use skills in a context that is so highly controlled.

The social interaction views of language acquisition discussed in Chapter 3 suggest that children learn to talk and to understand language because language is meaningful to them and because they need it to interact with others. It is difficult to contrive situations in pullout rooms that capture these qualities. Cognitivist views of language acquisition discussed in Chapter 3 suggest that children learn to talk and to interact with others because it is an integral part of learning about the world and how they relate to it. In this case as well, the context stripping that tends to accompany communication in pullout rooms can hardly be imagined to facilitate this type of language learning. Behaviorist views of language acquisition, also dis-

cussed in Chapter 3, suggest that children learn to talk the way they do because certain words and patterns are selectively reinforced as communicative, whereas noncommunicative language is not. Although stimuli and reinforcers can be controlled extensively in pullout rooms, using those rooms as contexts for natural reinforcement that encourages generalization is difficult. The kind of language encouraged in the contrived tasks often used and reinforced in pullout rooms more likely consists of isolated units of limited communicative value. Even linguistic theories of language acquisition (see Chapter 3) do not lead to the selection of pullout rooms as the best contexts for language learning. Such theories suggest that children learn language by exposure to a variety of linguistic evidence, from which they form hypotheses and infer linguistic regularities. The limited forms of evidence available in such contexts might tend to constrain, rather than extend, language-learning opportunities that contribute to language acquisition.

Although pullout rooms do have some advantages as contexts for providing language intervention, and children sometimes even prefer them to avoid embarrassment (see the section on children's preferences later in this chapter), they also have decided disadvantages. When pullout rooms are viewed solely as a context for pulling children out, taking them down the hall (or into any purely clinical area), fixing them, and putting them back, the risk is that any "fixing" will have limited relevance to children's lives. Changes may also be more likely to transfer to other contexts when those contexts are considered to be valid intervention settings. Although pullout rooms may provide one context for intervention, they should generally be used only in conjunction with attention to language use in other contexts.

Special classrooms in special buildings. Most often, children with severe and multiple handicaps are placed in special classrooms in special buildings. Many such "center" programs were developed during the 1970s to provide centralized services to children with low-incidence handicapping conditions in buildings specially designed to meet their needs (e.g., with ramps instead of stairs, bathrooms with access for wheelchairs, and therapeutic swimming pools). In some cases, the children served in such programs were just being returned to their home communities from state institutions, where (before Section 504 and the implementation of PL 94–142, 1977) they might have received limited or no education and special services.

In center programs, children might be bused long distances from several local districts within a cooperative or "intermediate" district to be brought together with children with similar impairments and educational and therapy needs. Within center programs, children may be pulled out of their classrooms to receive language intervention services, or those services may be provided as part of classroom programming.

The advantage of providing services to children in center programs is that facilities can be specially designed, and specialists can be gathered together to meet the needs of children with severe handicaps and to tailor activities to their levels of functioning. These same factors, however, can be listed as disadvantages. Interpretations of children's needs have shifted. Rather than emphasizing remediation of impairments in specialized environments, the focus has shifted to encouraging socialization and education of children with severe handicaps so that they may join the rest of society.

In some cases, attempts have been made to encourage integration of handicapped and nonhandicapped peers by building special facilities beside regular school education buildings. The results of such efforts in terms of peer interaction have not met expectations. For example, Mercer and Denti (1989) studied a 5-year effort to integrate regular and special education students on a campus where the students were housed in separate but adjacent facilities with separate administrators. When observational data and questionnaires revealed almost total segregation after the first 3 years, intensive efforts were undertaken to encourage integration further but without enduring effects. The authors concluded that "Physical, social, and psychological barriers created by the two-roof school erect almost insurmountable obstacles to integration. Future efforts should concentrate on building one-roof schools with a single facility and administration" (p.30).

Special classrooms in regular buildings. In some cases, children with language disorders are placed in special classrooms in regular buildings. The nature of service delivery in such classrooms depends not only on where the rooms are located but the teacher's orientation. Most teachers of special classrooms are special education teachers with credentials to teach children with handicaps such as mental retardation or learning disabilities. Many children with mental retardation and most children with learning disabilities need language intervention as well as other special education services. Such needs may be met partially within the special education classroom and partially within language intervention pullout rooms. Some children attend special education resource rooms that may function more as pullout rooms than as special classrooms, and these may be in addition to other pullout rooms where they receive speech and language intervention services (see Personal Reflection 5.5, where "Barbie" describes this situation from a student's perspective). Occasionally, speech–language pathologists serve as classroom teachers or co-teachers and assume the responsibility for teaching all or most of the curriculum to children with severe language impairments in self-contained classes (L. P. Hoffman, 1990; N. W. Nelson, 1981a). Approaches used in such classrooms are discussed in later chapters of this book.

Although children are often placed in special education classrooms based on their category of impairment, the services provided in different types of categorical rooms may not be distinguishable. In one study (Algozzine, Morsink, & Algozzine, 1989), interactions were analyzed in 40 self-contained special classes for children classified with learning disability, emotional handicap, or educable mental retardation. The results showed few differences in the teacher

---

Personal Reflection 5.4	"They're always trying to 'fix' Marti—as if they can't accept the fact that she's handicapped. They spend all their time working on things she *can't* do without giving her a chance to enjoy the things she *can*." *Carol Knibbs*, mother of a 14-year-old daughter who is retarded, quoted by Simons (1987, p. 48).

communication patterns, learner involvement, and instructional methods used in the three types of classes. The researchers commented that this outcome raised questions about the appropriateness of categorical grouping of students for instruction.

Regular classrooms. School-age children with language disorders may spend the majority, or only limited parts, of their days in regular classrooms. What these children are expected to do in such settings may vary widely, however, depending on how the professionals involved view the role of the regular classroom in the child's educational development. As in the preceding discussions, whether features of regular classrooms act as advantages or disadvantages for particular children depends on complex interactions among the variables of settings, people, and scheduling.

Regular classrooms may be integral to service provision, whether children's impairments are relatively mild or severe. When children can almost but not quite succeed in the regular classroom and the regular curriculum, service provision can focus on that setting, with language intervention designed to help children process the language of education. Pullout sessions may be used intermittently primarily to foster the process of curriculum-based language intervention (N. W. Nelson, 1989b), but the child is viewed to be a full member of the regular classroom. Whether the classroom itself is considered to be a language intervention context depends on the philosophy and attitudes of the entire educational team, including the building principal and, particularly, the classroom teacher. Even when conditions are less than ideal, however, the development of regular classrooms as intervention contexts can be influenced by using collaborative consultation, particularly when the language specialist-consultant approaches the classroom teacher with the question "How can I help you do your job?" rather than "How can you help me do mine?"

Traditionally, children have been "mainstreamed" into regular classrooms only in curricular areas where it was felt that they could be academically competitive (e.g., L. P. Hoffman, 1990). After full-integration policy shifts, however, children with more severe language impairments and associated handicaps may be placed in regular classrooms for all or major parts of their days, even when educators suspect that they may not be able to handle all aspects of the regular curriculum.

Beukelman and Mirenda (1992) have written about the educational integration of students with severe disabilities and the need for augmentative communication. They distinguished three patterns of academic and social participation as (1) competitive, (2) active, or (3) included. In this system, *competitive* academic participation is observed when students with disabilities can meet the academic standards expected of all students, at least in some areas. Some students are competitive only with compensations from specialized technology, a teacher's aide, or a reduction in the amount of work. *Active* academic participation is observed when students can participate in regular education activities and learning but cannot meet the same academic standards as peer students. *Included* academic participation is observed when students spend time with their peers in regular academic settings but have minimal ability to compete academically at the level expected of their peers. Inclusion in regular classroom settings is valued for other reasons.

Descriptions of social participation patterns are parallel (Beukelman & Mirenda, 1992). Patterns of competitive social participation describe students who exert autonomy in choosing social participation areas and friends and who influence the social environment cooperatively. Patterns of active social participation describe students who benefit socially from involvement with same-age peers and who enjoy participation but who influence it minimally. Patterns of included social participation describe students who are present in the regular classroom and for other school events but influence social interactions minimally and participate little.

In some school systems, regular classrooms are modified somewhat to meet the special intervention needs of children with language disorders and other handicapping conditions. For example, Despain and Simon (1987) described an approach in which they identified children at the end of the sixth-grade year who were at risk because of weak language skills for failure in science, social studies, and English courses when they advanced to junior high school. These students were placed in regular junior high school classes with regular teachers, but with fewer students, where teachers (with consultant help) could concentrate on incorporating the development of communication and study skills into course content.

When mainstreaming does not work, it is generally because a child is included physically, but integrated minimally, although the child might be capable of more. This unfortunate situation tends to occur when children move in and out of regular education classrooms but are not really viewed to be part of the class. (This is what happened to Barbie, Personal Reflection 5.5.) Although the other children are reading or receiving instruction, the mainstreamed children might be completing coloring worksheets at their desks as a way of keeping them busy rather than helping them learn. When this happens, it usually represents a breakdown at the people level rather than the setting level. Teachers may simply not know how to make the curriculum accessible to the special needs child or they may not expect the child to be able to handle any of it. When language problems are present, before decisions are made to remove children from regular classroom contexts, or to isolate them further from regular curricular expectations, regular and special educators and language specialists might collaborate to find ways to make more of the regular curriculum accessible. Techniques for doing so are discussed in Chapters 8 and 9.

Home and family contexts. Parents are first and foremost parents. Professionals must be careful to avoid shifting that relationship by asking parents to be primarily therapists for their children (see Personal Reflection 5.7). When home and family contexts are targeted as language intervention settings (and they almost always should be, if only indirectly), they may be used to intensify natural language experiences and interactions—experiences that cannot be provided in pullout rooms and other settings. Asking parents to turn their kitchen tables into pullout rooms carries the disadvantage of potentially adding to parental burdens more than helping their children.

Some strategies have been suggested, however, for using homes as fairly structured language intervention settings. Fey (1986) reviewed the literature on homes as intervention settings for young children. He found more evidence supporting changes in parental behavior following training than evidence that parents implemented the procedures in the home. Fey reported that monitoring of changed interactions

---

Personal Reflection 5.5

In this conversational sample, 11-year-old, third-grade *Barbie* (B) and her clinician (C), Janet Sturm (to whom I am indebted for this sample), are talking about Barbie's feelings about school. Barbie began the topic after they started talking about what is hard about school.

B: I don't know about Mrs. Y. She doesn't even let me take my books (in in) anywhere.

C: Really?

B: Yeah, (she) she's my second teacher. I have three teachers. My first one is [pause] Mrs. B. (She) she's my real teacher. Mrs. Y., she's the resource room. Mrs. M., she's my speech teacher.

C: Oh.

B: So, it's hard. You have to go, hurry, and go back, uh uh uh [motioning with her hands while she makes sound effects to represent traveling back and forth] and get [unintelligible word].

C: Like you're coming and going all the time?

B: Yeah [laughs]. Like in eighth grade.

C: Like they do in eighth grade.

B: They do nuh nuh nuh nuh nuh nah [motioning hands as if they're going back and forth]. Say bye, hi, bye, hi.

C: Trading classrooms. See, you'll be ready for eighth grade then won't you because you're used to it?

B: But sometimes I have to in the same room so [laughs] it's hard [laughs]. Like, ugh, you're getting dizzy and your head ache.

C: Really?

B: And sometimes I don't even eat lunch. I just pass.

Personal Reflection 5.6	"In order to foster change in regular education, special educators need to reduce the current emphasis on classifying, labeling, and offering 'special' programs for students who do not fit within the present regular education structure. Instead, they should put more emphasis on joining with regular educators to work for a reorganization of or modifications in the structure of regular education itself so that the needs of a wider range of students can be met within the mainstream of regular education."
	William Stainback, Susan Stainback, Lee Courtnage, & Twila Jaben (1985, p. 148).

in the home has been rare but that "when such monitoring has been done, the results sometimes indicate that parents do not administer highly programmed steps as planned or trained" (p. 311). He also recommended that parents be consulted regarding their own preferences for using the home to perform primary intervention activities. That recommendation seems entirely consistent with the policy guidelines and regulations discussed earlier in this chapter.

When considering home contexts, other options for using home-like settings beyond the family's home might also be considered. For example, if infants with handicaps are receiving extensive child care from someone other than their parents, such as their grandparents or day-care workers, that care setting might be considered as a possible intervention context. Here, also, the approach to be taken might be more successful if aimed at intensifying already available natural experiences rather than adding on unique therapeutic ones (see following section on people variables).

Modern families spend a lot of time in the car, which offers the advantage of providing a rich context that constantly varies but with tangible and meaningful language content opportunities. For example, one child learned to produce sentences with contractible

copulas (the verb *is*) and to extend her vocabulary riding in the car with her mother as part of the daily routine, playing the "There's a" game. In this activity, one person introduces the familiar game (after initial modeling) with a sentence like, "There's a barn." The other then responds with something like, "It's big," or "It's old," or "It's red." The game can continue for miles in town or country, and in a home-like context where neither parent nor child could do anything else.

Social contexts. Social contexts can vary widely and might include any setting in which the child participates other than home, school, or work. They also might include contexts within home, school, and work settings that are primarily social. For example, at home, language intervention might be set in social contexts involving interactions with siblings or neighborhood children. At school, it might be set in social contexts involving interactions with peers and non-teaching staff on the playground or in extracurricular activities, such as athletic events or club meetings. Other social contexts might include religious events, meals at fast-food restaurants, or shopping trips to the mall.

Anywhere the child participates or would like to participate (sometimes as a parental preference if the

Personal Reflection 5.7	"The speech therapist says, 'Do half an hour of therapy after dinner.' The physical therapist says, 'Do 30 minutes of therapy in your spare time.' What spare time?! I have two other kids and a husband! I finally said 'no' to all that therapy. I had to choose between being my child's extension therapist and being his mother. And I chose being his mother."
	Parent of a child with multiple needs who had multiple needs herself (we all do), quoted by Simons (1987, p. 51).

child cannot yet state preferences) may provide a social context for language intervention. The advantages of social contexts are their potential for encouraging generalization of newly acquired language skills, their natural reinforcers, and the provision of richer contexts and content for fostering those skills than available in most structured settings (Jenkins, Odom, & Speltz, 1989).

The disadvantages of social contexts as intervention settings is that they are typically less available to language specialists, planning trips to the mall or the principal's office is time-consuming, and the child may be embarrassed or distracted by having to meet language intervention expectations during natural social interactions. Evidence also suggests that simply placing children together in social contexts will not ensure that they will interact socially. For example, when Jenkins, Speltz, and Odom (1985) studied children with handicaps placed in integrated preschool settings (with normally developing peers) and in non-integrated preschool settings, they found that although physical integration occurred, social integration did not.

Varied solutions are available. Some involve people strategies, discussed later. These include consulting with others who have natural opportunities for social interactions with the child or directly facilitating social interactions between handicapped and nonhandicapped children. Other solutions involve setting up role-play activities designed to emulate social contexts. Simulations are designed to give children practice using new language skills in more sheltered contexts with the hope of transferring them later to true social contexts. For example, Hoskins (1987) designed a program in which the language specialist (in the role of "coach") sets up conversational groups for adolescents in special contexts.

When simulating social contexts, it is important to remember to guide actions with good questions. For example, as O'Brien and O'Leary (1988) asked, regarding mentally retarded youngsters, "Does learning to identify a picture of a hamburger and use the word in a sentence help them order a Big Mac? Does sequencing pictures really help them put their socks on before their shoes? Does labeling of empty grocery containers help them shop for healthful, economic meals?" (p. 356).

Vocational contexts. Historically, more lip service has been paid to working on language and communi-

cation skills in vocational settings than real service. However, as new options open up for integration in supported employment situations, and with the requirement established by PL 101–476 (1990) for transition plans to be included in IEPs, that may change. Supported employment involves the placement of handicapped workers in real-life job settings in the competitive marketplace but with consultants ("job coaches") who come in to assist them in completing the work competitively. Language specialists may, in turn, consult with supported employment consultants or other vocational rehabilitation specialists to analyze communicative contexts and to help adolescents and young adults develop the language and communication skills they need to succeed in vocational contexts.

If competitive employment seems unrealistic for some individuals, they may participate in sheltered work settings. If sheltered work settings are not appropriate, individuals still must have adequate communicative skills to gainfully occupy their time.

People Variables

Language intervention service providers either interact with the children directly to help them develop more mature language skills, or they consult with others who have direct interactions, or both. Language specialists often are educated as speech–language pathologists, with extensive coursework and practicum experiences in language, speech, and communication development and its disorders, and with master's degrees. They may or may not be certified as teachers as well, but teacher certification is generally required when speech–language pathologists teach varied curricular areas to children with severe language disorders in the classroom. Increasingly, speech–language pathologists view their intervention roles as including the development of literacy as well as oral language ability, but their background and inclinations vary (Casby, 1988).

Psychologists also may contribute actively to language assessment and intervention activities, having expertise in the areas of psycholinguistics and language processing as well as other aspects of learning and development. Also contributing are special education teachers and teacher consultants with expertise in uses of written and oral communication for learning, including specialists in learning disabilities and other areas.

The skills and attitudes that individuals in any of these professions bring to service provision to children with language disorders may vary widely depending on when, where, and how they were educated and the kinds of experiences they have had since ending their formal education. Transdisciplinary teams generally include other specialists, including regular educators, and health-care professionals such as occupational therapists, physical therapists, nurses, and physicians—in addition, of course, to parents and children themselves. When these teams work well, they develop flexible interactions, adjusting and changing to take advantage of each member's experience and interests as they consult with each other to share information across professional boundaries.

Provider roles and relationships.   *Language specialist providing direct service.*   When language specialists provide direct service, they work with children in deliberate ways in scheduled sessions. This is the most common role assumed traditionally by language intervention specialists. Within this general framework, specialists vary widely in the services they provide. The content and methods related to direct service provision are covered in greater depth in Chapters 7 to 9.

Language specialist as consultant.   The role currently receiving the greatest attention, and already touched on previously in this book, is the role of consultant. By this point, you should be familiar with the definition of collaborative consultations as

> an interactive process that enables teams of people with diverse expertise to generate creative solutions to mutually defined problems. The outcome is enhanced, altered, and produces solutions that are different from those that the individual team members would produce independently. (Idol, Paolucci-Whitcomb, et al. 1986, p. 1)

Although thus far I have emphasized the elements of mutual goal setting among transdisciplinary teams as a way to understand the essence of consultation, consultation often is interpreted to mean that the consultant provides service indirectly (i.e., through another person's contact with a target individual). In its broadest definition, consultation involves "an outside (the agency or profession) expert engaged in a voluntary relationship with primary interventionists (parents, teachers, caretakers)" (Marvin, 1987, pp. 4–5). Within this broad framework, consultant roles can be divided into two types: (1) collaborative models,

in which consultants facilitate the process of change (perhaps by asking good questions), but in which the actual intervention is carried out by other individuals, and (2) expert models, in which consultants provide more unidirectional services, including prescriptions, recommendations, and inservice suggestions, to individuals responsible for implementing them (Schein, 1978). Within the category of expert models, several variations are possible. Marvin (1987) listed three. The consultant as expert may (1) serve as short-term specialist to perform diagnostic and intervention activities that can then form the basis of recommendations to other potential interventionists; (2) serve as a prescriptive diagnostician, performing assessment, which will lead to prescriptions for forms of treatment implemented by others; or (3) serve as an information expert to those who bear the primary responsibility for delivering service.

Although the consultant role is currently receiving a great deal of attention, little research supports its efficacy. More reports are available regarding how it is done, in part possibly because so many variables influence consultative service provision. (e.g., Dublinske, 1974; Frassinelli, Superior, & Meyers, 1983; Fujiki & Brinton, 1984; Martin, 1974; Marvin, 1987, 1990; Pickering & Kaelber, 1978). Three that have stood out to me repeatedly as influencing success of my work as a consultant are (1) source of authority, (2) clarity of goals (and absence of hidden agendas), and (3) time available for the process.

By *source of authority*, I refer not only to the question of who has issued the official invitation to consult but also who has granted emotional entrance to the problem arena. I have been much more successful as a catalyst for change when multiple participants in a problem have invited me to join them in addressing it. When the source of authority has been granted initially by only one participant (it might be a parent concerned about current services or an administrator who invites assistance in evaluating a program or a professional), I know that my initial efforts will need to be spent in convincing the other participants that I am there to join them in problem solving, not to evaluate them or to tell them what to do.

For example, when parents initiate a contact regarding a school-age child, one way that I have sought to broaden the source of authority for my involvement is by asking parents to phone the school principal first, to let him or her know about the parents' request for my involvement. I then phone the principal, acknowledging his or her importance in the

Personal Reflection 5.8   "The job of the consultant is to make the other person look good."

Barbara Hoskins (Hoskins and Nelson, 1989).

problem-solving process and requesting assistance. As a speech–language pathologist, I also work closely with other speech–language pathologists who serve the child, being careful not to usurp their own authority. In developing a relationship with the child's teachers, I arrange observations at their convenience and give them feedback immediately after my visits (rather than after a delay). In feedback notes, I acknowledge our mutual concerns about finding the best ways to educate this child, share some of my observations about potential interactions of the child's language problems with the expectations of school language, and also indicate that the next step will be one of joint problem solving (not a set of recommendations from me).

When addressing a new problem, a consultant generally first works with the participants to clarify the goals for the consulting activities. Otherwise, consultants may work toward one type of goal, while other participants may work on another. That problem may be avoided by a frank discussion of goals, and writing them down, at the beginning of interactions.

When addressing goals, the consultant should try to determine whether any of the participants are harboring hidden agendas that might undermine the problem-solving activity, turning it into competitive, rather than cooperative, goal setting (see Chapter 1). If this occurs, the consultant may use a phenomenological perspective to attempt to understand the varied "truths" associated with the situation from the eyes of its participants. Then the consultant may work with the participants to refocus their attention initially on the areas in which they can agree, before tackling the more difficult confrontational issues. For

example, the group might be asked, first, to focus on what they want for the child. When discussions of how needs will be met are reserved until after this step is accomplished, the confrontational nature of many *how* discussions tends to be defused.

Finally, participants should know that using a consultative model in delivering services, at least in the early stages, is more likely to take time than to save time. Although the benefits to individual children, including those of keeping them in less restrictive environments, may be substantial, the consultative process requires time of the consultant and of the other participants. Activities that require time include (1) meeting to establish goals, (2) engaging in onlooker and participant observation activities, (3) conducting formal evaluation activities, (4) meeting again for joint problem solving, (5) establishing an intervention plan, (6) attempting implementation of intervention activities, (7) monitoring the evidence that the activities are successful, (8) meeting again to adjust the plan, (9) and providing extended follow-up.

Published accounts of language specialists serving as consultants have varied. Fujiki and Brinton (1984), in one of their earlier articles, suggested that the role of the language specialist in relationship to classroom teachers should be to "[provide] the classroom teacher with suggestions to complement a child's program of therapy" (p. 98). They indicated that language specialists might use a combination of inservice opportunities and recommendations related to individual children to enlist the teacher's collaboration in the language intervention process. Their work followed that of Pickering and Kaelber (1978) and others (Dublinske, 1974; Martin, 1974), who developed prin-

Personal Reflection 5.9   "The consultation program is not to be considered second best or to be used when direct intervention by the speech–language pathologist is not possible, but rather selection of this program should be based on the communication needs of the student. It should be the program of choice and not of desperation."

ASHA Committee on Language, Speech, and Hearing Services in the Schools (1984, p. 54).

ciples of consultation that include analysis of what teachers need to know about language development and how to encourage it. Frassinelli, Superior, and Meyers (1983) differentiated consultative service based on whether it involved (1) ongoing direct contact, (2) one-time or periodic contact, or (3) no direct contact with the client. Damico (1987) viewed it as a multidimensional process in which a speech–language pathologist assigned to a school might serve as its language specialist in a role broader than that traditionally assumed.

These are a few of the ways that consultation might be combined with other intervention approaches. It is difficult to imagine the success of any intervention program for a child with a language disorder without some level of consultation by a language specialist with the other important people in the child's life.

Language specialist as teacher. When language specialists serve as teachers, they assume responsibility for conveying the curriculum to children whose language problems make it largely inaccessible to them under ordinary circumstances. This professional's attention necessarily extends beyond students' ability to use language for various social and academic purposes to include the learning of information and skills targeted in the regular curriculum. The language specialist–teacher also must be willing to assume primary responsibility for academic development and behavior management.

Language specialist as co-teacher. Language specialists sometimes assume teaching roles with children with language disorders on a temporary or part-time basis. They co-teach with other professionals, who assume a major responsibility for teaching the regular curriculum. L. Miller (1989) described three variations of the team-teaching format: (1) The language specialist teaches a portion of the regular curriculum in the regular classroom with a regular classroom teacher (e.g., Norris, 1989). (2) The language specialist shares teaching responsibilities with another specialist (usually a teacher of reading, of students with learning disabilities, or of students with behavioral disorders) (e.g., O'Brien & O'Leary, 1988). (3)The language specialist in a resource setting shares supplementary teaching responsibilities (e.g., Simon, 1977, 1987).

Mixed models. Children do not have to be served in unitary models, and professionals do not have to

practice in only one model at a time. It is possible to mix strategies and delivery-model variables in programs individualized to meet children's needs.

Peer roles and relationships. Children's peers may play a variety of roles in the delivery of language intervention services. They may serve as models, assist in setting a stimulus context, or deliver natural reinforcers (L. Paul, 1985). Peers who participate in the language intervention process may or may not have handicaps themselves. They may be the same age as the target child, older, or younger. L. Paul (1985) has suggested that, when designing service-delivery options involving peers, the specialist needs to ask three essential questions: (1) Do peers provide appropriate models? (2) Do they provide sufficient opportunity for interaction? (3) Do they reinforce the child's attempts at communicating?

Peers in social interaction relationships. Numerous social advantages have been cited for integrating children with disabilities with nondisabled peers. As noted previously, however, simply placing these children together in the same classroom does not necessarily result in high-quality social interaction (Jenkins et al., 1985).

A study of the verbal productions of nonhandicapped preschool children in an integrated preschool showed their verbalizations to be less complex, less frequent, and less diverse when addressed to playmates with more severe handicaps than when addressed to children with mild handicaps or no handicaps, in both instructional and in free-play settings (Guralnick & Paul-Brown, 1977). These findings may simply reflect the normal pragmatic abilities of nonhandicapped children to judge the reduced comprehension abilities of their handicapped peers. It is of concern, however, if nonhandicapped children in integrated settings either "talk down" to their handicapped peers unnecessarily or fail to interact with them when left to play freely.

Recognizing these tendencies, Jenkins et al. (1989) designed a study of both integrated and segregated preschool settings. The authors established two kinds of interactions, called *social interaction* and *child-directed play*, which differed in degree of adult direction. In the *social interaction condition*, teachers organized four children with heterogeneous abilities into small groups and directed the children's play in 30-minute periods by (1) suggesting play ideas, (2) modeling appropriate play behavior, and (3) prompting appropriate social interaction among the children as necessary. In the child-directed play interactions (which were modeled after those of the High/Scope Preschool Cognitive Curriculum; Hohmann, Banet, & Weikert, 1979), children were also grouped heterogeneously, but they had more freedom of choice within the activities of the 30-minute time period. In the child-directed condition, children selected an activity and stated their plans to their classmates, carried out their activity in a work-play time with little assistance from the teacher, engaged in cleanup, and participated in a recall group in which they described what they did during work-play time. The heterogeneous groups of four children in the integrated classes were made up of one or two children without and two or three children with handicaps. In the segregated classes, one or two socially more skilled children were grouped with two or three socially less skilled children, but all had handicaps. The results showed a higher proportion of interactive play and higher language development in the more adult-directed social interaction conditions than in the less controlled child-directed play conditions in both settings. Children in the social interaction condition in the integrated classes, however, received significantly higher ratings of social competence than did the children in the segregated classes. Both teacher-direction and normal peer models appeared to play a role in achieving positive social interaction results for these preschoolers.

Problems associated with facilitating quality social interaction do not lessen as children advance in age, and children with less obvious handicaps, such as those with language and learning disabilities, may have as much (or more) trouble being accepted by their peers as do those with more obvious handicaps. C. L. Fox (1989) reviewed the evidence that students with learning disabilities are socially rejected more often by their peers than are nonhandicapped students and that mainstreaming does not automatically help handicapped students become more accepted by their peers. Fox reported that two kinds of techniques have been used to attempt to influence social acceptance of handicapped children: (1) attempts to teach specific prosocial behaviors to handicapped children through modeling, shaping, coaching, and cognitive problem solving and (2) attempts to influence the attitudes of nonhandicapped children through role playing, peer tutoring, reinforcement, enabling training, education, and sociodrama.

In a study of the second kind of approach, C. L. Fox (1989) paired 86 low socially accepted students with learning disabilities in fourth, fifth, and sixth grades

with 86 high socially accepted, same-sex, nonhandicapped students for 8 weeks of special activities, conducted once per week in 40-minute sessions. Student pairs were assigned randomly to one of four conditions: (1) In mutual interest groups, children were taught how to interview each other and to use information from their interviews to construct mutual interest booklets about each other using techniques described by C. L. Fox (1980) in *Communicating to Make Friends.* (2) In cooperative academic task groups, children were asked to make, play, and evaluate together math games that would be used with first- and second-graders. (3) In Hawthorne effect control groups (the Hawthorne effect is the potentially influencing effect of receiving experimental attention), pairs of children spent time in the same room with the other groups but worked independently of each other on the math games. (4) In control groups, pairs of children were identified but did not work cooperatively in any way and were not withdrawn from the regular classroom for special attention. The findings showed that social acceptability ratings for the students with learning disabilities in the first group rose over the 8-week period, the ratings for children in the second two groups did not change, and the ratings for the children in the control group actually declined.

Eichinger (1990) also employed cooperative techniques to encourage greater social interaction between 8 fourth- and fifth-grade regular education student volunteers (who had viewed a "Special Friends" slide and tape show that depicted students with and without disabilities playing together) and 8 special education students who had severe handicaps, such as severe cognitive impairment, autism, severe speech impairment, vision impairment, and extreme physical impairment. Four pairs shifted between a baseline condition and one in which they worked individually to complete some type of preassigned game or art activity, and four pairs shifted between a baseline condition and one in which they worked cooperatively, with the same set of materials to complete the game or art activity. The results showed that the disabled students in the cooperative pairs expressed significantly more positive facial affect, higher cooperative play levels, and frequent vocalizations when working cooperatively. No changes were noted during free-play sessions.

The results of all of these studies suggest that, although specific social and communicative benefits can come from integrating children with handicaps with normally developing peers, benefits are unlikely without specific adult intervention. These inter-actions, however, have focused mostly on social out-comes. The next section discusses the use of cooperative peer interactions to influence other learn-ing outcomes.

Peers in cooperative learning relationships. Coop-erative learning techniques have shown promise in reg-ular and special education for enhancing the learning process and building a sense of community among learners (Aronson, Blaney, Stephan, Sikes, & Snapp, 1978; Augustine, Gruber, & Hanson, 1990; D. W. Johnson, Johnson, & Holubec, 1988; S. Kagan, 1990). Tateyama-Sniezek (1990), however, carefully analyzed 12 published studies on the effects of cooperative learning on achievement by children with handicaps of varied types (7 with mildly handicapped students, 1 with hearing impaired students, 1 with severely hand-icapped students, and 3 with varied other kinds of experimental controls) and found equivocal results. Only six of the studies (50%) reported any significant effects on achievement favoring cooperative learning. Based on this analysis, Tateyama-Sniezek reported that "the only firm conclusion is that the opportunity for students to study together does not guarantee gains in academic achievement" (p. 436).

In spite of these rather discouraging results, bene-fits other than those related to increased academic achievement might result from cooperative learning activities for children with language disorders. A pri-mary question should be not only whether children advance academically but also whether cooperative learning approaches might provide more opportuni-ties for children to practice effective listening and speaking skills. Although research results are limited in this area, descriptions of cooperative learning activ-ities can offer some insight into their potential as lan-guage intervention contexts.

Cooperative learning activities vary in their imple-mentation, but in general, they involve the establish-ment of heterogeneous groups whose members are responsible for seeing that everyone in the group learns and understands the material. A student is not considered to have learned something until he or she has taught it to someone else (Johnson, Johnson, & Holubec, 1988; Slavin, 1983).

Some cooperative learning activities are appropri-ate for large groups, even as large as whole class-rooms. S. Kagan (1990) pointed out some of the differences between whole-class question-answer, which is the competitive structure used traditionally

for large-group discussion by classroom teachers, and something he dubbed *numbered heads together*. In traditional, competitive whole-class question-answer, (1) the teacher asks a question; (2) students who wish to respond raise their hands (usually, the high-achieving students do this, while the low achieving students sit on the sidelines); (3) the teacher calls on one student (causing others to lose the competition for the teacher's attention); and (4) the student attempts to state the correct answer ("winning" if correct, and "losing" if not). By contrast, S. Kagan (1990) described numbered heads together as fol-lows: (1) The teacher forms several groups of four students, each with heterogeneous abilities, and has the students number off within each group from 1 to 4. (2) The teacher poses a question. (3) The teacher tells the students in each small group to "put their heads together" to make sure that everyone on the team knows the answer (and how to explain it). (4) Then the teacher calls a number (1, 2, 3, or 4) to indi-cate that only people with that number are eligible to raise their hands to respond. The group gets credit for answers of its individual members.

The cooperative structure has the advantage of encouraging high achievers to share answers be-cause they know that their number may not be called. Thus, they are invested in helping to prepare their less proficient group mates to be ready to answer. Low achievers know they must pay attention be-cause they may have the opportunity to add to the score for the whole group, and they have been en-couraged by their group mates to do so. Using this ture, individual accountability is built in by confining the helping discussions to the group process. When individuals' numbers are called, they are on their own.

Other cooperative strategies can be used in small groups, with sizes as small as individual pairs. Again, S. Kagan (1990) contrasted traditional techniques and those of cooperative learning. In group discussion, according to Kagan, the teacher asks a low-consen-sus question, and the students talk it over in groups. Typically, with this approach, participation is unequal, with some students not participating at all, no individ-ual accountability, and only a small number of stu-dents getting an opportunity to talk. This structure, however, is particularly good for brainstorming and for reaching group consensus. Group discussion can be contrasted with the cooperative three-step interview approach in which students (1) form pairs within their teams of four and conduct one-way interviews in pairs; (2) reverse roles so that interviewers become interviewees; and (3) end with a roundrobin, in which each takes a turn sharing information learned in the interview. Kagan noted that the three-step interview is far better than the traditional discussion model "for developing language and listening skills as well as promoting equal participation" (p. 13).

Certainly, the use of cooperative learning activities as language intervention contexts for increasing the communication skills of children with language disorders deserves further attention. The language development benefits of such activities may be enhanced by providing intermittent direction from language specialists as consultants in the regular classroom. If children are already organized into small groups of four or fewer students by their regular classroom teachers, language specialists can participate with minimal disruption to the classroom routine by using some of the techniques developed by Hoskins (1987), acting as a sidelines coach to facilitate the interactions.

Other uses of peers to work with children with language disorders have been suggested. Larson and McKinley (1987) noted that peers could be enlisted as tutors by using a four-step process: (1) gaining educators' support, (2) recruiting and selecting potential tutors, (3) training, supervising, and supporting tutors, and (4) selecting students with language disorders who could benefit from this type of approach. Murray-Seegert (1989) reported on a program in a tough inner-city high school that paired severely disabled and nondisabled students in social contexts for the benefit of both.

The final word is not in. As in other areas, cooperative learning groups and peer tutors are probably good for some students, when organized in some ways, some of the time. There are no universal answers for students with language disorders, and some strategies for using peer support may not yet have been tapped. For example, older students who are at risk for dropping out of school because of academic failure might be recruited as volunteers to tutor younger ones. Reading and discussing books on the younger children's grade level might strengthen the skills of both (without insulting the older students) and could increase their motivation for participating in educational activities. Creative solutions will continue to be developed as professionals look at the best ways to meet children's needs.

Family roles and relationships. As mentioned, home contexts can be used in a variety of ways to provide services to children with language disorders.

The roles of family members in the intervention process can also vary widely, depending on sociocultural variables, the family's culture, and prior experiences of the adults in the family with health-care and educational agencies. Other influential variables are the age of the child with the language disorder, the severity of the disorder, and its association with other handicapping conditions.

For children of all ages and ability levels, families are primary contributors to incidental learning about the world and their place within it. As a general rule, however, parents of children with more severe and more obvious handicaps are aware earlier of their children's difficulties and are involved more extensively in language intervention and other special education and habilitation activities for their children. Often, the younger the child, the more extensive the family's role in the intervention process, simply because younger children spend more time in the family.

Parents have a special perspective on their child's needs at all age levels, and that perspective should be respected. Personal Reflection 5.10 is an example of a school system learning to listen better to what one parent had to say. It is a reminder to professionals of the requirements in the IDEA (PL 101–476) that parents must be given the opportunity to participate as active members of the IEP team.

Fey (1986) divided parental roles into two basic types: (1) parents as aides and (2) parents as primary intervention agents. I add a third role of (3) parents as incidental intervention agents. As you read this section, you might also extend the group of family participants that you are thinking about to include other members, such as siblings, grandparents, and grandparent surrogates.

Family roles as language intervention aides. When parents serve language intervention roles as aides, they may use the same objective and provide their children with the same kinds of intervention activities that are being used in the clinical or school intervention (pullout) setting, but in the home environment (e.g., Sandler, Coren, & Thurman, 1983; Zwitman & Sonderman, 1979). Parents can also participate by providing intervention directed at helping their children transfer newly acquired language skills to more natural contexts after they have reached a certain criterion in the more clinical setting (Gray & Ryan, 1973; Hughes, 1985; Mulac & Tomlinson, 1977).

Parents and other family members also can function as aides in less formal ways. Fey (1986) noted

Personal Reflection 5.10   "You listen to me politely, but you never write it down!"

Cathy Shortz, parent of a child with severe multiple impairments (SXI) in Jackson, MI.

These were the words of a frustrated parent describing her experiences with an Individualized Educational Planning (IEP) process in which her ideas about her son's needs for literacy development had not been taken seriously. This time, the message was heard. Speech–language pathologist *Mary Ann Berthiaume* asked Shortz to write down her thoughts and provide them to the team, including her son's classroom teacher, special education teacher, teaching assistants, occupational therapist, physical therapist, school psychologist, and principal.

The informal memo that Cathy Shortz wrote when the sincere invitation was issued, said:

"I'd really like to see beginning reading included in J's IEP this year. Hopefully by the end of the year he'll be able to do some sight reading—his own full name, family names—bathroom—drink—miscellaneous needs. Plus sentence structure, and how to group sentences to tell a story or have a conversation by choosing his words. I'd like to see some math. If only 1–50 and the awareness of 3 digits and up. This is a secondary desire—reading is my biggest concern.

I know this is a major request, but it's really time for academics to start showing up on his IEPs as a REAL goal. Maybe he won't be able to grasp it and at year's end it will be continued or declined, *but* either way I'd like his records to show the effort was made. Thanks for asking for my input. I'll get with you soon to work out our game plan.—C"

that "We often bring family members into the clinic sessions to serve as models, to heighten the child's attention, to help the clinician to motivate and reinforce the child, to help create more naturalistic intervention contexts, and, generally, to assist the clinician in any way possible" (p. 295). In our university clinic, this is what we did with a child "Stephen" who, at the age of 3 was nonspeaking and showed many symptoms of autism. We knew that Stephen's sisters played "house" with him at home, so we brought them in to play house in a play kitchen in the language preschool area at the university clinic. As they made pretend cupcakes and played dolls, we encouraged Stephen's sisters to include him in their play. We also taped some of Stephen's favorite songs and taught his sisters the accompanying motions so that they could repeat them with him at home. Then, when the activity was conducted in the clinic, Stephen watched his sisters closely, imitating their actions and interacting with them.

The involvement of siblings as tutors for adolescents with language disorders has also been described (Larson & McKinley, 1987). In deciding when such an approach might be appropriate, Larson and McKinley suggested that the sibling should (1) have the necessary skills and patience to work with the adolescent with the language disorder, (2) have the desire to participate, (3) be willing to be trained and supervised in carrying out assignments, (4) be willing to spend the necessary time and energy to do so, and (5) be older to maximize the potential of the interaction.

Several advantages may be realized from using family members as language intervention aides. Fey (1986) noted that such strategies can promote generalization across contexts and may allow parents to feel more involved in their children's programming. Hughes (1985) also commented that, "If parents are present during language teaching and are taught to provide stimuli (verbal or nonverbal) for eliciting the target language, then they are part of a 'common stimulus'" (p. 162), and they can also play a role in providing consequent events.

Potential problems may also be associated with this approach. Fey (1986) noted dependence on clinicians for direction, potential confusion, and frustration accompanying inadequately explained "homework," as well as lack of efficacy data about parents' abilities to serve as language intervention aides.

Roles of parents as primary language intervention agents. When parents are asked (or when they decide) to assume primary roles as intervention agents (see Fey, 1986, and Hughes, 1985, for reviews of this literature), they become the primary providers of direct intervention. This role is generally assumed after parents are trained to set up activities, recognize appropriate language behaviors, reinforce them, and keep records documenting progress. Often parents are expected to encourage language development indirectly and also to conduct formal intervention sessions several times per week.

Such approaches can vary widely. In his description of language intervention, Fey (1986) differentiated "trainer-oriented" intervention strategies from "child-oriented" strategies and added a third set of "hybrid approaches." The distinction is based on the degree of control that the adult or the child assumes over the selected activities and materials. Child-oriented approaches are similar to those used when parents are incidental intervention agents, but they differ slightly. When parents are primary intervention agents, they must constantly be aware of that role and must be prepared to document that procedures are working. When parents act as incidental intervention agents, they assume a more assistive role; they learn to use opportunities that occur naturally in the home, but they do not seek them out as aggressively or view themselves as trainers so much as parents.

Some of the positive results of studies in which parents served as primary intervention agents (summarized by Fey, 1986) have included success in reaching clinician-designated goals for the child and in general improvements in the parents' adjustments toward their children and ability to deal with their children's special problems. Fey also cautioned, however, that most of the evidence about the success of these programs comes from work with children with severe impairments who were learning early words and simple language structures. There is less support for parents' serving as primary intervention agents when working on more complex morphological and syntactic structures. Generalization results after parent-training programs also have not been as encouraging as might be expected.

Roles as incidental intervention agents. A third level of parental (and other family member) interaction is that of incidental intervention agent. Parents and others are taught to be vigilant and to use naturally occurring opportunities to foster language development in their children with language disorders. When using incidental strategies, however, parents do not serve as formal teachers or as intervention aides. Rather, they watch for brief episodes, precipitated by the child (B. Hart, 1985), in which they might intervene (incidental teaching techniques are discussed further in Chapter 6). Fey (1986) categorized this role as child-oriented intervention; no specific language structures are selected as goals, and no direct teaching of specific language behaviors is attempted.

Because of its informal nature, and because of individual differences among families and children, the effectiveness of this role is especially difficult to evaluate. The evidence reviewed by Fey (1986) and Hughes (1985) suggests, however, that simply encouraging intervention as a part of opportunities incidental to the process of daily living (rather than those that are formally planned) may not give parents sufficient information about how to intensify their own language-facilitating skills and how to provide multiple language-learning opportunities. Parents may need more direct training.

As one approach to parental training, Ruder, Bunce, and Ruder (1984) developed a rating sheet for parents to encourage them to monitor their use of such strategies as (1) getting their child's attention before they talked, (2) talking about the here-and-now, (3) labeling objects and talking about actions, (4) pausing to give the child opportunities to talk, (5) responding meaningfully, (6) expanding the child's utterances, and (7) asking appropriate questions. Videotapes and associated training materials are sometimes used to assist parents to identify opportunities and strategies that might occur incidentally in their interactions with their children.

Hubbell (1981) characterized the goal of this kind of involvement as being "not to teach the parent to teach the child. Rather, it is to establish transactional patterns that maximize opportunity for language growth within the child" (p. 275). Hughes (1985) identified changing "parents' language and nonlanguage behaviors in such a way as to facilitate language development" as "the clinician's ultimate goal" (p 163).

The need for sensitivity. As in other areas, the "best" approach for family involvement may differ widely from one family to another, and decisions must be made individually. Fey (1986) noted that language specialists must be sensitive to family differences. Parents may harbor widely different attitudes regarding their possible roles as causative agents in their children's language learning difficulties (recall the discussion on phenomenology from Chapter 1). Thus, although some parents may greet with relief efforts to involve them directly in the intervention process, feeling glad that they finally have professional guidance for doing something, others may regard such efforts as confirmation that they are somehow responsible for their child's difficulties. Fey (1986) cautioned that "clinicians must be aware of parents' sensitivities and take steps to ensure that their well-intentioned efforts to integrate parents into the intervention process reduce rather than exacerbate the parents' feelings of guilt, anxiety, and frustration" (pp. 292–293).

Scheduling Variables

To improve their language, children must have opportunities to use it. Therefore, a major concern in planning services is to maximize the time available for children to use language when talking, listening, reading, writing, and thinking. Scheduling also establishes times when children can be guided productively by language interventionists and others as they use their language skills and knowledge. Scheduling variables are intimately tied to setting and people variables and the number of children on a caseload at any one time (see Table 5.1 for caseload sizes recommended for speech–language services in the schools by the ASHA Committee on Language, Speech, and Hearing Services in the Schools). Scheduling is used to establish frequency of sessions, length of sessions, and duration of periods when special services will be provided.

Session frequency variables.   The amount of time the child should spend in sessions designed specifically for remediating a language disorder depends on the degree to which the child's other activities encourage his or her language development. Spe-

cialized intervention sessions can be less frequent when the child's language development needs are met in other contexts.

Adoption of the twice-weekly scheduling, traditional in many school and clinical settings, may be tempting. This schedule, however, may be established more because of convenience than because a deliberate plan to meet the child's needs requires it. Research support for selecting one schedule over another generally is not available. Scheduling decisions therefore must be made by considering what will best allow professionals and family to meet the child's language development needs (while not interfering with other needs) and to provide maximum opportunities for the child to participate in desired contexts. These decisions will likely vary depending on the child's age and other factors.

If the child is an infant at risk for a language disorder, the child's parents and other care givers play the primary role in encouraging the child's communicative development. The frequency with which a language specialist works with an infant and family to facilitate language acquisition is determined as part of the IFSP process. Generally, when children are in frequent and close contact with parents and other adults who know how to facilitate their language and communication development, language specialists do not need to be involved as frequently. When these adults have extensive needs for knowing how to interact with the child, greater time commitment from a language specialist may be required initially but may be reduced later.

As mentioned, some school-age children with language disorders are mainstreamed for all or part of the day in general education classrooms and are pulled out for language intervention sessions and other special education activities. For these children, decisions about session frequency should consider not only needs for language intervention but also needs to participate in important events in other academic, social, physical, artistic, and musical contexts.

TABLE 5.1
Recommended caseload sizes for delivering speech–language services in school settings

	8 Consultation Program (Indirect Service)	9 Itinerant Program (Intermittent Direct Service)	10 Resource Room Program (Intensive Direct Service)	11 Self-Contained Program (Academically Integrated Direct Service)
1 Cases served	12 —All communicative disorders —All severities (mild to severe)	19 —All communicative disorders —All severities (mild to severe)	26 —All communicative disorders, particularly language and articulation —All severities	33 —Primary handicap: communication —Severe/multiple disorders particularly language and articulation
2 Services provided	13 —Program development, management, coordination —Indirect services	20 —Program development, management, coordination, evaluation —Direct services —Coordination w/educators	27 —Program development, management, coordination, evaluation —Direct service self-study aide —Coordination w/teacher(s) —Teacher has academic responsibilities	34 —Program development, management, coordination, evaluation —Direct services plus academic instruction
3 Group size	14 —Individual or Group (indirect service)	21 —Individual or small group (up to 3 students/session)	28 —Individual or small group (Up to 5 students/session)	35 —Up to 10 students/speech-language pathologist —Up to 15/speech-language pathologist w/supportive personnel
4 Time per day	15 —Variable; Possible range ½ hr. (mild) to ¾ hrs/day	22 / 23 —½ to 1 hour/day	29 / 30 —1 to 3 hours day	36 —Full school day
5 Times per week	16 —1 to 5 times/week	24 —2 to 5 times/week	31 —4 to 5 times/week	37 —Full time placement
6 Rationale for caseload size	17 —Time necessary by organization —Variable needs	—Complex cases demand lower caseloads —Approximate national average	—Cases require intensive services —Consistent w/regulations	38 —Consistent w/regulations —Provides for intensive services
7 Caseload* maximums	18 —Up to 15–40 students	25 —Up to 25–40 students	32 —Up to 15–25 students	39 —Up to 15 students w/aide —Up to 10 students w/out aide

Draft prepared by the Committee on Language, Speech, and Hearing Services in the Schools August 1981. Final revision July 1983.
*NOTE: Maximums are not additive across programs and do not account for travel time.

Note. From "Guidelines for Caseload Size for Speech–Language Services in the Schools" by the ASHA Committee on Language, Speech, and Hearing Services in Schools, 1984, Asha, 26(4). p. 56. Copyright 1984 by American Speech-Language-Hearing Association. Reprinted by permission.

It can become a scheduling nightmare, but if children with language disorders have strengths that make them successful in other activities, their opportunities to participate should be protected and not automatically considered "less important" and available as time slots for special education activities.

Other particularly negative effects of traditional scheduling on students noted by students, parents, and school staff include the following: (1) being held responsible for material presented in pullout sessions in addition to material taught in regular classes; (2) pullout-session content irrelevant to regular education needs; (3) being held responsible for activities of general education classroom that occur while out of the room; (4) lack of time in the regular classroom to do seatwork and receive feedback; (5) missing teacher explanations and information about how to study for tests and do assignments; and (6) receiving reduced direct instruction and teacher assistance relative to peers (G. M. Anderson & Nelson, 1988).

One way to address these needs without adding on another kind of curriculum in patchwork fashion (as described by Barbie in Personal Reflection 5.5), is to establish the language intervention schedule to include an alternative experience that replaces some other regular part of the curriculum rather than adding to it. This scheduling approach works particularly well at middle school, junior high, and high school levels, where children change classes hourly. Language intervention sessions then can be provided daily in a regularly scheduled hour slot, for a small class of students who need assistance in gaining access to the language of instruction and using language to organize their approach to education (e.g., G. M. Anderson & Nelson, 1988; Buttrill, Niizawa, Biemer, Takahashi, & Hearn, 1989). A similar scheduling approach was taken by Despain and Simon (1987), by using regular science, social studies, and English classes as the context for building stronger communication and study skills, but with reduced class sizes and additional consultative assistance to the teachers.

Session length variables. Decisions about session length are related to what can be accomplished with a particular child within various time frames and what the child might miss in other contexts during special intervention. When children are placed in self-contained classrooms so that the language of instruction can be tailored to fit their needs and so that they can

achieve maximum talking time within small group interactions, they may attend all day every day. Preschoolers may be scheduled only for half-day periods. In one case (Mroczkowski, 1988), however, a self-contained language class was offered for kindergartners in blocks of time that included full-day classes 5 days per week.

Alternative classrooms for older students may be offered for hour-long periods (with one half hour for group instruction and one half hour for individual practice) (G. M. Anderson & Nelson, 1988). Resource room activities with specialists in learning disabilities may be scheduled for various lengths of time, and sessions with speech–language pathologists tend to be scheduled for 20 to 30 minutes in schools during school hours and 50 to 60 minutes in clinics outside of school hours. Remember, however, that although these time periods are usual, they are not necessarily optimal. We simply do not have the evidence to know, and so many variables operate in each situation that evidence would be very difficult to obtain.

In one study (Rich & Ross, 1989), however, students' time on learning tasks was measured in various educational settings, including regular class, resource room, special class, and special school. The sample included 230 elementary-age students, who were classified as mildly mentally retarded, moderately mentally retarded, emotionally disturbed, or learning disabled. As expected, variation was noted in the types of children served in the various settings, with more learning disabled and mildly retarded children spending time in regular classrooms and resource rooms, more moderately retarded and emotionally disturbed children spending time in special classrooms, and primarily moderately retarded children spending time in special schools.

The analysis (Rich & Ross, 1989) showed significant advantages in terms of in-class learning time for the resource room over any of the more restrictive settings. In regular classrooms, handicapped students spent approximately the same time on-task as did nonhandicapped students, matching earlier reported data that showed that regular elementary students spend approximately 4 hours in class, are allocated learning time of about 3 hours, and are on task about 2 hours (Denham & Lieberman, 1980).

We do not have data regarding the amount of time children can spend engaging in active language processing of various types in the various settings. For example, if a child has trouble using oral language expressively, that child needs time to practice talking in a facilitative context. We do know that children spend much more of their time in regular classrooms listening than talking. Elementary students spend over one half of their day listening to teachers talk, and estimates for high school students range as high as 90% (Bellack, Kliebard, Hyman, & Smith, 1966; Griffin & Hannah, 1960).

When scheduling language intervention services, the specialist must individualize decisions, taking into account as many variables as possible for a particular child. When determining session length, for example, an important factor to keep in mind is that the kinds of activities that occur within a particular timeframe can vary widely. Generally, younger and more cognitively limited children cannot work as long on a single activity as can older, more mature children. Ironically, however, younger children and those with greater limitations may need more repetitions of the same material before it makes sense to them or before they acquire a new skill. These needs can be met by scheduling more sessions of shorter duration, or by repeating similar activities several times in short blocks within the same sessions, interspersed with other different activities.

It is sometimes worthwhile for language specialists to analyze directly the amount of time that children with language disorders have the opportunity to communicate in social and academic contexts during a schoolday. Certain children in certain contexts may be particularly at risk for having insufficient opportunities to interact. For example, Capper (1990) analyzed how three severely handicapped children placed in mixed special education classrooms in three different economically disadvantaged, rural school districts spent their time. She found some disturbing evidence about how much time the three children spent alone, with no opportunity for social or communicative interaction or instruction. As illustrated in Figure 5.2, Capper found conditions in which

> Elizabeth was physically separated from her peers, assigned to a corner of a room that was blocked by low bookshelves and cabinets. Elizabeth and Tiffany had no learning activities with peers, but were with them primarily at recess and meals. Although Roseann spent nearly 28% of her day with classmates in group learning activities, no interaction took place. (p. 340)

Language intervention service-delivery decisions in situations such as these should include some collaborative problem solving aimed at identifying ways to increase students' opportunities to participate (review the discussions in Chapter 1).

Program duration variables. Public Law 94–142 requires that IEP content include a statement of "The projected dates for initiation of services and the anticipated duration of the services" (1977, §111a.346). Identical wording is used in the statement that outlines content for IFSPs required by PL 99–457 (1986, §677.(d)). Professionals have interpreted the duration requirement for IEPs in different ways (IFSPs are just beginning to be written). In general, they have not interpreted it as a requirement for a statement of prognosis as to how long the child might need special education services (including speech–language intervention). Rather, they have tended to use it to project the year or less that a particular IEP can be in effect before it must be revised.

As professionals plan with families for service provision to children with language disorders, they should be as flexible as possible in attempting to meet the child's needs. If the child and family appear to need a short period of intense direct contact, followed by more intermittent consultative contacts, the written plans should reflect that need. If children are likely to need language intervention services throughout most of their school careers, parents should informed of the possibility early, but with sensitivity, and plans should be revised as needs, abilities, and opportunities shift throughout the child's school career.

Preferences of children and their parents. *Children's preferences.* Children are rarely asked whether they would prefer one type of service-delivery model over another. That is not too surprising, given children's limited experiences with different kinds of models that might give them the opportunity for comparison. In one study (Jenkins & Heinen, 1989), however, 686 second-, fourth-, and fifth-grade children were asked about service-delivery preferences. Half of the children were currently receiving services for mild impairments (primarily learning disabilities) in either pullout or in-class settings, and the other half were their regular education classmates who had observed the special service models of their peers but had not participated in them. These chil-

FIGURE 5.2

Relative time spent on school-day activities and with peers by three girls with severe developmental disabilities in a poor rural school district

SCHOOL DAY ACTIVITIES OF THE STUDENTS

PERCENTAGES OF SCHOOL DAY WITH PEERS

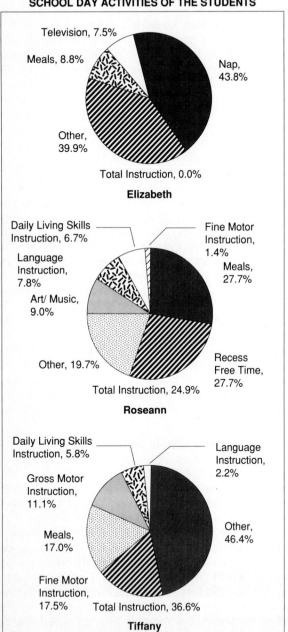

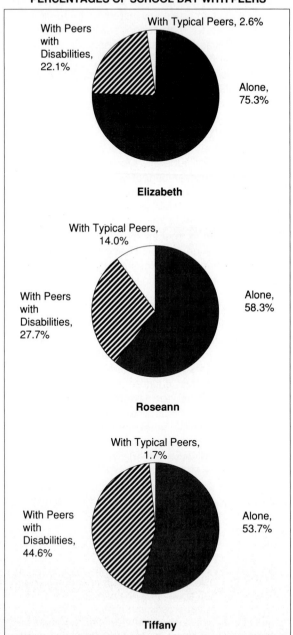

Note. From "Students With Low-Incidence Disabilities in Disadvantaged Rural Settings" by C. A. Capper, 1990, *Exceptional Children, 56*, p. 341. Copyright 1990 by The Council for Exceptional Children. Reprinted by permission.

dren were asked both about where they would rather have help if they were having problems with reading (pullout room or in class), and who they would rather have help them (their regular teacher or the building reading specialist).

The findings were interesting. Children who had experience with pullout services (either for themselves or their classmates) indicated a preference for that model over in-class programs, whereas children with in-class experience did not show a significant preference for one model or the other. Grade level also played a significant role in influencing choices, with older children indicating preference for pullout services significantly more often as a way of avoiding embarrassment. However, avoidance of embarrassment was listed as a reason both for preferring the pullout model and the in-class model. Other reasons given for preferring the in-class model were the convenience of not having to walk to another room and preferring to stay with classmates. Another reason for preferring the pullout model was the perception that specialists can give more and better help in a pullout room (Jenkins & Heinen, 1989).

When children were asked about the person from whom they would prefer to receive service if they were having trouble with reading, the vast majority indicated a preference for receiving help from their own classroom teacher, although responses varied somewhat based on children's current services and their grade. The reason "given most often by all students was that the classroom teacher 'knows what I need'" (Jenkins & Heinen, 1989, p. 522). Secondary reasons related to the impression that it is less stigmatizing to get help from the classroom teacher than from a specialist. In stating these preferences, Jenkins and Heinen (1989) noted that the children seemed to be indicating an awareness of the need to weigh the advantage "of obtaining help from some-one who is familiar with their problem (the classroom teacher) against the advantage of obtaining help from someone who has the time to provide it (the specialist)" (p. 522).

Although these results cannot be generalized completely to situations involving language intervention and language specialists, they do provide added insights that can be brought to the decision-making process. Elementary school children with mild handicaps are primarily concerned with getting help relevant to their needs to succeed in the regular classroom, but they wish to avoid embarrassment while doing so. They are not averse to going to pullout rooms if it can be done without embarrassment and if the help provided is relevant to their needs to succeed in their regular classrooms.

Parents' preferences. There are probably as many parental preferences for types of service delivery as there are parents. Because of the heterogeneity of children's language impairments, associated handicapping conditions, family histories, and community options, it is difficult to generalize about parental preferences. In addition, if professionals cannot agree on which service-delivery models are best, and if research has not offered clear-cut answers as to which models work best, how can parents be expected to agree on a preference for one kind of model over another?

Parents are experts on their own children. They are usually the most sensitive observers of the intervention setting's influence on their children's self-perceptions, and sometimes they assume strong advocacy roles to obtain services that they feel their children need. When their role as experts on their children is respected, they are valuable members of the team.

Hanline and Halvorsen (1989) studied parental preference by investigating parents' perceptions about

---

Personal Reflection 5.12	"Sometimes I feel overwhelmed. How can I evaluate this program? How do I know this is best? Then I remember that it's a team approach. I'm not in it alone. It's just my job to get the specialists I trust to talk to each other about it. I remind myself that they know the programs and I know Wilson. . . . Thinking of myself as Wilson's 'case manager' makes it easier to ask for the things that he needs."
	Barb Buswell, talking about her relationships to professionals and school systems, quoted by Robin Simons (1987, p. 54) in her book *After the Tears*.

their children's transitions from segregated to integrated educational placements. Parents of 14 children from 13 families in the San Francisco Bay Area were interviewed regarding their perceptions of the experience. The children ranged in age from 4 to 22 years and exhibited a variety of impairments (e.g. Down's syndrome, cerebral palsy, communicative handicap with motor delay, and multiple handicaps), with 11 children classified as severely handicapped. In two families, both mother and father were interviewed as primary advocates for their children, having fought for the change. In two other families, mothers were primary advocates; and in two others, fathers were primary advocates. Two additional mothers were interviewed about their children's moves from infant programs to integrated preschool settings, which had been initiated by the district planning team. The final four mothers were interviewed about their children's moves that were made as part of districtwide transitions.

Parents in these last two categories were most satisfied with the process. Parents who fought for their child's integration against opposition were the least satisfied, and they were resentful that they had had to play such a major role in the process. "As one parent asked, 'Why wasn't it done by the people whose job it is to do it?'" (Hanline & Halvorsen, 1989, p. 489).

When asked about their perceptions of the advantages and disadvantages of the integration model of service delivery for their children, five parents stated that there was no disadvantage to integration, and none of the parents reported regret about placing their child in an integrated setting. Parents' concerns were related to worries about their children's reduced ability to establish friendships within the community of persons with disabilities (who might serve as role models), about whether they would establish friendships with their nondisabled peers, and about their lack of experiences to prepare them for the social demands of regular schools. When asked about advantages, most parents spoke about skill enhancement, particularly in the area of social skill development, about their children's enhanced self-esteem and confidence, and about the presence of normally developing role models and increased stimulation in integrated settings that would prepare them for living in mainstream society (Hanline & Halvorsen, 1989).

Parents also reported that their own expectations for their children had been raised, along with their "admiration" for their children, and that they now had hopes that their children would lead more interesting and independent lives as adults. Parents of half of the children reported that their children had established friendships with nondisabled peers that extended outside of school hours, and several parents also noted the benefits in increased understanding of disability by nondisabled students. An added benefit to families mentioned by two parents was reduced concern about long-term care expressed by nondisabled siblings (Hanline & Halvorsen, 1989).

SUMMARY

When designing programs for individual children, the specialist should consider public policy at federal, state, intermediate, and local levels. Public policies are intended to guide service provision to children with special needs in positive ways, but it is up to professionals to see that they work. When service provision is ineffective, professionals must work together with parents and other professionals to ensure positive changes.

No one answer can apply to difficult questions about establishing a service-delivery context for an individual child. Answers can only come out of the collaborative process involving parents, teachers, health-care professionals, and other individuals. Multiple good answers may be possible for individual children. Comprehensive planning includes consideration of the multiple contexts in the child's life. The caution in putting together patchwork schedules, however, is that children like Barbie (see Personal Reflection 5.5) may get lost in the shuffle.

Finally, one more caution. In this chapter, I have considered only the obvious variables related to context. As S. F. Warren (1988) noted, "Context is more than who is present, when, with what objects, and in what environmental setting" (p. 295). In addition, context includes the linguistic context established not only in a current piece of specific discourse but also in the discourse history shared by the partners. Context also includes the social, emotional, and event interactions that become a part of the system that evolves when two or more people interact. Those are the variables that daily occupy the attention of language interventionists and are the variables that occupy much of the discussion in Part II.

6

Making Assessment and Intervention Work for Children

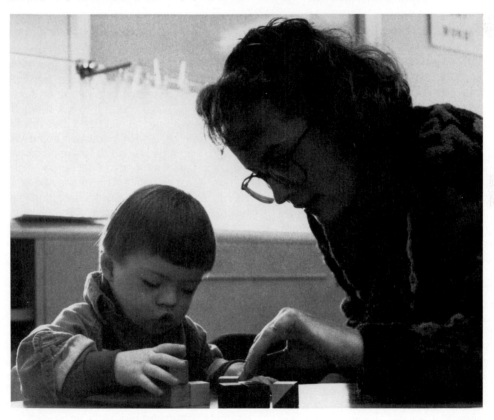

A Sequence of
Questions

Theoretical
Perspectives Guiding
Assessment and
Intervention Practices

Assessment and
Intervention as
Integrated Processes

❏ How should children with language disorders be identified, described, and treated?

Nowhere is it more important to ask good questions than when engaging in assessment and intervention for childhood language and communication disorders. Chapter 1 considered the importance of asking questions not only about what might be wrong (and right) about a particular developing individual's communicative abilities but also what that person's needs might be relative to the communicative expectations of important contexts and the opportunities for participation that those contexts afford. Chapter 5 considered perspectives regarding policy and service delivery. This chapter considers the more specific questions and strategies of language assessment and intervention across the age span from infancy through adolescence. In Chapters 7 to 9, assessment and intervention approaches are made even more specific for children in the early, middle, and later stages of language acquisition.

A SEQUENCE OF QUESTIONS

Different questions are appropriate at different stages of the assessment and intervention process. The flowchart in Figure 6.1 offers a summary of the main decision points and assessment and intervention activities for children of all ages and with all degrees of language and communication disorders. The details of this flowchart are the subject of Chapters 7 to 9. In particular, the content and contexts of the activities represented in the rectangular boxes will be discussed more thoroughly in those chapters as they relate specifically to early, middle, and later developmental stages and ages. The general principles that guide the decision-making processes of assessment and intervention are the focus of this chapter.

The intervention and assessment process starts with screening or referral activities that identify children with a problem (or risk of one) that potentially involves language and communication. The process has several possible exit points, depending on the outcome of events and decisions, at which participants may decide that special intervention for language and communication development is no longer needed. Even when exit decisions are made, however, follow-up checks conducted later may indicate that further assessment and intervention are warranted if a child's developing skills and the communicative demands of important contexts are too far out of synchrony.

The sequence of decisions that must be made in the process of providing services to children with language disorders involves designing procedures to answer a series of questions. The answers determine the broad course to be taken through the flowchart of procedures for a particular individual, and they lead to the formulation of new, more specific questions that relate to the unique needs of that person. Although the sequence may vary somewhat, the set of questions critical to the assessment and intervention process typically includes at least some of the following:

1. Does the child have a problem that might be related to a language disorder?   The first question leads a child into the language assessment and intervention system. It generally arises either during screening or referral. One reason for preferring an entry system based on referral rather than screening is that it is usually important to ask the general question about whether a child has a problem first, before asking the more specific question about whether the problem might be related to language disorder (rather than vice versa, as tends to happen with screening).

This question relates to unmet needs specific to certain contexts. It is designed to find out whether the child's ability to participate in critical contexts is hampered by an inability to do some of the things a person must do to succeed in that context. Another dimension of this question is that, by asking it of a variety of different people, in a variety of different contexts, the specialist may be able to determine if the child is perceived as handicapped, that is, if the child is at risk for social disvalue, even if not labeled as handicapped.

If a child scores below age norms on a screening test designed to assess language knowledge or language processing, but no one in the child's environment thinks the child has a problem, and if the child is functioning well when observed closely within those contexts, little of productive value can come from labeling the child as having a language disorder. Whatever wobbly language skills or processing behaviors are evident in formal assessment contexts, the child and participants in real-life situations must be compensating well enough to enable the child to function normally without special assistance. Premature introduction of assistance might remove the child from a natural context where he or she is apparently functioning well, and it might foster lowered self-expectations and lowered expectations by the adults in the child's environment. The ultimate result could be the "Pygmalion effect," in which lowered expectations are associated with lowered opportunities until the self-fulfilling prophecy comes true (Rosenthal & Jacobson, 1968).

An example of a situation in which it might be best to leave well enough alone is when a school-age child demonstrates a disorder of auditory processing when screened with a single test of an isolated function. For example, The Selective Auditory Attention Test (Cherry, 1980) requires children to point to pictures representing words presented over one headphone while an interesting story is presented through the other. Unless a child having difficulty on this test also demonstrates difficulty handling any of the oral or written language expectations of the regular classroom, it makes no sense to label this "problem" a problem. Auditory processes are a means to an end. They are not an end themselves.

On the other hand, low scores on screening tests that are appropriately standardized and implemented might be interpreted as indicators that children should be monitored, and in some cases, preventative services (possibly in the nature of consultation or ongoing monitoring) should be offered. Decisions may depend on a variety of factors, including possible causative influences, stages of development, contextual expectations, and multicultural influences.

The group for whom services should be provided before a problem may be clearly apparent is the group of infants and toddlers known to be at risk for developing problems. This is the group for whom many of the requirements of Public Law 99–457 were written (see Chapter 5) and is discussed in greater detail in Chapter 7. Preschool children are also often screened for language disorders and potential learning problems when they are ready to enter kindergarten.

2. Is the problem better explained as one of language difference rather than language disorder? Before it can be determined that a language disorder is involved, a critical question is whether the linguistic expectations of the context in which the problem is identified match the language abilities that the child would be learning if language acquisition were proceeding normally. It must be determined whether this is a case of language disorder (the child's not learning the language of important contexts normally), of language difference (the child's learning one type of language skill and the context's demanding another), or both.

Valid assessment procedures cannot be selected until professionals identify whether those standardized on mainstream cultures and linguistic systems are appropriate. If a child has limited English proficiency because his or her family's cultural or linguistic backgrounds differ from those of formal testing procedures and tools, alternative methods and tools must be used to answer the remaining questions of assessment and intervention.

3. Does the child have a language disorder (possibly related to some other condition)? If this is an initial assessment, one of the first questions that must be addressed is whether the communicative problems that have been identified might justifiably be attributed to a disorder of language development and whether some other causative condition might be active as well as or instead of a language impairment. Although discussions about the advisability of labeling impairment are swinging into full force in many states and nations at this writing, labels are often needed before services can be provided and reimbursed. (For example, see Wang & Reynolds, 1985, for a discussion of a successful intervention program involving declassification of students that was terminated because it resulted in a net loss of revenue for the school district.)

Regardless of the ultimate influence of philosophical discussions on policy, discovering whether problems are related to a language disorder or to some other factor will help to plan positive intervention for children, their families, and their teachers. Diagnosis (and labeling) of impairment is one of the primary purposes of assessment, but as discussed later in this chapter, defining language disorder operationally is difficult. Two kinds of criteria frequently used to answer the question about disorder type are *discrepancy criteria* and *exclusion criteria*. Both are discussed in greater detail later in this chapter.

4. Does the child qualify for special services? When judging whether a child qualifies for special services, the specialist not only must identify language disorder but also usually must determine whether the child meets eligibility criteria established by some public or private agency (e.g., a state department of education or a third-party payer). Eligibility criteria may involve not only judgments about characteristics of the impairment (possibly including discrepancy and exclusionary criteria) but also procedures for diagnosticians and decision-making groups, even including the specific makeup of those groups.

FIGURE 6.1
A decision-making flowchart for the primary steps of the language assessment and intervention process.

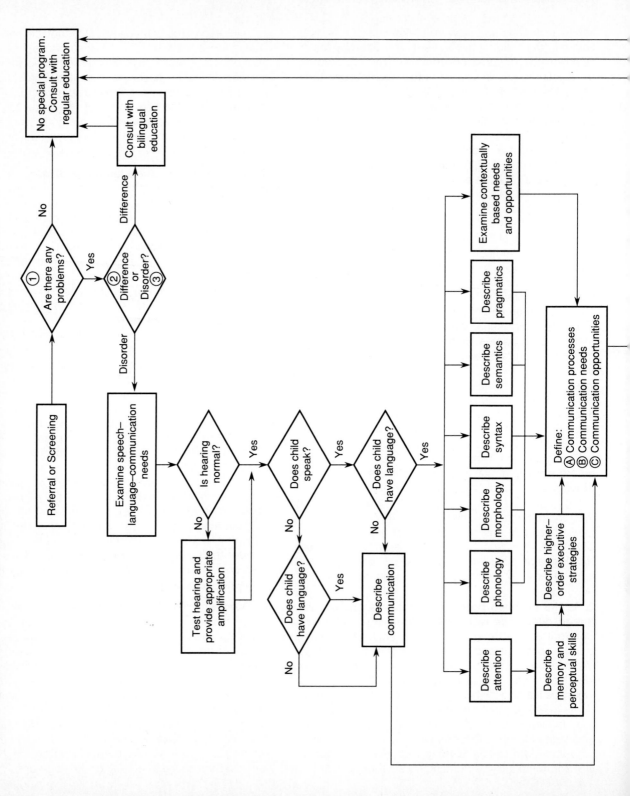

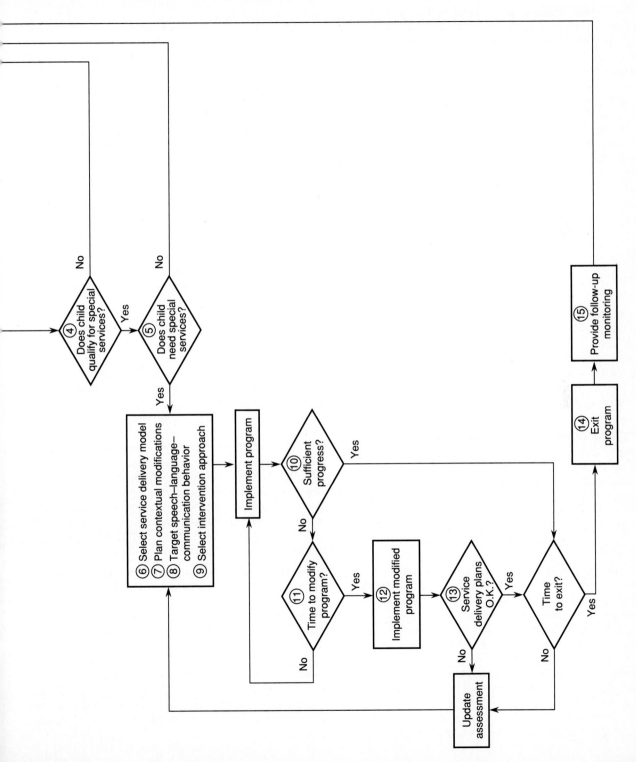

5. Does the child need special services? The question of whether a child needs special services may not always be asked, or it may be asked only in the context of the question about whether the child qualifies for special services, but the two questions are not exactly the same. Because a student qualifies for special services does not necessarily mean that he or she needs them. Conversely, some have suggested that the question about need should be asked without spending so much time, effort, and money on whether those children qualify. This could happen if regular, special, and bilingual education were not viewed and funded as separate entities but as cooperative ways to meet the needs of all students having difficulty achieving, no matter what the cause, and as a result, bias against youngsters from minority cultural or linguistic groups might be reduced (Reynolds & Wang, 1983; Rueda, 1989; J. E. Ysseldyke et al., 1983).

6. What kinds of services does the child need? This question was a major topic of the discussion in Chapter 5. Decisions about settings, people, and scheduling variables are used to select service-delivery models as part of transdisciplinary planning. Later in this chapter, the emphasis is on creating appropriate matches between the problems and strengths identified in assessment and the purposes, types, content, and contexts of intervention.

7. Should specific contexts be changed or introduced? Answers to questions about appropriate service are integrally tied to answers about whether specific contexts should be modified during intervention. When a child cannot function well enough to be competent in a particular environment, the two obvious choices are to change the environment or to change the child. Most intervention programs involve a little of both. In schools, a historical difference between speech–language pathology and other special education services has been that pullout speech–language services have aimed primarily to change the child by working directly to change specific behaviors. Classroom-based special education services have aimed primarily to change the educational environment, providing a special curriculum. Those distinctions tend to blur as school systems take a more deliberate look at how they might best meet the needs of all of their students.

When the ultimate goal is to assist children to have the skills, strategies, and motivation they need to par-ticipate successfully in society, education, and work as adults, it is important to identify contexts that may help them to develop those characteristics. The idea is to foster a closer match between the communicative demands of situations and the communicative abilities of children in the long run as well as in the short run. Sometimes this match can be achieved through a special modified context that can gain students access to learning not available in the regular classroom (e.g., G. M. Anderson & Nelson, 1988; L. P. Hoffman, 1990; N. W. Nelson, 1981a). Increasingly however, intervention planners are seeking ways to modify natural contexts with same-age peers to allow children with impairments greater opportunity to participate with peers who may or may not have impairments (e.g., N. W. Nelson, 1989b; W. Stainback et al., 1985).

8. Which speech, language, and communication behaviors and strategies should be changed? The other side of the intervention coin involves changing the child. When children's knowledge, skill, and strategies are insufficient to meet their communicative demands, intervention efforts involve targeting those areas that seem most in need of change and that would make the most difference to the child. The outcome of this part of the decision-making process is a set of operationally defined objectives targeting specific changes. To some extent, the choices made in writing objectives are guided by theories of language acquisition, which are discussed in the next section of this chapter. More direct influences on choices result from individualized assessment, which may involve comparing the youngster's abilities with those of normally developing peers. Communicative behaviors and strategies typically acquired in the early, middle, and later stages of language acquisition during childhood are presented in Chapters 7 to 9.

9. What intervention approach should be used to change targeted skills and knowledge? Not only the targets of intervention but procedures of intervention need to be selected. As discussed later in this chapter, selection and implementation of intervention methods are theory driven (whether or not that is always recognized), but an eclectic approach (N. W. Nelson, 1981a)—in which professionals select one or more methods that seem best suited for a particular purpose—stands the best chance of meeting the needs of individuals with special language development concerns.

10. Is progress occurring? Integral to intervention is the ongoing measurement of change. The plan for measuring progress is established as an integral part of the written individualized objectives. Each objective includes a criterion statement indicating how participants will know when it has been accomplished. Participants also must regularly obtain a broader view of the child. Federal policy determines the timing of this process to be at least twice a year for Individualized Family Service Plans (IFSPs) (as required by Part H) and at least once a year for Individualized Education Plans (IEPs) (as required by Part B, IDEA, PL 101–476, 1990).

11. Has enough change occurred in one area that it is time to modify the plan? To some extent, good plans become obsolete sooner than poor ones. If a plan works, the changes it specifies are made without taking forever, and thus, new targets are justified sooner. Of course, it is possible to write a plan targeting trivial changes that are easy to accomplish but make little difference to the child. The likelihood of this occurring is reduced if the progress-measuring plan includes measurement of several changes in several contexts determined to be relevant during earlier discussions of the child's needs.

12. If not enough change is occurring, what modifications are needed? If no change is occurring, or very little, modifications are also needed in the plan. Perhaps the targets were too ambitious. Maybe they do not meet contextually based needs. The mismatch between the communicative expectations of the child's environment and the communicative abilities of the child simply may be too great. The procedures being implemented may not be appropriate for the kinds of changes sought. Regardless, if positive change is not occurring, the plan must be changed.

13. Does the current service-delivery model remain best suited to meeting the child's needs? At some point, the specialist may decide that a basic change in the service-delivery model is needed. The occasion for this question may be a system-wide look at how the needs of all children with special problems are being met as a part of program accountability evaluation, or it may be asked on an individual basis. Parents of children served under the IDEA (PL 101–476, 1990) have a right to ask for a formal review of service delivery plans any time that they think that their children's needs are not being met. Part B spec-

ifies that at least once every 3 years, children must undergo comprehensive reevaluation and their need for special education services must be reconfirmed. This is usually interpreted to mean that children must again meet local eligibility standards based on current formal assessment results.

One of the most difficult problems facing professionals occurs when they think that a child continues to need special services but formal test results indicate that the student no longer qualifies. In such cases, primary options are (1) to conduct further testing specifically to tap the remaining areas of impairment, (2) to conduct different kinds of assessment to determine whether the student can actually apply newly acquired skills in the classroom, or (3) to decide that the professional is being overprotective and that the student is actually ready to be more independent of specialized intervention services than thought, particularly if given sufficient support in the regular classroom. At one time or another, all three of these options may be needed.

14. Is it time for the child to exit formal intervention services? At some point, it may be decided that a particular child is ready to exit formal speech and language intervention services. Federal policy set by the IDEA specifies that this cannot be a unilateral decision by a single professional but must be part of the IEP or IFSP process.

15. Does follow-up monitoring indicate a need for more direct attention to needs? A major point made in the discussion of causes, categories, and contributing factors in Chapter 4 was that disabilities evolve over time, not only as a result of changing abilities of children but also as a result of changing expectations of contexts. Results presented by Scarborough and Dobrich (1990), which were reviewed in Chapter 4, showed in particular that there is a danger that children who receive language intervention as preschoolers may appear to catch up with their peers when they first enter school but may run into problems later when language and literacy demands of school contexts again exceed their abilities. This situation was also illustrated by Damico's (1988) case study, reviewed and discussed in Chapter 1.

A little recognized requirement of the IDEA is that follow-up monitoring is required after children leave special education. As professionals become more skilled in using the strategies of collaborative consultation, and as natural contexts are used as an integral part of intervention, the student's transition from special contexts to home, school, and work may be smoother. In systems where the concept of a continuum of services is a reality, the view of service provision as an all-or-none decision can become more flexible, because the mechanism is in place to provide more intensive services if needed.

THEORETICAL PERSPECTIVES GUIDING ASSESSMENT AND INTERVENTION PRACTICES

Whether or not it is clearly recognized, one or more theoretical perspectives always guide language assessment and intervention practices. Even when a professional does not custom design a program but "buys" a ready-made approach, that professional is assuming that the theoretical basis of the "store-bought" approach is consistent with the child's needs. This may be the case. The position taken here, however, is that professionals must make choices that are deliberate and individualized in the context of collaborative interactions with others who know the child well and that are not based on chance, dogma, or prepackaged decision making.

Biological Maturation Theory Influences

Contributions of biological maturation theories. Language specialists sometimes make assumptions about the child's brain activity as they assist a child to learn language. Clinicians who have active models of neurolinguistic processing may draw on those to encourage children to make connections among different kinds of linguistic and other information.

Neurolinguistic theories, however, are much less likely to drive language assessment and intervention efforts with children who have developmental disabilities than with adults or even with children with acquired disabilities. Carrow-Woolfolk (1988) described the influences of neuropsychological theory on language assessment and intervention based on the theory that disordered language represents a condition of the central nervous system, particularly the brain. Therefore, intervention based on neuropsychological theory "is directed to improving the function of that part of the brain that is damaged or developmentally immature and/or encouraging other parts of the brain to 'take over' the function of the disordered part" (Carrow-Woolfolk, 1988, p. 66).

Assessment and intervention based on neurolinguistic theory rests partially on assumptions that various parts of the brain work in modular fashion and that certain areas may be more or less affected by particular kinds of impairments. For example, Broca's area, in the frontal lobe cortex of the left hemisphere, is known to play a role in using phonological, syntactic, and morphological rules to formulate and produce clearly articulated grammatical sentences. Wernicke's area plays a vital role in recognizing familiar phonological patterns as having meaning and in broader aspects of word recognition and language comprehension and contributes to word retrieval. The arcuate fasciculus, Broca's area, and Wernicke's areas all must be operational for a person to repeat another's linguistic production. However, a person may repeat without apparent understanding (as in echolalia) when those three components are operational but disconnected from broader association areas of the brain (Goodglass, 1981; Goodglass & Kaplan, 1983). Much evidence points to the right hemisphere as playing a major role in pragmatic areas such as interpreting nonlinguistic and paralinguistic communication devices such as gestures, facial expression, and prosody, and connected discourse events such as social conversation, narration, and humor (Springer & Deutsch, 1985). The importance of subcortical concentrations of gray matter and intact fiber association tracts to the development and support of complex linguistic skills such as literacy is just beginning to be appreciated (Aram, Ekelman, & Gillespie, 1989).

Assessment efforts that have the ulterior motive of subtyping or differential diagnosis of children with specific language impairment tend to use neurolinguistic and neuropsychological models consistent with an adult model of aphasia. For example, in their early subtyping study, Aram and Nation (1975) used formal and informal language tasks designed to tap comprehension, formulation, and repetition of selected phonologic, syntactic, and semantic aspects of language. Assessment tasks based on neuropsychological theory have also been generated to test relationships of dyslexia to linguistic dysfunction (e.g., Kamhi & Catts, 1989; Kamhi, Catts, Mauer, Apel, & Gentry, 1988; Vellutino, 1979), phonological processing problems (Kamhi & Catts, 1986; Lieberman & Shankweiler, 1985), speech production deficits (Catts, 1989), and even spatial conceptualization problems (Kamhi et al., 1988). Although research reports associated with such studies do not necessarily include discussion of assessment and intervention implications for individual students, clinical application of their methods remains a possibility.

Batteries of tests designed to measure central auditory processing are also based on neuropsychological theories. According to one view of specific language-learning disabilities, delay or deviation in language development is, with only a few exceptions, due to disordered brain function (Ferry, 1981). For example, such problems may represent lack of hemisphere dominance of language; inability to localize sounds; difficulty separating, synthesizing, or integrating sounds presented to the two ears; or difficulty separating a foreground message from background noise. Extending this view, Keith (1981) noted that, "In situations where the neurological structure is inadequate for processing a complex acoustic signal in an imperfect listening environment, language learning problems may result" (p. 63). Specially designed central auditory assessment tasks have been constructed to assess particular neuropsychological functions (the overlap with information processing theories should be readily apparent).

Even without formal assessment results, neurolinguistic theory may contribute to planning intervention activities for children. For example, we found a neurolinguistic perspective helpful in providing assessment and intervention for Sarah, the child with postleukemia encephalopathy whose description and magnetic resonance image appeared in Chapter 4. You may recall that Sarah's MRI scan showed massive reduction in white matter across wide areas, with damage particularly concentrated in posterior temporoparietal cortical and subcortical regions. Her clinical symptoms included significantly reduced language comprehension abilities, with better language expression abilities, particularly when she was allowed to initiate topics. Sarah also demonstrated immediate echolalia fairly regularly, particularly echoing direct questions rather than answering them. We interpreted the echolalia as a processing aid that might help Sarah move linguistic input from her relatively more impaired auditory comprehension system to her relatively more intact language production system and thus did not try to discourage it. We did, however, try to reduce the numbers of direct questions asked of her at first, and we made a concentrated effort to provide meaningful contexts in which Sarah might do most of the initiating or use modeled comments to stay on topic. For example, while looking at one of Sarah's favorite books, instead of saying, "What will the bunny do next, Sarah?" the clinician would say, "I wonder what that bunny is going to do." Gradually, we were able to reintroduce direct questions, and Sarah began to be able to answer them. The echolalia reduced in frequency as her other productive language abilities increased (Sturm & Nelson, 1989).

Biological maturation theories, on a broader scale, have implications for comprehensive treatment of children with all kinds of conditions. In particular, many conditions associated with frank impairments of biological systems peripheral to central nervous system language processing areas justify transdisciplinary intervention strategies to address those peripheral impairments. Perhaps no problem needs more immediate attention than hearing impairment, both in the earliest stages of language acquisition and beyond. A combination of services from professionals in varied fields should be provided early and consistently to ensure that the biological hearing mechanism is the best that it can be, that compensatory technology, in the form of personal hearing aids and other amplification devices are used whenever appropriate, and that the child learns to use the hearing system. Similar kinds of attention are needed when visual, anatomical, or motor problems are evident. Children with craniofacial anomalies such as cleft palate and other branchial arch syndromes are particularly at risk not only for speech acquisition difficulties but for hearing loss and feeding and social interaction problems. Children with these problems justify early attention and ongoing follow-up by transdisciplinary teams, including attention to language acquisition concerns.

One question based on biological maturation that may arise during assessment is whether to refer children for pediatric neurological evaluation when language disorder appears to be the primary concern. Every child should have access to good general health care of all types, auditory, visual, and dental. Whether or not a specific neurological evaluation is warranted is generally part of decision making by an entire health team and the family. Neurological referral is critical when a child is observed to lose previously acquired language abilities, and it is justified when the child might be having seizures. Most often, however, medical assessment is not called for when language disorder is suspected but no evidence of immediate neurologic pathology is present. A magnetic resonance scan, for example, can cost about $1,000, and its contribution to clinical decision making is limited in the absence of suspected treatable pathological processes.

Limitations of biological maturation theories. A primary limitation of basing language assessment and intervention on biological maturation theory is that the central nervous system as a biological mechanism is basically inaccessible to direct treatment. Attempts to directly fix a problem of biological maturation are limited by the modifiability of the system. Medical-surgical techniques may be used to treat such peripheral conditions as conductive hearing loss and anatomical anomalies and to address the neurological problems associated with tumors and traumatic brain injuries. For profound sensorineural hearing loss, cochlear implants may be used to stimulate the auditory nerve and the brain. In addition, drugs may be prescribed for children with seizure disorders and those with attention-deficit hyperactivity disorder (ADHD). Such treatments, however, are designed more to provide a system accessible to learning, rather than to modify any part of the language learning system directly. Compensatory techniques, aids, and devices used to augment hearing, oral communication, or writing all function in similar ways. For the most part, the central nervous system is modifiable only indirectly, through learning processes, and any of the other theoretical models contributes more to understanding how to foster learning than does the biological maturation model.

Another limitation of neuropsychological and biological theory for guiding assessment is that most assessment tasks designed to tap particular kinds of brain functioning are only guesses about what might be happening in the brain. As U. Kirk (1983) pointed out (see Chapter 2), most neuropsychological models of brain functioning are limited in their ability to explain "the consistency and variability that characterize the developing system, the matured system, and the system that is recovering from damage" (p. 23). Many tasks for assessing neuropsychological processing were developed first for adults with known lesions. When such individuals cannot perform a particular activity, it is inferred that the damaged area must make a critical contribution to performing that task. The child's developing brain, however, may not be organized in the same way. Other areas of the brain also may make a greater contribution to accom-

plishing the assessment activity than suspected. There is no way to clearly isolate the functioning of one part of the brain from contributions of other parts.

Nowhere is this problem more evident than in the assessment of central auditory processing skills. Tasks designed to measure selective auditory attention, short-term memory, auditory sequencing, and dichotic listening cannot prevent an intact language system, or even a disordered one, from playing a role in the outcome. Rees (1973, 1981) pointed out that causal relationships are not clear. Even if it were possible to associate reliably certain kinds of task dysfunction with certain brain lesion sites in children, such information would likely be of little value in designing remediation programs. On the contrary, the greater danger is that, based on specific skills testing, clinicians might be tempted to return to old approaches, such as therapy based on the results of the Illinois Test of Psycholinguistic Abilities (S. A. Kirk, McCarthy, & Kirk, 1968), in which assessment tasks were transformed directly into intervention tasks, such as requesting answers to questions like, "Do bananas telephone?" or prompting expressive language like, "It's a cup, it's pink, it's plastic, you drink out of it." (Recently, I was told about a teenager with autism whose favorite question is, "Can you swim in a bowling alley?" I shudder to think that this piece of apparent delayed echolalia might have come from a language intervention session, but it had a reminiscent ring about it.) As Hammill and Larsen (1974) found when they conducted a review of 38 studies of attempts to train children in specific psycholinguistic skills, not only were such approaches generally ineffective in changing communicative behaviors, but when behavioral change did occur, it had little relevance to the communicative needs of children.

Linguistic Rule-Induction Theory Influences

Contributions of linguistic theories. When based primarily on linguistic theory, the overriding goal of assessment is to represent a child's underlying grammar or knowledge of the rules of language. The primary goal of intervention is to develop that grammar further, which is done by setting up conditions so that children are led to induce the rules that they have not acquired naturally.

Although not based exclusively on linguistic theory, the assessment and intervention approach designed by L. Bloom & Lahey (1978; Lahey, 1988) is grounded largely in linguistic theory. The approach surpasses linguistic theory in its most limited focus on grammar (content-form interactions) to include language use and places language use in a social context. The following four assumptions, however, as outlined by Lahey (1988) illustrate the high consistency of the approach with a linguistic theoretical perspective: (1) Language involves interactions among the three components, content, form, and use. (2) The emphasis should be on language and communicative behaviors regardless of the cause of the disorder. (3) Information about normal language development should be used as the basis for the sequence of intervention goals. (4) Goals should be expressed in terms of language production explicitly and language comprehension only implicitly.

Linguistic approaches to language assessment and intervention have evolved as linguistic theory itself has evolved. As indicated in Lahey's outline of basic assumptions, assessment and intervention focus on observable aspects of language performance as a way to infer what children know about the rules of language (i.e., children's nonobservable language competence). Children are also seen as active participants in language acquisition, not as imperfect little adults whose primary developmental efforts are directed toward making fewer and fewer errors. Because the things children say and do during language acquisition permit glimpses of their hidden generative hypotheses about language, spontaneous samples of linguistic behavior are particularly important tools to clinicians who base their work on linguistic theory. Because oral language acquisition is considered primary to written language development, and because language expression is easier to observe than language comprehension, assessment and intervention efforts based on linguistic theory have also tended to involve speaking more than other communication modes.

When linguistic rule-induction theory guides language intervention practices, the primary target of intervention is knowledge of varied kinds of linguistic rules. A history of language assessment practices (Launer & Lahey, 1981) shows that, following the introduction of Chomsky's revolutionary linguistic theory (1957, 1965), assessment efforts focused primarily on analyzing children's ability to demonstrate knowledge of language form rules, particularly syntactic and morphological rules produced in spontaneous language and in response to structured language elicitation tasks. Then, "If the child missed a certain language structure on a test, that structure was listed as a goal of intervention. If the child responded correctly to a given language structure, the clinician assumed that the child 'knew' that structure, and it was not a target for intervention" (Launer & Lahey, 1981, p. 16).

Although early efforts to apply Chomsky's theory of transformational generative grammar (TGG) to language assessment and intervention practices included the admonition for clinicians to view "language as a linguistic structure having phonemic, semantic, syntactic, and morphological features" (Lee, 1966, p. 311), in operation, the focus tended to be more on form than meaning. Pragmatics was not yet a part of the picture.

The application of linguistic theory to language assessment and intervention began to change as developmental psycholinguistics contributed to its evolution. A particularly important influence was L. Bloom's (1970) focus on the need for a rich semantic-grammatic interpretation of children's early two-word utterances. Bloom also emphasized that context was an essential part of determining meaning. These two contributions foreshadowed the blending of linguistic, cognitive, and sociolinguistic elements into the content–form–use model of language development and disorders that Bloom & Lahey introduced in their influential text in 1978 (see Figure 6.2). Even earlier, L. Bloom (1967) had pointed out that clinical techniques based on unidimensional aspects of linguistic theory, such as those developed by Lee (1966) for analyzing the form of utterances in spontaneous language samples without considering

---

Personal Reflection 6.1	"Goals of intervention and assessment must include information about the interactions among content, form, and use." *Margaret Lahey, Ph.D.* (1988, p.179), describing her "three-dimensional" approach, based primarily on linguistic theory, but integrating elements of context and pragmatics as well.

FIGURE 6.2
The model for interaction of content, form, and use in language.

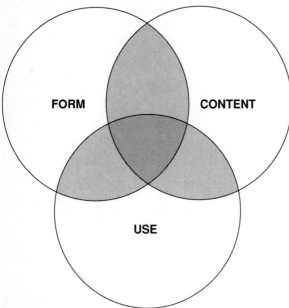

Note. Reprinted with the permission of Macmillan Publishing Company from *Language Disorders and Language Development* (p. 22) by Margaret Lahey. Copyright © 1988 by Macmillan Publishing Company.

their communicativeness, were limited and even distorted by their lack of contextual information.

Recognizing the multidimensional and interactionist nature of the L. Bloom and Lahey (1978) approach to assessment and intervention, Fey (1986) identified it as a separate approach from one based on TGG. In this book, however, Bloom and Lahey's approach is categorized as the best example of clinical application of more recent modifications of linguistic rule-induction theory. It remains to be seen whether even more recent linguistic theory developments—particularly contributions from government binding (GB) theory (Chomsky, 1981) and language learnability notions (Leonard & Loeb, 1988)—will work their way into assessment and intervention practices for children with language disorders.

Limitations of linguistic theories. Probably the greatest limitations of linguistic theory for directing language assessment and intervention practices are associated with the most limited interpretation of the theory. Although TGG, and especially GB theory, include some rules related to semantic and phonological representation, they primarily explain the syntac-

tic rules for forming single sentences. Rules related to pragmatics and to producing and understanding connected discourse are conspicuously missing.

In presenting his theory of multiple "relatively autonomous" intelligences, Gardner (1983) made explicit the view that some aspects of language are closer to representing the core essence of language than others. "The syntactic and phonological processes appear to be special, probably specific to human beings, and unfolding with relatively scant need for support from environmental factors. Other aspects of language, however, such as semantic and pragmatic domains, may well exploit more general human information-processing mechanisms and are less strictly or exclusively tied to a 'language organ'"(Gardner, 1983, p. 81).

Unlike theoreticians, clinicians cannot afford to ignore some aspects of language development to focus exclusively on others. In fact, a problem of some of the language intervention programs that were available in the 1970s was their focus on syntax at the expense of other aspects of language and communication. The theory that language is learned by inducing its regularities from linguistic evidence led to the construction of approaches that involved presentation of multiple exemplars of a particular syntactic formation rule (e.g., *is* + [Verb]*ing*), often in single isolated sentences presented to correspond to a stack of pictures, under the assumption that the child would eventually induce the rule of focus (e.g., Gray & Ryan, 1973).

These programs risked missing the needs of children who had language disorders not isolated to the area of language form (N. W. Nelson, 1981a). As the discussions of Chapter 4 indicated, all children with language disorders are not alike. In his 1987 paper, Leonard noted that even the profiles of children all labeled as having "specific language impairment" show "a great deal of variation in terms of relative strengths and weaknesses" (p. 30) (see Chapter 4).

As a hybrid approach, the three-dimensional interactional system proposed by L. Bloom and Lahey (1978), and developed further by Lahey (1988), permits description of children as having relatively more difficulty in any of the three areas, content, form, or use, or in integrating them into a whole system. To a great extent, this extension counteracts the primary limitation while maintaining some of the strengths of an approach based primarily on linguistic theory. As Fey (1986) pointed out, it is more an interactionist approach than one based strictly on linguistic theory.

Thus, it remains helpful to view language acquisition as a process by which children internalize the rules of language but with the newer view that children acquire rules by exposure to language regularities within meaningful, communicative contexts (Wells, 1986). In fact, by adopting the view that children with language learning difficulties nevertheless use language acquisition processes similar to those of normally developing children, intervention can be designed to keep children in more natural language-learning contexts with their peers. Rather than presenting different kinds of experiences, clinicians may concentrate more effort in consulting with others (particularly parents and teachers, but also peers) to intensify normal experiences and to present the kinds of scaffolding of experience (as explained in Chapters 7 to 9) that will give children access to the construction of meaning.

A second limitation associated with narrow clinical applications of linguistic theory is the potential narrowing of focus to a single stage of linguistic development, the preschool years, which I identify as the *middle stage of language acquisition*. It is only one of three important stages. Most professionals now recognize that although the majority of syntactic and morphological rule acquisition activity occurs during the years 3 through 7, some extremely important communicative events precede that period. Events occurring during the *early stage*, the prelinguistic communicative interactions of infancy, are now viewed as important in and of themselves as well as for their role in establishing a foundation for language acquisition. The *later stage* of language acquisition also includes developments now recognized as significant, particularly in metalinguistics, abstract language use, and sophisticated strategies for using connected discourse of different types.

Thus, the linguistic-induction strategies that seem so important for supporting certain aspects of language acquisition in a particular stage seem not so important for supporting other aspects in other stages. When the goal of an intervention program is to encourage children to induce the rules of language covertly, the strategies of nonlinguistic communication may be overlooked (as in the early stages), and the specialist may consider overt talk about language (as in the later stages) to be inappropriate.

The object of intervention programs based exclusively on linguistic theory is to enable children to learn the rules of language without talking directly about those rules. What are the limitations of this viewpoint relative to a more comprehensive picture of language acquisition, particularly one that includes academic uses of language, the development of literacy, and nonliteral language uses and comprehension? In its avoidance of metalinguistic discussion of the rules and in its emphasis on language expression over comprehension, the linguistic-rule approach (especially when it concentrates on rule production in single sentences) also risks missing the needs of older children, particularly those having difficulty meeting the complex language demands of school. Recognizing this limitation, Lahey (1988) included information about working on narrative discourse with children after they had reached a certain level of proficiency in smaller units.

In discussing broader issues of language competence, van Kleeck (1984), posed the question "How, if at all, does the notion of language awareness change our current thinking about language disabilities in children?" (p. 179). She then proceeded to answer the question by indicating several specific ways that metalinguistic factors might influence language assessment and intervention practices.

Before considering those points, let us review the meaning of the term *metalinguistics*. Like pragmatics, *metalinguistics* is a broad term. Any task that requires the participants to focus consciously on language as an opaque object with properties of its own, rather than as a transparent medium of communication, is metalinguistic. A metalinguistic act requires conscious awareness of language, particularly awareness of language on more than one level simultaneously. Many assessment tasks are metalinguistic. Examples are those requiring children to judge word pairs as same or different, to rhyme words, to segment words into syllables, to blend phonemes into words, to understand figurative language uses, or even to repeat questions rather than answering them.

Van Kleeck (1984) pointed out that language assessment commonly involves a combination of formal testing with informal language sampling, usually with the intention of using the results from the two types of activities to support each other in finding out what the child knows about language. It could be argued, however, as van Kleeck suggested, "that, rather than supporting each other, these two data sources tap *different* aspects of the child's knowledge of language and that they are, therefore, not truly comparable" (p. 187).

One type of test is not necessarily good and the other bad, they are simply different. The point is to recognize those differences and to take advantage of them. Children need to be able to use language as a tool of social interaction, but they also need to be able to use it reflectively, particularly in school and during literacy acquisition. Indeed, as they grow older, to be socially appropriate, children need to be able to tell jokes, recognize puns, and use slang and double entendres, all of which have metalinguistic elements.

An intervention approach that extends beyond primary linguistic uses of language to include metalinguistic ones may also be justified. Van Kleeck (1984) noted two ways to do this. First, intervention methods might be used to help children acquire linguistic rules that they have been unable to acquire naturally by using metalinguistic strategies to help them notice a previously ignored linguistic unit, such as a plural ending or an auxiliary verb form. Second, metalinguistic awareness itself might be a legitimate target of intervention. Either approach suggests some value in extending beyond the confines of decision making based solely on linguistic rule-induction theory.

Behaviorist Theory Influences

Contributions of behaviorist theories. Behaviorism offers a technology for designing procedural approaches to language assessment and intervention that is more developed than that provided by any other theoretical perspective. This characteristic prompted Fey (1986) to note that, "Since the early 1960s, operant theory, or behaviorism, probably has had a greater impact on intervention practices than any other theory" (p. 3).

One of the most basic tenets of behaviorism is that nothing is hidden or mysterious. Everything that needs to be known can be observed by analyzing the effects of antecedent and consequent events on behavior. In addition, the stimulus–response–reinforcement paradigm of behaviorism offers a ready-made plan to modify a person's behavior. A recognized need for change is, after all, the reason that intervention is sought.

The tools of behaviorism include elements of both analysis and control. Duchan (1984) pointed out that "Language, in a behaviorist framework, is a response that is either triggered by a stimulus or produced in anticipation of a subsequent reinforcement" (p. 63). According to B. F. Skinner's (1957) view of radical behaviorism, language is treated either as a response

to a presenting stimulus (a *tact*) or as an operant (a *mand*) that is either strengthened or weakened by subsequent reinforcement.

In the therapeutic milieu, the analysis techniques of behaviorism are used to define observable and measurable behavioral targets. Hidden, central processes, such as those representing mental states or motivational elements are considered to be beyond the purview of the observer and not critical to the outcome of interactions. In behavior modification approaches, context is never ignored, but it is often engineered. Environmental influences are considered to be of paramount importance in determining whether a certain desired behavior will be emitted, and once produced, whether it will be more likely to occur again in the future. Thus, the behaviorist often sees the control of context as an important tool in intervention and may write highly structured programs specifying all critical dimensions for sequences of interactions (e.g., Costello, 1977; Gray & Ryan, 1973; Sloane & MacAulay, 1968).

The basic tenets of a behaviorist perspective on language assessment and intervention were outlined by Craig (1983):

> (1) all behavior, including language, can be observed, described, and characterized in peripheral terms without involving the mind or central behavior; (2) complex behaviors are the sum of a set of simple behaviors; and (3) learning is the relationship between time and response strength. (pp. 103–104)

The view of complex behaviors as the sum of a set of simple behaviors invites the breakdown of language into steps that can be mastered one at a time. In behaviorism, the assessment process not only involves analysis of current levels of functioning, it also involves the use of task analysis procedures to outline learning goals. Under this theoretical umbrella, when deciding what to teach next, developmental level may be considered less important than task simplicity, and functionality may be viewed as more important than linguistic sophistication. In contrast with traditional linguistic-based or cognitive-based approaches, determination of whether children meet developmental prerequisites may play little role in programs designed by behaviorists (e.g., Guess, Sailor, & Baer, 1974). Early examples of such programs especially "placed no 'entrance requirements' on the learner" (L. McCormick, 1990a, p. 188).

The technology of behaviorism involves control of antecedent and consequent events to shape responses and sometimes to encourage children to initiate behaviors. A variety of strategies can be used, some of which may also be employed in programs based on theories other than behaviorism with slight modifications of procedure and terminology:

Attention training. This involves an initial intervention objective in which a child is trained to "look at me," or to "look at this," to receive a reinforcer just before the presentation of a new target stimulus (L. Kent, 1974).

Modeling. In modeling, a demonstrative model is presented, and then the child is reinforced for attempts to reproduce it. The adult produces the model with a clear intention of presenting the child with an example, essentially indicating, "Here's how it's done."

Imitation training. Imitation is the other side of modeling. It is the behavior produced by the child rather than by the trainer (L. McCormick, 1990b, p. 218). Imitation may be directly taught if the child has difficulty reproducing the behavior of another. This is usually done in a series of steps:

1. A period of mutual imitation; the trainer imitates a behavior produced spontaneously by the child.
2. The trainer models behaviors the child has produced earlier in the same session.
3. The trainer models behaviors the child has produced in the past.
4. The trainer models a modified behavior close to one in the child's repertoire with the hope that the child will be able to imitate the modification (using reinforcers at every step to strengthen the child's attempts at responding).
5. Gradually, the child is able to imitate completely novel behaviors.

Reinforcement strategies. Reinforcers are defined by their effect on behaviors, not by a preconceived notion of whether they might be positive or aversive (L. McCormick, 1990b). Although all reinforcers serve to strengthen the behavior they follow, not all reinforcers are positive: *Positive reinforcers* are positive events whose presence increases the probability that a response will recur. For example, the act of requesting desired objects (called *manding* by behaviorists) may be reinforced with the objects requested. *Negative reinforcers* are aversive events whose removal increases the probability that a response will recur. For example, a child with tantrums may be

placed in a "time-out" booth until the tantrum subsides, at which point the child is removed from the booth. Negative reinforcers are sometimes also viewed as "escape factors" that work to sustain undesirable behavior. Carr, Newsom, and Binkhoff (1980) described two children for whom aggressive behavior seemed to be negatively reinforced (i.e., increased in frequency) because it resulted in their being removed from undesired work situations whenever it occurred. Donnellan, Mirenda, Mesaros, and Fassbender (1984) recommended that care givers infer from this type of behavior the communicative message, "Leave me alone! I don't want to do this!" (p. 202).

Varied reinforcement schedules are used in different stages of behavioral training. Reinforcement schedules of 100% (i.e., a positive reinforcer presented after every desired behavior) are often used initially, but frequency of reinforcement may be gradually reduced as new behaviors are stabilized. Eventually, only intermittent reinforcement, or only naturally reinforcing environmental consequences are used to maintain the behavior. Planners generally try to avoid removing reinforcement entirely or too abruptly, for fear that a newly acquired behavior will be extinguished entirely (unless the intended outcome of intervention is that an undesirable behavior, which has been inadvertently reinforced, be extinguished), but they try to avoid a situation in which a desired response can only be maintained through the application of artificial reinforcers.

Punishment strategies. If the desired outcome is the reduction of an undesirable behavior rather than the recurrence of a desirable one, punishment strategies may be used. Like reinforcement, punishment is defined by its effect on the behavior it follows (not by a preconceived notion of what might be aversive). Any consequence that reduces the frequency of a preceding behavior is considered to be punishing for a particular individual.

For example, echolalia may be defined as undesirable by behaviorists. In such cases, a behaviorist solution might be to shout, "Don't echo!" as a punishing consequence for echolalic responses. This approach would generally be accompanied by measurement in changes in the frequency of the behavior. However, as Duchan (1984) has pointed out, such a theoretical stance fails to recognize the potential communicative value of the echolalia. In this case, charting only reduction in the "undesirable" behavior of echolalia may miss a concomitant suppression of other types of communication as well.

Aside from this example, a hot debate is now raging among parents and professionals as to whether aversives should ever be used either in the form of punishment or negative reinforcement for individuals with severe disabilities. Some parents and professionals feel that only strong aversive punishments, such as those involving administration of electric shock or water or vinegar squirted in the face, are effective in reducing self-injurious behaviors, such as hand biting or head banging. Others feel that extreme use of aversive measures, such as physical restraint or ongoing isolation, is abusive and is never justified. This position is summarized in Box 6.1 in a *Resolution on Abusive Treatment and Neglect* passed in 1988 by the Board of Directors of the Autism Society of America.

Prompting and cuing.   When a child is not giving sufficient attention to a stimulus or to a particular part of a stimulus, cues may be used to highlight its salient features (e.g., through gesture or exaggeration, such as touching a child under the chin to indicate the need for the final velar consonant /k/ at the end of the word *book*). The terms *prompt* and *cue* may be used interchangeably (L. McCormick, 1990b), but some prefer to reserve the term *prompt* to refer to direct efforts to guide a person into making a particular response (e.g., by guiding a person's hand or touching him on the elbow to initiate a response). *Putting*

through and *hand-over-hand* prompts are used to physically assist a motor response. Such prompts are difficult to use for tasks involving oral communicative responses.

Fading.   When cues and prompts are successful, the usual approach is to begin to try to fade them. This is done by reducing their intensity or their frequency and reinforcing the child when the desired behavior continues to occur. The idea is to remove prompts entirely, so that natural stimuli alone result in the desired response; that is, the response is under *stimulus control.*

Shaping.   The basic strategy of operant conditioning, shaping involves selective reinforcement of responses that are increasingly close to the target. A parent of a nonverbal child might be encouraged to respond by providing a desired breakfast cereal, accompanied by the phrase, "Oh, you want some cereal" first, when the child looks at a cabinet where a favorite cereal is kept; next, only when the child uses a whole-hand reach as well as a look; after that, only when the child points; then, only when the child points and vocalizes at the same time; and finally, when the child produces increasingly close approximations of words and then phrases.

Discrimination training.   A basic part of behavioral training involves teaching children which responses to provide to which stimuli. For example, when a word is spoken, a child might be expected to discriminate that word from others with which it might be

---

Box 6.1   Autism Society of America: Excerpt from Resolution on Abusive Treatment and Neglect

The Society calls for a cessation of treatment and/or intervention which results in any of the following:

1. Obvious signs of physical pain experienced by the individual;
2. Potential or actual physical side effects, including tissue damage, physical illness, emotional stress, or death;
3. Dehumanization of an individual with autism by the use of procedures which are normally unacceptable for non-handicapped persons in all environments;
4. Ambivalence of discomfort by family, staff, and/or caregivers regarding the necessity of such extreme strategies or their involvement in such intervention; and
5. Revulsion or distress felt by handicapped and non-handicapped peers and community members who cannot reconcile extreme procedures with acceptable human conduct.

Note. "Resolution on Abusive Treatment and Neglect" by the Autism Society of America, July 16, 1988, *The Advocate,* 20(3), p. 17. Reprinted courtesy of the Autism Society of America.

confused to select a particular object or picture the word represents. Later, the child might be expected to discriminate objects on the basis of their function. For example, a child might be asked, "What do you use to fix your hair?" or "What do you use to sweep the floor?"

Chaining.　One way to build complex behaviors from simpler ones is through chaining. Chaining is particularly useful for training behaviors where sequence is important (e.g., washing hands independently). Either backward chaining or forward chaining approaches may be used. Both approaches take advantage of selective limits on short-term memory. Backward chaining takes advantage of the "recency effect," which represents the finding that the last item of a sequence is usually the most easily recalled. Using backward chaining, a speech–language pathologist might teach a child to produce a multisyllabic word like hamburger, by asking the child to imitate each of the following syllabic combinations in sequence:

-ger

-burger

hamburger

Forward chaining takes advantage of the primacy effect of short-term memory (STM), and starts by modeling early elements in a chain, adding on later elements as success is experienced.

Stimulus and response generalization.　The object of a behavior training program is to extend the newly trained behavior beyond the immediate context. Stimulus generalization occurs when the child learns to use a new label, such as *hat,* to go with many types of headgear, some of which the child has never seen before, as well as with a picture of a particular kind of hat. The technical explanation is that varied stimuli begin to take on controlling properties for that same response. Response generalization occurs when the conditioning of a particular response results in increased probability of other responses similar to the original. This happens when varied responses are in the same response class. An example is when a child learns to use plural morphemes in response to a set of pictures of duplicate items and then asks for "two pretzels" at snacktime.

Repeated trials.　Because responses are thought to be strengthened through practice and with each reinforcement, behavioral programs are designed to elicit a high number of target responses of a particular type. Part of the behaviorist approach is to subdivide behaviors into discrete units so that effects can be measured without being confounded by uncontrolled events. Discrete trial learning is typical of intervention programs based on behaviorist principles. However, not all trials are presented in the same format. Three different possibilities were described by Mulligan, Guess, Holvoet, and Brown (1980): In the massed trial format, trials are presented one right after the other, with no time for other responses between trials. Using this format, children's attempts to make spontaneous contributions are usually actively discouraged. In the spaced trial format, repeated trials of the same type are grouped together, as they are in the massed trial format, but a rest period or pause is interspersed between trials. In the distributed trial format, trials are interspersed with other activities, and related and new responses are permitted or even encouraged between presentation of trials.

Limitations of behaviorist theories.　Perhaps the greatest limitation of basing assessment and intervention strictly on behaviorist theory is that such approaches tend to be reduced to a technology without a content. Without a theory that encompasses internalized language structure and development, and without a theory that proposes active roles for language learners, task analysis becomes almost the sole basis for making intervention decisions. It is then difficult to know what to work on first.

Interestingly, although humans are good at acquiring and using communication under most circumstances, we are not particularly good at analyzing language into small pieces that can be put back together in a functional whole for individuals who fail to learn it normally (perhaps it cannot be done). For example, one part of language learning that seems to be critical is the knowledge of words as symbols. When children fail to learn words naturally, the task might be broken down to involve repeated presentation of words to correspond to limited sets of objects placed in front of the child. Then a trainer could prompt the child to point to an object named. Later, discrimination training might involve requiring the child to answer "yes" or "no" appropriately when asked, "Is this a brush?" or "Is this a shoe?" Massed trials might be used to increase the frequency of response reinforcement during a particular time period, with the intention to increase its strength.

After a period of time, the child might be able to point to objects or perform label verification tasks to criterion (or might not; if you were to sit in front of a set of objects and be asked repeatedly, "Is this a brush?," you might begin to wonder after a while). However, even when reaching this point, the child may be no closer to a concept of what a brush can be used for or how to request one or what conversation is all about than before the training started.

The crux of this problem is that language seems to be too complex a system for some children to master on their own, but breaking it down into manageable pieces does not make it simpler so much as different. Thus, many children taught with behaviorist methods find it difficult to generalize newly learned behaviors back to complex real-life situations. Some behaviorists have attempted to address this problem by focusing on the functionality of language and other behaviors (L. McCormick & Schiefelbusch, 1990).

Functional responses are natural and necessary in children's everyday interactions and produce immediate, specific, and potentially naturally reinforcing consequences (Guess, Sailor, & Baer, 1978). For example, instead of using handclapping as the target of imitation training activities, the specialist might teach a child to imitate bringing a cup to the mouth to get juice or pointing to a cookie to get a bite of it. In these situations, the reinforcers are received as natural consequences of the child's actions.

Another problem is that, although definition of contextual events is a critical part of behaviorist theory, the definition of intervention contexts tends to be trivialized through behavioral analysis that involves reduction into discrete units and results in focus on pieces of behavior rather than interactions among people. The principles of behaviorism generally have been demonstrated in the laboratory and in small-scale experiments. Progress is measured only in terms of specific pieces of behavior targeted for intervention and not in terms of broader situational outcomes.

Studies that have attempted to assess generalization from training contexts to natural environments (e.g., Hughes & Carpenter, 1983; S. F. Warren & Rogers-Warren, 1983) or to teach it directly (e.g., Stokes & Baer, 1977) have shown poor or mixed results. Broad-scale efficacy of strict behaviorist-oriented approaches across multiple aspects of children's lives is difficult to demonstrate.

Additionally, by denying the relevance (or even existence) of internal processes and emotional states such as interest and motivation, reductionistic behaviorist programs fail to take advantage of the rich opportunities that encouragement of self-directed exploration and desire to communicate might afford. The behaviorist perspective also reduces children's behaviors into categories as either appropriate (thus justifying reinforcement to increase their frequency) or inappropriate (thus justifying punishment or ignoring to reduce their frequency) (Duchan, 1984). Reasons that might explain children's behavior have traditionally not been considered. For example, echolalia has been treated as a behavior to be extinguished rather than as an indication of internal processing that might be facilitative or communicative, perhaps representing inner states such as frustration or discomfort.

The past limitations of many behaviorist-oriented programs can be overcome. More recent approaches analyze possible communicative functions of aberrant behavior and design intervention approaches in which such behaviors might be treated as communicative (Donnellan et al., 1984).

Modified behavioral approaches have also been designed to reduce the passivity that frequently results when children are taught exclusively in stimulus–response–reinforcement modes. Children tend to become prompt dependent and thus never to learn to recognize the assertive and communicative possibilities of language use. (Behaviorists explain this as too much reinforcement of tact behaviors and not enough of mands.) Mirenda and Santogrossi (1985) devel-

---

Personal Reflection 6.2   "Although reinforcement may explain food searching in rats, it has failed to explain the average human child's search for communicative competence."

John Neil Bohannon, III, Butler University, and *Amye Warren-Leubecker*, University of Tennessee at Chattanooga, writing about theoretical approaches to language acquisition (1989, p. 209).

oped a "prompt-free" approach for starting over with an 8½-year-old nonspeaking girl, Amy, who only pointed to pictures on her communication board when an adult or peer asked "What do you want?" or "Show me what you want." In the revised program, the number of symbols available for selection was reduced back to one, and Amy was only reinforced when she spontaneously touched the symbol picture (a can of pop), first, accidentally, and then, intentionally, while engaging in other activities. In this approach, spontaneous use was defined as "the ability of the learner to identify the need for, locate, and indicate or produce the correct communication symbol in response to naturally occurring cues *only*" (Mirenda & Santogrossi, 1985, p. 143).

Others have overcome some of the limitations of behaviorism by using naturally occurring, not highly structured, learning contexts; keeping interaction events whole rather than breaking them down into component parts; using topics initiated by children, not by adults; using naturally occurring, not contrived reinforcers; and using dispersed, not massed, trials. These approaches have been called *incidental teaching*. The principles of incidental teaching were first reported by B. Hart and Risley (1968) and have since been expanded (B. Hart & Risley, 1975, 1986; B. Hart & Rogers-Warren, 1978; Kaiser & Warren, 1988; S. F. Warren & Kaiser, 1986; S. F. Warren & Rogers-Warren, 1985).

Although the rubric *incidental teaching* may be used to apply to several variations of approach, it basically refers to the "interactions between an adult and a child that arise naturally in an unstructured situation, such as free play, and that are used systematically by the adult to transmit new information or give the child practice in developing a communication skill" (B. Hart & Risley, 1975, p. 411). The techniques of incidental teaching borrow from other theoretical perspectives, particularly social interaction theory, but they also maintain some of the technology of behaviorism. Four primary strategies include the following:

1. *Modeling*. Models of desired responses are presented in environmentally appropriate contexts.
2. *Mand-model*. When children show interest in a particular item or activity, they are directly prompted (e.g., "Tell me what you want to do") and may even be prompted to "Give me a whole sentence." If further modeling is needed, it is provided, and when a satisfactory response is

obtained, it is reinforced with the desired object or activity.
3. *Time delay*. This technique is used to avoid prompt dependence. Rather than prompting, the adult arranges the environment to elicit the child's interest. When the child looks at the object and then the adult, the adult seeks to establish and maintain eye contact. If the child does not speak, the adult may model a response twice (with adequate time between models), and then, if the child still does not speak, the object or activity is provided nevertheless.
4. *Incidental teaching as a specific procedure*. Each episode starts with an initiation by the child. Adults attend to the child's interest and help the child to make more elaborate requests or comments through modeling and reinforcement within the natural contexts of the events.

Although incidental teaching approaches use natural learning contexts, they are not particularly naturalistic. Kirchner (1991) commented that "milieu teaching may be the most 'naturalistic' of the behaviorally derived approaches, but can hardly be considered pragmatic" (p. 83).

Information Processing Theory Influences

Contributions of older information processing theories. Information processing is sometimes considered a subcomponent of general cognitive processing rather than a theory on its own. When information processing theory influences decision making, however, the focus of assessment and intervention shifts. Rather than targeting developmental abilities or linguistic rule knowledge, assessment and intervention target the processes associated with input and output and with centralized processing of information. According to this model, a mixture of peripheral and central processes are used to sense new information, to recognize it, to hold it in memory, to make sense of it, to compare it with prior experience, to formulate new information, and to express it. Ironically, the current emphasis on information processing theory in the language acquisition literature (e.g., Bates & MacWhinney, 1979, 1987; Bates, Bretherton, & Snyder, 1988) is, in some ways a return to an earlier period when information processing theory exerted a strong influence on clinical practices. Some key elements of the theory have changed considerably, however.

Information processing theory has been around a long time. Carrow-Woolfolk (1988) noted that "the single-path serial model of cognitive processing (sensation → perception → cognition → memory) has existed since the time of Aristotle" (p. 10). Helmer Myklebust (1954, 1957) popularized this "bottom-up" model of information processing for modern clinical purposes with children, adding the concept of "inner language." He applied the model to discussions of auditory disorders and to the differential diagnosis of the causative basis of language and learning disorders. Subsequently, with Doris Johnson, Myklebust introduced the idea of learning style into the literature. The D. J. Johnson and Myklebust (1967) text *Learning Disabilities: Educational Principles and Practices* was particularly influential in urging clinical identification of primarily auditory or primarily visual strengths and/or deficits in children with language learning problems and contributed to intervention plans based on those patterns. Johnson and Myklebust emphasized assessment of specific processing skills, including "perceptual skills" such as attention and figure–ground discrimination and "language skills" such as verbal memory, sequencing, integration, and formulation. Teaching methods based on these efforts circumvented areas of deficit rather than attacking them directly. For example, if a child had trouble with auditory sequential processing skills and was having trouble with a phonics approach in the initial stages of learning to read, the common wisdom was to avoid phonics altogether and to teach the child to read via a more visually based whole-word "sight" approach.

The 1960s also brought a more complex version of the sequential processing model in the version designed by Osgood and colleagues. Osgood intended to integrate the major psycholinguistic functions of speaking and listening with aspects of the stimulus-response theory of B. F. Skinner (1957; Osgood, 1967, 1968; Osgood & Miron, 1963). This move was consistent with efforts to develop neuropsychological theory to correspond with processing deficits associated with brain damage and aphasia (Wepman, Jones, Bock, & van Pelt, 1960) (see Figure 6.3). The Osgood and Miron and Wepman models became the blueprint for the construction of the Illinois Test of Psycholinguistic Abilities (S. A. Kirk et al., 1968). This test exerted a major influence on assessment and intervention. It was often directly translated into a "psycholinguistic" approach that involved practice performing the same sort of tasks as those used in the test. Processing models were then popular for representing written language processing as well. Gough (1972) presented

a detailed sequence of processing events that must occur during "one second of reading." (Other models are reviewed by H. Singer & Ruddell, 1985.)

Limitations of older information processing theories and contributions of new ones. After this surge of activity, the pendulum swung the other way. For a while, it was unfashionable to talk about processing and perceptual skills. This was probably a function of the burst of information about normal acquisition of language rule systems that resulted from Chomsky's (1957, 1965) influence, and also disenchantment with the clinical promise of "psycholinguistic methods." Attention turned to other issues as the broader field of psycholinguistics emerged, including studies like those of Roger Brown (1973) and his colleagues, which offered new targets for language assessment and intervention (Lee, 1974). In this climate, what children knew about language began to be viewed as much more important than how they processed it, particularly because language acquisition was now viewed as being driven largely by innate sets of competencies.

It also became apparent that the term *psycholinguistics,* as used in the title of the Illinois test and the intervention activities based on it, was far too limited. Studies were beginning to shed doubt on whether the so-called "psycholinguistic approach" to language intervention was effective (Hammill & Larson, 1974). Soon thereafter, L. Bloom and Lahey (1978) also questioned the efficacy of a "specific skills" orientation, and in addition, they offered an alternative theoretical perspective with application implications.

During the same period, scientific evidence was reported that focused on a processing impairment as a central feature of specific language impairment. Several studies conducted by Paula Tallal and her colleagues pointed to an auditory sequential processing deficit, particularly for detecting and remembering sequence for stimuli produced in rapid sequence (Tallal, 1980; Tallal & Piercy, 1978; Tallal & Stark, 1976). Meanwhile, audiologists were investigating other techniques for measuring central auditory processing capabilities, both in adults and children, and were attempting to understand their clinical applications (Keith, 1977, 1981; Lasky & Katz, 1983).

The potential collision of two disparate theories made for some interesting publications (e.g., K. G. Butler, 1984a; Cromer, 1981; Duchan, 1983; Lasky & Katz, 1983; Rees, 1973, 1981; F. Smith, 1973), and

FIGURE 6.3

A model of levels of function in the central nervous system that includes interconnections among central and peripheral processes and hypothesized sites of disruption for some neuropathologies.

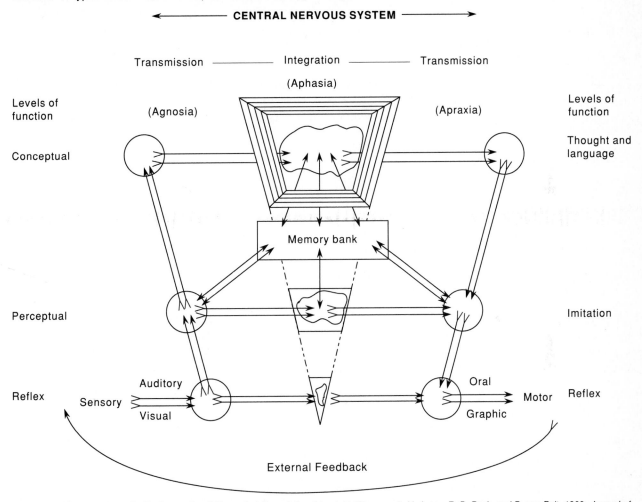

Note. From "Studies in Aphasia: Background and Theoretical Formulations" by J. M. Wepman, L. V. Jones, R. D. Bock, and D. van Pelt, 1960, *Journal of Speech and Hearing Disorders*, 25, p. 326. Copyright 1960 by American Speech-Language-Hearing Association. Reprinted by permission.

the discussions are not over yet. During this period of intense conflict, however, a new view of information processing began to emerge that had the potential to integrate elements from both camps. Duchan (1983) used the metaphor of the older view of auditory sequential processing as an elevator, commenting that "A prevailing idea then was that processing language was something like sending a linguistic package up and down a freight elevator in a multilevel, rectilinear building" (p. 83). She summarized the dis-

tinctions between older and newer models of information processing, noting that

> typical language processing models have deficiencies because they incorrectly assume that listeners begin by hearing the signal and then, in a step-like manner, continue through and passively process until an interpretation is made. Instead, perhaps even before the signal is introduced, there is an active higher order processing going on which selects the relevant signals and process their contents in parallel fashion. The listener uses both

signal and higher order knowledge in the effort to make sense of what is going on and to fulfill particular needs. (p. 89)

These revised theories of information processing included several new elements missing from earlier versions. First, higher level processes were now viewed as potentially exerting influence on lower ones, and second, multiple processes were now viewed as operating simultaneously. Both of these elements were part of the shift from a serial "bottom-up" model to a parallel "bottom-up–top-down" model of processing. Also, both were consistent with views of language as rule-based behavior and of cognition as organized schemata. Thus, successful processing became viewed as a result of two-way, combined influences, including influences of knowledge sources on attention and perception, as well as vice versa.

A third new element was that language learners were viewed as active participants in language processing tasks rather than as passive receptacles in which things happened. They had reasons for talking and listening, reading and writing, which could help them fine-tune their attention and make sense in contextual frameworks. In Rumelhart and McClelland's (1981) interactive model of written language processing, a reader comes to a text with a set of expectations about the visual input likely to be encountered. Such expectations are based on prior knowledge of the structure of letters, words, phrases, sentences, and larger pieces of discourse, as well as aspects of the nonlinguistic context. According to this interactive model, reading is a series of hypothesis-testing moves that are used to construct meanings. During this process, visual information from the page is used to strengthen some hypotheses, to weaken others, and to formulate new predictions. Comprehension is defined as the state reached when the accumulated evidence most strongly supports one hypothesis (Rumelhart & McClelland, 1981).

A fourth new element is recognition of the importance of the context in which the information is presented (both linguistic and nonlinguistic) and of the clarity of the information signal. Snyder and Downey (1983) pointed out that attention allocation depends on at least two things: (1) the information available and (2) the amount of resources (processing capability) that can be allocated to the task. A task lacking sufficient information for the processor to complete it is *data limited*, and a processor lacking sufficient skill

to carry out a task is *resource limited*. Part of interactive processing models is the recognition that such conditions are relative to each other. More competent processors rely more on top-down processing skill to fill in information that may be missing from the signal. When prior knowledge is weak, processors become increasingly dependent on signals that are very clear.

Continued limitations of newer information processing theories. Interactive models did not resolve the difference in viewpoint between linguistic, cognitivist, and information processing views about whether language is best conceptualized as a set of relatively independent *modules* filled with certain kinds of *knowledge* (which are also relatively independent of the rest of cognition), each with its own vertical structure, or as a set of *processes* that are not particularly unique to language but operate *horizontally* across a variety of areas of cognitive functioning. This difference remains to be resolved. If the first viewpoint is more accurate, language intervention programs should target grammatical rules and lexical relationships. If the second is more accurate, language intervention programs should target comprehension and expression, short-term memory, and perception.

The argument is not especially pertinent to current clinical discussions, because neither the linguistic nor the information processing view has a particularly strong set of intervention procedures. I have already noted the lack of a well-developed instructional technology for moving linguistic induction forward once information has been gathered about a child's current limited language knowledge. Similar problems are associated with knowing how to use data gathered from assessment of auditory processing for planning intervention programs. Although it is relatively easy to gather abundant data about children's ability to process various auditory signals, these data do not lend themselves readily to constructing intervention plans relevant to children. Books about auditory processing in children typically devote many more passages to assessment than to intervention (e.g., Keith, 1981; Lasky & Katz, 1983; Willeford & Burleigh, 1985).

Certainly, no one proposes a return to the time when children practiced repeating series of digits as ways to strengthen their short-term auditory memory skills, and no one has yet proposed that elements of parallel distributed information processing (PDP) theory (such as node activation) can be translated directly into intervention activities. The computer models used to test PDP theory (Bates & MacWhinney, 1987; McClelland, Rumelhart, & PDP Research Group, 1986) tend to focus only on a tiny part of the system at a time and hence do not lend themselves well to clinical design for teaching language in all its complexity.

What then are the alternatives? Approaches designed to target language processing (rather than language knowledge) tend to rely heavily on metalinguistic sound discrimination and segmentation tasks (Lindamood & Lindamood, 1969; Sawyer, Dougherty, Shelly, & Spaanenburg, 1985; Semel, 1976; Sloan, 1986). Such tasks may have some relevance to the early development of reading decoding skills, or to performing academic tasks in the elementary grades, but their relevance to primary language development and to the ability to read for meaning is less clear.

Other approaches integrate aspects of several different theoretical perspectives within top-down and bottom-up processing models (K. G. Butler, 1981, 1984a). Some even include the need to consider the influence of varied contexts (acoustic as well as linguistic) on children's abilities to process complex auditory-linguistic signals (Lasky & Cox, 1983; N. W. Nelson, 1985, 1986). The influence of top-down processing models can be seen in efforts to teach children to use higher order knowledge to compensate for assessed limitations in signal-processing capabilities and to continue to add to that organizational knowledge and motivational system. The influence of bottom-up models can be seen in efforts to make signals clear enough, loud enough, slow enough, and simple enough that children will have a chance of making sense of them. Aspects of such interventions may even extend to measuring the acoustic characteristics of key learning environments, such as classrooms of hearing impaired and language-learning impaired children, and providing sound treatment to make them more conducive to learning (P. J. Hart, 1983; Ross, 1978).

Cognitivist Theory Influences

Contributions of cognitivist theories. Influences of cognitivist theories on assessment and intervention practices are related to the idea that sequence and rate of language development are influenced by sequence and rate of cognitive development. This leads to a heavy dependence on developmental scales in deciding what knowledge and skills to target as part of intervention. Earlier acquired behaviors may also be seen as prerequisites for later ones, and cognitive advances may be seen as prerequisites for linguistic ones.

For example, as discussed in Chapter 2, research has provided some evidence that the appearance of first words is associated with children's awareness that other people may serve as agents. The use of words like *allgone* (indicating disappearance) is also highly correlated with children's ability to demonstrate object permanence (Bates, 1976; Bates, Benigni, Bretherton, Camaioni, & Volterra, 1979; Bates & Snyder, 1985; Corrigan, 1978). When intervention programs use this information, they involve efforts aimed not only at communicative development but at general cognitive development as well. This might result in an emphasis on peekaboo games, using both people and objects, and on cause and effect activities designed to demonstrate ways in which people can affect their environment.

Assessment and intervention based exclusively on cognitivist principles are not prevalent. This may be partially because cognitive theory comprises several versions (see Chapter 3 for a review). Cognitivist principles also tend to be blended in with other approaches, particularly those based on information processing theories. Some aspects of cognitivist theories, however, have specific implications for designing language intervention.

One significant influence is the view that children actively participate in their own development. This

| Personal Reflection 6.3 | "We remember and process what we understand and find pertinent, not what our memories can span."

Judy Duchan, speech–language pathologist, and *Jack Katz*, audiologist, writing in a chapter called, "Language and Auditory Processing: Top Down Plus Bottom Up" (1983, p. 36). |

view is common to both linguistic and cognitive theories. Whereas behaviorist theories tend to present children as passive participants whose behavior is modified by external conditions, cognitivist theories present them as active learners whose cognitive processes shift as they pass through a series of qualitatively different developmental stages, each of which depends on advances of the prior one. The most frequently applied view of developmental stages comes from the work of Piaget (e.g., 1926, 1970; see Chapter 3).

The general goal of programs influenced by cognitivist theory is to assist children to advance through Piaget's stages and to develop the language and communicative behaviors that accompany them. In a developmental approach, assessment aims to identify a child's current level of functioning in multiple cognitive domains so that intervention can start at the child's current level of functioning. Because cognitive development is viewed as a tightly linked process, even though skills in some domains may lag somewhat behind those of others, developmental domains are viewed as being basically interrelated. Based on the outcome of assessment and looking at the next step on developmental scales, intervention is then implemented by arranging environmental experiences to encourage children to expand their schemas about how the world works through their experiences with it. Items on developmental scales may even be translated directly into intervention objectives.

Another contribution of cognitivist theory is to look at behavioral outcomes as evidence of inner activity. Unlike behaviorist theory, cognitivist theory acknowledges a rich and active set of inner processes. This leads to a different view of developmental "errors" when committed by children. Cognitivist influence leads clinicians to analyze errors as rich evidence about the child's evolving theories and schemas about language and other phenomena. Such evidence can then be used to fine-tune intervention efforts.

Cognitivist theory, in its emphasis on self-directed learning, also contributes to the development of intervention approaches designed to teach older children and adolescents to adopt metacognitive strategies. In its simplest definition, *metacognition* is thinking about thinking. Similar to metalinguistic behavior, metacognitive behavior involves a conscious awareness of processes that have primary functions that are ordinarily transparent. Strategies training is particularly important for students with language-learning disabilities in upper elementary and secondary grades be-

cause they seem to have difficulty acquiring such strategies on their own. Examples of strategy-training approaches are discussed more thoroughly in Chapter 9. Briefly, they involve teaching students to adopt conscious strategies of problem solving, to teach them to direct their own learning (Buttrill et al., 1989; Deshler, Alley, & Carlson, 1980; Lloyd, 1980; Schumaker, Deshler, Alley, & Warner, 1983; Torgesen, 1982).

Linguistic and cognitivist approaches have in common their view of children as active learners, who form, test, and revise their hypotheses about the world as they develop. However, the approaches also have some distinctions. A primary distinction relates to issues of *modularity* (Fodor, 1983). Analysis methods guided by linguistic or neuropsychological theory tend to focus on the relative separability of language and the rest of cognition and also on the relative separability among the various rule systems of language (e.g., phonological, grammatical, and lexical). A cognitivist viewpoint tends to be more interactionist, based on the premise that "Language is an interactive system that depends crucially on processes and representations from a number of cognitive domains" (Bates, Bretherton, & Snyder, 1988, p. 11). In the interactionist view, processes such as perception, storage, recognition, and retrieval of information act as a common stock of mechanisms that can be used across cognitive domains, including language. In this way, cognitivist and information processing theories are linked.

Limitations of cognitivist theories.   Some of the problems associated with a strictly developmental approach have been discussed in preceding chapters. Although perspectives from normal development across cognitive domains do provide an essential part of the framework for language assessment and intervention, they also have some limitations. Primary among these is the tendency for a strictly developmental approach to result in children being restricted to environments and activities designed for developmental age peers rather than chronological age peers. The "readiness" issue, particularly when extended across domains, can also result in limited access to disparate activities (e.g., the child with physical impairments, mentioned in Chapter 1, who was not taught to read because he could not yet zip his pants).

Cognitivist theory is aimed primarily at explaining normal development when it unfolds spontaneously.

It does not offer a strong technology for encouraging development when development is delayed. From a strict Piagetian (Piaget, 1964) viewpoint, developmental advances occur only when a state of disequilibrium occurs within children. However, as Case (1985) pointed out, others have questioned this limited view and have shown that it is possible to design teaching strategies that can help children advance from one stage to the next. Pascual-Leone's (1984) solution was to combine Piagetian theory with aspects of behaviorism and information processing theories to explain how both intrinsic and extrinsic factors could help children activate new schemas through interaction of the four factors: (1) cues from the internalized scheme itself, (2) field effects that might make particular features of stimuli stand out for attention, (3) logical cues regarding structural relationships, and (4) mental power or attention. Case's (1985) addition of executive control structures is also consistent with strategy-training approaches based on elements of cognitivist theory.

Rice (1983) commented that few training studies based on cognitivist theory have been reported. The existing studies fail to support the idea that prior cognitive understandings are a prerequisite for training (Rice, 1980) or that training certain cognitive structures will necessarily facilitate communicative behaviors (Steckol & Leonard, 1981). Rice (1983) summarized that "the cognition hypotheses have not fulfilled their early promise, but they have spawned a range of explanations that contribute helpful perspectives" (p. 355). For example, she identified an ongoing clinical danger as stemming from the lack of recognition of what she called the *mapping problem*. Although children may not enter the therapeutic interaction with a fully developed nonlinguistic concept of things such as cup-like objects, clinicians may assume that children do and that all that is needed is teaching the child to associate the label *cup* with that notion.

Some recent attempts have been made to blend a rich interpretation of cognitive theory with young children at risk for having language disorders, with aspects of social interaction theory. One such approach is called *Transdisciplinary Play-Based Assessment* (TPBA; Linder, 1990). Linder described TPBA as "both an assessment and intervention process" (p. 4). It provides a structure to observe across cognitive, social-emotional, communication and language and sensorimotor development domains during play interactions. The procedure differs from more formal developmental assessments in its use of child-initiated actions and general assessment questions (rather than specific assessment tasks implemented as prescribed). It also involves the observation of play in different contexts and with different partners.

Social Interaction Theory Influences

Contributions of social interaction theories. Assessment and intervention approaches based on each of the preceding theories are missing a system for blending the content and procedures into a unified intervention approach. Biological maturation theories emphasize anatomical structure without offering much regarding target content or procedures. Linguistic theories focus on content and say little about procedures. Behaviorist theories offer a well-developed set of procedures but with relatively undefined content. Information processing theories focus on a content that is not really content and offer procedures that can support other intervention efforts but do not stand well on their own. Cognitivist theories cross wide expanses of content and offer little except developmental expectations as procedural guidelines.

Two of the major contributions of social-interaction theory are its focus on *function*, suggesting that children learn to talk and to practice their communication skills when they have a reason to do so, and *context*, suggesting that form–content language structures are determined not only by communicative function but by contextual factors. Functional elements offer an area of content to target in the intervention process, and contextual elements offer a philosophy on which assessment and intervention procedures can be based.

Recognizing the limitations of earlier form-based linguistic approaches, Lucas (1980) recommended looking at children with language disorders as potentially having a general disruption in one of four areas, which she defined based on speech-act theory. The potential areas of difficulty were in:

> (1) developing the rules; (2) establishing a desire or motivational cause for having an intent to linguistically express; (3) having a need to communicate to a hearer; and/or (4) being capable of participating in the active process. (p. 45)

Any difficulty in language that can be observed as a communication deficiency can be considered to be a legitimate target within the social interaction paradigm. An important distinction between programs based on this and other theoretical perspectives, however, is that even when linguistic rules or cognitive behaviors are targeted, they are not taken out of context, either for assessment or intervention.

Context is considered to be a critical feature of programs based on behaviorist theory as well, but contexts may be rigged in behaviorist approaches to be artificial. Although exceptions do exist, in the form of such behaviorist-originated approaches as "milieu" (B. Hart & Rogers-Warren, 1978) or "incidental" teaching (B. Hart & Risley, 1968; S. F. Warren & Kaiser, 1986), such approaches are not necessarily required by behaviorist theory, they only happen to be allowed by it. On the other hand, social interaction approaches to language assessment and intervention by definition require the use of naturalistic contexts and interaction strategies.

Within the broad realm of programs based on social interaction theory, variation can be found along the naturalness continuum. The common elements of such programs are intervention in everyday contexts and the emphasis on the importance of communicating with real partners in sincere communicative interactions that serve a real purpose. This suggests that professionals must assume a different kind of role in the process. Muma (1978) described the role of clinicians in traditional direct-teaching programs as being of the "jug and mug" variety. The clinician's role is to pour language into the waiting child. In programs conceptualized within a social interaction framework, however, Muma (1983) identified three quite different basic intervention components: (1) peer modeling, (2) parallel talk, and (3) parent participation.

When organizing intervention approaches based on social interaction theory, the roles of language specialists vary from those played in more traditional approaches. They must recruit active communicative partners from among other people important to the child (e.g., parents, teachers, and peers) and must consult with them as they learn to conduct maximally effective interactions, eliciting high-quality communication from the child. In addition, clinicians may participate as communicative partners.

Craig (1983) contrasted the role of clinicians in behaviorist and mentalist (here called linguistic-induction) therapy models. She noted that, "In contrast to the 'teacher' and 'facilitator' roles of the other major paradigms, within pragmatic approaches the clinician should serve as a 'trouble shooter' for the child—locating and eliminating the source of trouble in any

communication flow and thereby maximizing the child's communicative potential" (p. 114).

This role requires that clinicians function in a *child-centered* mode, with the child initiating. Norris and Hoffman (1990a) pointed out that this mode is essentially related to a whole-language view in which naturalistic strategies are used that involve "a more socially oriented, child-initiated and child-controlled interaction style of treatment. . . . The child-initiated style of interaction assumes that language is indivisible from a context of shared meaning and social use, and that children discover the properties of language through immersion in the communicative process" (p. 28). Arwood (1983) labeled such an approach "pragmaticism."

These models may seem aimed exclusively at the early or middle stages of language intervention (infancy through preschool years), but some have attempted to interpret contextually based language intervention for the school-age years. For example, Norris (1988, 1989) showed how small reading groups within classrooms could be used as the context for language intervention with children in early elementary grades. In the approach she dubbed *communicative reading strategies* (CRS), Norris described how language intervention specialists can use the reading group context in a three-step process to (1) organize some linguistic unit for the child (e.g., a sentence within the text, a phrase within a complete sentence, or a concept within a word, phrase, or paragraph); (2) give the child an opportunity to use language to communicate the information by reading the relevant text to the group; and (3) provide feedback to the child (e.g., in the form of an acknowledgment, request for clarification, or extension of the idea) based on the information communicated to the group.

For school-age students of all ages, N. W. Nelson (1989b) described how curriculum-based language assessment and intervention could be grounded in the various aspects of the curriculum that children are supposed to master. The critical dimension of this and other approaches is that relevant content and contexts from the child's world guide assessment and intervention. In addition, the professional assumes the role of *participant* to guide the student, rather than functioning in the usual teacher role, as the *student* attempts to master the language of the curriculum. This is essentially the "troubleshooter" role described by Craig (1983), except that it is aimed at older children.

Elements of programs based on social interaction theory have existed at least since clinicians began trying to integrate language function into intervention. In discussing approaches based on the other theoretical perspectives in this section of the chapter, I have pointed out the influence of social interaction theory in modifying many of them, such as the linguistic-based content–form–use model developed by L. Bloom and Lahey (1978; Lahey, 1988), Linder's cognitive-based TBPA model (1990), and the behaviorist-based incidental teaching model (e.g., B. Hart & Risley, 1968; S. F. Warren & Kaiser, 1986). The current focus on the importance of social interactions in the development of child language competencies has the potential of becoming dogma. It is time for caution.

Limitations of social interaction theories. When specialists began to interpret pragmatic issues for clinical application, they expressed a concern that clinicians might view pragmatics simply as a fifth linguistic rule system (added to phonology, morphology, syntax, and semantics), to be inserted into the general linguistic rule-induction framework (Craig, 1983; Gallagher & Prutting, 1983). To simply add pragmatics as a new set of intervention goals, perhaps coupled with modification in carryover strategies, would not do the theory justice. As Craig emphasized, the broader perspective of pragmatics, which is tied closely to the concept that "language is acquired and used in a social context" (Bates, 1976, p. 412), does more than influence the choice of intervention *targets*. It leads to a paradigm shift that dramatically influences choices about language intervention procedures.

Most of the more recent practical interpretations of this theory involve rich interpretations of its broad implications. Even in such cases, however, potential limitations remain. Because approaches based on social interaction theory tend to place a priority on targets involving language use and pragmatics, potential targets involving language content–form interactions may receive less attention than they need. Not all children have exactly the same kind of language disorder, and not all children need exactly the same kind of intervention. Fey (1986) noted that an uncritical implementation of a "natural is better" assumption leads some clinicians to

select activities that do not allow the implementation of effective procedures. Consequently, intervention sometimes provides little more than what the child would ordinarily get from the natural environment. History has demonstrated the extreme difficulty which many of these children have in extracting conventional patterns of communication from such natural contexts. For example, children who are reasonably good communicators but who have marked difficulty with language form often seem oblivious to many of the structural details of language. Since their own efforts to communicate are reasonably effective, the need to attend and master the use of language form is often not readily apparent. In my experience, a clinician can often facilitate growth in the child's vocabulary and perhaps pragmatic and cognitive skills by providing highly natural and enriching experiences. The rate of development of syntax and morphology, however, often continues to lag. (p. 65)

Social interaction theory provides a strong rationale that combines aspects of several other perspectives with the view that children are whole people whose development is influenced by internal as well as external variables. Because social interaction theory provides a strong philosophical basis for selecting procedures (although with a relatively unstructured environmental technology), it translates fairly well into intervention models. It is now popular for this reason among others. Like any other model, however, it should not be adopted uncritically for all children without considering their needs as individuals (Cromer, 1981).

Integrating Influences From Six Theoretical Perspectives

How can elements of each of these six theoretical perspectives be used to make choices that are best for individual children? Is the solution to adopt one theory and to base all assessment and intervention decisions on it, or is there a better way?

Consider the premise further that different children have different needs and that some theoretical perspectives are better suited to meeting some needs than others. For those who accept such a premise, the problem of decision making shifts from one of selecting the best theory to serve all children's needs to selecting the best theory (or theories) to serve a particular child's needs.

Some theories may also be better suited to addressing needs associated with particular aspects of the language intervention process than others. The stimulus–response–reinforcement elements of a behaviorist paradigm are a part of any human interaction, whether controlled by design or not. Yet, the application of this technology might be so much richer if guided by aspects of theories that view children as active information seekers and that view the language system as complex. Information processing theory might also contribute ideas about how to build the attention needed for further learning. Rather than viewing attention as a set of specific behaviors to be learned, one might view it from the cognitivist perspective, as a set of "questions being asked by the brain" (F. Smith, 1973, p. 28). Adopting this viewpoint can also introduce metacognitive elements that can guide the intervention process toward teaching the child to use new self-questioning strategies (this is the "question transplant" idea introduced in Chapter 1). This approach might blend disparate views that define learning as the strengthening of a stimulus–response relationship (behaviorism), as "remembering what you're interested in"(social interaction; Wurman, 1989, p. 137), and as "relative to something you understand" (cognitivism; Wurman, 1989, p. 167).

As a metatheory, system theory offers a framework for problem solving that allows integration of multiple theoretical perspectives. When children are viewed as integral members of larger systems and as comprising a network of interactive subsystems, decision makers have a framework for juggling sets of varied concerns and activities to meet varied purposes. Different theoretical explanations can be viewed not as competitive alternatives but as mutual contributors to the decision-making process. Specialists can then design intervention to assess a particular situation using the tools most suitable for identifying its critical features and can use strategies matched to particular needs. Careful thought and collaborative goal setting are required.

The best way to characterize a practice that blends the most desirable aspects of multiple theories is *eclectic*:

> **eclectic**, ek·lek'tik, *a.* [Gr. *eklektikos—ek*, and *lego*, to choose.] Proceeding by the method of selection; choosing what seems best from others; not original nor following any one model or leader, but choosing at will from the doctrines, works, etc., of others. (Thatcher, 1980, p. 274)

As this dictionary definition indicates, one should not confuse eclectic with disorganized or random practices. An eclectic approach involves careful, deliberate selection from among several choices. Selecting the best involves neither lack of theory nor devotion to any one theory. Rather, it involves making intentional choices that vary as purposes vary, and is an important part of the matching process discussed in the following sections.

ASSESSMENT AND INTERVENTION AS INTEGRATED PROCESSES

Using Team Contributions Effectively

When children are seen as members of whole systems, they cannot be treated in isolation. When whole systems are the focus, assessment and intervention cannot be viewed as isolated processes.

Contributions of members from several professional disciplines may be needed, depending on the particular child, but most certainly, contributions are needed from parents and the children. When children are of school-age, or even preschool-age, members of the educational community are essential members of planning and intervention teams, and when children near the end of schooling, vocational planners may be appropriate team members.

How should teams be organized, and how should they function? Calling a group of people together does not ensure that it will function as a team. Understanding the various ways that teams can function will contribute to the development of a more effective team.

Recognizing different models. Not all team processes work in the same way. L. McCormick (1990c) defined a team as "a group of persons who have a shared goal and required actions to perform in order to reach that goal" (p. 262). Beyond that basic similarity, at least three different team approaches may be taken.

Multidisciplinary. A multidisciplinary team is merely a team composed of representatives of different disciplines. The term implies nothing more about mode of organization or functioning. Related to the lack of intentional interaction, V. Hart (1977) identified several problems that might stem from a multidisciplinary approach in which a group of individuals works independently. Primary among these are the possibilities for conflicting recommendations, neglect of important information, and presentation of separate implications not reconstructed into a whole picture. The multidisciplinary mode also is more likely to result either in the kind of "competitive goal setting" or "independent goal setting" (D. W. Johnson & Johnson, 1975) discussed in Chapter 1.

Interdisciplinary. An interdisciplinary team is distinguished from a multidisciplinary team by the formal communication channels between disciplines and a case manager to coordinate services (McCormick & Goldman, 1979). Interdisciplinary models also often involve consultative relationships between professional "experts" and the individuals who spend the most time with target children. Because consultation of this sort tends to flow only in one direction (e.g., from the consultant to the teacher), the team may have no mechanism for the teacher to play an equal role in decision making and for providing the input necessary for establishing the validity and reliability of assessment and intervention outcomes (L. McCormick, 1990c).

Transdisciplinary. A transdisciplinary team encourages active sharing of information and skills across disciplines in multiple directions. The term *transdisciplinary* was introduced by Hutchinson (1974) to describe the collaborative nature of the relationship in a project for atypical infants and their families. The model was described further by Lyon and Lyon (1980) as having three key features: (1) *joint functioning*, team members perform service-delivery functions together whenever possible; (2) *continuous staff development*, members train and receive training from each other in reciprocal interactions; and (3) *role release*, team members not only share information with each other, but assist each other to perform functions usually reserved to their own disciplines. L. McCormick (1990c) summarized the relationship as follows:

> Team members are accountable for seeing that the best practices of their respective disciplines are implemented, monitoring program implementation, training others if necessary, and revising programs when evaluation data indicate that procedures are not working as well as intended. (p. 269)

The concept of role release was developed further by Woodruff and McGonigel (1988) to include the following dimensions: (1) *role extension*, members learn from each other; (2) *role enrichment*, members teach each other; (3) *role expansion*, members assume

aspects of each others' professional roles, and (4) *role support*, members provide the necessary backup support for each other as they assume the roles of other disciplines.

Focusing on cooperative goal setting. A truly transdisciplinary team cannot function unless members participate in cooperative goal setting. A program implemented as a single integrated service is less fragmented and potentially more effective than a team comprising a set of separate appointments with separate goals.

The transdisciplinary team process is not without its critics. Some have questioned whether teams can make better decisions than individuals and whether they are cost-effective (Yoshida, 1983; J. R. Ysseldyke & Algozzine, 1982). Efforts to conduct research on team process are also complicated by the fact that different labels do not always represent clear distinctions among kinds of functional relationships (Golin & Ducanis, 1985). Unidisciplinary approaches sometimes may be desirable, particularly at some points of development and when the child seems to have a relatively isolated impairment. Cooperative goal setting by individual professionals with important family members remains desirable and is critical if programs are to be relevant to children's individualized needs.

Using Assessment to Diagnose Disorder

Defining disorder. An operational definition of language disorder is required for diagnosis. An operational definition can be applied to potential exemplars to rule them in or out of a particular category.

In Chapter 4, I argued the need for a broad view of language disorders, including conditions beyond those known as "specific language impairment." Bashir's (1989) definition is repeated here:

> *Language disorders* is a term that represents a heterogeneous group of either developmental or acquired disabilities principally characterized by deficits in comprehension, production, and/or use of language. Language disorders are chronic and may persist across the lifetime of the individual. The symptoms, manifestations, effects, and severity of the problems change over time. The changes occur as a consequence of context, content, and learning tasks. (p. 181)

Although this definition has many strengths (discussed in Chapter 4), it is not specific enough to be used for diagnosing a child as having a language disorder without further information. It begs the question "What are deficits in comprehension, production, and/or use of language?"

Another definition, proposed by the American Speech-Language-Hearing Association (ASHA) Committee on Language, Speech, and Hearing Services in Schools (1982), has similar problems being operationalized without further detail:

> A language disorder is the impairment or deviant development of comprehension and/or use of a spoken, written, and/or other symbol system. The disorder may involve (1) the form of language (phonologic, morphologic, and syntactic systems, (2) the content of language (semantic system), and/or (3) the function of language in communication (pragmatic system) in any combination. (p. 949)

This definition uses the form, content, and use ("function") categories suggested by L. Bloom and Lahey (1978), which are cross-referenced with the five systems, phonology, morphology, syntax, semantics, and pragmatics. It also mentions "comprehension and/or use" of these systems, and specifically refers to "spoken, written, and/or other symbol systems." The element of heterogeneity that Bashir (1989) emphasized is only hinted at in the phrase, "in any combination."

A third definition, suggested by Lahey (1988), clarifies the expectation that the disorder occurs while learning one's native language and that it involves discrepancy from developmental expectations based on chronological age:

> Thus we can use the term *language disorder* to refer to *any disruption in the learning or use of one's native language as evidenced by language behaviors that are different from* (but not superior to) *those expected given a child's chronological age.* (p. 21)

Many questions remain after all of these attempts at definition. The primary question concerns the meaning of phrases such as "any disruption in the learning or use" (Lahey, 1988, p.21), "impairment or deviant development of comprehension and/or use" (American Speech-Language-Hearing Association Committee 1982, p. 949), and "deficits in comprehension, production, and/or use of language" (Bashir, 1989, p. 181). Exact meanings may be ignored when language disorders are defined in the abstract, but they must be addressed in some way when answering the question "Does this specific child have a language disorder?"

When establishing operational criteria for determining language disorder, questions of deviance, disruption, or deficit are often defined by comparing observed abilities of one child against expected abilities for some comparison group of children. The comparison group may vary. Most commonly, a child's language development (usually measured with formal testing procedures and perhaps the mean length of utterance (MLU) of a spontaneous language sample) is compared with that of a group of children (1) at the same chronological age (CA) or (2) at the same mental age (MA). Although the IDEA requires nonbiased assessment, with the expectation that the comparison group of children will come from the same linguistic and cultural conditions as the child (PL 101–476, 1990), in practice this requirement is often ignored (Taylor & Payne, 1983).

Tallal (1988) expressed the rationale for using MA referencing as well as CA referencing in diagnosing specific language impairment this way:

> It is essential that in addition to demonstrating that language abilities of a child are significantly below what would be expected based on the child's chronological age, it is important to establish that they are also significantly discrepant from what would be predicted based on the child's mental abilities. (p. 211)

Using discrepancy criteria to define disorder. A problem arises in practice because children's language abilities usually are not compared directly with those of local peers of either the same CA or MA. Rather, indirect comparisons are made psychometrically with a remote normative group of "peers" (a different group of remote peers is used for each test) by administering standardized tests and applying a set of discrepancy criteria. Children are given one or more language tests to determine their language age (LA), and one or more intelligence tests (usually one) to determine their MA. Then, the scores earned on those different measures are compared to see if they are discrepant enough to meet a standard established by a qualifying agency (as discussed later). Less commonly, comparison measures might be made against achievement test scores, or other grade-level measures.

Several problems arise from this approach. First, psychometric problems are associated with attempting to directly compare scores earned in relationship to two different normative samples. Even standard scores are not directly comparable (Seashore, 1955). This problem is compounded by the fact that, in multicultural pluralistic societies, the children included in normative samples may be from cultural and linguistic communities different from the child being tested. Few tests have been standardized on children from diverse sociolinguistic groups, and simply averaging the scores of a small proportion of minority group children into the norms of a test designed to measure majority culture and linguistic knowledge does not remove this element of bias.

One reason for the lack of culturally fair tests may be the costly nature (in terms of both time and money) of test standardization. Another is that it would be difficult to establish national norms appropriate for all of the diverse geographic, ethnic, and socioeconomic demographic combinations in the United States, let alone other parts of the world.

An alternative is to establish local community norms. This is one of several possible solutions mentioned by Vaughn-Cooke to reduce bias in testing (1983). In practice, local norms are rarely established. Of course, there is good reason for this. A lot of time and a thorough knowledge of psychometric procedures are required to gather adequate samples of one child's language behavior to obtain an accurate picture of functioning level. Practitioners cannot perform a community-based normative study every time they need a set of scores for comparative purposes. (However, Sabers & Hutchinson, 1990, provide a software package to gather local norms on frequently used tests.)

Even if appropriate norms are available, scores earned on cognitive functioning tests cannot be assumed to be independent of scores earned on language functioning tests. The confounding of LA and MA scores is another source of possible bias in assessment designed to determine the presence of a language disorder. The problem is threefold. First, some cognitive assessment tools use tasks very similar to those used in language assessment. Thus, two ostensibly different scores compared for discrepancy may reflect the same impairment (this is particularly a problem with full-scale IQ scores). Second, other cognitive assessment tools, although designed specifically to measure nonverbal cognitive skills, may tap only a limited aspect of nonverbal cognition, particularly at certain ages. For example, Johnston (1982a) found that the test items for children under age 8 from the Leiter International Performance Scale (Leiter, 1959) represented primarily their ability to recognize the physical characteristics of visual stimuli and may not have adequately tested other aspects of

nonverbal cognition. Similarly, Kamhi, Minor, and Mauer (1990) used an item analysis of the 50 items on the Test of Nonverbal Intelligence (TONI; L. Brown, Sherbenou, & Johnsen, 1985) and showed that 15 items (30%) required perceptual rather than conceptual processing. Furthermore, almost all of the perceptual items occurred early in the test, making it possible for most children up to the age of 11 to obtain normal range IQs without passing any of the conceptual items. Third, even when cognitive assessment tools use nonverbal stimuli and responses and even when they require more complex forms of cognitive processing, still there is no way to be sure that a child with a language disorder may not be disadvantaged. The unavailability of verbal mediation strategy may make it more difficult for children with language disorders to encode key features of nonverbal stimuli. Yet, their scores are compared with the normative sample scores that may have been enhanced by the normal ability to use verbal strategies to identify, retain, and manipulate nonverbal symbols. To appreciate this possibility, consider the matrix problem that appears in Figure 6.4. Notice how this and similar items from the TONI might lend themselves to linguistic encoding of forms and relationships that might facilitate selection of correct choices.

Not all discrepancy criteria involve LA–MA comparisons. Another approach to identifying language disorder is to use a set of discrepancy criteria specifying intralinguistic comparisons (Fey, 1986). Several different measures of different aspects of language are compared. Thus, children's scores on one test that measures one aspect of language might be compared against scores from another test that measures another aspect of language. The rationale behind this approach is that it can reveal scattered patterns of developmental accomplishments, which have been reported for children with specific language disability (e.g., the "patterns of frequency of usage" differences, Leonard, 1980, discussed in Chapter 4). By looking for patterns within children that indicate the co-occurrence of some more developmentally advanced behaviors along with some earlier developing behaviors that have apparently failed to evolve, professionals may find an important piece of the puzzle. It is a piece that tends to be missing when overall scores are compared without looking at what they might represent.

In fact, identification of this type of scattered pattern represents an example of an inclusionary criterion for determining who belongs in the group of

FIGURE 6.4
Matrix problem from the Test of Nonverbal Intelligence.

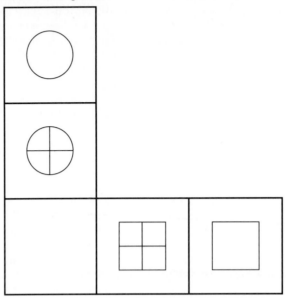

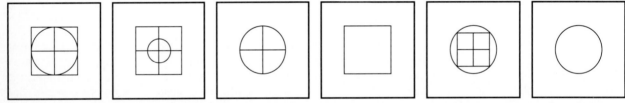

Note. From *Test of Nonverbal Intelligence* (p. A24) by L. Brown, R. J. Sherbenou, and S. K. Johnsen, 1985, Austin, TX: Pro-Ed. Copyright 1985 by Pro-Ed. Reprinted by permission.

children diagnosed as having a language disorder. Alan Kamhi (1990) suggested that perhaps more time should be spent looking for inclusionary criteria and less for exclusionary criteria and that perhaps criteria used for defining language disorder should shift with the child's age.

Using exclusionary criteria to define disorder.
Exclusionary criteria are established to determine whether the child's language-based symptoms are related to a specific language impairment or perhaps to some other disorder that includes language difficul-

ties as only one part of a more complex picture. In some ways, this is a question about cause. To identify a child as having a language disorder, it is necessary to rule out that the child has some other kind of disorder. Or is it?

Maybe what is needed is an awareness that, in the heterogeneous category of children with language disorders, some have language disorders relatively isolated from other impairments, and others have language disorders thoroughly intertwined with other kinds of impairments. Both might need special education services related to their language disorders (a finding pertinent to the discussion of the next section). But only one group might meet the definition of language disorder if it is based on exclusionary criteria for determining specific language impairment.

Here, again, the question of purpose comes into play. If the purpose of diagnosing language disorder is to select subjects for a research project designed to study aspects of specific language impairment, then Tallal's (1988) comments are pertinent. In a presentation at the National Conference on Learning Disabilities, Tallal argued:

> The number one priority for research [is] the development of standardized inclusionary and exclusionary criteria and the encouragement of their uniform usage for subsequent federally funded or privately funded research in this area. (p. 206)

Stark and Tallal (1981) attempted to establish standardized exclusion criteria to define specific language impairment operationally for research and to differentiate specific disorders from possible mixed disorders. They produced the following:

1. *Hearing level*: failure to pass 250- to 6,000-Hz screening or to perform picture-pointing task at 25-dB hearing level.
2. *Emotional and behavioral status*: history of severe behavior or adjustment problems.
3. *Intellectual status*: performance scale IQ less than 85.
4. *Neurological status*: evidence of neurological deficit or lesion.
5. *Speech motor skills*: evidence of peripheral neuromuscular or speech articulation impairment.
6. *Reading level*: reading age-level score more than 6 months lower than composite LA score.

When considering this list, it is important to keep in mind its purpose. It was designed to determine whether children might qualify as subjects for a research project, not whether they might qualify for receiving clinical services based on language needs, which are two very different purposes. In the Stark and Tallal (1981) study, only one third of the 132 children originally identified by clinicians as meeting the loosely defined referral criteria for the study met the stricter operationally defined criteria for diagnosing specific language deficits.

Commenting on this 2:1 mismatch between clinicians' judgments and criteria-based determination of specific language disorders, Aram, Morris, and Hall (submitted) noted that something must be wrong with the current processes used to identify language-disordered children, either with clinicians' assessments, the use of assessment criteria, or both. I think the mismatch is not nearly so disturbing when one considers that identifying a narrow group of children as research subjects vastly differs from identifying a broader group of children to provide clinical services. "Specific language impairment" is not an established fact but a scientific hypothesis (Aram, et al., submitted; Leonard, 1987).

To return to the philosophical framework introduced in Chapter 1, no definition of language disorder is adequate from a clinical standpoint if it fails to ask more than whether psychometrically determined inclusionary and exclusionary criteria can be met. Although a psychometric approach might be instrumental in identifying certain kinds of impairment, it has little to say about whether a child has a disability that becomes evident when the child attempts to perform essential communicative or language-based tasks. To operationalize this part of a definition of language disorder, ethnographic as well as psychometric tools must be employed (Kovarsky & Crago, 1991).

As defined in this book, a psychometric approach involves sampling a child's behavior in multiple relevant contexts and basing an assessment of language disability on judgments of two types: (1) *judgments of degree*, children show more frequent inability to meet communicative demands than their peers, and (2) *judgments of kind*, children have language-based difficulty qualitatively different from that of their peers in similar contexts. In addition to asking psychometrically based questions about impairment and contextually based questions about disability, specialists should ask socially based questions about opportunity to participate (Beukelman & Mirenda, 1988) and about risk for social disvalue (Fey, 1986; Tomblin, 1983, 1989).

Using Assessment to Determine Eligibility for Service

The importance of eligibility criteria. A second purpose of assessment is to determine eligibility for receiving special intervention services. As noted, this purpose might seem indistinguishable from determining whether the child has a language disorder, but the two actually are separate.

Consider the possibility that a child's language skills might be delayed relative to CA but commensurate with abilities across other delayed developmental areas. The language disorder then is often considered to be a part of more general cognitive limitations. This child may or may not be identified as having a language disorder, depending on how the local community defines language disorder, but the child may still be eligible for language intervention services even if mental retardation is identified as the "primary" disorder. Conversely, it is also possible that a child may be diagnosed as having a language disorder according to some set of accepted professional criteria but still may not qualify for services based on a set of agency-specific eligibility criteria.

Rueda (1989) emphasized the importance of separating questions of eligibility from questions of need, particularly for students from language-minority groups who have "mildly handicapping conditions" such as communication disorders, learning disabilities, or mild mental retardation. Rueda's concern was that such individuals might either be over- or under-identified as handicapped when decisions were made only on the basis of psychometric measures of impairment:

> Even though underclassification has been a much less visible issue than misclassification, there is a danger of exclusion from needed services because low-achieving students cannot meet specific criteria even though they need additional academic assistance. (p. 124)

Rueda (1989) continued that such problems are particularly likely to occur when ability–achievement discrepancy criteria are used as primary eligibility standards. For example, when English-only IQ tests are used to measure cognitive "ability," the artifact of mismatch of student background with language and cultural test demands may result in students with limited English proficiency and language disorders being unable to demonstrate sufficient discrepancy to qualify for clearly needed services. As noted in the previous section, the confounding of language and cognitive abilities on IQ tests can have a similar effect on children from mainstream linguistic and cultural groups who are "low achieving" or "dull-normal," and who tend to fall through the cracks for receiving the special attention because "ability" and "achievement" measures both tap the same language-related weaknesses.

Assessment to determine eligibility usually requires reference to official policy guidelines, and as noted in Chapter 5, state education agencies are most often the source of such criteria (although criteria may be established at intermediate and local levels as well). In addition to a set of standards to identify the child's language impairment, criteria for determining intervention eligibility may include a variety of required procedures as well as assessment of specific areas of language knowledge and use. Required standards might include those based on discrepancy and exclusion criteria. Required procedures might include spontaneous language sampling and classroom observations. Specified areas of language knowledge and use might include requirements for demonstrated impairment in receptive and/or expressive language (based on an information processing theoretical model), or in one or more of the areas of language content, form, and use (or phonology, morphology, syntax, semantics, and pragmatics) (based on linguistic and social interaction models).

Using psychometrically sound practice to guide decisions. Even the use of CA (Lahey, 1988) as the standard for determining discrepancy between expected and observed abilities is not without controversy. The basic objection to such a criterion is that it might result in classification of children with general developmental delays as having language disorders. Beyond that concern, CA-based eligibility criteria still require an answer to the question "How different must a child's language be from that of same-age peers before it is considered a disorder?"

Answering this question requires both sound knowledge of psychometric principles and professional common sense. The psychometric relationships among several kinds of test scores are illustrated in Figure 6.5. The exact middle of a normal distribution for a particular age group can be expressed as a standard score of 100, a percentile score of 50, or a z-score of 0 (based on standard deviations from the mean). How far should a child be allowed to deviate from that exact middle score for her age to be considered to be outside of "normal expectations?"

Interpreting different kinds of scores. Raw scores, as numbers of correct or incorrect responses, by themselves mean nothing. Scores must be transformed before they can be used to compare children against a normative standard. This is usually done by using tables provided in test manuals to transform the child's raw score into (1) a standard score, (2) a percentile score, or (3) an equivalent score.

Standard scores and percentile scores function in similar ways. **Standard scores** may be expressed in several ways, e.g., as z-scores, T-scores, IQ-type scores, or stanines (see Figure 6.5). For example,

FIGURE 6.5

Chart illustrating normative relationships: The normal curve, percentiles, and selected standard scores.

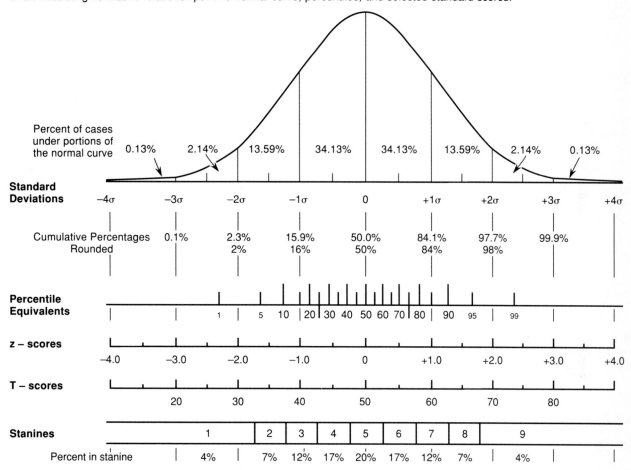

consider the use of standard deviations in eligibility decisions. When a child earns a raw score of 36 on a test, and the mean score for children of the same age is 48 with a standard deviation (*SD*) of 6, that child is scoring exactly 2 *SD* below the mean (48 − 36 = 12; 12 ÷ 6 = 2). This can be expressed as a *z*-score of −2.

Percentile scores indicate the percentage of children in the normative sample in a certain age range who earned a raw score lower than that of the target child. For example, when a child earns a percentile score of 30, this indicates that the child scored higher than 30% of the children in the same age range who took that same test (this is why you can never score higher than the 99.9th percentile on tests; it is impos-

sible to score higher than yourself). Percentile scores are not to be confused with percentage scores, which provide another way of expressing raw scores (i.e., as a proportion of items correct rather than as a straight frequency count).

Equivalent scores specify some level of functioning, usually grade level (often used in tests of reading or other academic skills) or age level (often used in tests of language to yield an LA or in IQ tests to yield an MA). To know how to interpret equivalent scores appropriately, it is important to know how they are derived. Equivalent scores represent average scores earned by a particular group of children at the same age or grade level. Thus, when you obtain a raw score for a child and look it up on a table provided with the test to assign an age-equivalent score, you are actually identifying which group of children earned that score as an average. When you report this score for the target child, you are then comparing the child to a different age group, not to his or her own age group.

Lahey (1988) pointed out the pitfalls of this approach. To illustrate the problems with it, she described a 7-year-old child whose raw score on a language test was equivalent to the mean score for 5-year-olds. Because a 2-year delay is often considered to be the standard for judging a child to have an impairment, such a result might lead to the conclusion that the child is indeed language disordered. Equivalent scores, however, are only central tendency measures; they represent mean scores for a particular limited age range. They do not represent the distribution of scores for that age group. Thus, depending on the test and the norm sample, distributions of scores across age levels may overlap considerably. In Lahey's example, when the distribution of scores for this test were considered for 7-year-olds (the same age as the child), his score was clearly within 1 *SD* of the mean for that group. When compared with his own age range, the child clearly falls within normal limits on this particular test. Any decision about the presence of a language disorder in this child would have to involve additional evidence, including the reason for referral and evidence about the actual performance of language-related tasks in the classroom.

When specialists use formal testing to support eligibility decisions, the inferences they draw are more likely to be appropriate when based on standard scores than on equivalent scores. Lahey (1988) made a rather strong recommendation that evaluation of assessment instruments should be based on whether they include sets of standard scores, or at least standard deviations as well as mean scores. She also commented that "measures that report standard scores are more useful than measures that report only age equivalent scores; and when there is a choice between both types of reporting for an instrument, standard scores should be utilized" (p. 162).

Using standard scores to make eligibility decisions.   How should standard scores be used to make eligibility decisions? Different agencies use different sets of criteria regarding standard deviations.

Sometimes, test authors also recommend cutoff criteria. It is fairly common to expect agencies to require that children must score at least 1 *SD* below the mean on some measure(s) to qualify for services. Others use a criterion of at least −1.5 *SD*. Still others recommend a criterion of at least −2 *SD*, but that is probably too stringent. Can you tell why by looking at the relationships illustrated in Figure 6.5?

To answer this question, notice (by referring to Figure 6.5) that when a test population is distributed normally, only 2.3% of the population scores more than 2 *SD*s below the mean. This suggests that only around 2% of a population of children would be expected to exhibit a language disorder.

What is the percentage of children actually expected to exhibit language delays significant enough to be considered disorders? You may notice that this is a circular question. It depends on the stringency of the inclusion criteria for the population of children studied, along with many other variables, such as the children's ages, their cultural and socioeconomic matches to a standardization sample, and the philosophy of those who are defining what is important for the children to know. Lahey (1988) summarized the results of eight different studies, some of which used more than one set of psychometric criteria (some lenient, −1 *SD*, and some conservative, −2 *SD*) to identify the prevalence of language disorder. Estimates ranged from below 1% to over 12% of the population, with variation both within and between studies. As expected, the lowest prevalence percentages were found in studies using −2 *SD* as a criterion (Randall, Rynell, & Curwen, 1974), as well as those referring children between 5 and 14 years of age to special clinics (Rutter, Graham, & Yule, 1970). In one of the largest and most recent of the studies, Beitchman, Nair, Clegg, and Patel (1986) conducted a two-tiered assessment of 1,655 five-year-old kindergarten-age children in the Ottawa-Carleton region of Canada. The results showed that 6.4% of the group demonstrated evidence of speech disorders alone, 8.04% showed evidence of language disorders alone, and 4.56% showed evidence of mixed speech and language disorders. Even if the group of children with speech disorders alone is eliminated from this set, these results suggest that 12.6% of all kindergarten children show evidence of language disorder and that approximately a third of these demonstrate evidence of speech impairments as well. These percentages are considerably higher than the 2.3% that represents the proportion of a normative sample scoring more than 2 *SD* below the mean. It suggests that the criterion is too stringent. Probably a criterion of 1.5 or 1 *SD* below the mean for the child's age group would be better, and probably more than one test or subtest should be used to support the child's need in this way.

It may also be helpful to use different criteria for defining varied levels of severity. For example, Wiig (1989) recommended judging "total language scores" on the Clinical Evaluation of Language Fundamentals—Revised (CELF-R) (Semel, Wiig, & Secord, 1987) based on the following criteria:

❑ Mild to moderate language disorder, between 1.0 and 1.5 *SDs* below the mean
❑ Moderate language disorder, between 1.5 and 2.0 *SDs* below the mean
❑ Severe language disorder, more than 2.0 *SDs* below the mean

The requirements for comprehensive evaluation established by the IDEA (PL 101–476, 1990) make it clear that more than one test score and more than one person must participate in the decision to place a child in a special education program. It is also required that tests be valid for the purpose for which they are used. Keeping this in mind, it is helpful to consider that the same standard scores may mean different things at different ages. Developmental curves vary in shape across age ranges for both language and other developmental advances (they usually decelerate, starting off steeply and then tapering off to near plateaus until old age at which time declines may begin), and certain kinds of skills also vary in their contextually based importance for infants, toddlers, young children, and adolescents (Bishop & Edmundson, 1987; Rescorla, 1989; Scarborough & Dobrich, 1990). For example, children who are significantly behind age peers in specific language skills at age 3 years may appear to catch up at age 5, only to fall behind again when literacy learning demands become significant in the school-age years (Scarborough & Dobrich, 1990). The significance of a 20th percentile score for an infant may be very different from the significance of a 20th percentile score for a high school senior.

Discrepancies among scores may also have different implications with different tests. For example, Aylward (1987) has described a problem associated with using discrepancy between verbal IQ (VIQ) and performance IQ (PIQ) scores on the Wechsler Intelligence Scale for Children—Revised (WISC-R; Wechsler, 1974) as the sole criterion for diagnosing learning disability. Research has thus far yielded inconsistent data regarding the size and direction of VIQ–PIQ discrepancies on the WISC-R for children with learning disabilities. Aylward commented that, "Although learning-disabled students may show great subtest scatter (i.e., differences in performance among the various subtests) and VIQ–PIQ discrepancies, there are many children without learning disabilities who also show these abnormal patterns, and there are many learning-disabled students who do not show these patterns" (p.48).

By comparison with the WISC-R, the more recently standardized Kaufman Assessment Battery for Children (K-ABC; Kaufman & Kaufman, 1983) has thus far shown more consistency in demonstrating a directional difference between its sequential and simultaneous scales for children with learning disabilities. Kaufman & Kaufman (1983) noted that children with learning disabilities "performed consistently well on Gestalt Closure, one of the purest measures of Simultaneous Processing" and "tended to score most poorly on the Sequential Processing subtests" (p. 139). The point is that "a statistically significant discrepancy is not necessarily an abnormal one" (Aylward, 1987, p. 51). On the K-ABC, the average scatter between sequential and simultaneous scale composite scores is 12.3 points. Kaufman and Kaufman (1983) have suggested that a 22-point discrepancy must be reached before being considered unusual and denoting "marked scatter" (p. 194).

All of this suggests that decisions to make children eligible to receive special services are very complex, indeed. To attempt to simplify these decisions may inadvertently trivialize them at best and may make them inappropriate or harmful to children at worst. The best way to guard against mistakes is for thoroughly educated professionals to collaborate with parents and others to make the best decisions possible to meet the needs of individual children. The age-related discussions of Chapters 7 to 9 provide some additional information to facilitate the process.

Selecting procedures that are valid for the purpose for which they are used. *Validity as a relative concept.* The concept of *test validity* refers to the "appropriateness, meaningfulness, and usefulness of the specific inferences made from test scores. . . .

The inferences regarding specific uses of a test are validated, not the test itself" (American Psychological Association, 1985, p. 9). This is an important concept that is often overlooked. Test validity is not absolute, no matter how extensive the original test validation information. Unless a test is used for the specific purposes for which it was intended, the inferences drawn from it cannot be considered valid.

In judging the validity of using a specific test for a specific purpose, several sources of validity information should be used. The three major categories follow:

1. *Construct-related evidence* indicates that the test is based on a sound theoretical construct embedded in a conceptual framework that makes it possible to interpret the meaning of the results. In judging a test's construct validity for a particular purpose, it is important to determine whether the test design is consistent with the theoretical perspective of the user who will interpret its results. For example, the inferences drawn from a test designed to measure aspects of information processing likely would not yield valid results for inferring knowledge of linguistic rules. Test results must be interpreted within the same theoretical framework in which the test was constructed.

2. *Content-related evidence* indicates that the test items, tasks, or questions represent a defined domain of content. Part of judging the content validity of inferences drawn from particular tests involves determining whether the test measures what it purports to measure. Any assessment involves sampling bits of behavior to judge the larger picture. No test can cover all of the content of a domain. The question is whether the bits chosen accurately represent the broader picture. In this regard, it may be helpful to conduct a task analysis of the actual demands of a particular test or subtest, rather than just taking its label for granted. For example, one of the (S. A. Kirk, McCarthy, & Kirk, 1968) subtests on the Illinois Test of Psycholinguistic Abilities is called auditory reception. One might think that this means that the test samples auditory reception of language, but it samples only a limited aspect of it. The items on this subtest are all of the variety, "Do airplanes fly?," and "Do ponies shave?" They assess comprehension of only one type of syntactic structure, but they do provide a chance to observe the child's knowledge of semantic relations between a variety of agents and actions of sentences.

3. *Criterion-related evidence* shows that the test scores are related to some measure of outcome, such as predicting school performance, or performance on some other kind of criterion measure. When judging a test's criterion-related predictive success, it is helpful to determine how frequently the test results in false-positive or false-negative decisions. A *false-positive* decision selects a person as special in some way who is not special in that way; a *false-negative* result fails to select a person as special in some way who is special in that way. For example, when using screening tests it is particularly important to assess the relative value of making false-positive or false-negative decisions. Lowering cutoff thresholds may result in more children initially being screened in than truly need special attention. Raising cutoff thresholds may result in the opposite.

In assessing the validity of a test for a particular purpose, the specialist must consider that purpose, the test construct and content, and the representativeness of the standardization sample relative to the needs and background of the child. Standardization data alone can suggest an illusion of validity that is not really there in a particular situation. The illusion of validity is particularly dangerous when assessing children from multicultural backgrounds, which is considered in the following discussion.

For a professional to feel confident that a test performance is a valid representation of a child's ability, it is also critical that the child exert optimal effort. Experienced evaluators recognize the importance of establishing rapport before attempting to administer a formal test and of arranging the sequence of a test session to obtain the best performance possible. Most of us know the temptation of giving a child a formal test and feeling certain that the child could demonstrate a particular behavior if only the task were modified slightly. Of course, we also know that if we want to use standard scores to interpret the test results relative to the normative group, we must follow the standard administration procedure as closely as possible, because any significant variation may invalidate those inferences. Usually, the test instructions provide some information about how much encouragement can be given, but some children are simply bigger risk takers than others (see Personal Reflection 6.4). Any other alterations of the task should be done only after the test is administered in the standard way and quantitative data have been gathered. Then, it may be possible to gather additional qualitative information by altering the demands of the task slightly. Just be careful to record what you do, and be sure to make your task alterations clear in your discussion of any qualitative differences that result.

The best approach may be to recognize the limitations and contributions of formal tests for what they are. They are highly structured observations of limited aspects of behavior in specialized contexts. Formal tests are useful to define a disorder's parameters relatively objectively. I use them minimally in my own practice, but I do use them, especially when diagnosing a child as having a language disorder and determining eligibility for service. They help me to validate my own less formal impressions of a child's functioning (I have found that spending a lot of time with children with special needs tends to result in warped internalized standards of "normal"), but I find the information that I obtain from informal assessment procedures much more useful in planning intervention efforts. I am also careful to use contextually based informal assessment information of varying types to assist me in judging the validity of the results from formal assessment.

Score reliability must be established. Knowing the variability frequently characteristic of children with language disorders, it is surprising how often we tend to treat a single score earned on a particular day as representing a child's "true" performance. Part of phenomenology involves recognizing the relativity of "truth" and the way the essential nature of a phenomenon varies depending on the tools used to observe it and the internal and external contexts in which it occurs.

Tasks vary in how "tight" they are. Informal tasks are informal partly because the evaluator exerts less control over the context, which can lead to considerable looseness from one observational occasion to another. As stated throughout this book, sometimes that is helpful, particularly if context is valued as part of the intervention process. However, one reason for giving a formal test is that the test maker may have established its reliability. This is usually done in two ways: (1) Test–retest reliability is established by giving the test more than once to the same group of children after enough time has passed that the first administration is not likely to influence the second, but the children are unlikely yet to have experienced much natural growth. (2) Split-half reliability is established by comparing scores earned on items on one half of a test with the other. Both comparisons are usually expressed as correlation coefficients. A third type of reliability that may be expressed this way is interscorer reliability. Particularly when much professional judgment is involved in assigning scores to items, interscorer reliability coefficients may be computed by comparing scores assigned by more than one evaluator for the same behaviors.

Besides having confidence in the reliability of a test procedure, evaluators need to be confident about the level of functioning that a score represents for a particular child. This is done by using information about the standard error of measurement. Standard error also provides a measure of reliability expressed as a range of score units within which a child's "true" score actually lies (the score that would emerge as the average of an infinite number of test administrations without any retest effects). Standard error varies for different confidence intervals, depending on how confident an evaluator wants to be that an actual score lies within a particular range. A confidence interval of 95% would therefore include a wider range of scores than a confidence interval of 85%. Some

Personal Reflection 6.4	"Take a chance. Sometimes the brain knows more than you think it does." *Gloria Zeal Davis* (1990, p. 4), Orton-Gillingham tutor, trying to urge a third-grader to take a risk after he had refused to attempt many test items. Davis used the analogy of expert skiers, racing beyond the edge of their ability as an analogy for what persons with language disorders must be encouraged to do. But for this child, on this particular day, Davis had to conclude, "No luck—the fear of failure was too painful. Far from extending his experiences beyond the edge, perhaps he would never even see the mountain snow." (p. 4)

test manuals report standard error values for different confidence intervals at different age levels. If it is not reported, standard error may be computed by subtracting the reliability coefficient from 1 and multiplying the square root of that value by the standard deviation (Lyman, 1986). One reason that the WISC-R (Wechsler, 1974) is used so extensively to measure intelligence is that it is considered to be one of the most reliable of all psychological instruments. It has a standard error of measurement of 3 points for a 68% confidence interval (the percentage of cases between ±1 *SD*) (Aylward & Brown, 1987).

Criterion-referenced testing. Not all quantitative assessment measures are norm referenced, some are criterion referenced. As previously discussed, norm referencing involves judging performance relative to some larger standardization group. Norm referenced tests generally are required to determine eligibility for services. Criterion referencing involves judging performance relative to some predetermined level of performance. Criterion-referenced tests are more frequently used to measure progress than to determine eligibility, but they also might be used to support eligibility decisions. For example, a child might be considered not to have a problem in reading if the child can read and can answer 85% of related questions correctly in a sample of grade-level appropriate curricular materials. Criterion-referenced testing is more closely related to answering the question about disability than impairment. When a criterion is set, it stands as someone's estimate of what a child must do to succeed in a particular context.

Criterion-referencing is the method used when assigning letter grades in most educational settings (unless grading is on the curve, which is norm referenced). Behavioral objectives constitute a form of criterion-referenced testing for judging progress during language intervention programs.

Curriculum-based assessment. When a criterion-referenced approach uses success in activities related to the academic school curriculum, it is curriculum-based. Idol, Nevin, et al. (1986) defined curriculum-based assessment (CBA) as "a criterion-referenced test that is teacher-constructed and designed to reflect curriculum content" (p. vii). Not all CBA is criterion referenced (Marston, 1989) or involves the construction of specific tasks (N. W. Nelson, 1989b). More generally, CBA is defined as the use of the student's progress in the local school's curriculum to measure success in education. Tucker used (1985) this definition, adding, "Curriculum-based assessment includes *any* procedure that directly assesses student performance within the course content for the purpose of determining that student's instructional needs" (p. 200). Other sources (Shinn, 1989) support this flexibility inherent within different CBA models.

CBA may be modified to be used primarily for curriculum-based language assessment. The focus then is not so much on whether the child is learning the course content but on whether the child is using language knowledge, skills, and strategies effectively when attempting to learn the course content. I have suggested that this approach be defined as the "use of curriculum contexts and content for measuring a student's language intervention needs and progress" (N. W. Nelson, 1989b, p. 171). Particular areas of language strengths and needs then can be identified without assigning a numerical value to the performance, or even a pass–fail judgment, although qualification is possible. Rather, the specialist uses the assessment information to select intervention target areas, intervention methods, and a way to observe qualitative changes in performance over time.

Multicultural perspectives for guarding against bias in assessment. It is fairly clear to all involved that the results of a test based on standard English (SE) would provide an invalid measure of true language ability for a child whose native language is not SE. Such tests are clearly not appropriate for a child who is either non-English speaking (NES), also termed non-English proficient (NEP), or who has limited English proficiency (LEP). Although less clearly recognized, the same bias may apply when a child is learning a variation of English based on rules of a system such as Black English Vernacular (BEV; sometimes called *ebonics*) or other nonstandard varieties of English, such as Appalachian English.

One area that has received considerable attention is the assessment of children learning BEV. More than 20 years have passed since serious challenges first addressed the validity of inferences drawn from administering standardized assessment instruments to children learning BEV (Baratz, 1969; Taylor, Stroud, Moore, Hurst, & Williams, 1969; Wolfram, Williams, & Taylor, 1972). Yet, alternatives in the form of culturally fair, nonbiased assessment tools are still not available (Taylor, 1985; Taylor & Payne, 1983; Reveron, in press; Vaughn-Cooke, 1989; Wiener, Lewnau, & Erway, 1983).

As S. L. Terrell and Terrell noted (1983), "the development of dialect-sensitive or culture-fair language tests has not kept pace with the development of testing materials designed to assess the speech and language of standard English speakers" (p. 3). Reveron (in press) commented further that "there currently exists a dearth of valid language tests for speakers of non-mainstream English dialects, particularly BE" (p. 2), and Vaughn-Cooke (1989) noted that the situation still had not changed by the end of the last decade. This is in spite of the fact that in 1975 PL 94–142 (1977) mandated that selection and administration of all test materials and procedures used to evaluate handicapped children must not be racially or culturally discriminatory. Partially because of the lack of tests to meet that mandate, Taylor and Payne (1983) commented that "If this stipulation were enforced today to its fullest intent, most school systems in the United States would be in violation of the law" (p. 8).

A variety of reasons can be hypothesized for the lack of appropriate measures, some of which relate to concerns about how such an instrument should be designed. Many alternatives for constructing culturally fair instruments are available, none are perfect. Vaughn-Cooke (1983) has listed and evaluated the following possibilities used to construct new tests:

1. Standardize existing tests on non-mainstream speakers.
2. Include a small percentage of minorities in the standardization sample when developing the test.
3. Modify or revise existing tests in ways that will make them appropriate for non-mainstream speakers.
4. Utilize a language sample when assessing the language of non-mainstream speakers.
5. Utilize criterion-referenced measures when assessing the language of non-mainstream speakers.
6. Refrain from using all standardized tests that have not been corrected for test bias when assessing the language of non-mainstream speakers.
7. Develop a new test which can provide a more appropriate assessment of the language of non-mainstream English speakers. (p. 29)

For several years, I have been working with Yvette Hyter (with consultation from Walt Wolfram) on an approach combining Vaughn-Cooke's (1983) recommendations 3, 4, and 7 in the development of Black English Sentence Scoring (BESS) (N. W. Nelson & Hyter, 1990a, 1990b). BESS is a tool for nonbiased

assessment of the language of BE-speaking children between the ages of 3:0 and 6:11. It is used in conjunction with Lee's (1974) Developmental Sentence Scoring (DSS) to award points for grammatical features in eight categories (see Chapter 8).

J. G. Erickson (1981) also urged that a broader view be taken of the language problems of bilingual bicultural children than that based on surface grammatical features alone and noted that the answer may not lie in new tests modeled after old ones. She described most traditional assessment tools as discrete point tests, which "reflected the thinking that language was a series of separate or discrete points which, when added up, made the whole. Language was not viewed as a synergistic and social phenomenon" (p. 4). Based on such thinking, some tests in English have simply been translated into other languages, a method that both violates the statistical support for the test and results in questionable cultural and linguistic relevancy of test items.

In addition, Heath (1984) and Wolfram (1983) have pointed out that not all children have the same frame of reference for taking formal tests, which we often assume they have. Heath noted that most formal tests are based on assumptions that normal language learners (1) know the routines of test behavior; (2) are information givers, interpreters of pictures, and narrators; and (3) know how to segment language into "words" and "meanings" and know how to identify the mainstream meaning of texts. In addition to possible problems associated with unfamiliar task characteristics, Wolfram pointed out that testing is a social occasion with many specialized game-like rules, but that all players may not use the same rules. For example, he noted that in some cultures, children may have learned the relative values of silence and withdrawal in the presence of more powerful adults. Cheng (1989) gave the example of Japanese children, who may say "yes" when they mean "no" because it is rude in Japanese culture to say "no" in some contexts.

Evaluating children from diverse cultures requires more than understanding the linguistic differences between the child's first language and standard English. An appreciation for the broader elements of cultural differences is required, including a self-awareness of how one's own cultural background influences communication as well as attributes one values as positive and evaluates as normal. G. A. Harris (1985) pointed to the need for "educators and other professionals, including language specialists, to come face to face with a new skill necessary for clinical competency—that of understanding the effects of culture on communication" (p. 44).

Cultural literacy has been described as the "broad working knowledge of the traditions, terminology, folklore, and history of our [a] culture" (Bjorkland & Bjorkland, 1988, p. 144). Of course, it is a practical impossibility for professionals to be culturally literate in all of the different cultures they might encounter among children with language disorders. Cultural diversity is rich even within "one" culture. For example, Cheng (1989) pointed out that hundreds of distinct languages and dialects are spoken in East Asia, Southeast Asia, and the Pacific Islands. G. A. Harris (1985) noted that Native American tribes in the U.S. Southwest are distinct and sovereign nations.

The professional can attempt to view the cultural milieu of a particular child or group from within the eyes of other group members. D. L. Taylor (1986) suggested that language disorder be defined for members of minority cultures when their communicative behaviors deviated sufficiently from the norms and expectations of that child's own language community. Other than gathering local norms on tests, the only way to find this out is (1) to ask people in the child's own community and (2) to observe the child's communicative behavior relative to that of other members of the child's own cultural group.

J. G. Erickson (1981) offered a model of language that differs from the discrete-point model on which most formal tests are based, one that is more consistent with the social interaction theoretical perspective discussed in this book. Erickson's model is based on the following four assumptions:

1. Language is a symbolic, generative process that does not lend itself easily to formal assessment.
2. Language is synergistic, so that any measure of the part does not give a picture of the whole.
3. Language is a part of the total experience of a child and is difficult to assess as an isolated part of development.
4. Language use (quality and quantity) varies according to the setting, interactors, and topic. (1981, p. 7)

Recognizing the contextual-based nature of many problems of second language learners, Garcia and Ortiz (1988) supported using referral criteria for language minority students that are grounded in observations by teacher assistance teams (TATs) formed exclusively of regular educators, with speech–

language pathologists or other special educators called in only as consultants. These teams would address a series of questions designed to prevent inappropriate referrals for special education services: (1) Is the student experiencing academic difficulty? (2) Are the curricula and instructional materials known to be effective for language minority students? (3) Has the problem been validated through the collection of several kinds of information? (4) Is there evidence of systematic efforts to identify the source of the difficulty and to take corrective action within the regular education system? (5) Do student difficulties persist? (6) Have other programming alternatives been tried? (7) Do difficulties continue in spite of alternatives? If at each of these steps, the answer is still affirmative, then students may be appropriately referred as having disorders that justify evaluation rather than simply having differences that should be addressed in other ways.

A study by Damico, Oller, and Storey (1983) also supported the use of pragmatic elements in everyday communication rather than surface grammatical criteria to diagnose language disorder among bilingual children. The children in their study were 10 Spanish–English bilingual children who had been referred by bilingual classroom teachers for a special education evaluation. The procedure involved collecting language samples in both languages and then scoring the samples in two ways: (1) using traditional morphological and syntactic structural criteria, and (2) using pragmatic criteria such as nonfluencies, revisions, and delays. As might be expected, criteria application identified two different subgroups of children. The children were reevaluated 7 months after they had all been mainstreamed in essentially monolingual English classroom settings. The results revealed that the pragmatic criteria were superior predictors of both academic achievement and teacher ratings. The authors concluded that traditional diagnostic criteria needed supplementation (not replacement) by pragmatic criteria. Based on discussions of the heterogeneity of language disorders in Chapter 4, and particularly the description of the symptoms of specific language impairment, we might expect that multiple criteria are needed to identify all children with language disorders.

The use of a set of contextually based social interaction assumptions with a strong pragmatic base obviously has some strong implications about assessment of culturally and linguistically diverse children.

As summarized by J. G. Erickson and Omark (1981), assessment should

> [sample] communication in a natural setting and [obtain] supportive information from integrative testing and interviews, including probes into specific functions and forms of language use. It is a model that encourages the use of criterion-referenced testing, and, when indicated, norm-referenced testing based on local data. (p. 7)

Using informal as well as formal procedures. Certainly, informal assessment procedures are critical when making decisions about the needs and abilities of children from nonmainstream cultural and linguistic groups, but informal procedures also can provide important validating insights and diagnostic information for all children with special needs. An overview of ecological and ethnographic principles consistent with a system theory view of complex behavior in complex contexts was presented in Chapter 1. The specific techniques are considered further as they apply to each of the three developmental ranges in Chapters 7 (early), 8 (middle), and 9 (later). The techniques include strategies for interviewing participants, using observational strategies, and gathering naturalistic samples and other artifacts.

Interviewing participants. To gather information relevant to a child's needs and reflecting the perspectives of the various persons in the problem situation, key individuals must be asked directly about their perspectives.

Shifting out of a traditional mode, which focuses almost exclusively on assessing and fixing impaired communicative processes within children, to a collaborative mode, which focuses on needs and opportunities as well as impairments, requires a new set of strategies. One is the participant interview. Borrowed from anthropologists, this ethnographic technique provides a way of looking at a culture (in this case, the varied cultures of a child's home and school)

through the eyes of the participants (Green & Wallat, 1981; S. Stainback & Stainback, 1988).

Although participant interviewing is related to the traditional practice of "gathering the case history," it is distinct in several ways. The interview is not just another method of gathering information. The interview discourse is part of intervention. It is also often a key to moving an interaction into the cooperative goal-setting mode. The types of questions the interviewer asks influence the kinds of discourse elicited from interviewees, and it is desirable to elicit more than one kind of discourse. When I interview participants in a problem situation, I find it helpful to ask questions of two types: (1) I ask participants to tell about the problem. This kind of questioning usually elicits expository discourse, including labels for key aspects of the problem and the hierarchical set of priorities as viewed by the participants themselves. (2) I ask participants to tell anecdotes to illustrate the problem. This usually elicits narrative discourse, including characterization of the interactions among the participants in a way that allows me to begin to form a more complete picture and to begin to apply my own labels and interpretations.

When interviewing participants, the interviewer's attitude is especially important. If the participants' perspectives are to be understood, the interviewer must remain nonjudgmental about participants' comments. For example, although I may not think it productive to label a child who avoids a situation in which he expects to fail as "lazy" (in fact, I might call that "smart"), it is important for me to know that this is how that child's problems appear to his teachers and parents. Accepting individuals' viewpoints as valid representations of how they feel about issues does not mean that the interviewer may not, at some point, wish to encourage participants to shift those views.

Where and when interviews occur may vary. In the early stages of assessment and intervention, sepa-

---

Personal Reflection 6.5 "The goal in interviewing is to have the participants talk about things of interest to them and to cover matters of importance to the researcher [professional] in a way that allows the participants to use their own concepts and terms."

Susan Stainback and *William Stainback* (1988, p. 52), writing about uses of interviewing in qualitative research with application to clinical interactions.

rate interviews with each of the important participants may yield clearer pictures of individuals' views of the problem. Group interviews, however, also have advantages, because the participants can learn from each other and can begin the process of cooperative goal setting as a natural outcome of identifying current abilities, needs, and opportunities. When a child has a patchwork schedule requiring him to spend time with several different special education and regular education teachers each day, just asking each teacher to describe the child's responsibilities in that setting may lead to teachers' spontaneous problem solving to consolidate aspects of several different curricular expectations. Even in ongoing programs, it is important to update the picture regularly because children and contexts change. Annual review IEP meetings can be used for this purpose, if they are small enough, but update interviews held before IEP meetings may be more productive. Then, the formal meeting can be used to summarize the priorities established in earlier interviews so that mutual goal setting and planning can proceed efficiently at the meeting.

Participant interviews can be used to satisfy several different assessment purposes. They can be as helpful in determining the presence of a problem in the initial stages of treatment as they are in monitoring progress in the later stages. Particularly when children have cultural differences that make the validity of standard assessment procedures more questionable than usual, I rely heavily on input from people in the child's own cultural and home environments for diagnosing language disorder. The evaluator can feel fairly confident that a child has a problem requiring attention when parents respond with immediate and definite confirmation when asked, "Have you noticed this child being different from your other children in when he began to talk, how he talks, or how much he talks?" The speed and quality of the verbal and nonverbal responses you receive to this type of questioning should allow you to tell whether this has been bothering interviewees or whether you have suggested a new possibility that they have to mull over. It is also helpful when participants offer to back up their evaluative judgments with specific examples. If they do not volunteer them, request examples. Although this kind of inquiry is particularly useful when questions of linguistic or cultural difference are involved, it can be just as useful for children from mainstream-culture homes.

If a parent seems hesitant to identify this child as being different in development, and if others who work with the child regularly seem to have no concerns until the possibility is raised to them, caution should be exercised in finding the child to have a language disorder, even if some formal test results support such a conclusion. Several options are available, including further testing, further naturalistic observation, or a scheduled recheck (usually at 6 months to 1 year, depending on the child's age, with younger children checked more frequently).

Using onlooker and participant observation techniques. Onlooker observation can be conducted in situations that participants feel are relatively natural and important. Of course, part of an ecological perspective is that, as soon as an outside observer enters a context, the context changes. Not only is the child probably different when being observed by an outsider, particularly in a strange environment, but the child's parents, siblings, teacher, or peers are probably different as well. This fact needs to be taken into account, but the primary objective of onlooker observation is to obtain a contextually bound view of the linguistic demands of those contexts and how the child uses language when intervention is not provided intentionally.

In participant observation, the language specialist begins direct contact with the child and with his communicative partners. This process has two purposes: (1) to find out how the participants interpret events during the events and (2) to determine how interactions might change if the variables are purposefully shifted.

Gathering naturalistic samples. Basing decisions about language disorders on naturalistic language samples is not a new phenomenon (see, e.g., W. Johnson, Darley, & Spriesterbach, 1952; McCarthy, 1930, 1954; Templin, 1957). Spontaneous language sampling was given a further boost after the publications of Chomsky (1957, 1965) and R. A. Brown (1973). Whole books and monographs (e.g., Barrie-Blackley, Musselwhite, & Rogister, 1978; Hubbell, 1988; Longhurst, 1974; Lund & Duchan, 1988; J. F. Miller, 1981) have since been written about gathering and analyzing naturalistic samples of language and communicative behavior, and I will not attempt to review them extensively here. Specific suggestions for analyzing spontaneous language samples relative to developmental expectations are included in Chapters 7 to 9, particularly, Chapter 8.

Some elements are basic to all types of spontaneous sampling. James (1989) identified the process as consisting of two basic steps, both of which require special considerations: (1) collecting and recording the sample and (2) analyzing it.

The choice of audio or video recording of the sample is important (generally, the younger the child, and the more nonverbal the communication, the more critical is the use of video equipment), but the primary concern is whether the collected sample truly represents the child's language ability. Because of the importance of gathering samples of children's best performances, it is helpful to know what kinds of conditions tend to foster those. Hubbell (1988) identified three major influences on children's talking; (1) their language knowledge and skill, (2) their purposes and motivations, and (3) the contexts in which they are talking.

Although adequate samples can be obtained by clinicians acting as conversational partners in clinic rooms (Olswang & Carpenter, 1978), children have been found to produce longer utterances in samples gathered by their mothers at home than in those gathered by clinicians in clinical settings (Kramer, James, & Saxman, 1979). Recognizing the influence of different environmental contexts and conversational partners, researchers often recommend (e.g., J.F. Miller, 1981; Lund & Duchan, 1988) that clinicians use multiple contexts and conversational partners to obtain more representative, contextually-based samples.

Emphasizing the importance of human factors in determining how much a child talks, Hubbell (1988) reviewed literature suggesting that three interrelated human relationship factors can work together to create a context that elicits maximum talking from children: (1) "Children are likely to talk more when they have equal or greater power in a relationship than the listener does," (2) "The more limits there are on children's behavior, the more their activities are constrained, the less freely they communicate," and (3) "Children talk more when the topic is of immediate interest to them" (p. 10).

The necessary length of samples has also been studied. Generally, samples of 50 to 100 utterances are adequate for most purposes (L. Bloom & Lahey, 1978). The amount of time required to gather the sample varies depending on the child. Younger or more reticent children may require longer than ½ hour to produce a sample of this length, but a gregarious child may produce a sample of more than 100 utterances in less than 30 minutes (James, 1989). To investigate several questions about length and number of language samples, K. N. Cole, Mills, and Dale (1989) used test–retest and split-half reliability techniques on language samples gathered from 10 children between the ages of 52 and 80 months. Cole et al. interpreted their results as having four implications: (1) Collecting more than one language sample yields more representative information about a child's productive language. (2) Contrary to traditional wisdom, "children do not necessarily produce more complex or longer utterances during the second half of a language sample due to a 'warm-up' effect." (3) "Two shorter examples taken on different days may yield slightly more information about a child's lexical production." (4) "A 50 utterance sample may yield 73–83% of the lexical information found in a 100 utterance sample" (1989, p. 266)

Different sampling strategies also work better for children of different ages. Toys with multiple pieces associated with well-known cognitive play scripts (such as playhouses, barns, and fastfood restaurants) tend to work better with younger children. Complicated or broken toys may also be more likely to elicit questions from some children. Some toys that do not work as well are stacks of pictures, which tend to elicit stilted language with little cohesion, and art or building activities such as clay molding, drawing, or blocks, which may lead children to get so involved in the activity that they are less likely to talk. School-age children and older preschool children are less reliant on props and are more likely to use narrative discourse as well as conversation in their samples. Sampling should include varied discourse as well as varied sentence structures to be representative.

Gathering elicited samples. Spontaneous samples sometimes do not allow sufficient opportunity to observe certain kinds of language behaviors. Relatively more structured elicitation techniques then can be used to try to draw forth particular behaviors. The most frequently used elicitation strategy is a direct request for imitation. Because of the control possible when using such a strategy, it has been a frequent choice on formal standardized tests. It also has been recommended for use as a nonstandardized assessment (Menyuk, 1968; J. F. Miller, 1981), but problems have been identified in the use of the technique. Some evidence suggests that it may underestimate spontaneous language performance (L. Bloom, Hood, & Lightbown, 1974; Connell & Myles-Zitzer, 1982; Prutting, Gallagher, & Mulac, 1975; Weber-Olsen, Putnam-Sims, & Gannon, 1983), whereas other evidence suggests that it may overestimate that performance (Kuczaj & Maratsos, 1975; C. Smith, 1970).

Recall the earlier discussion in this chapter about metalinguistic versus linguistic contexts and the different demands they make for processing by children. Elicitation tasks, such as patterning or puppet modeling, almost always involve some metalinguistic elements. Children must grasp that they are playing some type of language "game" to participate appropriately. (I remember one preschooler who went along with our requests for imitation just fine, until we came to a question such as "Say, 'Do frogs jump in the grass?'" She answered "no" and nothing we could do persuaded her that she was supposed to repeat the question rather than answer it.)

Other elicitation tasks that linguists and speech–language pathologists have developed to judge knowledge of linguistic rules are reviewed in Chapter 2. As illustrated there, elicitation tasks vary in their naturalness. Some fall so close to spontaneous language sampling on the naturalness continuum that they are hard to distinguish. For example, Dollaghan, Campbell, and Tomlin (1990) described video narration as a new context for sampling "spontaneous expressive language." They gathered these samples by having clients produce on-line descriptions of the cartoon events they observed on videotapes and found that the procedure had advantages in terms of increased consistency across samples.

Assessing comprehension informally. Most language-sampling techniques are aimed primarily at assessing language production rather than comprehension, although transcripts of language-sampling events can provide information about both processes. Because language comprehension is relatively more difficult to observe directly, it is often overlooked during informal assessment activities. Information about language comprehension, however, is critical to understanding a child's language abilities and needs. In contexts such as classroom participation, language

comprehension may play an even greater role in meeting children's needs than does language expression.

Perhaps the biggest problem associated with measuring language comprehension informally arises from the difficulty in separating the child's comprehension of a particular situation, based on nonverbal cues, from the child's comprehension of language, based on linguistic cues. James (1989) suggested use of the terms *communication comprehension* and *linguistic comprehension,* respectively, to recognize the distinction. Typically, formal testing procedures are more likely to measure linguistic comprehension because they are designed to present isolated examples of particular language structures out of context. The usual strategy is for the evaluator to read a sentence to a child who is looking at a set of pictures so that the child can select the picture that best matches the sentence. This strategy fails to provide a way to observe comprehension of discourse connected to other linguistic and nonverbal information. Using this approach, it is also quite difficult to estimate how well the child comprehends complex language of the type found in school curricular experiences.

Informal comprehension assessment measures vary with the client's age. With older children and adolescents, assessing language comprehension informally using CBA techniques is essential to understanding possible interaction of their language and academic difficulties. With younger children, comprehension usually can be assessed informally in play with the children as spontaneous language samples are gathered. With infants and toddlers, comprehension almost always must be assessed through observation of their interactions with their care givers during familiar routines.

A frequent problem that I have observed when speech–language pathologists and special educators assess comprehension informally is that they tend to overestimate children's linguistic comprehension abilities because these professionals are such facilitative communicators. Having learned well the strategies for helping children with limited language abilities to communicate, they often unconsciously use those strategies during assessment. They may sometimes employ nonverbal cues like pauses and eye gaze to facilitate their listeners' comprehension without being aware of using those cues. It is fine to vary the contextual cues consciously to observe their varied effects, but a problem occurs when language comprehension skill is attributed to listeners when the children actually are exhibiting communicative comprehension.

With younger children, these problems can be overcome if clinicians design some specific requests for either verbal or nonverbal behaviors that cannot be understood based on context alone and then refrain from using nonlinguistic or paralinguistic cues to augment the message. I almost sit on my hands sometimes to avoid gesturing when asking a child to retrieve a particular toy from a particular place in the room. With older children, comprehension may be measured by asking questions about a story they have heard or a text they have read. Another strategy that I have found to be particularly helpful in CBA is to ask students to paraphrase a sentence or short paragraph. That is a particularly good way to find out whether they have acquired traditional meanings of complex sentences. For math story problems, asking students to sketch what they think a problem means is another good way to see how they transform language symbols to other modalities.

Gathering other artifacts. When the language comprehended or produced is written, artifacts may be gathered. The difficulty in using written language artifacts, such as class assignments, or writing portfolios, such as journals, is that the evaluator is often uncertain of the context in which the assignment was explained and produced. This problem can be addressed by interviewing the teacher or child about the item as well as looking at it, and by combining these perspectives with participant observation. Other methods for gathering artifacts include audiotaping and videotaping of more naturalistic verbal and nonverbal interactions. The value of audio and videotapes is that they not only can help in analyzing current systems (or subparts of the culture) but also can provide a historical record for marking progress. Tapes sometimes can be made without an outside observer present and thus may provide a clearer picture of the influence of natural context.

Using Assessment to Establish a Prognosis

When using assessment to establish a prognosis for improvement, the specialist may need some different strategies. Accurate determination of prognosis in the decision-making process has considerable importance for children. It can influence decisions made in the present and the future.

For preschool children with specific language impairments, Bishop and Edmundson (1987) charac-

terized problems related to establishing prognosis as follows:

> On the one hand, it might seem desirable to initiate therapy as early as possible to give the child the best opportunity of overcoming the impairment before starting school. On the other hand, the disorder might resolve naturally, and treatment could create more problems than it solves by producing low expectations in teachers, anxiety in parents, and self-consciousness in the child. The parents of a language-impaired child want to know what the future holds, in particular, whether the child will be able to cope with regular schooling. Should one offer reassurance or a guarded prognosis? This is an area where even experienced clinicians find it hard to make decisions. (p. 156)

As these comments acknowledge, despite the importance of prognosis, establishing it is an inexact process, relying on a combination of professional expertise, experience, and knowledge of factors that influence language development among children with language disorders. Expertise is a broad concept; experience comes only with time and opportunity, but information about factors influencing language development can come from a review of the results of scientific inquiry.

Using prognostic data from longitudinal studies for children with specific language impairments. Longitudinal studies of change among children with language disorders provide one of the best sources of information about factors influencing prognosis. Several studies of this type have been conducted. Chapter 4 considered evidence from longitudinal studies and clinical reports suggesting that language disorders tend to persist as children grow older but may change in their expression (Aram, Ekelman, & Nation, 1984; Aram & Nation, 1980; Fundudis, Kolvin, & Garside, 1979; S. E. Maxwell & Wallach, 1984; Stark et al., 1984).

Consider the scenario in which symptoms of oral language deficit that are obvious when children are preschoolers become less evident during the school-age years. Then, the most obvious symptoms may be difficulty in learning to read. Although basic language impairments may persist, they may be hidden by the fact that children with early language disorders tend to make fewer errors in their expressive language as they grow older (perhaps partially as a result of development and partially as a result of intervention). When speaking, children can select among a variety of ways to express their ideas. When listening or reading, they have no choice. They must process whatever is presented. That is, children may choose to speak primarily in simple sentences, rarely using complex connectives, or even misusing them from a logical-semantic perspective (e.g., a language-impaired child might say, "I fell off my bike because I hurt my arm"), but still sound OK to teachers and adults whose ears are tuned to hear articulatory or syntactic errors. In the school-age years, and in academic contexts particularly, language comprehension needs are critical (perhaps even more critical than language expression skills). The difficulties that some language-impaired children experience in such contexts may be masked by their apparently error-free oral language productions. Thus, instead of language weakness being identified as the root of the problem for such children, other reasons may be invoked (e.g., not paying attention, not trying, laziness). A language specialist, by asking the right questions, can contribute to the process of sorting out the potential contribution of the language disability to the child's problems. Failure to consider the prognosis for academic risk that may persist after surface features of language improve is failure to learn from the case study presented by Damico (1988), which was reviewed in Chapter 1.

Evidence that can be used to make prognostic judgments has been gathered by many researchers in a variety of longitudinal studies. Table 6.1 summarizes the major characteristics of those studies in terms of sample size, time at longitudinal follow-up, and whether an evaluation or interview method was used to measure outcome. The results of the studies regarding prognostic variables are also summarized. Most of these researchers selected their samples using criteria to exclude conditions such as hearing loss, mental retardation, and frank neuromotor impairments. Readers should keep in mind that Table 6.1 generally represents findings regarding only a very narrow section of the entire realm of children with language disorders for whom they may need to establish a prognosis.

Another caution regards variables that may not be reported in Table 6.1 as being significant based on existing research but yet may be significant to a child. For example, environmental conditions such as socioeconomic status, child abuse, and neglect are not mentioned.

Schery (1985) investigated the usefulness of socioeconomic status variables in determining prognosis for children with language disorders. Noting that such

variables are "usually very strong predictors of performance in language and educational research with nonimpairied children" (p. 81), Schery was surprised to find that neither socioeconomic status nor socioemotional variables predicted initial levels of language functioning in her study of 718 children with specific language disorders in the Los Angeles County schools. (This public school sample population is important because it is probably more representative of the broader population than that group of children whose parents make special efforts to bring them to university or community clinics.) As Schery summarized, "Indeed, the children showed pervasive problems that were unrelated to family background characteristics such as parents' education, occupation, and cultural/ethnic ties" (p. 81). On the other hand, the improvement made by children in the 2- to 3-year study period was affected by many variables related to social status, including the children's own socioemotional status and personality characteristics, their mothers' levels of education, and the presence of physical discipline in the home.

Establishing a prognosis when language disorder is mixed with other conditions. When language disorder is mixed with other impairments (e.g., hearing loss, mental retardation), or when disorders stem from acquired brain injuries, the prognostic picture becomes even more complicated. As a general rule, the level of language functioning observed when children are first identified may be the best indicator of their ultimate outcome, perhaps in concert with levels of cognitive functioning in other areas, as well as consideration of causative factors (both past and ongoing).

When language disorder accompanies severe disabilities, including autism. The importance of level of language functioning in determining ultimate outcome for persons with severe disabilities has been repeatedly confirmed, particularly with regard to autism. Schreibman (1988) noted that "It is widely accepted that the single most important prognostic indicator (for autistic and other handicapped children) is language ability" (p. 147). Yet, the expectations for advanced language development among children with autism are usually quite limited.

One longitudinal study of children with autism involved a 7-year follow-up of 85 autistic boys and 34 autistic girls (with a control group of 36 children). DeMyer et al. (1973) found that only a few of the children with autism learned to use speech more complex than for making simple requests. Those who

TABLE 6.1

Prognostic factors identified in research studies associated with better and poorer outcomes for children wth speech and language disorders. (*Note.* These prognostic indicators are not organized by strength of prediction—initial language scores and nonverbal IQ measures tend to be the best prognostic indicators—some factors listed are rather weak.)

Better Prognosis	Poorer Prognosis
No family history of language and/or reading disability[a,b]	Significant family history of language and/or reading disability[a,b]
Low-risk birth[b]	High-risk birth[b]
Reported to be communicative as infant[b]	Reported to be noncommunicative as infant[b]
Younger (<6:6 years) when first identified[c]	Older (>6:6 years) when first identified[c]
Younger when still having difficulty[b]	Older when still having difficulty[b]
Less severe when identified[b,c,d]	More severe when identified[b,c,d]
Higher nonverbal IQ[a,b,d,e]	Lower nonverbal IQ[a,b,d,e]
No associated deficits (e.g., hearing, mental retardation)[b,d,e]	More associated deficits[b,d,e]
Fewer language components involved[b,d,e,f]	More language components involved[b,d,e,f]
Problems limited to articulation[f]	Problems with language or mixed articulation/language[f]
Able to retell story with picture at 5 years[d]	Unable to retell story with pictures at 5 years[d]
High score on exp. Northwestern Syntax Screening Test (NSST) as preschooler[e]	Low score on expressive NSST as preschooler[e]
Child prefers to participate in groups[b]	Child prefers to be alone[b]
Parents say positive things about child[b]	Parents rely on physical discipline[b]

Potential Problems for Children as They Grow Older

Persistent language and speech problems
> Proportions vary: 40%,[g] 50%,[f] 56%,[d] 80%[c]
> Continue to develop speech and language skills but at slower rate than peers[c,h]
> Broader problems tend to give way to narrower ones[b]

Difficulty learning to read/persistent reading difficulty
> Proportions vary: 40%,[g] 75%,[a] 90%[c]
> For some, severe reading problems may follow a period of illusory recovery at age 5[a]

Other limitations of academic achievement
> Proportions vary with inclusion criteria for study:
>> In one follow-up study[e] of preschoolers with nonspecific language disorders when they were adolescents, 20% were in classes for students with mild retardation, and 69% of the remaining needed tutoring, grade retention, learning disability classroom placement
>> In another study,[h] only 24% received grades below a B or C level, but 52% had some academic difficulties and needed some tutoring

Few or mild problems with social interaction
> One study reported only a small proportion of 8%[h] having significant social-emotional difficulties
> Parents may rate child as showing significantly less social competence, but comparable to normal adolescents in involvement in activities[e]

Potential for Excellence

(Few studies have investigated areas of excellence)

Some excel in communication-related activities (e.g., debate, organization leadership, drama activities)[h]

Some attend college, finish a BA or BS degree, and attend graduate school[f] (all of the 18 young adults in the Iowa study[f] either finished high school or were still attending)

---

[a] Scarborough & Dobrich (1990). 4 children, evaluated at 2:6 years; 5 years; end of grade 2.

[b] Schery (1985). 718 children, originally identified at 3:1–16:4 years. At 8 years, records reviewed. Correlates of improvement over 2- to 3-year period studied.

[c] Stark et al. (1984). 29 specifically language-impaired (SLI) children, identified at 4:6–8 years; evaluated at 8–12 years.

[d] Bishop & Edmundson (1987). 68 SLI children (19 more with low nonverbal IQs and "general delays"), evaluated at 4; 4:6; 5:6 years.

[e] Aram, Ekelman, & Nation (1984). 20 adolescents originally identified as preschoolers with language disabilities, evaluated +10 years later.

[f] Hall & Tomblin (1978). 18 adults with language impairments (LI) evaluated in early elementary years (compared with 18 adults with artic. imp. evaluated in early elementary years); 13- to 20-year follow up interviews with parents.

[g] Aram & Nation (1980). 63 children, identified at <5 years; evaluated at 9 years (included children with multiple problems).

[h] R.R. King, Jones, & Lasky (1982). 50 adolescents (did not exclude motor, hearing, intellectual deficits); identified as preschoolers; +15-year follow-up interviews with mothers.

remained seriously detached from their social environment and who were loners tended to have the worst prognosis. Other negative indicators were cognitive functioning below the educable level of mental retardation and the failure to develop functional language by age 5. (This cutoff of 5 years is commonly cited as the point beyond which speech is unlikely to develop in children with autism; this does not mean, however, that augmentative and alternative communication techniques should not be used with nonspeaking autistic children before the age of 5.)

In a review of other studies concerning prognosis for children with autism, Ornitz and Ritvo (1976) reported that 7% to 28% of these children develop seizures before age 18 and that 75% are likely to be assessed as mentally retarded throughout life. They also found that severe social and interpersonal problems were likely to continue even among those persons with autism who made considerable improvement.

The prognosis for other children with severe cognitive and multiple handicaps is also limited. DeMyer, Hingtgen, and Jackson (1981) summarized the results of six longitudinal studies of children with severe and multiple disorders (including autism) and found overall outcome judgments reported with the following ranges of proportions: 5% to 19%, "good outcome" (defined as borderline normal): 16% to 27%, "fair outcome"; and 55% to 74%, "poor outcome."

Not all sources agree that the picture is so bleak for children with autism. For the most part, the picture emerging from the literature is highly consistent with a limited prognosis determined largely by the individual's cognitive function level and especially by the language function level in the preschool years. Although most children with autism grow up with continued severe disabilities, some exceptions do occur (Lovaas, 1987). Reports of dramatic results of facilitated communication therapy for some individuals with autism (Biklen, 1990) also lead to new questions about establishing prognosis for this group.

When language disorder accompanies hearing impairment. The general prognostic picture for children with hearing impairments is also integrally tied to their prognosis for language improvement. Unfortunately, the picture is not too promising for many children with profound, congenital hearing losses in spite of recent advances in education, speech and hearing sciences, and communication engineering

(Osberger, 1986). For these children, a consistent finding has been the failure to reach a level of functional literacy (fourth-grade reading level) by the time they graduate from high school.

As for children with autism, language skill plays a significant role as a prognostic indicator for children with hearing impairment. Goldgar and Osberger (1986), in a multivariate analysis of 150 students (90 boys and 60 girls) from a state school for the deaf, found that "language, particularly expressive language, is the major determinant of academic achievement in the sample studied" (p. 87). Those authors also noted that receptive language plays a role as well, and that their study provided further statistical evidence for the interrelation of expressive and receptive skills. Nevertheless, expressive measures correlated more highly with academic achievement than receptive measures did. Interestingly, two results that were not highly correlated with academic achievement were speech intelligibility and degree of hearing loss. Visual perceptual skills were significantly correlated to academic achievement. Some children with profound hearing losses also have learning disabilities, but Goldgar and Osberger noted the difficulty of separating the influences of hearing loss and learning disability.

The prognosis may not be equally limited for all children with profound hearing impairments. In a separate study of adolescent children with profound losses, Geers and Moog (1989) confirmed that English language competence is the highest predictor of achievement in the acquisition of advanced literacy skills for students in oral/aural programs. In contrast with the generally accepted results for students with this level of hearing loss as reaching a plateau in reading at about the third-grade level (Schildroth & Karchmer, 1986), the mean reading level demonstrated by these students was eighth grade. Other positive prognostic indicators for this group included "at least average nonverbal intellectual ability, early oral education management and auditory stimulation, and middle-class family environment with strong family support" (p. 84).

One of the most significant questions facing families and teachers of children with profound hearing impairments is their prognosis for acquiring functional spoken language. For some families, decisions are guided by strong philosophical stances either for an exclusively oral or a total communication approach. Others seek professional guidance about methods that might be best for their child. To establish a prognosis for the acquisition of spoken language and to select the most appropriate communication modes for educating a particular hearing impaired child, Geers and Moog (1987) devised a Spoken Language Predictor (SLP) Index. They designed the SLP to overcome some of the limitations noted in the more commonly used Deafness Management Quotient (DMQ; Northern & Downs, 1984). To aid decision making, points are assigned in each of five areas: (1) hearing, further subdivided into ratings of speech reception capability and aided articulation index; (2) language, assigned a percentile ranking on a test standardized on hearing impaired children; (3) a nonverbal intelligence quotient; (4) family support, rated subjectively; and (5) the child's own speech communication attitude. Based on points assigned in these five areas, a recommendation is made either for speech emphasis, provisional speech instruction, or sign language emphasis.

When language disorder follows acquired brain injury. Another group of children for whom determining prognosis is difficult but important is the group with acquired brain injuries. As discussed in Chapter 4, the prognosis for children with well-defined lesions of cerebrovascular origin is usually quite good (although some children may have severe persistent reading difficulties). The prognosis for children with acquired seizure disorders, however, varies widely, and the picture for children with traumatic brain injuries is not clear at all.

Summarizing the literature regarding the prognosis for expressive language recovery following traumatic brain injury in childhood, T. F. Campbell and Dollaghan (1990) found it to be limited in several ways, including: (1) a lack of longitudinally gathered detailed data, (2) a relatively narrow range of verbal abilities sampled (usually in nonnaturalistic contexts), and (3) a lack of information about concomitant variables that may affect outcome such as age, cause, associated neurological disturbance, duration of coma, and preinjury cognitive and academic status. Campbell and Dollaghan, using multiple measures of language recovery, found that children and adolescents with severe brain trauma, as a group, improved on the majority of measures, but individual variability was considerable, and only a few reached the levels of their control subjects. The authors concluded that the prognosis for clinically significant improvement among children and

adolescents with severe acquired brain injuries is quite good, but some deficits in expressive skills may remain apparent up to at least 12 months following injury.

Remembering individual differences. The contrasts reported for children with various types of problems show that the apparent prognosis for a large group of children may not accurately represent the actual prognosis for a particular child. These contrasts also suggest that prognosis can be influenced by more than variables within the child. (Remember the refrain, problems are not just within children, and neither are the solutions.) In fact, a major question might be "How does the mode or frequency of treatment influence the prognosis for improvement for a particular child or group of children?"

The difficulty is that this question is much more readily answered for individual children than for groups of children. That is one reason why no large-scale research studies of treatment efficacy have appeared in the literature. As Bishop and Edmundson (1987) pointed out, it is virtually impossible to interpret research results from large-group studies that attempt to correlate amount of treatment with the degree of improvement. For example, consider how decisions are made about who gets how much treatment. In most cases, children with the most severe language problems receive more intensive language intervention treatment (except, perhaps, for children with severe multiple impairments, whose programs are discussed in Chapter 7). The children with the most severe problems also tend to have the worst prognosis. Therefore, it is easy to imagine how thoroughly confounded the two variables must be in most large-scale longitudinal studies. Therefore, and because of the questionable ethics associated with withholding a desirable treatment, demonstration of treatment efficacy will continue to rely primarily on individual and small-group studies with single-subject designs.

Parting advice. Establishing prognosis is more than a scientific endeavor, or even a clinical one. It brings a lot of emotional baggage, for both the professional and the family. Although establishing a prognosis is particularly challenging for new professionals, the significance of the process rarely escapes the attention of even the experienced practitioner. Even after many years of experience, I still view the establishment of prognosis as one of the most challenging parts of my professional practice, whether I am giving a legal deposition about a child who was head injured in a vehicular accident or talking privately with parents. Perhaps this is because I am aware of the potential that prognosis not only may predict the future but also may influence it.

I have had to examine my own philosophy regarding the more subjective elements associated with establishing a prognosis. I offer a bit of advice in two of those areas. Both relate to the broader advice for focusing on the overall picture and not only the close-up. The first has to do with hope and the second has to do with quality of life.

Whenever a person makes an educated guess about prognosis for a particular individual (and that is all it really is), the foremost concern should be sensitivity to the needs of the real people involved in a real-life situation. Perhaps one of the worst things you can ever do to people is take away their hope. Therefore, a portion of this parting advice is to use the data presented here for what they are, but not to give them more credit than they deserve. This requires a careful balancing of what we usually think of as "objective realism" with positive expectation. None of us knows for sure the outcome for a particular child or even an adolescent. It does no harm to acknowledge this, especially when one must convey a discouraging prognosis to parents. In those cases, I try to give parents the most honest picture I can in a way that leaves a window of hope. All of us can hope for a better outcome than we expect.

The same philosophy applies when children have mild-to-moderate disabilities. It is illustrated in this sample of clinical discourse that might be used when talking to the parents of a preschooler with moderate language difficulties:

> You asked about the future. Based on experience with other children like Jeremy, we find that at least half of them continue to have some problems with their language all the way through school. We also know that learning to read is especially difficult for many children who have had language disorders like Jeremy's, even when their speech starts to sound better. So we will have to watch out for that and try to do some things to prevent problems as much as we can.
>
> But you should also know that, even with continuing language problems, most kids like Jeremy can graduate from high school and some even go to college. A lot depends on the things that all of us, including Jeremy, do from now on. And the better Jeremy feels about himself, the more he'll be able to give all he has at each

step along the way. The challenge we all will face is to keep expectations high without placing unrealistic pressure on Jeremy. *The* most important contribution that parents can make to this whole procedure is to convey to their child a sense of their unconditional love. He also needs to know that you respect his efforts, no matter how small.

The problem is that too often professionals get the idea that they are being unprofessional unless they are absolutely objective (usually interpreted as conservative) about the prognosis for improvement, but they fail to notice that prognosis is a subjective process based on value judgments. It is a value judgment that prognosis usually is expressed in normative terms based on formal test results. It is a value judgment that leads "good outcome" to be defined as "normal functioning." Now, do not misunderstand these comments. I doubt that anyone would disagree that normal functioning (or above) is good in most cases. A problem results, however, when judgments of quality of life become so thoroughly intertwined with judgments of normal functioning that persons with severe limitations can never be expected to have a "good outcome." Outcome is a value judgment. Who is to say that the set of values used for judging outcome should not be redefined? Then a person who can act appropriately and participate in society (no matter how limited) might be judged as having a "good outcome"? Who is to say that values other than normative ones are important not only in some cases, but in all?

Using Assessment to Outline the Parameters of Impairment, Disability, and Handicap

The preceding questions about value judgments recall the purpose of assessment that relates to defining impairment, disability, and handicap for individuals (defined in Chapter 1). It is not easy to keep all three aspects in mind at once; it is far easier to slip into a more unitary focus, partially because the unitary focus on impairment is traditional in both clinical and special education practices. The medical roots of speech–language pathology were transplanted from clinics to schools in the early days of the profession (L. Miller, 1989). Thus, the traditional focus was based on the medical model—diagnosis and treatment, with cure the ultimate goal. Murray-Seegert (1989) described a similar focus among special educators regarding persons with multiple handicaps:

For reasons having to do with the history of mental retardation, medical and psychological theories dominate current thought on disability, shaping both our professional vocabulary and the goals of our interventions. Because of this heritage, the special education and rehabilitation literature tends to focus on problems within the individual child—encouraging teachers and therapists to "diagnose" difficulties and "prescribe" solutions—while largely ignoring the ways in which sociocultural elements of the child's environment may *make* an impairment into a handicap. (p. xi)

A comprehensive approach does more. It is guided by not just one, but three questions: (1) What is wrong (and right) here? (2) What are this person's needs? (3) What are the attitudes of others around this person that influence the person's opportunities to participate?

Describing impairment. Answering the first question—what is wrong (and right) here—is still one of the most important functions of assessment. Newer approaches generally build on old ones and rarely replace them.

Consider, first, the traditional approach. For the most part, the traditional practice of speech–language pathology, as mentioned, has been aimed as identifying, analyzing, labeling, and "fixing" (whenever possible) impairments within individual children. Based on this approach, context, if considered at all, is viewed as a set of confounding variables that must somehow be stripped away, or at least controlled, so that the "real" problem, which is assumed to underly the daily symptoms, can be treated.

Using this approach, the evaluation context must be standardized so that a particular child can be compared to a normative sample of children who have taken the same test under similar conditions. If the child being tested happens to speak a different language or a different dialect of English, we know that we are in trouble, but all too often, the only available solutions are inadequate. We end up either under-compensating, by attributing all variation from the norm to language disorder (failing to account for possible influences of language difference), or overcompensating, by attributing all assessed difficulties to dialect or language difference (failing to identify a language disorder when one actually exists) (S. L. Terrell & Terrell, 1983).

Once a child is identified, the next most important task is to gather information for planning intervention. When using the communication processes model (Beukelman & Mirenda, 1988), the specialist generally

assesses the various components of language to identify areas of relative impairment or strength, then targets the weakest areas (usually) for intervention. Assessment continues as the program progresses, until finally, targeted skills are judged close enough to developmental expectations that intervention is no longer needed.

How does one decide which "communication processes" to evaluate and target? The answer to that question differs based on the choice of theoretical model driving the program. For example, as discussed earlier in this chapter, if the primary theoretical model is linguistic, targeted areas will relate to language content, form, and use (or phonology, morphology, syntax, semantics, and pragmatics). Under a behavioral model, assessment will entail a search for behaviors that should be increased or decreased and for conditions that seem to be reinforcing for the child. In an information processing model, language comprehension and expression might be targeted (perhaps defined by modality into areas of listening, speaking, reading, and writing), as well as specific memory and perceptual processes. With a cognitive model, basic concepts might be targeted for a preschooler, or higher level thinking skills for an adolescent, but establishing developmental levels across several domains is likely to be a priority. If the driving model is a social interaction one, the targets will more likely be demonstrations of the child's ability to use language appropriately and flexibly in a variety of contexts.

The tools used to conduct these varied assessments will also vary depending on their purposes. A combination of formal and informal methods usually will be used. Remember that an eclectic model involves blending positive aspects from more than one approach into a whole that works best for the situation at hand, taking care to ensure that the approach is not fragmented. This is part of the danger Damico (1988) identified as the "fragmentation fallacy," discussed in Chapter 1. Norris and Hoffman (1990a) also expressed a concern with a "discrete communication skills" approach, noting that it tends to result in an adult (usually a speech–language pathologist) identifying "a specific communicative behavior and [providing] activities designed to elicit and reinforce the target skill" (p. 28).

Recent modifications in the communication processes model of assessment involve attempts to manage multiple pieces of information in different domains simultaneously. Context is the added concern during assessment. The key question becomes not just "What is wrong?" but "What is wrong (and right) with the way this individual's communicative processes function in these varied contexts?" Professionals working in the newer model still may form specific hypotheses about varied elements of an individual's neurolinguistic and neuromotor systems, knowledge of linguistic rules, stimulus–response–reinforcement patterns, information processing abilities, cognitive abilities, and social interaction attributes. They may even test aspects of those hypotheses in relative isolation from each other, but they recognize that doing so implies a special set of contextual concerns, and they never fail also to observe how the system works when it is integrated with contexts relevant to the client.

Describing disability. Remember that definitions of disability are relative to the demands of contexts. Therefore, any attempt to define disability must first involve an inventory of the contexts important to the child. Some consideration of ways to decide what contexts might be important for a particular child were discussed in Chapter 5. Taking natural contexts into account does more than simply extend the focus of language assessment efforts. It moves the process into a communication needs model (Beukelman & Mirenda, 1988) of assessment. Here, the definition of what communicative skills should be assessed becomes a function of the expectations of the contexts identified as important. Instead of treating "context as if it were the enemy of understanding rather than the resource for understanding which it is in our everyday lives" (Mishler, 1979, p. 2), it becomes an integral part of the assessment process.

When we evaluate children with an eye not only to ferreting out impairments, but also to identifying interactions of competencies with contextual demands to yield functional performance, we become more relevant.

For example, consider the needs of a child with wobbly language competencies and ADHD who is having difficulty comprehending what to do when faced with complex teacher language in a classroom full of acoustic, cognitive, and social-emotional "noise." The assessment of this child's needs might include an observation of interactions of curricular demands and the oral communication ecology of the classroom with what is known about the child's

impairments in other contexts. One goal of the assessment might be to look for factors that may particularly facilitate or disrupt successful processing, perhaps extending from linguistic complexity to acoustic clarity to what is known about the child's understanding of subordinating conjunctions. This example includes elements aimed at identifying areas of impairment that might be treated as well as areas of disability that might be reduced through intervention. It also relates closely to modifying attitudes that contribute to the level of handicap experienced by this child.

Describing handicap. The phrase *describing handicap* refers to the need to consider attitudes and opportunities when conducting an individualized assessment and to the subjective nature of "being handicapped." This aspect of assessment is probably better described as the search for ways to increase opportunities for participation.

This portion of assessment is motivated by the participation model described by Beukelman and Mirenda (1988). It aims to identify and modify levels of opportunity. In relation to previous examples, this means analyzing the contexts in which the child already participates and collaborating with others to try to identify how the child might participate more. It is highly consistent with a social interaction theoretical model.

For example, assessment might focus on increasing the child's opportunity to participate in successfully completing class assignments by designing a backup system to ensure that he gets the assignments and understands them. An assignment notebook (Pidek, 1987) could be provided for traveling between school and home, and a "buddy" strategy could be used to allow the student to check understanding of assignments in the classroom.

Selecting Goal Areas and Gathering Baseline Data

Assessment and intervention are thoroughly integrated processes. Evaluating language and communicative skills in contexts ranging from formal tests to naturalistic samples provides a wealth of information that can be used to establish goals. Sometimes such a comprehensive approach can yield so much information that it becomes overwhelming. I then remind myself that I do not need to know everything there is to know about a child to be relevant to his needs. I can also collaborate with others to pool our information. It is enough to have a clear idea of the child's present functioning in a variety of areas, to have a sense of the priorities of others who know the child well, and to have an idea of how much the child can participate in those contexts identified as important. At this stage of the process, knowing the priorities is more important than knowing the details

Shifting focus when writing goals and objectives. Difference in scope is one of the major distinctions between goals and objectives. Goals nail down the essential elements of the big picture. Objectives specify aspects of change targeted within it. To keep the scope appropriately broad when establishing goals, I often encourage speech–language pathologists to think of goals as *goal areas* (N. W. Nelson, 1988b) for laying out the horizontal scope of a program, whereas sequences of objectives define aspects of a program's vertical dimensions. Goals address the question "What should we work on?" Objectives address the question "How will we know the program is working?"

Goals are established first. Hopefully, they emerge as a result of the collaborative process encouraged throughout this book. Deciding on goal areas requires a group of people to meet to identify areas most in need of focus. The meeting may also validate areas that might have been identified by particular professionals as part of the more general assessment process.

A variety of strategies can be used for selecting goal areas. Decisions often involve selecting areas that are (1) most impaired, (2) most obvious, (3) earliest in a developmental sequence, (4) most amenable to treatment, (5) most functional, (6) most critically needed at the moment, or (7) identified as highest priority by the parent, teacher, or child.

Although the application of varied criteria may yield slightly different recommendations about potential goals areas, usually some fairly strong convergence results. Remember that it is fine to think about goals as relatively broad areas. Goals may be expressed as loosely as expecting "improvement" in a particular area (a looseness that would not pass muster for operationally defined objectives). For example, a group of participants might decide that a child needs to work on listening comprehension and direction following, vocabulary acquisition (relational terms in particular), and narrative organization. These then become the specific goal areas for the language intervention programs designed to complement comprehensive programming efforts to help this child become more successful in school.

Some goal areas may be more context bound than others; that is all right. It is a natural outcome of the three-dimensional framework discussed here. Although all of the goal areas may be heavily influenced by communicative and linguistic behaviors, some may be a little fuzzy around the borders that connect one professional discipline to another; that is all right, too. The language specialist most responsible for seeing that these goals are met is usually a speech–language pathologist, but considerable overlap with needs addressed by a variety of other professionals may occur.

The point to be remembered here is that when a collaborative process is used for mutual goal setting, the members perceive that they can obtain their goals if and only if other participants also obtain theirs. When professionals consult with each other in a truly transdisciplinary program, they are conscious of working toward the same goals (although they may divide the work up a bit). When issues of overlap and redundancy do arise, systems work best when a mechanism is in place to resolve them directly. As might be expected, this approach takes both time and work, along with an excellent set of people skills, but it can be extremely satisfying to all involved when it works properly.

Another reason that it is advisable to state goals simply is that they are easier to remember. I believe that clients with the potential to understand their own goal areas should know what those goal areas are. If possible, they will have participated in establishing them. I often ask clients, "Now what are we working on here?" "What are you trying to get better at?" Then, I help them to rearticulate their goals in a way that is meaningful to them. I find that this kind of metacognitive strategy helps them to feel a sense of control and responsibility for their own improvement.

In contrast with the loose way in which goals are stated, objectives must be stated more precisely. They are sometimes called behavioral objectives or performance objectives because they operationally define performance such that they can be used to measure change. Although some objective writing systems require as many as six or seven components, I find that three-component model usually suffices. Using this approach, each objective specifies

(1) what the child will do, (2) under what conditions, and (3) how well.

The *do* statement is especially important. It must be written in terms of the child's behavior (not the clinician's; it is not a description of procedure, although it may imply procedure), and it must be written in terms of observable behavior. Although writing a *do* statement in behavioral terms might seem to predispose the intervention process to a behaviorist model, the statement can be consistent with describing desired change based on any of the models. Even "hidden processes" can be targeted; if they are, some plan must be established to identify when they have occurred based on observable indicators. For example, a *do* statement may indicate that a child will "answer questions to demonstrate comprehension," or "keep his body and eyes oriented toward the teacher to demonstrate attention."

In a sequence of objectives, the *do* statements may be written to specify behaviors of increasing variety, length, fluency, complexity, abstraction, or sophistication as the program proceeds. The type of shift specified will depend on the type of knowledge, skill, or strategy being targeted. Sometimes, rather than shifting the *do* statement over time to indicate progress, the conditions statements or criteria statements are shifted to document change.

The conditions statement establishes the context in which the desired new behavior will be demonstrated. I have repeatedly emphasized the importance of context. When specified in a sequence of objectives, context may be a major element in determining whether or not a child will be able to demonstrate a desired behavior. Both linguistic (e.g., "in words," "in complex sentences") and social interaction contexts (e.g., "in social conversational with friends," "when reading aloud in the classroom") may be specified. The conditions statements in a series of objectives will likely reflect the outcome of assessment activities that have identified linguistic and social interaction contexts in which the child appears more or less disabled.

The usual procedure is to sequence objectives so that contextual demands become increasingly intense over time. Part of the influence of social interaction theory, however, has been to suggest that it is counterproductive to remove a desired behavior from natural contexts in the early stages of intervention with the intention of targeting it later in more natural contexts. Such a strategy contributes to widely recognized problems of generalization. Although some theorists might argue that a behavior should never be targeted outside its natural context, a less radical alternative is to specify a target behavior within its linguistic context, and then to identify several different social interaction contexts in which the desired behavior may be targeted at the same point of the program, that is, in a horizontal arrangement rather than a vertical one. This strategy, illustrated in Figure 6.6, may involve the expectation that the child will use the targeted communicative skill in an individual interaction with the language specialist, and in the same day, will use the skill when interacting socially with peers. This differs from the old approach of attempting to perfect a new skill in an isolated setting before sending the child out into the real world. Instead, the assistance of other participants is enlisted to monitor change beyond the walls of the isolated speech room.

The statement that quantifies how well a child will perform a particular skill, demonstrate knowledge, or use a strategy is the criterion statement. How it is written will depend on the nature of the targeted change and how much evidence the language specialist feels is necessary to be confident that the objective has been met. The criterion statement should be written with enough precision to allow the professional to identify when it has been met. Frequently used choices are (1) percentages, (2) ratios, (3) frequencies, and (4) duration. Each has its advantages for specifying different kinds of change.

Establishing baselines.   After identifying the goal areas, the language specialist should explore each in a little more detail than the initial evaluation may have permitted. In my experience, three goal areas are the right amount for most children. Of course, more areas, or less, may be targeted, and that is sometimes appropriate. I find, however, that four areas become a little hard to manage and that most children have more than one or two areas of need.

A baseline is established by carefully describing a problem area as it exists before intervention or before a particular phase of intervention. The description usually is both quantitative and qualitative. The qualitative description is parallel to the statements included in performance objectives, except the baseline statements specify *what is*, rather than *what is desired*. Baseline statements are written in terms of observable behaviors (again, possibly used as indices

FIGURE 6.6
A set of short-term instructional objectives.

LANGUAGE USE: CONVERSATIONAL DISCOURSE

CHILD: _____ AGE: _____ SCHOOL: _____ GRADE/LEVEL: _____ Date: _____

SPEECH-LANGUAGE PATHOLOGIST: _____ OTHERS IMPLEMENTING OBJECTIVES: _____

GOAL: The child will demonstrate skill for taking conversational turns, and for initiating, maintaining, changing, and concluding topics and conversations.

PRESENT LEVELS OF PERFORMANCE:

PART A. CONVERSATIONAL STRUCTURE

SHORT-TERM OBJECTIVES:

THE CHILD WILL:	CONVERSATIONAL CONTEXT											COMMENTS/ TECHNIQUES/ EVALUATION
	Practice Conv. with speech-language pathologist		Spontaneous Conv. with speech-language pathologist		Conv. with Adult Other than speech-language pathologist		Conv. with Peer		Conv. with Group of 2 or More Peers		
	Date In.	Date Accom.	Date In.	Date Accom.	Date In.	Date Accom.	Date In.	Date Accom.	Date In.	Date Accom.	
1. demonstrate ability to initiate, and to respond appropriately when others initiate *conversational openings*, by demonstrating each of the following skills (each behavior observed in 3 separate conversations):											
a. give attention when it is requested with verbal and nonverbal cues, by establishing eye contact, moving into proximity (if necessary and appropriate), and orienting body toward speaker;											
b. get attention from prospective listener by using appropriate verbal (such as *Hi! Got a minute? What are you doing?*) and nonverbal cues along with proximity and orienting strategies;											
c. maintain attention during a 2- to 3-turn exchange;											
d. maintain attention during conversation on several topics of 2 to 3 turns each;											
e. maintain attention during an extended conversation on a topic (at least 7 turns);											
f. maintain attention during a conversation in which the topic is changed at least 2 times.											

Note. From *Planning Individualized Speech and Language Intervention Programs* (p. 274), Revised and Expanded, by Nickola Wolf Nelson, copyright 1988 by Communication Skill Builders, Inc., PO Box 42050, Tucson, AZ 85733. Reprinted by permission.

of deeper processes), and they describe both linguistic and nonlinguistic context variables. Several different descriptions of the appearance of a targeted communication skill in several different contexts therefore may be required. The specialist should quantify the targeted knowledge, skill, or strategy.

Naturalistic observation is the only way to develop a baseline against which progress in "real-life" situations can be judged. Nevertheless, it is sometimes helpful to establish a more formal test–retest approach to measure progress, particularly when targeting a skill, such as sound–symbol association, rather than, for example, lexical knowledge or a metacognitive strategy for taking tests, which tend to be more contextually bound. When formal procedures are used, however, the language specialist must keep in mind psychometric concerns about how frequently the same test can be readministered. Contrived tasks should use a different set of stimuli than those used in the pretest format so that the specialist can determine whether generalization is occurring.

Professional judgment is required to decide how much time should be spent in gathering baseline information. Cost–benefit analyses must be made. Although scientific procedure dictates that baseline data should be gathered over several observation points until reliability (stability over time) can be established, it is usually neither feasible nor desirable to spend too much time gathering additional assessment data before beginning intervention. Some baseline information, however, must be gathered (usually in more than one context), and the data should make up a valid representation of the targeted behavior.

The method of gathering baseline information will set the stage for similar observations at the end of the intervention period. Perhaps at the end of a school grading period or as specified in an IFSP or IEP, the targeted behavior will be observed again under the same conditions to judge progress. The new description should compare favorably with the old in that the observed behavior will represent an advance, or it may appear under new more demanding conditions, or it may be appearing more frequently, or less, as specified.

Identifying the developing edge of competence. Part of the intent in gathering baseline information is to identify what I call the *developing edge of competence*. Finding it can assist the professional to know where to begin to focus, or how to arrange contextual

conditions, when attempting to facilitate change. In almost any goal area, children can already demonstrate some behaviors (or linguistic rules) that are so firmly established that they are unlikely to disappear even under the most demanding conditions. At the other extreme, some behaviors or linguistic rules in the same domain are simply beyond the child's current capabilities. Somewhere in the middle is a developing edge of competence in which abilities wobble. In this area of complexity, the child can either demonstrate only part of the desired behavior or can demonstrate it only under some conditions. It is highly contextually dependent performance. Remember Sheldon White's (1980) description of children with wobbly competencies (from Chapter 2):

> A child is not a computer that either "knows" or "does not know." A child is a bumpy, blippy, excitable, fatiguable, distractible, active, friendly, mulish, semi-cooperative, bundle of biology. Some factors help a moving child pull together coherent address to a problem; others hinder that pulling together and tend to make a child "not know." (p. 43)

In this region, the developing edge of competence, intervention efforts are most likely to bear fruit. It is part of a contextually based intervention program to identify factors that tend to help a child pull together a new behavior or set of behaviors and make them work and then to use those factors as part of the intervention plan.

Designing and Implementing an Intervention Plan

Matching purpose, type, content, and contexts of intervention. Designing and implementing an intervention plan requires a careful juggling of many factors. A major premise of this book is that no one type of intervention plan is right for all children. Chapters 7 to 9 are devoted to discussions of assessment and intervention content and contexts that are specific to early, middle, and later stages of language acquisition. This division is motivated primarily by a developmental perspective, but each of the other theoretical perspectives can be used as well when planning and implementing activities, depending on a particular child's individualized needs.

To achieve flexible programming to fit children's needs, it helps to remember that objectives and activities are not in a one-to-one relationship. Several different activities may be used to work on the same objective and the same activity can be used to work on several different objectives.

Remember also that in normal development children do not often (if ever) set out on a path to master one morphological or syntactic rule at a time and then practice that particular structure until they master it. For example, when acquiring irregular forms, normally developing children may go through a phase, first, of correctly producing irregular plurals like "feet," apparently as unanalyzed imitations. Then they seem to recognize them as plurals and produce overregularized forms like "foots" or "feets," before finally learning the exceptions to this rule and settling back into "feet." Meanwhile, children may be moving toward maturity in using other forms and structures while working this form through its stages. They may seem to stay at one level for weeks before making the next linguistic discovery.

Recognizing the cyclical nature of this normal developmental process, Hodson and Paden (1983) designed cyclical scheduling for their phonological intervention approach. Although this technique has been used less frequently to introduce other linguistic goals in therapy, Fey (1986) suggested that a similar cyclical approach might be used for other interventions.

Almost any intervention program includes both horizontal and vertical elements (see Figure 6.7). As discussed in the section on establishing goals and objectives, when more than one goal area is targeted at the same time, those areas constitute a horizontal focus. Within each area, however, clinicians generally plan a set of objectives they wish to accomplish as they move vertically through that goal area (federal monitors usually look for two or three). Vertical program sequences are determined by gradual incre-

FIGURE 6.7
Combined horizontal and vertical organization of goals and objectives.

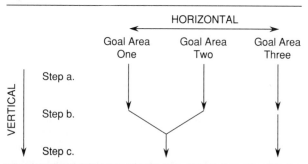

ments based on factors such as developmental order, linguistic complexity, or linguistic abstraction. Objectives from each of the horizontal goals areas may also be integrated with those from other targeted areas in the same intervention contexts to encourage "carryover" into natural settings.

Another set of concerns when balancing intervention plans involves relationships between standards and work. Because language intervention specialists have traditionally introduced a speech and language curriculum in addition to the school curriculum and often do not give grades, academic standards have been less a matter of focus for speech–language pathologists than for other special educators. Standards become an important issue when the language specialist consults with the classroom teacher or assumes responsibility for teaching some of the academic curriculum to the student (e.g., G. M. Anderson & Nelson, 1988; L. P. Hoffman, 1990; Simon, 1987).

Often in the past when children have been "mainstreamed" into regular classrooms, the overriding concern has been keeping them busy. Either children were given a special set of busy work activities with little relevance to the activities of the rest of the class, or they were expected to do all of the regular class work but not to be too successful at it. In contrast, Beukelman and Mirenda (1992) suggested that the goal for competitive participation for students who use augmentative and alternative communication (AAC) systems in regular classrooms should be to meet the standards using modified activities and workloads, not to meet modified standards based on the same workload as peers. This option might be more appropriate for many children with special needs, not just those with physical impairments.

Fostering a better match between children and contexts (making choices about methods). Reducing the amount of work expected of a student with motor, cognitive, or linguistic abilities, but keeping standards for quality high is one way to foster a better match between children and contexts. Part of helping children to succeed in the important contexts of their lives involves attempts to change them, for example, by helping them to acquire new lexical knowledge, new ability to use particular linguistic rules, or new strategies for using knowledge they already have. Another part involves attempts to change the context to foster a better match.

Box 6.2   Decision-making continua that influence the choice of intervention methods, targets, and contexts when designing programs for children

Task analysis ↔ Developmental sequence ↔ Contextually based needs

Adult-centered ↔ Child-centered

Highly structured ↔ Nurturant-naturalistic

Direct ↔ Indirect

Discrete skills ↔ Holistic

Pullout ↔ Integrated

Decisions may be easier to make when they are visualized as moving in one direction or another on a continuum. Box 6.2 summarizes several different continua that involve decision making about service provision. The interrelation of these elements on the continuum are discussed more fully in the following sections.

Direct control of task complexity.   Special education and language intervention approaches have tended to develop as separate pullout experiences partly because separation creates greater opportunity to control task complexity than that in integrated settings, where children presumably have experienced difficulty. Several variables that can be manipulated directly to make a task more or less complex are illustrated in Figure 6.8. It is important to remember, however, that setting up communicative events with specially engineered contextual characteristics may remove events so much from their natural contexts that newly acquired behaviors may depend totally on those special contexts and may fail to generalize. Working within natural contexts, keeping experiences as intact as possible, and monitoring targeted changes within those more naturalistic experiences therefore are desired techniques.

Using mediated experiences and scaffolding.   The use of more naturalistic experiences is an alternative to designing special tasks for intervention. These experiences should be mediated for the child to intensify aspects targeted in the intervention plan. Intervention strategies of this type have been modeled, to some extent, on the parents' role in normal language acquisition.

Bruner (1978, 1983) described ways in which parents build scaffolds by controlling linguistic and nonlinguistic contextual variables to make new information and behaviors accessible to their children.

Snow (1983) noted that parents use similar interaction techniques when guiding their children through early book reading and other literacy experiences, including semantic contingency strategies for staying on topics the child introduces, scaffolding for structuring and constraining the demands of the activity, accountability procedures for requiring that a child contribute to or complete tasks at the child's level of capability, and routines for presenting new content within the structure of highly predictable interaction patterns. Teachers also sometimes use mediation and scaffolding strategies when they help children individually with problems in completing assignments or when they read a passage from a textbook, by asking leading questions and by emphasizing particular content before having children read the passage themselves (Applebee & Langer, 1983; Cazden, 1988).

The mediated approach moves away, however, from the structured stimulus–response–reinforcement paradigm typical of formal behavior modification sessions and classroom teaching. In mediated learning, the adult approaches the interaction with specific objectives in mind, but acts as a participant or co-learner in problem solving with the child, rather than as a traditional "teacher." The adult intentionally looks for opportunities within naturally occurring contexts to frame aspects of events and to focus the child's attention and efforts to elicit targeted behaviors that enable the child to master these behaviors.

Mediated learning strategies (Feuerstein, 1979) are based largely in the social interaction theory contributions of Vygotsky (1978). Vygotsky said that children learn all psychological function through interaction with a more competent member of their culture who controls tasks to be consistent with what he called the child's "zone of proximal development" (similar to what I call the developing edge of competence).

FIGURE 6.8
Task variables that can be controlled in direct treatment approaches.

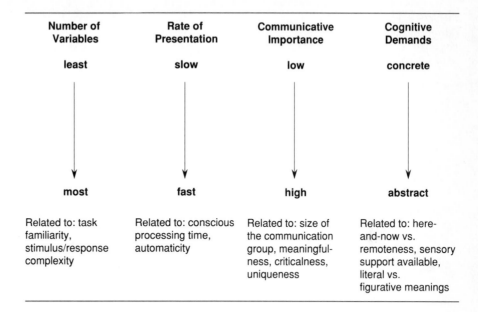

Number of Variables	Rate of Presentation	Communicative Importance	Cognitive Demands
least	slow	low	concrete
↓	↓	↓	↓
most	fast	high	abstract
Related to: task familiarity, stimulus/response complexity	Related to: conscious processing time, automaticity	Related to: size of the communication group, meaningfulness, criticalness, uniqueness	Related to: here-and-now vs. remoteness, sensory support available, literal vs. figurative meanings

This adult, or a more competent peer, initially provides a great deal of support to ensure the child's successful participation at an optimal level but gradually relinquishes control as the child assumes greater self-regulation capability for mediating his own behavior. Vygotsky defined this shift as transfer from interpsychological to intrapsychological functioning.

An advantage of the mediated approach is that it does not require analysis of tasks into small bits so that they can be presented in discrete units, later to be rebuilt into wholes. Instead, the adult may enter a naturally occurring holistic context with the child and make it manageable by framing certain aspects for the child's immediate attention and getting the child to begin to ask himself questions about what to do next.

When using this strategy, rather than preselecting all content for an intervention session, the adult follows the child's lead, making the approach more child initiated (Norris & Hoffman, 1990a, 1990b). For preschoolers, the adult may provide an interesting play setting with varied materials and areas and then let the child choose where to play. For school-age children, the adult may use the regular curriculum to provide the content and contexts for target skills work.

Using different kinds of methods for different kinds of problems. In their content–form–use model, L. Bloom and Lahey (1978; Lahey, 1988) provided a way to organize language intervention efforts based on children's specific needs. They argue that it makes more sense to consider individual differences based on needs and abilities in these three interacting systems of content, form, and use than to treat children differently based on their presenting conditions.

Different needs may justify different intervention methods. In their transactional model of child language, McLean and Snyder-McLean (1978) schematically illustrated (see Figure 6.9) the interactions of different motivating factors, contextual experiences, and elements within those experiences with the developing subsystems of language content, form, and function.

It is difficult to imagine a child with problems focused in language use progressing in a program that does not use social interactions as a primary intervention context. Language content problems signify a need for meaningful experiences as a way of developing world knowledge. Pulling language out of context likely would be counterproductive for these children. Other children—like Fey's (1986) active communicators and many children with the profile of specific language disorders, learning disabilities, and dyslexia (overlapping, not mutually exclusive categories)—have relatively more difficulty with language form than with its content and use. Some of these children seem to go merrily on their way, communicating fairly well although with a preponderance of content words supplemented by gestures, with syntax, morphology,

FIGURE 6.9
A transactional model of child
language, showing the interactions
of language content, form, and
function, with motivations and
contexts.

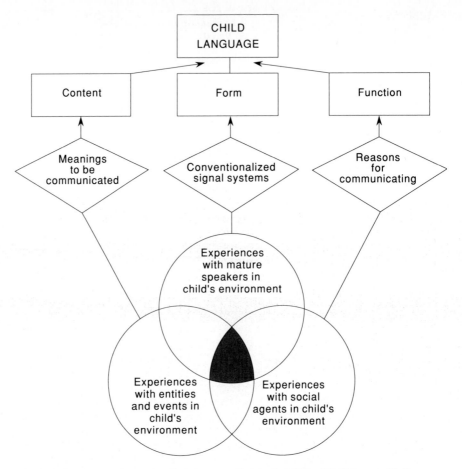

Note. From *Transactional Approach to Early Language Training* (p. 213) by J. E. McLean and L. K.
Snyder-McLean, 1978, Columbus, OH: Merrill-Macmillan. Copyright 1978 by Merrill-Macmillan. Reprinted
by permission of the authors.

and phonological maturity lagging far behind. For
these children, language intervention entirely in the
context of intact communicative situations may not
be the most efficient way to help them acquire
needed skills. Proficiency in language form seems to
require more practice than language content or use.

Somewhere along the line, however, *drill* became
a dirty word, mostly for good reasons but not necessarily for reasons that apply in all situations. Drill
is counterproductive when children have difficulty
understanding language and communication, learning
how to express their meanings and intentions, and
learning to understand the meanings and intentions
of others. When children have difficulty with motor
control of word articulation, when they need to

become more fluent and automatic in the inclusion of
certain morphemes or syntactic structures, or when
they have limited opportunity to practice those skills
in natural contexts, then specialized, highly structured
activities may be an important part of their intervention programs. In my experience, children with intact
cognitive abilities but specific expressive language
impairments particularly may benefit from more focused and intensive practice sessions. The decision of
whether to include practice sessions need not be of
the either/or variety. Remember that an eclectic approach might allow combinations of procedures, so
that when highly structured practice does seem in the
child's best interests, it can be combined with more
child-centered, naturalistic activities. Slobin's (1979)

Personal Reflection 6.6   "I am concerned about whether my 4-year-old daughter is getting the right kind of service. She can't talk (I've been told that she has developmental apraxia), but she can play quite well. Still, no one works directly with her speech. All they seem to do is work on teaching her to play."

Mother of a nonspeaking child expressing concerns about whether her daughter's needs are being met in her special education classroom.

observation that new forms are first used for old functions and that new functions are first served by old forms may guide intervention practices in this regard.

Keeping purpose clear. It will be easier to decide how to adjust a program for a particular child along each of the continua outlined in Box 6.2 if the purpose of intervention for that child is kept in mind. Chapter 1 considered a broad purpose for language intervention; changes are targeted in the communicative systems of individuals and in the important contexts of their lives, relevant to their needs for social appropriateness, acceptance and closeness; formal and informal learning; and gainful occupation (whether paid or unpaid).

Although the general long-term outcome goal may be communicative competence, many differences are based on individual factors, such as age, family constellation, associated causative conditions, needs, and abilities that differentiate the programming decisions for individual children. Wilcox (1989) noted that some of the differences also center whether the purpose of intervention is remediation, prevention, or compensation.

Traditionally, most goals of speech and language intervention and special education programs have been remedial. The usual strategy in a remedial program is to identify one or more areas of impairment, often by measuring delay or disorder in development against normative expectations, and then to design activities to help the child either acquire a new desirable behavior, eradicate undesirable behavior, or mitigate the effects of some long-term impairment that cannot be corrected. When mitigation is the intention, the program takes on the role of tertiary prevention (see discussion of prevention in Chapter 4).

Sometimes, particularly in infant programs, the major focus of the intervention is prevention. A preventive focus is most likely to be appropriate when some unalterable biological condition, such as brain

damage, Down's syndrome, or sensory or motor impairment places the infant at risk for developmental delay. Then, even though a disorder may not yet be apparent, services may be provided to influence other alterable aspects to reduce the likelihood that problems will develop or to lessen their severity (Wilcox, 1989). This focus might also be appropriate for preschoolers and kindergartners with specific language impairments who are at risk for reading disability, by intensifying their prereading "print literacy" (van Kleeck, 1990) experiences (e.g., by giving additional experiences with story structure and by deliberate exposure to print and writing, and perhaps by urging parents to watch Sesame Street with them, Mason, 1980).

Aspects of an impairment sometimes cannot be directly altered no matter how early services are provided and no matter how appropriate they are. For example, some persons with severe oral-motor deficits and some with profound hearing losses may never learn to speak intelligibly. These individuals, perhaps in addition to other remedial and preventive intervention efforts, need to be assisted to compensate for the areas of impairment. Compensatory efforts might include devices and strategies to meet needs in alternative ways. For example, an augmentative communication device for the child with cerebral palsy and an interpreter for the deaf child might enable them to participate in regular classrooms.

When the specialist considers all the ways that children's disabilities, handicaps, and impairments might be reduced, planning is more likely to involve more than one of these purposes. It is also more likely to be relevant to their lives and those of their families and teachers.

Monitoring Progress During Intervention

Many methods are available for marking progress during intervention. Progress is measured differently for different purposes. As part of the philosophical framework introduced in Chapter 1, I recommended taking both wide-angle and close-up views to build a comprehensive picture of effects in the child's life during intervention. This section further considers methods for measuring progress.

Keeping an eye on the forest. The big picture will stay in focus if the language specialist uses questions about disability (i.e., whether contextually based needs are being met), handicap (i.e., whether the right kinds of communicative opportunities are being provided), and impairment (i.e., whether specific communicative processes are changing) to guide progress measurement.

Relevant change. Professionals occasionally need to stand back and ask whether the changes occurring are relevant to the overall purposes of assisting clients to make changes relevant to their needs (needs to be socially appropriate and to have social closeness, to use language and communication skills for formal and informal learning, and to gainfully occupy their time). These questions are best addressed in collaboration with others in daily contact with the child and who know him well. The techniques used to answer these questions are usually interview and observation. It is difficult to use formal measurement techniques to get answers about relevance.

Functional outcomes. Another part of relevance can be assessed by documenting functional outcomes. (Functional outcomes are improved functioning in a natural context.) The concept of functional assessment entered the field of special services through the practices of specialists in rehabilitation and long-term care. "Simply described, functional assessment is a measure of a person's ability to function in his or her environment despite disease, disability, or social deprivation" (Frattali & Lynch, 1989, p. 70).

The concept is less firmly a part of habilitative and educational services provided to infants, toddlers, children, and adolescents. Yet, it can be useful. When functional outcomes are mentioned for persons with severe disabilities in multiple domains, people often think immediately of such activities of daily living (ADLs) as dressing, bathing, toileting, and feeding, but there is much more to being functional in life than having minimal physical care needs met. Although these needs are important, and communicative

improvements may contribute significantly to improved ADL functioning, other functional outcomes also should be measured. For example, following are other functional outcome questions that might be asked about individuals with severe communicative impairments that can never be corrected: "For business or social purposes, can they attract the attention of someone other than persons who have been assigned to work with them, and can they maintain and terminate such transactions appropriately? Can they use language to get information and to give it (whether or not topics are complex or abstract)? Can they use communicative and thinking skills well enough to keep themselves busy and entertained or for getting the resources they need to do so?"

For students in school who can "almost but not quite" (ABNQ) succeed in the regular curriculum, a different set of functional outcomes may be sought. If changes in language and communicative behavior are significant and relevant, they should influence improvement in many areas only indirectly related to speech and language. For example, functional outcomes might be measured as increased participation in activities in the classroom and on the playground or in other extracurricular activities.

More objective measures also can represent functional outcomes for such students. Grades earned on report cards and on individual assignments, projects, and tests can serve as criterion-referenced measures to demonstrate functional improvements. CBAs can do the same. For norm-referenced evidence of functional outcomes, achievement test scores may be used.

Perhaps the most important thing to keep in mind when attempting to get the big picture is that more than one kind of evidence is needed. Also remember that more than one perspective is needed to build a multidimensional picture of truth.

Keeping an eye on the trees. When children have significant needs, broad evidence of progress may not appear quickly. When a whole system does begin to change, it also may be difficult to sort out the factors contributing to that change. System theory suggests that attempts to assign credit to individual components of a comprehensive collaborative program would be artificial, because the synergistic force of multiple subsystems is more than the sum of the parts. Nevertheless, it is important to gather evidence that elements of measurable change are occurring in specific targeted areas. Although some social interactionists argue that whenever a complex skill such as communication is analyzed into discrete parts, it is trivialized, merely setting a goal that a child will become more communicatively competent is not enough. More specific indices are needed. Progress in specific areas can be monitored in several ways, discussed in the following sections.

Keeping log notes.   After each direct or consultative contact regarding a particular child, it is helpful to keep dated notes on what happened. The log notes can provide a running commentary about progress in several goal areas and associated qualitative comments. Generally, they should take no more than 5 minutes to write and should require no more than one fourth of a page. Otherwise, they likely will not be written immediately and become a chore rather than an aid. In addition to qualitative comments, log notes can be used to quickly record quantitative data in the form of frequency information, percentages, or proportions to be entered on a progress chart later.

Charting data.   The old adage that a picture is worth a thousand words is certainly true for monitoring progress. Almost any behavior that can be observed in natural (or formal) contexts can be quantified in some way, and quantities can always be charted. Charts provide a clearer picture of growth than numbers presented in isolation (readily available computer programs make the charting process easy).

The thought of charting data may bring to mind highly structured approaches with massed instructional trials of stimulus–response–reinforcement. In this type of approach, the percentage correct may drop every time a criterion is met and new, more demanding conditions are introduced. For example, Gray and Ryan (1973) used stacks of pictures and a highly imitative approach to get children to produce utterances of increasing length and complexity, after which the support of the imitative models was gradually removed. In this approach, all responses were charted, and if a child plateaued at a level under 80% correct for 3 days straight on this program, it was taken as a sign that branching was needed, and alternate prompting and cuing strategies were recommended.

Charting also can be used for communicative behaviors occurring in much more naturalistic contexts. Rather than shifting conditions as a child moves through a sequence of programmed objectives, yielding an expected sawtooth pattern, a segment of communicative behavior is viewed in an intact context within a particular time-frame. These samples usually are not taken every session but may be taken once a week or once a month, depending on their purpose. More than one behavior can be quantified, either on-line or from audio or videotapes. An example might be the number of times a child looks in the direction of an adult who calls his name as a proportion of opportunities within a standard block of time.

Figure 6.10 presents charted data from a communication sample gathered in a session with a child with autism (L. Watson, Lord, Schaffer, & Schopler, 1989). It illustrates how a single chart may record naturalistic observations coded for context and the actual linguistic and nonlinguistic forms the child produced to make qualitative judgments about the functions and semantic categories encoded and to categorize aspects of the sample for subsequent use in quantitative analyses.

Keeping running language samples.   Another way to keep a more qualitative running record is to keep a separate piece of paper at hand to record on-line bits of language samples (with essential contextual information) that arise naturally in interactions with a child. This is not a formal language sample, and it cannot be used for formal analysis, such as for computing MLU, but it is very useful for keeping track of unusual things the child says. I usually enter a new date at the beginning of each contact and write down any utterances, as the child says them, that are especially long and complex or that demonstrate a peculiar use of a linguistic rule or unexpected evidence of miscomprehension. This can also be used to keep track of new vocabulary for children in the early stages of language development. Writing down only exceptionally good or unusual productions certainly biases the sample, but over time, a pattern of increasing length, complexity, and appropriateness of utterances hopefully will emerge. The examples of restricted language also can provide a window into the child's current language processing, can assist in keeping assessment up to date, and can contribute to planning for future sessions with the child.

Noting when objectives are accomplished.   Well-written instructional objectives include criteria for knowing when they have been accomplished. When a sequence of objectives is arranged vertically, dates can be entered whenever a new objective is initiated or accomplished in a particular context. Figure 6.7

FIGURE 6.10

Illustration of a charting method that combines qualitative and quantitative observations of a naturalistic communicative interaction between a teacher (observer) and a student with autism.

Student: Ralph
Observer: Warren
Date: 1/17
Time began: 9:30
Time ended: 11:30

CONTEXT	WHAT STUDENT SAID OR DID	Request	Getting Attention	Reject	Comment	Give Information	Seek Information	Other	Object	Action	Person	Location	Other
① Makes mess while making breakfast	towel (signs)	✓							object wanted				
② Work-folding clothes	finish (signs)			✓						own action			
③ Free time-R. walks into kitchenette	touches teacher's arm		✓										
④ "	hands teacher a cup	✓											
⑤ T: "What?"	drink (signs)	✓							object wanted				
⑥ T. hands R. orange juice	pushes jar away			✓									
⑦ R. opens refrigerator	drink (signs)	✓											
⑧ T: "Drink what?"	R. picks up cola bottle												
	+ signs drink	✓							object wanted				
⑨ R. stands up T.: "What do you want?"	bathroom (signs)	✓										own location	
⑩ R's shoe untied; to T.	shoe (signs)	✓							object acted on				
⑪ " "	shoe (signs) + holds								object acted on				
	up untied shoe	✓											
⑫ finishes playing with comb	finish (signs)			✓						own action			

FUNCTIONS | SEMANTIC CATEGORIES

Note. From *Teaching Spontaneous Communication to Autistic and Developmentally Handicapped Children* (p. 29) by L. Watson, C. Lord, B. Schaffer, and E. Schopler, 1989, Austin, TX: Pro-Ed. Copyright 1989 by Pro-Ed. Reprinted by permission.

illustrates a combination of vertical and horizontal aspects of programming (N. W. Nelson, 1988b).

Using Exit Criteria to Decide When to Quit

At some point, a decision may be made that enough treatment has been provided and that the child should be dismissed from the language intervention specialist's active caseload. It is not always easy to know when to quit. Treatment, therefore, not uncommonly continues beyond the point when it is no longer in the child's best interest.

Fey (1986) noted that decisions about exiting are usually made because one of three situations has occurred:

1. The child has reached all stated objectives and is no longer considered to be at risk for social disvalue (i.e., the child can no longer be viewed as language impaired [or language handicapped]).
2. The child's progress toward stated goals has plateaued and efforts made to modify the intervention plan, including goals, procedures, activities, and goal attack strategies . . . have not lead to notable gains in the child's performance.
3. The child exhibits continued progress toward basic goals, but there is no evidence that the intervention program is responsible for these gains. (p. 47)

These situations can be identified by answers to three questions: (1) Is more change needed? (2) Is more change possible? (3) Is the attempt to bring about more change through special services justified by a cost–benefit analysis?

The question "Is more change needed?" may be answered by using some of the previously discussed strategies to identify a language disorder in a child, justifying a need for special services. Public Law 94–142 requires that this question must be asked at least once every 3 years for school-age children as a part of their comprehensive 3-year reevaluations.

The question "Is more change possible?" may be answered by using the goals and objectives and progress-monitoring techniques of individualized programming. When I gather data failing to support progress in the child, showing a plateau effect rather than a positive slope, my first question is not whether the child might no longer need service. Rather, it is, "What am I doing wrong?" That is followed by the question "How can I find out how to do things better?" The child may need a different service-delivery model or service provider rather than to be released from treatment entirely. Think about what it must mean to families with children in special education who have the same teacher or speech–language pathologist year after year. No matter how wonderful the teacher or clinician is, the parents and child rarely experience that special sense of hope that comes each fall with regular education when meeting the child's new teacher. Even worse, think about what it means to families when the only teacher or clinician with the right kind of credentials to work with their child is not so good or is not so good for their child. That must be discouraging, indeed. Effective administrators work to prevent this by moving staff and children when the need is apparent. Other concerns also influence choices. Least restrictive environment requirements cannot be violated. The philosophy of including more children with severe and multiple problems in regular education experiences may also reduce this problem.

Nevertheless, children who still need special education sometimes may no longer need speech and language intervention services. For example, a child with cognitive limitations might need a boost to get going in communicating, but when growth in speech, language, and communication level off and are commensurate with other developmental domains, he may no longer need direct service. In Chapter 7, a Michigan Decision-Making Model (N. W. Nelson et al., 1981) is suggested for determining occasions like this. It advocates a need for a strong language component in every child's regular or special education curriculum, but it suggests different levels and modes of service to be delivered by language intervention specialists.

The costs implied in the question "Is the attempt justified by a cost–benefit analysis?" are not usually monetary. In fact, the regulations of PL 94–142 clearly state that decisions must be based on the child's needs rather than what a district can afford. There are other costs to consider. It may be judged as too costly to a student's need to be in the regular classroom to pull him out twice a week or more, or it may be judged too costly to a child's need for consistency to design a patchwork schedule with a variety of settings and interventionists. Cost is always relevant to the expected benefits. If potential benefits are high enough, more cost is acceptable, but if the benefits have been shown to be minimal, a child's time may be better spent in other ways.

Exit decisions are not easy. They can be guided by asking the three preceding questions, but they should never be made without using the kind of collaborative processes (required by federal policy in United States) discussed throughout this book.

Judging Program Accountability

In an earlier discussion on establishing prognosis, I acknowledged the difficulty of judging program effectiveness on a large scale. Program accountability may be judged in more than one way, however.

In a complex program serving multiple kinds of children using multiple kinds of service-delivery models, it may not always be feasible to measure the effectiveness of the program as a whole. All professionals, however, at least need to have well-organized strategies for keeping data on the number of their clients and sessions, as well as session type and length. They also need to keep categorical data about assessment and intervention outcomes (e.g., in terms of numbers of individuals evaluated and diagnosed as needing service, numbers referred, numbers receiving follow-up monitoring, etc.) Most agencies have a specific method for collecting these data and a regularly scheduled period for reporting.

Numerical accountability is important, and usually is required, but increasingly agencies also want evidence of quality assurance. A danger of simple number crunching is that it may obscure efforts to demonstrate that children are indeed making progress as individuals. Regardless of an interest in quality assurance when assessing program accountability, program monitors and administrators may fail "to see the trees for the forest" (just the opposite of the danger sometimes facing individual clinicians working alone). Administrators may seem to focus exclusively on the question "Can we afford it?" when professionals wish they would ask, "Does it work?" Professionals may find that administrators are more likely to find a way to afford a program if they can be given some hard evidence that it works, and even more so, that it works better than old, or different, or less expensive methods.

When a treatment approach is experimental and differs dramatically from accepted practices, a traditional experimental design may be best to assess its effectiveness. Lovaas (1987) took this approach in his study of the intensive, comprehensive behavior therapy treatment program for children with autism. Most practicing professionals usually do not use carefully controlled experimental designs to demonstrate program effectiveness. Sometimes, however, it is essential to gather more precise and representative data, and other times it is advisable to do so.

It is essential to prepare a plan to demonstrate that a project is effective in meeting its objectives efficiently (i.e., it meets efficacy requirements) when advocating for a grant from a third-party agency. More than one method usually is described to measure the accomplishment of objectives. A test–retest plan or a set of criterion measures might be used with an accounting of how many individuals in the special program reach criteria established in several areas. It might also be helpful to show that clients are either progressing farther or reaching desired goals faster than they did under an old approach. Qualitative measures, such as interviews, also can document program effectiveness, and functional outcome measures are critical for demonstrating program relevance. I know of one group who assembled a·slide-tape show to demonstrate the continuing need for a classroom for severely language impaired children. Perhaps its most effective elements were audiotaped language samples of children in the program illustrating their significant needs (of course, with their own and their parents' permission and not identifying them as individuals). Board members heard those needs better than they could see them, and they maintained the program.

SUMMARY

This chapter has covered a lot of ground, beginning with the steps required to meet the needs of an indi-

vidual with language disorders. I also considered how six different theoretical perspectives influence decision making, either program-wide or daily. My own best sense of overall theoretical perspective is that none of the six individual perspectives meets all of the needs of all infants, toddlers, children, and adolescents with language disorders. Therefore, I advocate a strategy that involves making thoughtful choices on an individual basis. It is an eclectic approach but not a disorganized one.

In implementing an eclectic approach, you may find that some perspectives work better for guiding practices with certain individuals. I have discussed, particularly, the importance of keeping elements of a social interactionist perspective in the program, no matter what other elements are part of it. Children need reasons to talk and to understand, to read and to write, and to use language for thinking. They also need to practice those skills in real social contexts that can make reasons for communicating apparent. Professionals also need techniques for assisting change and for ensuring that it will stick. Behaviorist principles can be used to influence the exchanges between specialist and child and the choices about presentation of stimuli, responses, and reinforcement, regardless of the other theoretical perspectives used. Effective programming means recognizing that outwardly observable behavior depends on the workings of inner aspects of a system involving physiological as well as psychological processes. Ensuring that children have access to information, and assisting them to process it actively and to understand it at multiple levels is part of ensuring that children will have tools and strategies for continuing to learn and communicate on their own. Biological and psychological processes such as reception, attention, perception, memory, and recall are best seen as means to an end, not as an end in themselves. Linguistic theory offers a way to conceptualize what children must learn, and cognitive theory suggests how children might be led to integrate the various domains of knowledge, skill, and strategies by using developmental sequences as blueprints.

These are the elements of effective programming and the outline of strategies for using them. Chapters 7 through 9 examine the varying implementation of these strategies, depending on the developmental needs of infants, toddlers, children, and adolescents in early, middle, and later stages of language acquisition.

PART TWO

Balancing Ages and Developmental Stages

This section provides specific information and strategies for working with infants, toddlers, children, and adolescents with language disorders and communication deficits. Of course, ultimately, we do not work with groups but with individuals. The view of clients as individuals participating in broader systems is central to successful practice. To a large extent, the successful practitioner can call on past experience and general knowledge about language disorders and related conditions, while never losing sight of the need to learn about the present client, an individual with unique abilities, needs, and opportunities.

Questions of organization of topics related to ages and stages of development assume more than technical importance in Part 2. These chapters convey information about the content and contexts of early, middle, and later stages of language acquisition. Each chapter provides information about developmental expectations, typical partner interactions, and usual communicative contexts. Also included are suggestions for using the information in assessment and intervention with youngsters at that particular stage of language acquisition. This strategy raises a major question. Where should one discuss older children who stay at earlier stages of language development?

In the past, youngsters were automatically grouped with others in the same developmental stage. For example, a 13-year-old student with profound cognitive and multiple other impairments functioning at a presymbolic level would be assessed as functioning at an early stage of language acquisition and would be viewed primarily in the context of what is known about infant and toddler development. When a 13-year-old is functioning at a 13-month-old level, it does, after all, make sense to start at that child's level when planning intervention. Such a unidimensional approach, however, misses the other two facets of comprehensive programming discussed throughout this book—contextual demands and opportunities.

The questions "What abilities does this child need to participate in the important contexts of his or her life?" and "What communication opportunities should the environment provide?" cannot be answered by focusing on a single developmental dimension. The child's language system may have remained at a 1-year-old level, but his or her body and social interaction needs may not. Even the child's language and speech behaviors may not be accurately characterized by describing them as similar to those of a 1-year-old. The normally developing 1-year-old changes rapidly. Every day brings new exploration and shifts of experience and ability. The 13-year-old with profound impairments may have behavioral routines that are much more closely tied to particular contexts and people.

An alternative organizational strategy is to discuss individuals in sections with their chronological age peers rather than with their developmental stage peers. This strategy is consistent with the position argued by many parents and advocates and by organizations such as The Association for Individuals With Severe Handicaps (TASH), the Autism Society of America (ASA), and the Association for Retarded Citizens (ARC). Yet, discussions of issues such as complex sentences and complex literacy activities appropriate to the needs of normally developing 13-year-olds may be irrelevant to the needs of adolescents with profound impairments (for an alternative view, see discussions on Facilitated Communication Therapy, e.g., Biklen, 1990, 1992; Crossley & McDonald, 1984). Where does this individual fit in? On a broader scale, that is exactly the question facing society today.

The 13-year-old with early-stage abilities is an extreme case, but similar questions could be asked about individuals with mild or moderate impairments. Should they be placed in activities with their developmental age peers or with their chronological age peers? Should they be discussed in this book with their developmental age peers or with their chronological age peers?

Fortunately, although we do not always recognize the possibility, we can take an eclectic approach to solving problems such as this. We are not forced into an either/or position unless we allow ourselves to be. Studying the interactions of parents and 1-year-old infants advancing to symbolic communication can be useful in working with the 13-year-old with profound multiple impairments. For example, the adult's ability to "read" the individual's behavior as communicative even when it is not intended that way, or as representational even when it is not formed with words, may provide a key to helping profoundly impaired adolescents become maximally functional. It is also useful to see the 13-year-old as a person moving into puberty, who may be more interested and communicative when included occasionally with same-age peers than when stacking rings on a toy.

Questions of need and opportunity are equally important for the 8-year-old with language skills at a 6-year-old level as they are for the profoundly impaired individual. No one wants to put children in situations where they are sure to fail. Yet, removing children from contexts with their peers to ensure success on a short-term basis may, in the long-run, ensure failure in adulthood.

Juggling many important concerns is the business of multidisciplinary and transdisciplinary teams, including students and parents, as well as professionals. The organization of Chapters 7 to 9 is designed to facilitate perspective juggling that will permit consideration of children's needs within the contexts of one or more developmental levels, while not forgetting the contexts of their chronological levels. This is done by including commentary on older children with earlier stage abilities in multiple sections. My hope is that this approach will seem not redundant but, rather, will facilitate decision making that will work for children of all kinds of ages and abilities.

Considerations of other special concerns are also woven throughout the chapters rather than being consigned to special chapters or sections of their own. Topics such as the need for multicultural sensitivity and uses of augmentative and alternative communication technology and strategies are discussed throughout Part 2. The purpose of this approach is to encourage the use of mutual goal-setting and problem-solving methods that are consistent with a collaborative model of consultation rather than an expert one. Although varied participants bring varied expertise to problem solving, aspects of problems cannot be ignored or passed on to someone else if the child is to be treated as a whole person participating in a whole system. The philosophy that *problems are not just within children, and neither are the solutions* continues to guide the discussions of this book.

7

Early Stages

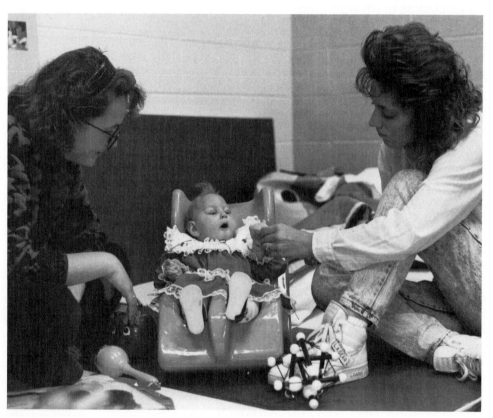

Children Needing
Intervention Aimed at
Early-Stage
Developments

Measuring Early-
Stage Abilities,
Needs, and
Accomplishments

Methods and Targets
of Early-Stage
Intervention

❑   Who may need treatment for early-stage problems?

❑   What tools can be used to measure early-stage needs and abilities?

❑   What kinds of intervention targets and methods are appropriate?

Infants and toddlers accomplish amazing feats in the acquisition of communicative ability by the 3rd year of life. But they do not start at zero. This chapter considers the developmental abilities and expectations associated with the earliest stages of language acquisition, along with possible disruptions and what to do about them. For the most part, this period can be marked from birth, when most children already have communicative potential and some foundation skills, and extends into the 3rd year of life, when normally developing children can reliably combine two words to express varied linguistic meanings but do not yet build full syntactic constructions.

This chapter provides information on developmental expectations and potential intervention targets that can be used with children in the early stages of language acquisition whether they are in the birth to 3-year age range or have passed that level chronologically but still have early-stage needs. The focus for the first group is on prevention and on intervention as a process primarily to foster normal development (whether disorders are congenital or acquired). The focus for the second group may be more on remediation and compensation (e.g., by providing an augmentative device to compensate for inability to speak) as well as prevention. All children and their related adults may benefit from approaches that involve redefinition and reeducation (in addition to other efforts). Definitions for processes of remediation, redefinition, and reeducation were suggested by Sameroff and Fiese (1990): (1) *remediation* is the process of helping children with identified delays or disabilities to develop skills that more closely approximate behavior expected at a given chronological age within their cultural system; (2) *redefinition* is the process by which professionals enable care givers to redefine their perceptions of their children's abilities by helping them to reevaluate their children's strengths and weaknesses; and (3) *reeducation* is the process by which professionals help parents learn better ways of raising their children.

For example, redefinition and reeducation might be appropriate in mothers' verbal interactions with their hearing impaired infants. S. J. White and White (1984) observed that maternal language may be "an overt reflection of the mother's feelings and judgments about her child's level of functioning" (p. 43) as much as a way of communicating, because direct information sharing is not a true part of the earliest maternal–infant dialogues. Thus, when parents have trouble matching their input to their infants' needs, professionals may assist by helping parents redefine their perceptions of those levels of functioning. White and White also suggested that children whose age or hearing status interferes with their ability to understand words respond more to the affective information behind the words. "Children respond to facets of the mother's emotional status perhaps more than to what mothers say" (p. 46). Part of the reeducational process for preventing maladaptive interaction patterns involves helping mothers learn not to pour words into their babies but to engage their babies in interactive dialogues that can best foster communicative (and emotional) development.

For a developmental perspective to contribute to any of the possible intervention approaches, the specialist needs information about developmental targets. As discussed throughout this book, however, a focus aimed exclusively at the "trees" of developmental expectations risks missing the "forest" of children's most critical real-life needs. Questions about need, opportunity, and participation must constantly accompany questions about ability and impairment. Developmental expectations provide a blueprint for intervention targets, which is probably the best blueprint available, but it is not the only one.

The integrative education movement asks which contexts should be available to the child with early-stage communicative skills based on chronological age as well as developmental concerns. Intervention methods also vary, depending on many special concerns beyond either developmental or chronological age. Other factors influencing intervention methods include associated causative conditions, family support, community and school district attitudes and resources, and the participants' theoretical and philosophical views. This chapter considers multiple factors and places the content and methods of early-stage language intervention into varied, meaningful contexts.

CHILDREN NEEDING INTERVENTION AIMED AT EARLY-STAGE DEVELOPMENTS

Children with only mild-to-moderate language acquisition delays may not be much older than their normally developing peers when they pass through similar stages. Strategies for identifying children during early stages of development who have "milder" developmental problems, including specific language impairments, are still emerging. Thus, many children at risk for language disorders are not identified until their preschool years (ages 3 to 5). These are the children who can "almost but not quite" (ABNQ) meet the developmental expectations of their normally developing peers. Other children who have conditions with established but relatively moderate developmental risk (e.g., some children with Down's syndrome) may be better characterized as "OK now but risky later." These children may pass through some early developmental stages almost on time (A. M. Wetherby, Yonclas, & Bryan, 1989) but may run into more trouble as contextual expectations become more complex.

On the other hand, some children have frank, multiple, severe impairments easily identified at birth. These problems tend to be long-lasting and to severely limit ultimate development. Some children who have severe disabilities, particularly those with severe cognitive impairments, may never master any but the earliest stages of language or communication, even in adulthood. This limited prognosis, however, does not reduce their right to receive appropriate attention to their communicative needs.

IDENTIFYING INFANTS AT RISK FOR DEVELOPMENTAL PROBLEMS

Risk Factors and Early Identification

Risk factors in infancy are often differentiated into three categories: (1) *established risk*, related to a diagnosed medical disorder of known cause, such as Down's syndrome or deafness; (2) *environmental risk*, related to life experiences, such as abuse or neglect, that place an infant who otherwise may be biologically sound at risk for developmental delay; and (3) *biological risk*, related to a history of prenatal, perinatal, neonatal, and immediately postnatal events that might insult the developing central nervous system, compromising further development, but the effects of these events are yet to be established (Liebergott,

Bashir, & Schultz, 1984; Ramey, Trohanis, & Hostler, 1982; Tjossem, 1976). These categories are not mutually exclusive, and the same child may demonstrate more than one kind of risk.

Factors related to established and environmental risk were discussed in Chapter 4. Biological risk may be associated with prenatal and perinatal factors such as environmental toxins and infections such as cytomegalovirus (D. A. Clark, 1989). The concerns about infants born with acquired immunodeficiency syndrome (AIDS) from their infected mothers continue to grow (Odom & Warren, 1988). In addition, the first wave of "crack" cocaine babies born of addicted mothers is now entering schools in the United States. Although their risks for demonstrating particular communicative impairments are not yet clear, children born of drug-addicted mothers can be expected to be at risk in multiple ways. Other factors associated with biological risk at birth include prematurity, asphyxia, and intracranial hemorrhage.

Premature infants are those born at less than 37 weeks of gestation, with the percentage of prematurity in the United States remaining constant at around 7% to 8% of all newborns over recent years (D. A. Clark, 1989). Not all premature infants are at equal risk. The birth weight of 2,500 g is frequently cited as a threshold of risk based on size. Babies below that weight may be at greater risk than premature infants who weigh more. Other babies who are full term but small for gestational age, possibly as a result of fetal alcohol syndrome, are also at risk. A birth weight of less than 1,500 g is considered to be very low birth weight. Additional risk factors, such as sensory deficits or adverse environmental factors, multiply the risk of developmental difficulty. "Sick" premature infants—who experience complications such as asphyxia, respiratory distress syndrome, metabolic disorders, and intracranial hemorrhage—therefore are at greater risk for developmental problems than "healthy" premature infants (Field, 1979).

Infants and toddlers with special needs or risks for developmental disorders usually enter the service-delivery system through medical referral, some after extended care by medical professionals. Ensher (1989) noted that very premature infants (born at 24 to 28 weeks of gestation) typically require hospital stays of at least 3 to 4 months and are often discharged with such technological dependencies as oxygen assistance. When an infant leaves the neonatal intensive care unit (NICU), or even while still in it, a speech–language pathologist may evaluate the neonate's current status and consult with the family about their concerns such as feeding and the best ways to encourage initial communication and to enjoy social interactions with their infant.

In addition, the infants should undergo auditory screening assessment before leaving the hospital, with follow-up whenever hearing status is in doubt. A few states require hearing screening of all newborns, and others require screening and follow-up for any infant who meets criteria of a high-risk register (see Box 7.1), but any child whose birth is associated with any of the previous risks should undergo careful and early assessment of hearing status.

Hearing sometimes is screened merely by using a special sound-generating device to present sounds of known frequencies and intensities under semicontrolled conditions. The infant's ability to hear these sounds is inferred by a physician or nurse observing the eyeblink response (called the *auropalpebral response* [APR]). However, this method relies on fairly subjective observation, and it is not highly reliable. More objective methods are available but not universally; they are also more expensive. One relatively objective method uses a "Crib-o-gram," a specially designed crib with sensors connected to a polygraph recorder to measure changes in newborns' movement patterns from before introduction of a 92-dB complex tone to immediately afterward (for at least 20 trials) (Kinney, Ouellette, & Wolery, 1989). Another objective method, auditory brain stem response (ABR) audiometry, uses surface electrodes placed on an infant's head during a normal sleep state (no sedation required) to sense potentials evoked by controlled auditory stimuli (Amochaev, 1987). When there is any doubt about an infant's hearing sensitivity, early hearing assessment should be conducted and interpreted by an audiologist. Even among audiologists, agreement is not universal about how extensive screening and diagnostic measures must be to assess the hearing of infants at risk (Turner, 1990).

It is widely agreed, however, that informal means such as parental report, hand clapping, and noise makers are simply not sensitive enough. They are too easily contaminated by uncontrolled circumstances and may lead to false-negative decisions about hearing risks (Kinney et al., 1989). Furthermore, intact peripheral hearing is too critical to the infant's further development, particularly in the area of language, to risk delaying identification of a hearing loss, especially because early amplification can make an important difference in ultimate auditory and linguistic functioning.

Some infants may have developmental risks that are not identified while they are still in the hospital but show up later in infancy. Referrals from public health facilities and well-baby clinics to other service agencies often provide an important avenue for identifying infants with risks such as these. Part of the strength of the amendments of Public Law 99–457 is that they require interagency agreements so that health, educational, and other social service agencies

---

Box 7.1   Criteria recommended by the American Speech-Language-Hearing Association (Joint Committee on Infant Hearing, 1991) for identifying infants at risk for hearing impairment

1. Family history of childhood hearing impairment.
2. Congenital perinatal infections.
3. Anatomical malformations of the head and neck.
4. Birth weight less than 1500 g.
5. Hyperbilirubinemia at a level exceeding indications for exchange transfusion.
6. Ototoxic medications.
7. Bacterial meningitis.
8. Severe asphyxia, which may include infants with Apgar scores of 0 to 3 who fail to institute spontaneous respiration by 10 minutes and those with hypotonia persisting to 2 hours of age.
9. Prolonged mechanical ventilation.
10. Findings associated with a syndrome known to include sensorineural hearing loss.

may be more likely to communicate with each other. Unfortunately, this does not always mean that such agreements will work, or that parents will necessarily have the knowledge, emotional and financial resources, or transportation to take advantage of all available opportunities. It takes time to adjust to having a new baby, let alone having a baby with unexpected problems.

Nursing professionals who tend to have early contact with families after a baby is born with risks may provide a particularly important link in this network because their knowledge crosses both medical and family systems concerns. One study that spanned eight disciplines (Bailey, Simeonsson, Yoder, & Huntington, 1990) showed that nurses and social workers tended to receive more specific information about family assessment and intervention than professionals in any of the other disciplines studied. Part of a transdisciplinary service-delivery model calls for role release and the funneling of information through one professional acting as case manager. Often, particularly when physical care needs are involved, the case manager may be a nurse. When a case-manager approach is used, families are less likely to be overwhelmed by a set of fragmented and possibly conflicting interactions with many different professionals. Of course, many factors enter into decisions regarding what kind of person qualifies best as case manager for a particular child. As always, such decisions should be individualized.

Child-Find Efforts and Screening

Although they do not always work extremely well, all states are required by the Individuals with Disabilities Education Act (IDEA, PL 101–476) to identify children who might need special services but who might not otherwise come to the attention of service agencies. *Child Find* is a "systematic process of identifying infants and children who are eligible for enrollment in intervention programs, tracking those individuals and making them known to appropriate service providers" (Wolery, 1989, p. 120). Serious Child-Find efforts are complicated, involving many components, such as defining the target population, screening and prescreening, public awareness, and referrals, to keep track of children and to provide services.

The need for *public awareness* cannot be taken for granted. When I was employed in the schools, I once had to explain to my own supervisor why a speech–language pathologist should be involved in the inter-disciplinary team seeing infants. He could not imagine such a professional being of any use before a child began to talk! One of the things I learned from that experience was that "public" awareness efforts conducted on several levels would be needed to make appropriate early intervention services available to all children who needed them.

Screening in the Child-Find programs consists of activities used to answer the question "Should this child be given a thorough diagnostic assessment?" Many screening efforts involve preliminary assessments of large groups of children using published screening instruments designed to identify children who might have impairments or who are at risk for demonstrating disabilities.

Formal screening instruments should meet all of the psychometric standards discussed in Chapter 6, and they should yield as few false-positive (overreferrals) and false-negative (underreferrals) errors as possible. It is also helpful if screening procedures for young children are appropriate for serial use. Wolery (1989) noted that serial screening during the preschool years is useful because it "allows delays that occur later in the toddler and preschool years to be identified, allows better decision making because of the multiple data points, and assists in providing parents with information about child development and rearing" (p.129).

Sparks (1989b) also recommended serial assessment, based on the rationale that infant behavior changes so strikingly, particularly during the first 18 months of life, that multiple observations permit better inferencing about environmental influences, and that serial observations can reveal whether the child is developing faster in one domain than in another (e.g., motor skill faster than language or vice versa). However, because no instrument has yet been shown to predict with much certainty which infants will exhibit developmental delays—even when their births have involved seemingly overwhelming complications—Sparks also recommended that professionals should not rely on neonatal screening results to predict later behavior for babies who have difficult beginnings. The picture is relatively hopeful for the majority of survivors of NICUs, because the majority are found not to demonstrate severe or even moderate handicaps (M. C. McCormick, 1989).

Several kinds of screening tools appropriate for use with infants and toddlers are identified in Appendix A. They vary in their standardization characteristics and also in whether they are appropriate for screening comprehensive developmental domains or are intended for identification of communication problems primarily. Two of the instruments used most frequently for general assessment of neonatal status were developed by T. Berry Brazelton, M.D., and his colleagues. The Neonatal Behavioral Assessment Scale (NBAS) (Brazelton, 1984) is credited with heightening the awareness in the medical community of the newborn's behavioral capabilities and individual differences when it was introduced in its first edition in 1973. The instrument included the traditional evaluation of neurological reflexes and developmental milestones but extended beyond it (O'Donnell & Oehler, 1989). Widespread use of the NBAS over subsequent years demonstrated that small-for-gestational-age and premature infants were less well organized than their full-term peers. This led to the development of the Assessment of Preterm Infant Behavior (APIB) (Als, Lester, Tronick, & Brazelton, 1982) to assess low-birth-weight infants (Sparks, 1989b).

IDENTIFYING CHILDREN WITH SEVERE COMMUNICATIVE IMPAIRMENTS WHO NEED LANGUAGE INTERVENTION AND AUGMENTATIVE AND ALTERNATIVE COMMUNICATION SERVICES

Children who have severe disabilities such as moderate-to-severe cognitive impairments and autism are at risk to remain at early stages of language acquisition for some time after their same-age peers have moved on. Severe sensory and motor deficits, particularly in combination with other problems, also increase the risk for significant delay. For these children, it is important to identify the extent of central cognitive and linguistic deficits and to separate those deficits as much as possible from more peripheral sensory and motor deficits. Intervention may involve provision of compensatory methods and technology, such as acoustic amplification and augmentative communication, along with environmental modifications and adaptations.

In the early stages of normal language acquisition, children move from prelinguistic interactions, with others interpreting their behavior (including vocal behavior) as communicative (the *perlocutionary* stage), through a phase when they communicate intentionally but only nonverbally (the *illocutionary*

stage), into a phase when they use verbal symbols to communicate and to express increasingly wide ranges of meanings (the *locutionary* stage). These gross landmarks in early communicative development can provide part of the map needed to establish early-stage intervention plans (Table 7.1 outlines these major developmental shifts). Children whose development is impeded by severe sensory, motor, and/or cognitive deficits may find some aspects of this process of developmental shifting more accessible than others.

When considering the needs of children whose development is severely impeded, it is important to recognize that not all nonspeaking individuals are severely language impaired. The distinction is important. As discussed originally in Chapter 2, differentiation of factors related to language, speech, and communication can assist in identifying children who need varied special services and in planning appropriate intervention strategies. Nonspeaking children may have varying degrees of communicative and linguistic abilities. Some nonvocal individuals are quite verbal; they can use linguistic symbols in meaningful, productive, and conventional ways. Other communicative individuals who vocalize their needs and frustrations may be nonverbal. Because the terminology associated with these conditions may be confusing, professionals in augmentative and alternative communication (AAC) have attempted to clarify it (Fried-Oken, 1987; Vanderheiden & Yoder, 1986). Those efforts are summarized in Box 7.2.

This chapter considers the needs of individuals with severe communication impairments related to conditions such as autism, cerebral palsy, and mental retardation, but readers should be clear about the reasons for inclusion. Only individuals who are using prelinguistic communication and who are in the earliest stages of verbal interaction are discussed here. Some individuals with any of these causative conditions can enter middle and later stages of language acquisition. In particular, a diagnosis of cerebral palsy predicts nothing about the state of a child's language system. Language intervention services needed by nonspeaking individuals should be matched to their language function levels with consideration of their chronological ages and not only of their speech impairments.

A premise underlying the treatment of all severely communicatively impaired children is that, just as no child is untestable, no child is incapable of achieving some level of communication. As some researchers

TABLE 7.1
Stages of additive intentional and linguistic communicative development

Approximate Age (Months)	Stage	Characteristics
0–8	**Perlocutionary**	Communicative intention is inferred by the adult
	Proactive perlocutionary	Active environmental exploration Vocal and gestural signals not directed at others Anticipates no contingent social outcomes No evidence of linguistic comprehension
8–12	**Illocutionary**	Child communicates intentions
	Primitive illocutionary	Signals directed at others expecting specific outcomes Signals may be subtle and only interpreted by immediate caregivers Signals apparently goal directed, as indicated by persistence or frustration if goal not reached Early apparently linguistic comprehension, but only in highly context-bound routines
	Conventional illocutionary	Evidence of clear concept of communication Conventional use of gestures and vocalizations to achieve specific outcomes Prelinguistic signals interpreted by wider range of people Greater persistence if communicative goals not met More evidence of linguistic comprehension, particularly in context, but some multi-word utterances and some object labels may be understood out of context
>12	**Locutionary**	Child communicates intentions using conventional linguistic forms
	Emerging locutionary	Linguistic forms (words or signs) beginning to be used consistently for communication Word use is decontextualized Forms are conventional and understood by many others Some forms may be idiosyncratic and understood only by those close to the child Nonverbal devices (gaze, vocalizations, and gestures) may remain major part of repertoire Increased comprehension of single and simple multiword utterances, both in and out of context
	Locutionary	Language is primary means of sending and receiving messages Language knowledge (both receptive and expressive) extends beyond early multi-word utterances to include varied sentence types, grammatical morphemes, and some complex sentences Language is used to talk about things that are temporally and spatially removed from the current context Most language is understood, except for some abstract and nonliteral uses

Based on Bates, Camaioni, & Volterra, 1975; Prizant, 1984.

have noted (Watzlawick, Beavin, & Jackson, 1967), it is impossible *not* to communicate:

> No matter how one may try, one cannot *not* communicate. Activity or inactivity, words or silence all have message value: they influence others and these others, in turn, cannot *not* respond to these communications and are thus themselves communicating. It should be clearly understood that the mere absence of talking or

of taking notice of each other is no exception to what had just been asserted. (p. 49)

Children in different stages of language development need different kinds of services, whether or not they can speak. (The needs of children with severe speaking and writing impairments functioning at middle and later stages of language acquisition are discussed in Chapters 8 and 9).

Box 7.2   **Terminology associated with augmentative and alternative communication**

Aided communication technique. Any augmentative and alternative communication (AAC) technique using some type of physical device or object (e.g., communication board, chart, mechanical or electronic aid).

Augmentative and alternative communication system. The total integrated network of techniques, aids, strategies, and skills an individual uses either to supplement (augmentative) or to replace (alternate) inadequate natural speaking capability. It includes (1) one or more communicative techniques, (2) a symbol set or system, and (3) a variety of communicative–interactive behaviors.

Communication. Process by which information is exchanged between individuals using both verbal and nonverbal behaviors.

Communication aid. A physical object or device that helps a person communicate (e.g., communication board, electronic aid, voice output communication aid).

Communicative mode. One of the several different major channels or forms of communication (e.g., speaking, listening, reading, writing, gesturing).

Nonspeaking person. Anyone whose speech is temporarily or permanently inadequate to meet all of his or her communication needs and whose inability to speak is not primarily due to a hearing impairment.

Nonverbal communication. Communication that does not involve the use of words (spoken, written, or signed); it does use nonverbal communicative behaviors such as kinesics (communicative posturing and bodily movements); paralinguistics (pitch height and range, stress, intonation, vocal intensity, articulatory control); proxemics (interpersonal distance); and chronemics (timing factors).

Nonvocal verbal behavior. The communication of information through some physical structure other than the vocal tract and oral musculature (e.g., written language, sign systems, and rule-governed graphic symbol systems, e.g., Blissymbols).

Skill. An ability developed over time and with practice (both strategies and skills, e.g., pointing or spelling, contribute to the relative competence a person exhibits when using AAC system components).

Strategy. A specific way of using aids or techniques more effectively for specific purposes (e.g., when communicating under time pressure, a more telegraphic style may be used; different strategies may be used for group communication).

Symbol. An abstract but recognized object, mark, or graphic design that stands for or represents something else (e.g., Rebus, picture, Blissymbol, word, American Sign Language sign, gesture, or speech morpheme).

Technique. A method for transmitting ideas (e.g., linear scanning, row–column scanning, signing, common gestures, natural vocalizations, facial expressions, eye pointing).

Unaided communication technique. Any AAC technique that does not require a physical aid (e.g., manual, gestural, manual–visual sign, facial communication).

User interface. The physical means a person uses to control a communication aid (involves matching the most functional anatomical sites and positions for the person with a communication aid through, e.g., pointing, adaptive switches, touch panels, joysticks, or lightbeams and sensors).

Verbal communication. The use of words in written, spoken, and/or signed modes (synonymous with *linguistic*).

Vocal verbal behavior. The communication of information expressed with functional oral speech (synonymous with *speech*).

Based on Fried-Oken, 1987; Vanderheiden & Yoder, 1986.

MEASURING EARLY-STAGE ABILITIES, NEEDS, AND ACCOMPLISHMENTS

The most valid and comprehensive assessments of children in the earliest stages of language acquisition are based on multiple methods of data gathering, including observations of communicative interactions in multiple contexts with more than one partner. As noted, for infants at risk, serial assessments may be conducted to monitor and document changes over time. Neisworth and Bagnato (1988) argued that outcomes are more comprehensive, reliable, and valid when based on a multidimensional assessment model that employs multiple measures, derives data from multiple sources, surveys multiple domains, and fulfills multiple purposes.

CONTEXTS FOR EARLY-STAGE ASSESSMENT AND INTERVENTION

Hospital

When established risks, biological risks, and marked environmental risks are evident at birth, assessment and intervention are appropriate while the infant is still in the hospital. Sparks (1989b) listed essential assessment components: (1) the prenatal and perinatal birth history, (2) factors that seem to influence the infant's ability to maintain physiological organization (called *homeostasis*), (3) oral–motor status and feeding needs, and (4) the infant's hospital environment, including the amount and kinds of stimulation to which the infant is exposed (e.g., ambient noise), as well as nurturing opportunities for communication. Specific characteristics to look for in each of these areas are discussed in conjunction with potential targets for intervention later in this chapter.

Home

In the broadest sense, home-based services are defined simply as services delivered in the home of a target infant or toddler rather than in a center. Bailey and Simeonsson (1988) noted that the rationale for providing assessment and intervention in the home is twofold. First, homes can provide natural contexts for facilitating the roles of parents as primary interventionists for their children. Second, homes may be preferred for assessment and intervention, based on practical considerations such as increased access to

children in rural areas and the relative economy of providing services in homes compared to the expense of setting up a large center-based facility.

Furthermore, communication specialists may find that periodically seeing children, parents, and siblings interacting in their own home, with the materials and within the contexts available there, may yield a better understanding of home routines and ways to best use them during intervention. Clinical recommendations then may be expressed in ways relevant to everyday opportunities in the standard routine at home. The specialist should emphasize assisting parents not only to improve things for their children but to make things easier for themselves. A professional might assist a mother to position her child in an infant swing (in which the infant rarely fusses or cries) so that the mother can see the child's face (and vice versa) while she folds laundry, talking to her child about the clothing—whose they are, their size, and their softness—while folding them.

Disadvantages of providing home-based assessment and intervention services also may be evident. These include the reluctance of some parents to be cast in the role of primary teacher for their young children, limited access to different professional specialists, limited opportunities of children for social and communication interactions with peers when isolated at home, and limited access to a wide range of toys and specialized equipment in many homes (Bailey & Simeonsson, 1988).

Infant Center or Clinic

Advantages and disadvantages are also associated with assessment and intervention in center-based programs. Among the advantages, Bailey and Simeonsson (1988) mentioned the availability of early childhood education teachers with proficiencies for facilitating learning, communication, and development; the availability of related service personnel such as speech-language pathologists, occupational therapists, and physical therapists; and opportunities for infants to engage in social and communicative interactions with handicapped and nonhandicapped peers.

In addition, Wieder and Findikoglu (1987) mentioned that their urban infant center allowed mothers with special needs to experience a responsive and nurturing environment. The center also offered individualized therapeutic programs for both infants and care givers; therapy groups for mothers and children; workshops on nutrition, birth control, toys, and driver's education; a high school equivalency program; trips; and celebrations of birthdays and holidays.

Disadvantages associated with providing services to infants and toddlers in center-based programs concern the potential reduction of parental time spent with their infants and opportunities to establish attachments in one-to-one interactions. In addition, advances made in center-based programs may not generalize back to home environments, and travel to centers may be impractical for some families (Bailey & Simeonsson, 1988).

Classroom

When older children remain at earlier stages of development, assessment and intervention in special and regular education classrooms may be appropriate. The focus should be on the communicative demands and supports of contexts as well as on the intrinsic abilities of the child and the potential interactions between them. Both intervention needs and progress can be determined best when children are assessed within the school and home, where they are expected to participate. When conducting ecological assessments of children with handicaps in classrooms, Carta, Sainato, and Greenwood (1988) suggested that specialists should ask questions not only about the effects of static environmental features, such as materials, spatial arrangements, teacher/pupil ratio, and ratio of handicapped/nonhandicapped children, but also about dynamic features regarding the effects of teacher behavior. Those authors also suggested that ecological assessments consider not only the current placement but how the current environment helps children develop survival skills they might need in the "next environment" (p. 225).

The relative advantages and disadvantages of placing children with severe disabilities in regular education classrooms versus special education classrooms in either regular education buildings or center-based special schools have been discussed at several points throughout this book. No single answer is best for all children and for all purposes. Rather, decisions must be made about what is best for individual children by considering multiple factors. In a later section, varied models are presented for assessing older children

with early-stage abilities. (In Chapters 8 and 9, further information is presented about conducting ecological assessments of classroom contexts.)

A FAMILY SYSTEMS APPROACH TO EARLY-STAGE ASSESSMENT

The influence of context should be considered whenever assessment and intervention services are provided to children with language disorders. Context should be considered during planning for every child, but it is particularly important when planning for infants, toddlers, and older individuals with severe communicative impairments, in part because communicative partners must bear a disproportionate share of the communicative burden when interacting with these children.

The system theory perspective (developed in Chapter 1) is ideal for working with infants in the contexts of their families. A family systems perspective of the assessment process addresses many factors that influence the availability of family resources for dealing with the problem, not only in the present but over the long haul (Barber, Turnbull, Behr, & Kerns, 1988). These factors include characteristics of the exceptionality; characteristics of the family (e.g., family size and form, cultural and religious backgrounds of the members, socioeconomic factors, and geographic location); and personality characteristics of the individual family members. Family interactions are influenced not only by the parental subsystem of the mother–child dyad, which has been studied most extensively, but other family subsystems, such as the marital and extrafamily subsystems.

How individuals cope with infants with disabilities may also be influenced by where families are in the "family life cycle." Family life cycles are typically divided into six or more stages defined in terms of the ages of children, particularly the oldest child. Six common stages are (1) birth and early childhood, (2) elementary school years, (3) adolescence, (4) young adulthood, (5) empty nest, and (6) elderly years (Barber et al., 1988). Stepfamilies and single-parent families can bring added complexities to family life cycles as well, sometimes resulting in repeats and recycling through the stages.

No matter when babies with special needs arrive in their families' life cycles, they can be expected to foster significant stresses that surpass those normally associated with having a baby (which does not suggest that families cannot enjoy a child with special needs and feel positively influenced by the experience) (Barber et al., 1988). However, when parents have special needs themselves, suggesting influences of environmental risk factors in conjunction with established and/or biological risk factors, it is particularly important for the specialist to consider parental mental health concerns and the parents' possible need for support in caring for and interacting with their infants.

For multirisk families, the picture may be even further complicated by the parents' lacking the organizational skills, trust, or motivation to seek professional assistance. Wieder and Greenspan (1987) found that the staff of their clinical infant development program had to develop special techniques for engaging and working with such families (see Personal Reflection 7.1); the staff needed to be persistent, respectful, and sensitive when offering services to multirisk families who had never been able to take advantage of special services, but who clearly needed them.

Assessments in infancy should address the infant, primary care givers, and interactions between them (Sparks, 1989b). When assessing parental resources and the potential need for services to support parental efforts, Wieder and Greenspan (1987) recommended thinking in terms of primary and secondary maternal functions. As primary maternal functions, they included "the ability to provide physical care and protection, the basic ability to read an infant's signals of pleasure or displeasure, and the minimum emotional basis for a human attachment between mother and infant" (p. 11). As secondary maternal functions, they included "the ability to discern a child's changing developmental needs during the course of the first two years of life and the capacity to respond promptly, effectively, and empathically to the signals" (p. 11).

MODELS FOR ASSESSING OLDER CHILDREN WITH EARLY-STAGE ABILITIES

When older children have severe communicative impairments making it difficult for them to advance past early stages of language acquisition, they probably also have multiple handicaps that justify intensive special education services, and they may have been part of a special education services network for some time. Thus, these children do not need to be "found" in the same sense that infants and toddlers at risk do. However, they may need to be viewed from a fresh perspective.

Periodically, difficult decisions must be made about the extent to which these children should be included in regular education buildings, classrooms, and activities and about the kind and amount of services they should receive from a speech–language pathologist. For example, "Should services be consultative or direct? Should they be daily or intermittent?" In addition, the specialist should locate and reevaluate children who may have been underserved because no one had considered that they might be able to communicate better with an AAC system than unaided (or with a more effective AAC system). These children may need intensive, specialized services for relatively short durations to determine whether they need an AAC system, and if so, what kind.

As noted previously, the questions about whether older children with severe handicaps should be integrated into regular school buildings and classrooms are highly complex, and they can be answered only by teams of professionals and parents on an individual basis. The specialist may find it helpful, however, to have a system for thinking about these children in the context of more than one level of participation. The major steps in Beukelman and Mirenda's (1992)

| Personal Reflection 7.1 | "In most cases, continued reaching out by an interested person willing to hear about and try to understand the difficulties a mother, father, or family was experiencing eventually met with a response, however slight, indirect, or cautious it might be. We learned that each family, like each baby, could respond if our overtures were persistent, respectful, and sensitive." |

Serena Wieder, Ph.D., and *Stanley I. Greenspan, M.D.* (1987, p. 11), writing about the staffing, process, and structure of a clinical infant development program developed to provide preventive intervention for infants in multirisk families.

participation model of assessment are diagrammed in Figure 7.1. Notice that two kinds of barriers to participation may be identified as this model is implemented. The first involves limits on levels of opportunity available to the child. A focus on removing policy and traditional practice barriers and on assisting participants to acquire new knowledge and skills for working with children with severe disabilities may contribute to reducing levels of handicap. A second kind of barrier concerns limits on levels of access. When conducting activities on this limb of the model, a focus on increasing natural ability may contribute to reducing levels of impairment, and a focus on the potential for environmental adaptation and the use of assistive technology may contribute to reducing levels of disability.

The outcome of all of the efforts illustrated in the flowchart in Figure 7.1 is a decision about participation. The standards for deciding who can participate in various settings may vary with the levels of participation expected. As noted in Chapter 5, Beukelman and Mirenda (1992) distinguished three patterns of academic and social participation. They suggested that, in either domain, children can be (1) competitive, (2) active, or (3) included. Children who remain at early stages of language development would not be expected to be competitive, or even active, in regular classroom academic or social contexts, but they might be included in at least some regular education or extracurricular activities during a school day. If the child is included, the specialist should conduct a contextually based assessment of how to best match the environment and the child.

Within this overall framework, questions about relative ability levels across several areas of development are appropriate. That was the purpose of the Michigan Decision-Making Model, originally developed by N. W. Nelson, Silbar, and Lockwood (1981) and described by N. W. Nelson (1989a). This approach focuses more on communicative processes rather than on communicative needs or opportunities. This model includes four components: Two of them, a reference chart (see Appendix B) and a summary chart (Appendix B and Figure 7.2) are used to integrate information from a variety of formal and informal assessment activities. The other two components are a service-delivery decision-making chart (Figure 7.3) and an AAC decision-making chart (Figure 7.4).

The Michigan summary chart is used to estimate and compare a child's current levels of functioning across the four domains—cognitive bases, receptive language, expressive language, and social interaction and play. No single assessment tool is recommended for making the background judgments for shading in this chart, but the methods developed by Linder (1990), Norris and Hoffman (1990a), and A. M. Wetherby and Prizant (1990) (described later) are particularly well suited for conducting multidimensional observational assessments that include compensation for sensory and motor deficits. For example, Linder (1990) described how a motorically involved child demonstrated age-level conceptualization of dramatic play even though her results on a standardized intelligence test indicated that she was mentally retarded. The more positive results were obtained because, in the play context, the girl was able to direct a facilitator's actions through a sequence of dramatic play events using her eyes and vocalizations to demonstrate a higher level of maturity.

The summary chart accompanying the Michigan Decision-Making Model (Figure 7.2) is a condensation of the reference chart that appears (with slight modifications from earlier versions) in Appendix B. The reference chart may be used to help fill in the summary chart by conducting interviews with parents and other participants to try to gain the most accurate picture of a child's best levels of functioning in real-life settings. For example, when parents are given clues as to what kinds of behavior represent development in a specific area and contexts that might elicit it, they may be able to provide specific examples of their child's demonstrating that behavior. Check-off boxes on the reference chart may be filled when this evidence is available. Remember that no matter how the information is gathered, allowances must be made for sensory and motor deficits that may interfere with demonstration of a particular level of functioning, and tasks should be modified as appropriate. The previously discussed (see Chapter 3) limitations of the Piagetian model for explaining contextually based cognitive development variations should also be kept in mind when using this system, because it is tied most closely to that model.

Following is a case example demonstrating use of the Michigan Decision-Making Model in developing services for Andrea, a 4-year-old student with suspected cognitive and related impairments functioning at a presymbolic level expressively. The summary chart shown in Figure 7.2 is shaded in to illustrate Andrea's function profile. It is helpful, while sitting

FIGURE 7.1
Participation model.

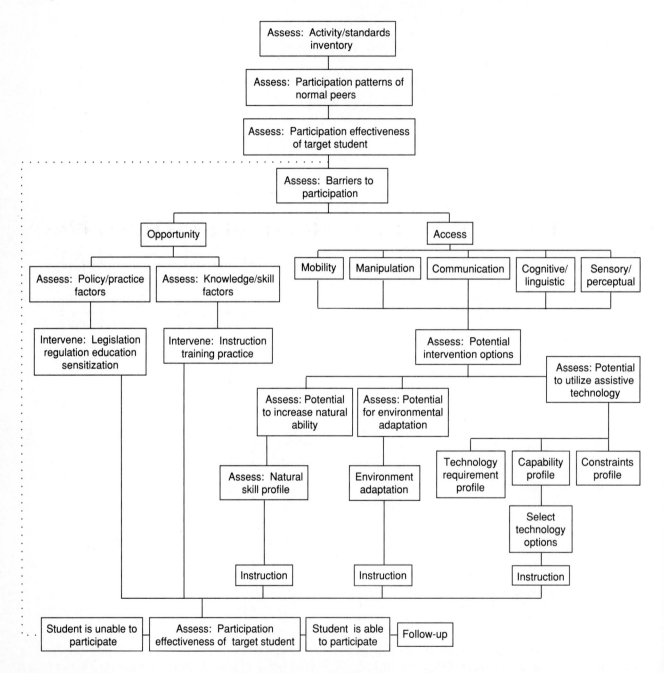

FIGURE 7.2

Summary chart shaded to illustrate Andrea's profile.

Name: _____ BD: _____   Speech-Language Clinician: _____

Date: _____   Classroom Teacher: _____

COGNITIVE BASES	RECEPTIVE LANGUAGE	EXPRESSIVE LANGUAGE	SOCIAL INTERACTION & PLAY
Preintentional (Birth to 8 months) *Sensorimotor I, II, III* __ Infant moves from being purely reflexive to showing the initial beginnings of goal-oriented behavior __ Developing object permanence	__ Startles to sound __ Turns to sound __ Reacts to human voice __ Responds to tone of voice	__ Cry __ Reflexive Vocalizations	__ Engages in interaction __ Maintains interaction __ Initiates interaction __ Indicates preference for familiar people and objects
Early Intentional (8 to 12 months) *Sensorimotor IV* __ Uses familiar means to achieve novel ends	__ No word comprehension yet __ Imitates on-going action __ Looks where parent looks	__ Differentiated cries __ Syllabic babbling	__ Plays nursery games __ Plays with toys
Late Intentional (12 to 18 months) *Sensorimotor V* __ Invention of new means to achieve familiar ends	__ Responds appropriately to single words in context	__ Hi/bye routines __ First words __ Words used as "performatives" (to manipulate environment)	__ Solitary or onlooker play __ Hugs doll, pulls toy
Representational (18 to 24 months) *Thought* *Sensorimotor VI* __ Begins symbolic thinking	__ Understands words without context (points to pictures) __ Follows 2-word commands	__ Novel one-word utterances __ Asks "What's that?" __ Onset of 2-word utterances	__ Parallel play
Early Preoperations (2 to 3½ yrs) __ Thought is preconceptual __ Inference is sometimes but not always correct	__ Begins to understand Wh-questions __ Answers yes/no questions	__ Two-word utterances __ Basic sentences develop __ Morphological markers develop	__ Symbolic play
Late Preoperations (3½ to 7 yrs.) __ Beginning of intuitive thought __ Problem solves by trial & error (not always correct)	__ Points to pictures representing sentences __ Uses word order to understand agent-object relationships	__ Uses compound and complex sentences __ Uses language to relate experiences __ Talks about remote experiences __ Adequate voice, articulation, fluency	__ Plays in small groups
Concrete Operations (7 to 12 yrs.) __ Classifies on 2 characteristics	__ Understands conditional causal sentences	__ More clauses per sentence __ Uses language to converse, persuade, tease	__ Genuine cooperative play

Instructions:

1. Place a check mark beside characteristics demonstrated (reference chart or other evaluation tools may be used as necessary)
2. Shade in areas which describe functioning (areas may be partially shaded)
3. Refer to program decision chart

Recommendations:

Note. From *The Michigan Decision-Making Strategy for Determining Appropriate Communicative Services for Physically and/or Mentally Handicapped Children* by N. W. Nelson, J. C. Silbar, and E. L. Lockwood, November 1981, presented at the annual conference of the American Speech-Language-Hearing Association. Los Angeles. Copyright 1981 by N. W. Nelson, J. C. Silbar, and E. L. Lockwood. Reprinted by permission.

FIGURE 7.3
Placement and program decision chart.

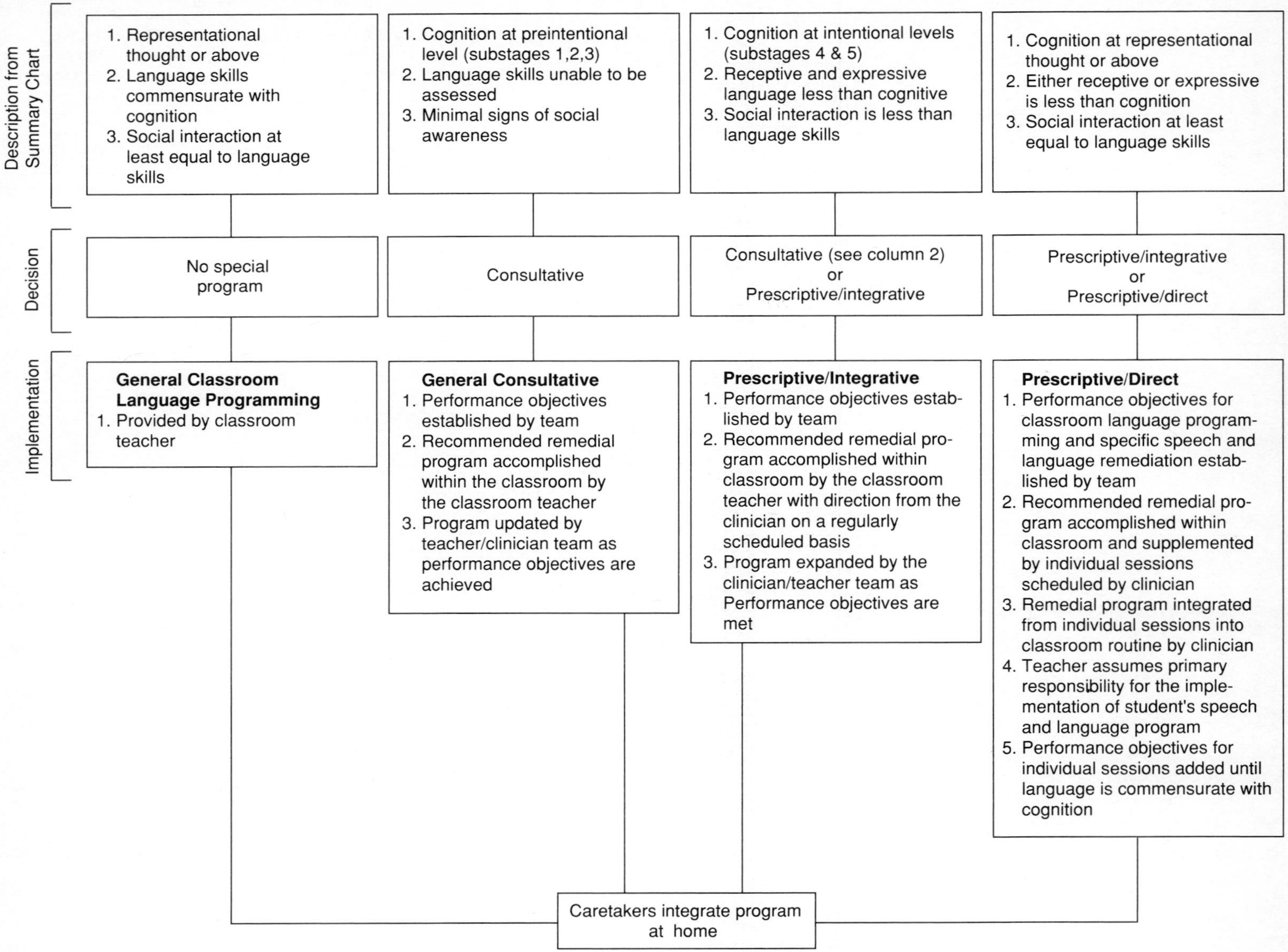

Description from Summary Chart	Decision	Implementation
1. Representational thought or above 2. Language skills commensurate with cognition 3. Social interaction at least equal to language skills	No special program	**General Classroom Language Programming** 1. Provided by classroom teacher
1. Cognition at preintentional level (substages 1,2,3) 2. Language skills unable to be assessed 3. Minimal signs of social awareness	Consultative	**General Consultative** 1. Performance objectives established by team 2. Recommended remedial program accomplished within the classroom by the classroom teacher 3. Program updated by teacher/clinician team as performance objectives are achieved
1. Cognition at intentional levels (substages 4 & 5) 2. Receptive and expressive language less than cognitive skills 3. Social interaction is less than language skills	Consultative (see column 2) or Prescriptive/integrative	**Prescriptive/Integrative** 1. Performance objectives established by team 2. Recommended remedial program accomplished within the classroom by the classroom teacher with direction from the clinician on a regularly scheduled basis 3. Program expanded by the clinician/teacher team as Performance objectives are met
1. Cognition at representational thought or above 2. Either receptive or expressive is less than cognition 3. Social interaction at least equal to language skills	Prescriptive/integrative or Prescriptive/direct	**Prescriptive/Direct** 1. Performance objectives for classroom language programming and specific speech and language remediation established by team 2. Recommended remedial program accomplished within classroom and supplemented by individual sessions scheduled by clinician 3. Remedial program integrated from individual sessions into classroom routine by clinician 4. Teacher assumes primary responsibility for the implementation of student's speech and language program 5. Performance objectives for individual sessions added until language is commensurate with cognition

Caretakers integrate program at home

Note. From *The Michigan Decision-Making Strategy for Determining Appropriate Communicative Services for Physically and/or Mentally Handicapped Children* by N. W. Nelson, J. C. Silbar, and E. L. Lockwood, November 1981, presented at the annual conference of the American Speech-Language-Hearing Association. Los Angeles. Copyright 1981 by N. W. Nelson, J. C. Silbar, and E. L. Lockwood. Reprinted by permission.

with parents and others in the planning group, to shade in sections of the form while talking about the accomplishments they represent and gaining validating confirmation from parents and others that the profile accurately reflects the child's abilities as they see them. Later, the specialist may use this chart to mark progress by shading in new achievements with a different color or marking pattern.

Andrea shows evidence of being almost up to expectations for her 4-year-old chronological age in three of the four developmental domains, but in the area of expressive language, she lags considerably behind. In nonverbal communicative attempts, Andrea demonstrates "hi–bye" routines and other forms of gestural, nonverbal communication deliberately to make her intentions known, and she can imitate a few signs taught to her by her parents, but she does not yet clearly use symbols spontaneously for communication. Thus, only a portion of the expressive language box at the 12- to 18-month level is shaded. When this profile is then used as input to the service-delivery decision-making chart (Figure 7.3), Andrea fits the needs profile of the fourth column. That is, she has one area (expressive language) significantly lower than others in combination with evidence of early preoperational thought, basically intact language comprehension, and symbolic play and social interaction skills that are close to age level. Andrea therefore is judged to need some fairly direct language and speech intervention services. In particular, because Andrea's problem seems to involve severe developmental oral–motor and speech apraxia, she may benefit from intensive direct focus on speech production as well as language use.

In addition, the fact that Andrea is 4 years old and cannot yet speak intelligibly in even the most limited way clearly indicates that she needs an augmentative communication system. It is increasingly rare to find AAC specialists who recommend waiting for 2 or 3 years to see if speech will develop, and Andrea probably should have been served in this way earlier. Every individual needs a way to communicate now, and all normally developing individuals use many different techniques and strategies to communicate their messages. The AAC system is now viewed primarily as an option added to a child's communication network rather than as a replacement for speech or as a sign that professionals have given up on assisting the child to acquire speech (although the danger that an alternative mode may result in reduced efforts to help a child learn to speak naturally is real and should not be ignored).

For Andrea, all four indicators suggesting a need to consider AAC options are present (see Figure 7.4). She clearly communicates intentionally, her receptive language skills and cognitive abilities are considerably more advanced than her expressive language, her expressive speech and language attempts are limited and unintelligible, and yet her social interactions suggest a desire and underlying ability to communicate much more. Even if Andrea demonstrated only one or two of these indicators, the need for AAC still should be deliberately considered. Furthermore, the communicative needs of children even more limited than Andrea, who do not yet show signs of intentional behavior, should be considered similarly. Remember that *no* nonspeaking child is considered to be too impaired for attention to his or her communicative needs.

The recommendations differ based on the child's abilities. In the earliest stages of communicative development, more of the burden is on the communicative partner. With children in the preintentional (perlocutionary) communication stage (review Table 7.1), the specialist focuses on nudging the child into

FIGURE 7.4
Augmentative and alternative communication decision making chart.

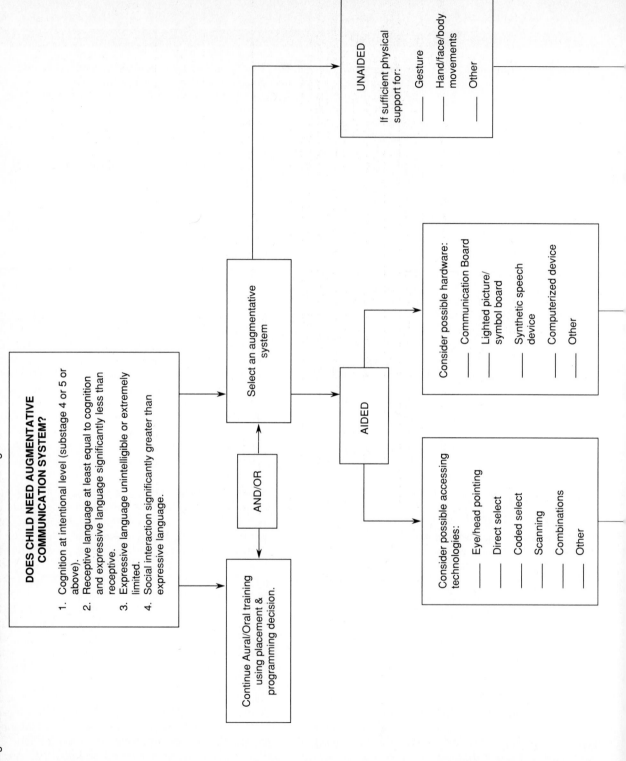

DOES CHILD NEED AUGMENTATIVE COMMUNICATION SYSTEM?

1. Cognition at intentional level (substage 4 or 5 or above).
2. Receptive language at least equal to cognition and expressive language significantly less than receptive.
3. Expressive language unintelligible or extremely limited.
4. Social interaction significantly greater than expressive language.

Continue Aural/Oral training using placement & programming decision.

AND/OR

Select an augmentative system

AIDED

UNAIDED

If sufficient physical support for:

____ Gesture
____ Hand/face/body movements
____ Other

Consider possible hardware:

____ Communication Board
____ Lighted picture/ symbol board
____ Synthetic speech device
____ Computerized device
____ Other

Consider possible accessing technologies:

____ Eye/head pointing
____ Direct select
____ Coded select
____ Scanning
____ Combinations
____ Other

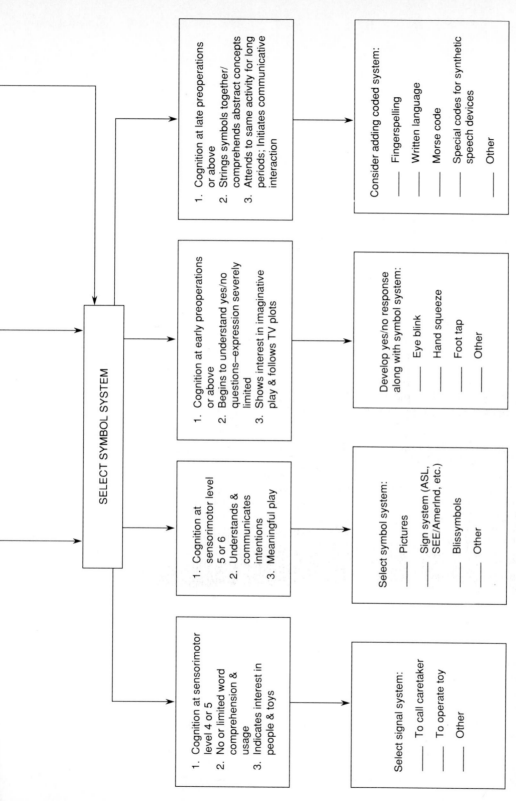

Acknowledgement: The development of this chart was influenced by the work of David Yoder.

Note. From *The Michigan Decision-Making Strategy for Determining Appropriate Communicative Services for Physically and/or Mentally Handicapped Children* by N. W. Nelson, J. C. Silbar, and E. L. Lockwood, November 1981, presented at the annual conference of the American Speech-Language-Hearing Association. Los Angeles. Copyright 1981 by N. W. Nelson, J. C. Silbar, and E. L. Lockwood. Reprinted by permission.

intentional (illocutionary) communication. The specialist responds to current behavioral signs as if they were communicative and explores options that may encourage the child to begin to be aware of the possibilities of goal-directed communication, encourages the expression of intentions, and then assists the child to express those intentions more clearly and by using more conventional means. Andrea has already moved beyond the earliest parts of this sequence. She is ready to acquire more conventional means of expression.

The AAC decision-making chart (Figure 7.4) can assist in this process by contributing to the selection of a symbol system, a display method, and accessing techniques (see the following section on early stage word–symbol acquisition for a further discussion of the symbol-assessment process). Andrea's levels of symbolic play suggest that picture symbols might be explored for use in her preschool classroom. Furthermore, if she had a device with voice output, she could participate in activities such as circle time and reporting the weather audibly to her classmates. Because she has the cognitive development necessary and good general motor control, she can probably indicate yes–no responses with a combination of natural gestures and natural speech attempts, and she can use direct selection with her augmentative device by pointing or pressing a fairly small switch with her fingers.

The primary disadvantage of a communication device for Andrea would be that she would have to carry it around, and it might not be the most practical mode of communication for physically active Andrea in less formal settings. Therefore, her parents might be encouraged, in addition, to continue their efforts to learn a more sophisticated sign language system along with Andrea and to use it always in conjunction with speech. The advantages of this system within the family are that it may allow more flexibility of vocabulary acquisition (because the only limits are imposed by human memory and knowledge of signs and not by physical storage and display capacity of a low-tech or high-tech device). It is also available wherever family members and others know the system, without the need for a physical communication device. Of course, Andrea's parents are aware of the limitation that sign language is not generally intelligible to the public, but their acceptance of it, their awareness of Andrea's need to be able to express herself linguistically now, and their previous independent attempts to use such a system with her make it a good option to consider in conjunction with others. Whatever expressive language modalities Andrea uses, her level of receptive language also suggests that she should be encouraged to combine symbols expressively into at least two-word utterances. The specialist also should reassess her needs continually, because they are likely to change. Finally, the specialist should continue to give direct attention to Andrea's need for intelligible natural speech.

TOOLS AND STRATEGIES FOR EARLY-STAGE ASSESSMENT

Some measurement methods appropriate for children in the earliest stages of development are designed to diagnose disorder, but many instruments act more as gross screening devices and are so imprecise that they fail to differentiate among children diagnostically, particularly at the youngest ages. For example, a 3-month delay, which might be ignored for a 4-year-old, could be highly significant for a 5-month-old child.

Very young children therefore should be eligible for services when they are at risk and not only when it is possible to diagnose a frank disorder. Some assessment instruments designed for screening and diagnosis in the earliest stages of language acquisition are presented with brief abstracts in Appendix A. A select few are discussed more fully in the following sections.

Formal Assessment Tools

Some tools focus on general developmental concerns, and some are aimed more specifically at the assessment of communication and related developmental advances. The Transdisciplinary Play-Based Assessment approach (TPBA) (Linder, 1990) is an example of the first kind of approach, and the Communication and Symbolic Behavior Scales (CSBS) (A. M. Wetherby & Prizant, 1990) is an example of the second. These two approaches are described here to illustrate some of the principles of assessment appropriate to the prelanguage and early language stage of development. Other strategies useful for describing abilities in specific areas and for specific populations are described in the following section on methods and targets of early-stage intervention.

Transdisciplinary Play-Based Assessment. The TPBA (Linder, 1990) was mentioned in Chapter 6 as an example of an approach that represents combined elements of cognitivist and social interaction theoretical perspectives. It is designed for children functioning developmentally between the ages of 6 months and 6 years, using a play interaction context to provide opportunity for developmental observations in four domains: (1) social–emotional, (2) cognitive, (3) language and communication, and (4) sensorimotor. This truly transdisciplinary approach involves a team of parents and representatives of disciplines who release their varied professional roles to a single play facilitator who works directly with the target child while the others observe, in arena fashion. During the 1 hour to 1½ hour of videotaped play interaction, the team also observes the child interacting with her parents and a peer. No standardized scores are computed with the TPBA, but the outcome is an analysis of developmental level, learning style, interaction patterns, and other relevant behaviors that can become an integral part of intervention planning. Linder reports that "Communication between the parents and other team members, prior to and during the assessment, is the key to ongoing dialogue that will continue throughout the child's involvement in an intervention program" (p. 1). The outcome of assessment using the TPBA might be a description of current levels of performance and a set of recommendations such as those illustrated in Box 7.3.

Communication and Symbolic Behavior Scales. The CSBS (Wetherby & Prizant, 1990) has some features in common with the TPBA, but after field testing is complete, it will be standardized. The CSBS also differs from the TPBA in that, although it includes items addressing cognitive and social–affective behaviors, it primarily aims to assess communicative behavior. This test is currently available in a research edition while being standardized, but it now includes pre-standardization data gathered on 34 normally developing children and 27 children who were either language delayed or exhibiting delays in social communication as well as information about reliability and validity. The CSBS is designed to be used with children whose functional communication ages are between 9 months and 2 years.

A "standard but flexible format" (A. M. Wetherby & Prizant, 1990, p. 1) and a variety of procedures are used to gather the data used in CSBS analysis. The procedures include a care-giver questionnaire, direct

---

Box 7.3	An example of results and recommendations based on the TPBA

An evaluation determined that Melody enjoyed and initiated dramatic play. She was capable of putting together a 3-step sequence of activities with objects in relation to a doll. She poured "milk" in a cup, fed the doll, and burped it. The evaluation also found that Melody had difficulty taking turns with adults and peers. Her language was intelligible about half the time and was limited to 2-word approximations ("a o," for "want more"). Melody was able to label familiar objects, but did not attempt to imitate new words.

Program recommendations for Melody should include:

1. Encouraging Melody's dramatic play and modeling 3-step sequences in new behaviors with the doll, in order to promote generalizations (washing the doll's hair, drying it, and combing it);
2. Expanding her existing 3-step schemes by adding one more step (after burping the doll, putting it to bed);
3. Helping Melody to generalize her vocabulary by presenting variations of common objects (different shaped and colored combs, brushes, socks, etc.) every day. Also, adding one common object not presently in her expressive vocabulary each week was recommended (deciding with the parents which common objects are most relevant in her life). (p. 18)

Note. From *Transdisciplinary Play-Based Assessment: A Functional Approach to Working With Young Children* (p. 18) by T. W. Linder, 1990, Baltimore, MD: Paul H. Brookes Publishing Co. Copyright 1990 by Paul H. Brookes Publishing Co. Reprinted by permission.

sampling of verbal and nonverbal communicative behaviors, and observation of relatively unstructured play activities. In the manual, Wetherby and Prizant indicate that the care-giver questionnaire can be completed before the assessment, which takes about 1 hour and is videotaped for analysis and scoring (videotaping is optional for TPBA). The videotape scoring is also reported to take a little more than 1 hour for trained evaluators.

The sampling procedures of the CSBS resemble natural, ongoing child–adult interactions, using a continuum from structured to unstructured contexts. The procedures start with a warm-up, followed by a series of "communicative temptations" based on earlier work by A. M. Wetherby and Prutting (1984). For example, the temptation with the wind-up toy includes steps to (1) activate a wind-up toy and then let it run down, allow the child to pick it up (or hand it to the child), and wait for the child to signal for the adult's help; (2) reactivate the toy after the child's first communicative signal, then let it run down, allow the child to pick it up, or hand it to the child and wait for the child to signal for help; (3) reactivate the toy again after the child's second communicative signal, again let it run down, and again allow the child to pick it up or hand it to the child and wait for the child to signal for help; (4) after the child's third communicative signal, put the toy within the child's reach without reactivating it and wait; (5) after the child's fourth communicative signal, hold up the toy and label it or comment on it without reactivating it, then put it on the table and wait; and (6) after the child's fifth communicative signal, reactivate the toy, and then remove it from the table, saying, "Bye, bye, turtle [penguin]." In addition to the communicative temptations, the CSBS also provides a preliteracy activity in the form of a book-sharing event as well as materials and strategies for a set of symbolic play probes, language comprehension probes, and combinatorial play probes. At the conclusion of the CSBS session, care givers are asked to help validate the results by rating their child's behavior in several areas in terms of how typical it was during the session.

Box 7.4 is an outline of the sampling procedures and instructions used in the CSBS. Scoring of the CSBS is accomplished by assigning a rating of 1 to 5 for each of 20 separate scales, including 16 communication scales (subdivided into the four areas, communicative function, communicative means, reciprocity, and social-affective signaling) and four scales for rating symbolic behavior (subdivided into two areas).

The CSBS has many psychometric strengths combined with a firm foundation in current social interaction theory of how language develops. It maintains a holistic framework for the assessment process, while allowing professionals to analyze subcomponents of language to assist in planning and measuring progress. Preliminary results suggest that the test can be administered reliably in serial fashion, at about 3-month intervals, to measure progress in multiple communicative areas as well.

A limitation of the CSBS's research edition is that it gives little assistance to evaluators for using the qualitative and quantitative results in planning programs. It is expected that the field testing will result in information that can be used for multiple purposes, including diagnosing disability, monitoring developmental changes, marking progress augmented by intervention, and deciding which areas to target in the intervention progress. Even in its current form, the test offers rich possibilities for description and quantification of a child's early communicative behaviors relevant to the child's everyday needs.

Informal Procedures: Blurring the Boundaries Between Assessment and Intervention

Whenever children are suspected of having language disorders, formal assessment procedures should be augmented by informal ones (Roberts & Crais, 1989). For many reasons, however, informal procedures, and procedures blending assessment and intervention goals beyond labeling, are especially appropriate in the early stages of communicative development. First, a diagnostic label may not be an appropriate or a fruitful goal of infant and toddler assessment because children change rapidly in the first months and years of life; a label assigned one month may not be appropriate the next. Second, policies that encourage preventive intervention approaches enable the specialist to postpone the differential diagnosis of specific disorders in very young children without jeopardizing the family's access to services. Third, more can be learned about the child's abilities and needs through working with the child to encourage further development, and noting how the child learns, than by presenting isolated tasks and assessing whether a particular kind of skill or knowledge is already present.

This process-oriented assessment is not new. In 1977, DuBose, Langley, and Stass identified the following assumptions underlying a process-oriented approach to assessing children with severe handi-

Box 7.4   Outline of sampling procedures and instructions

I. Warm-Up (10–15 minutes)
I am going to begin by asking you some questions about how [child's name] communicates. You can hold [child's name] on your lap or let him [her] play on the floor.

II. Communicative Temptations (10–20 minutes)
We want to get a sample of how [child's name] communicates with sounds, gestures, or words. First, I am going to present some situations that will encourage [child's name] to communicate. Please try not to direct [child's name] or tell him [her] what to do. Also try not to ask him [her] questions. Wait for [child's name] to initiate. If [child's name] communicates to you, try to respond naturally, by helping him [her] or noticing what he [she] is playing with. Remember, don't tell [child's name] what to do.

1. Wind-Up Toy
2. Balloon
3. Bubbles
4. Peek-a-boo
5. Walk Mouse, Creep Mouse
6. Blocks in Box
7. Jar
8. Toys in Bag

III. Sharing Books (5 minutes)
Now we want to see what [child's name] does when looking at books. Try to avoid telling [child's name] what to look at or asking [child's name] to label the picture. Follow [child's name]'s lead by noticing or labeling the picture that he [she] directs your attention to.

IV. Symbolic Play Probes (10 minutes)
Now we want to see how [child's name] plays with different sets of toys. Again try to avoid telling [child's name] what to do or asking [child's name] questions. Follow [child's name]'s lead by commenting about what [child's name] is doing.

1. First Toy Set (Feeding Set or Grooming Set)
2. Verbal Instructions and Modeling
3. Second Toy Set

V. Language Comprehension Probes (5 minutes)
1. Comprehension Response Strategy
Now we want to see how [child's name] understands words by asking him [her] to point to body parts. What body parts does [child's name] know?
2. Body Parts
3. Agents
4. Possessor–Possession Combinations

VI. Combinatorial Play Probes (5 minutes)
Now we want to see how [child's name] combines objects in play. Again try to avoid telling [child's name] what to do or asking [child's name] questions. Follow [child's name]'s lead by commenting about what [child's name] is doing.

1. Blocks
2. Stacking Rings
3. Nesting Cups

VII. Caregiver Perception Rating Form

Note. From *Communication and Symbolic Behavior Scales Manual* (Table 2.1) by A. Wetherby and B. Prizant, 1990, Chicago, IL: The Riverside Publishing Company. Copyright © 1990. Reproduced with permission of The Riverside Publishing Company, Chicago, IL.

caps: (1) Children are "active agents" operating on their environments. (2) The learning process can be measured and modified within the contexts of the assessment. (3) Children's learning potential is best assessed by observing their performance in learning tasks, for which corrective feedback can be provided.

A major distinction between formal and informal assessment procedures is the degree to which an adult evaluator controls the sequence of events, selects the stimulus materials, and prescribes the responses. Norris and Hoffman (1990a) differentiated adult-initiated approaches from child-initiated strategies for interacting with children at prelanguage stages of development (see Table 7.2). Although the approach advocated by Norris and Hoffman was relatively informal, it was not without direction. Their Infant Scale of Nonverbal Interaction, which is provided as an appendix to their article (Norris & Hoffman, 1990a), outlines target behaviors in the three domains of vocalization, limb actions, and facial and body postures. Based on observations in these three areas, Norris and Hoffman rate children's levels of interactive behaviors as being at one of five levels designed to characterize shifts at 3-month developmental intervals:

Level I (1–3 Month Rating). These behaviors occur in response to general stimulation, and are usually in *reaction* to the adults' actions or the general environment.

Level II (4–6 Month Rating). These behaviors occur in response to play between people, generally reflecting turn taking but not specific control over others.

Level III (7 to 9 Month Rating). These behaviors occur when the infant initiates control in the interaction, by imitating actions and reacting as participants share interactions with objects.

Level IV (10 to 12 Month Rating). These behaviors include imitations of actual *functional* actions and conventional gestures or vocalizations; their meaning is usually clear in context.

Level V (13 to 18 Months Rating). These behaviors are directed at getting the adult to share objects, or to control the game so the adult keeps playing. (pp. 34–35)

The results of the research conducted by Norris and Hoffman (1990a) using these techniques supported the use of child-initiated strategies for assessment and intervention with children in the early stages of development. The child-initiated approach yielded both a greater frequency and higher developmental levels of communicative behaviors than the adult-initiated approach did (but see further discussion on the effects of context on varied intentional communicative acts in the following section on early intentional communication).

Some informal assessment tools for early stages of communicative development have been devised specifically to look at the interactions between care givers and their children. One of these, the scale for Observation of Communicative Interactions (OCI)

TABLE 7.2
Differences between adult-initiated versus child-initiated interactions

Adult-Initiated	Child-Initiated
Specific semantic, phonological, syntactic or pragmatic skills are targeted.	A level of communication is targeted: content, form, and use are indivisible.
Adult designs an activity to elicit targeted behaviors with high frequency.	Activity is designed to allow for a variety of communicative behaviors to occur; adult interprets.
Specific forms are taught receptively (pointing to exemplars) and expressively (shaping productions).	Adult imparts meaning on child's behavior by interpreting it as a request, comment, protest, and so on.
The adult form is used as the standard for an acceptable response.	Adult adds complexity to spontaneously occurring behavior.
A one-to-one relationship is established between a word and its referent.	Communications are interpreted variably to create novel effects with limited communicative behaviors.
Imitation and shaping are used to elicit closer approximations to a target behavior.	Adult provides models; the highest communicative behavior the child produces is responded to each moment.
Nontargeted behaviors are considered irrelevant and interfere with elicitation of targeted responses.	Any behavior interpretable as communication; adult imparts contextually appropriate meaning.
Adult feedback focuses on the correctness of the child's response.	Adult responds with contextually appropriate action and words to indicate what child had communicated.
Secondary reinforcers (claps, praise, tokens) reward the occurrence of target behavior.	Behaviors are reinforced through their effects—controlling the actions of the adult and toys.

Note. From "Comparison of Adult-Initiated vs. Child-Initiated Interaction Styles With Handicapped Prelanguage Children" by J. A. Norris and P. R. Hoffman, 1990, *Language, Speech, and Hearing Services in Schools, 21*, p. 29. Copyright 1990 by American Speech-Language-Hearing Association. Reprinted by permission.

(M. D. Klein & Briggs, 1987), was designed specifically to measure care-giver responsivity to the infant's communicative cues. It includes a continuum of 10 categories of responsiveness, ranging from basic care-giving responses to more sophisticated efforts to facilitate language and conceptual development. It can also be used to guide intervention efforts. Another scale that can be used for combined assessment and intervention is the Parent-Infant Interaction Scale (G. N. Clark & Seifer, 1985). The areas this scale addresses include care-giver interaction behaviors, care-giver and child social referencing, reciprocity, and care-giver affect. It can be used to rate the care giver's relative sensitivity to the infant's cues along a continuum in which physical restraint or forced head turning by parents are rated as least sensitive and most intrusive, and expansion or elaboration of a child's behavior, such as comments on the child's focus of attention, are rated as most sensitive.

Another consideration is whether the procedures used in assessment offer broad enough samples of early language, speech, and communication to provide evidence (in the prelinguistic or one-word stage) that a child might need intervention services. Broader views of communicative processes are needed, particularly to illuminate uneven profiles associated with specific difficulties in language acquisition (review information in Chapters 4 and 6 on scattered ability levels as evidence of language-learning disability).

Recognizing this need, A. M. Wetherby, Yonclas, and Bryan (1989) explored the possibilities for using a varied set of indicators in the early stage of language acquisition. They tested the procedures with children who demonstrated three different kinds of causative conditions (using some of the techniques that later became part of the CSBS, described previously), including: four children with Down's syndrome (ranging in age from 30 to 35 months), four children with specific language impairments (19 to 29 months), and three children with autism (30 to 52 months), all of whom functioned in the prelinguistic and one-word stage. Wetherby et al. used indicators in the following four categories: (1) communicative functions, (2) discourse structure, (3) communicative means, and (4) syllabic shape (note that these categories relate closely to the observational categories of the CSBS by A. M. Wetherby & Prizant, 1990, outlined previously).

The results of the measures in these four areas varied for the different groups of children. Outcomes for children with Down's syndrome fell in the normal range in all four areas; those for children with specific language impairment demonstrated deviance only in the area of syllabic shape; and results for children with autism fell outside the normal range in all areas except adequate rates of communicating (A. M. Wetherby et al., 1989).

Based on their results, A. M. Wetherby and her colleagues (1989) made some preliminary recommendations for using information about these four parameters in making clinical decisions about children's relative needs in language, speech, and communicative development. They also noted that the prognosis for a particular child might be worse if more parameters are affected and if certain parameters are affected (e.g., the absence of consonants might be less worrisome than the absence of joint attention acts). Another important factor in establishing prognosis may be the amount and rate of change observed in a child's profile with advancing age.

METHODS AND TARGETS OF EARLY-STAGE INTERVENTION

The methods and targets of intervention for the earliest stages of language acquisition are integrally tied to the relationships between children and the important adults in their lives. The following discussion is intended not to constitute a "curriculum," or a set of organized program objectives (see N. W. Nelson, 1988b, for sets of goals and short-term objectives; see N. W. Nelson & Snyder, 1990, for a computerized version of those goals that can be edited). Rather, it is intended to guide language specialists and others interested in early communicative development to some possible areas to target in intervention, and based on current theories and research, to provide characteristics to look for and methods to use to facilitate development.

Many organized curricula are available to encourage development of communication and other domains among infants and toddlers at risk. Because home settings are more likely to be used in early infancy, they are also more likely to be used in cases of established risk, such as with infants with early-identified hearing impairments. Several available curricula have been specially designed for working with infants with severe hearing losses and their parents, for example, the Ski–Hi curriculum (T. Clark & Watkins, 1985) and many others (e.g., Northcott, 1977; Sitnick, Rushmer, & Arpan, 1982; Statewide Project for the Deaf, 1982). Some curricula are designed to cross disability (and risk) categories (e.g., The Carolina Curriculum for Handicapped Infants and Infants at Risk, Johnson-Martin, Jens, & Attermeier, 1986). The INSITE Model (T. Clark, Morgan, & Wilson-Vlotman, 1984) is designed specifically to provide home intervention services to infants with sensory impairments and multiple handicaps. The ECO Model, developed by MacDonald and his colleagues at the Nisonger Center in Ohio (described by MacDonald, 1989), focuses on establishing interactive communicative partnerships with infants and toddlers, no matter what their presenting conditions. Curricula vary in organization and relative focus on certain aspects of development, but most now represent an awareness that early development does not represent only acquisition of a set of isolated skills but reflects the nurturing and encouragement of communication as a cohesive, meaningful, and functional process.

GETTING THE BASICS TOGETHER

Organization and Early Sensing of Care and Safety

Any physical problems that interfere with an infant's respiratory system, vocal tract, or feeding capabilities have implications for the development of speech and possibly of language. They also have implications for many complicated expectations facing parents and the emotional bonding between the adult care giver and the child with special needs. When parents must deal with technology to maintain their infant's health (e.g., tracheostomy tubes for breathing through a neck stoma or suctioning equipment for keeping the airway clear), the demands on parental time, patience, and stress levels multiply. Quality communication efforts may seem secondary to getting through the day with a baby whose life is at risk.

Part of the early assessment of infants at risk relates to how well they can organize themselves. Thus, an important part of early intervention is to

assist parents to provide a secure and stable environment that can support children's abilities to organize themselves. Some of the questions addressed by the Assessment of Preterm Infant Behavior (APIB) (Als, Lester, Tronick, & Brazelton, 1982) can be instructive toward planning these earliest stages of intervention. Sparks (1989b) summarized the questions of the APIB that have implications for developing intervention objectives for neonates:

❏ When, and with what help, does the infant function smoothly?
❏ How much and what kinds of stress and frustration are seen in the infant?
❏ How much handling can the infant tolerate before losing control?
❏ Is the infant's homeostatic balance easily disrupted?
❏ What strategies does the infant exhibit to avoid losing control?
❏ What support is necessary to help the infant maintain self-control? (p. 47)

The joint process of answering these questions constitutes some of the mutual goal setting and collaborative problem solving of early intervention. This kind of questioning may be used to guide initial IFSP discussions of child and family needs and strengths (see Chapter 5). It is also consistent with recent hypotheses about the earliest internal and external goals that seem to drive infant behavior (Tronick, 1989). For example, Tronick described early internal goals as being aimed at maintaining physiological homeostasis, establishing feelings of security, experiencing positive emotions, and controlling negative emotions. Early external infant goals include interacting with others, maintaining proximity to care givers, engaging in positive reciprocal interactions, and exploring objects. In Greenspan's (1988) view, as parents assist their infants to achieve physiological and emotional regulation, they contribute to their children's ability to focus energy on the animate and the inanimate world, paving the way for them to establish emotional attachments and to develop in other ways.

Establishing Mutual Communicative Efficacy and Reciprocal "Dialogues"

The earliest forms of communication have been called *behavioral state communication* (Dunst & Lowe, 1986). In this preintentional stage of 0 to 3 months of age, whether an act will be considered communicative depends more on the interpretive abilities of adult care givers than the expressive abilities of children. The signals emitted by some infants are more "readable" than others', however, and the abilities of parents to read their infants' needs may vary as well. These mutual interactional abilities may become early targets of intervention efforts.

To create a better match between the communicativeness of prelinguistic children at risk and the receptiveness of their parents or other caregivers, Prizant and Wetherby (1990) suggested using the transactional model of dynamic transactional interrelationships among the three variables of child characteristics, care-giver characteristics, and environmental influences (Dunst, Lowe, & Bartholomew, 1990; Sameroff & Chandler, 1975). Part of the power of transactions is that, over time, care-giver–child interactions build a sense of mutual efficacy, in which bidirectional, contingent social responsiveness of care-giver and child together develop patterns of future communicativeness. Thus, an important part of the intervention process is to assist care givers to accurately interpret their child's early social and communicative behavior so that the care giver's response can meet the child's needs or support social exchange, contributing to this sense of mutual efficacy (Prizant & Wetherby, 1990). Contingent responsiveness of care givers may also serve to teach the child the signal value of specific behaviors, such as crying and noncry vocalizations (Owens, 1988).

Schaffer (1977) described mother–infant influence on each other's behaviors during early infancy, with mothers looking for clues as to the amount of stimulation their infants can tolerate based on signals of infant attentiveness. By 3 months, because most infants can maintain fairly constant internal states (Owens, 1988), infants also can be attentive for longer periods. As Owens described it, "At any given moment the caregiver must determine the appropriate amount of stimulation based upon the infant's level of attention" (p. 165). At some points, infants may appear to be overstimulated (and need to be given time without stimulation), and at other points, they appear to be understimulated (and need enhanced input).

During this stage, the specialist may aim intervention to assist mothers and other care givers to become more accurate in identifying the infant's internal states and being responsive to them (Brazelton, 1982). Lynch-Fraser and Tiegerman's (1987) book *Baby Signals* is designed to help parents learn to recognize their infants' states and varied learning styles and to encourage those, even at very young ages and when communicative styles are very different. As noted in Chapter 4, efforts to teach synchrony, rhythm, and sensitivity to infant signals may be particularly important when infants have physical impairments or autism that make them respond to stimulation in unexpected ways. During intervention, the specialist should assist care givers not to be discouraged by initial lack of infant responsiveness. The specialist also may assist parents to look for opportunities to become synchronous with their infants in communicative cycles (Brazelton, 1982; Tronick, Als, & Adamson, 1979) that include the following phases:

1. Initiation,
2. Orientation, which establishes the partner's expectations regarding interaction,
3. Acceleration to a peak of excitement,
4. Deceleration, and
5. Turning away. (Brazelton, 1982, p. 51)

Research in normal development has shown mothers to assist their infants to maintain attention and to engage in these early mutual "dialogues" by using a set of techniques (Schaffer, 1977):

1. *Phasing techniques*—care givers monitor infant signals to time stimulation input to be most effective.
2. *Adaptive techniques*—care givers use highly ordered, predictable input sequences to assist infants to assimilate new information.
3. *Facilitative techniques*—care givers structure environmental routines to ensure infant success.
4. *Elaborative techniques*—care givers allow their infants to indicate an interest and then elaborate on it gesturally, vocally, and verbally.
5. *Initiating techniques*—care givers direct their infants' attention to objects, events, and persons, and then monitor that attention.
6. *Controlling techniques*—care givers tell and show their infants what they want them to do directly (emphasizing key words with pauses and gestures) and then assist them to comply.

In normal development, care givers use modifications such as these to increase their infants' opportunities to participate in mutual dialogues, with those prelinguistic dialogues reaching a peak of frequency at around 3 to 4 months of age (Owens, 1988). Similar strategies might be targeted directly for working with care givers in the intervention process (N. W. Nelson, 1988b).

MacDonald (1989) presented many suggestions for helping care givers and other communicative partners become more responsive to young children. He related them to a set of five principles for developing social and communicative partnerships: (1) Based on the partnership principle, parents should question whether they are sharing their child's learning in a balanced, give-and-take relationship. (2) Based on the matching principle, parents should question whether they are interacting and communicating in ways that their children can also do and that allow them success. (3) Based on the sensitive responsiveness principle, parents should question whether they are responding to those subtle behaviors that represent their children's developmental steps. (4) Based on the child-based nondirectiveness principle, parents should question whether they are allowing their children sufficient control over their own learning and are permitting them to express themselves. (5) Based on the emotional attachment principle, parents should question whether their social attitudes are effective in helping their children to be social. MacDonald then presented a series of steps from the ECO model that parents can use to become play partners, turn-taking partners, communicating partners, language partners, and conversation partners with their children.

Early Vocal and Phonological Behavior

When normally developing infants begin to engage in mutual social interactional dialogues with their care givers and move toward expressing communicative signals with increasing intentionality, they simultaneously exercise their vocal tract mechanisms in other ways. Along with extending the reflexive oral–motor abilities available at birth for sucking and swallowing into more sophisticated abilities under increasing voluntary control, they also begin to shape their vocalizations into productions that sound increasingly phonological, including greater proportions of varied consonants in their vocalizations from prelinguistic to multiword stages. As they move through these stages in the normal pattern, an increase first appears in the use of isolated vocal acts and vocal acts combined with gestures, then verbal acts predominate (rather than gestural or nonvocal acts) (Carpenter, Mastergeorge, & Coggins, 1983; A. M. Wetherby, Cain, Yonclas, & Walker, 1988).

For some infants with motor impairments or medical complications, the process may not be as simple as it appears in normal development. Hill and Singer (1990) wrote about the problems facing infants for whom upper airway obstruction mandates the need for tracheostomy tubes to allow them to breathe but that interfere with their ability to vocalize. For some, the tracheostomy tubes may need to stay in place for up to 30 months, with this period of mechanically impaired vocalization extending far into the linguistic development stage. Results of long-term follow-up studies of children who were tracheostomized as infants are mixed. Some evidence indicates that expressive language delays may appear as these children advance into their elementary years (Hill & Singer, 1990). Results of earlier studies (G. S. Ross, 1982) also suggested that children with limited cognitive abilities are particularly at risk. Communicative specialists therefore should work closely with medical personnel to minimize duration of intubation procedures as much as possible without jeopardizing the health and safety of children and perhaps should be prepared to provide language intervention for expressive language difficulties as children with early tracheostomies advance in age.

Other kinds of intubation also may be problematic. Jaffe (1989) described the use of tubes for nonoral feeding sometimes required to prevent aspiration, malnutrition, and fatigue in biologically at-risk infants. The two major categories of feeding tubes are (1) those inserted down the pharynx and esophagus into

---

Personal Reflection 7.3   "Getting a first language going well cannot be approached like other school subjects; it must happen through close interactive living."

James D. MacDonald, Ph.D., Director of the Nisonger Center of The Ohio State University, talking about the essential involvement of parents in early language intervention in his book *Becoming Partners With Children: From Play to Conversation* (1989, p. 199).

the stomach through the nose (called *nasogastic* [N-G] tubes) or through the mouth (called orogastric tubes) and (2) those inserted directly into the stomach by means of minor abdominal surgery known as *gastrostomy*, implanting a gastrostomy tube (G-tube) or esophagostomy tube. Although physicians and parents may find it easier to accept N-G or orogastric tubes than gastrostomy tubes (at least until long-term eating problems are identified), the insertion of these tubes is associated with some clearly negative influences on early communicative development. Among these are negative social and emotional implications, preclusion of the association of oral eating with positive sensory experience, and the difficulty of encouraging feeding, nonnutritive sucking, and oral-motor stimulation and functioning (Jaffe, 1989).

Vocalization problems are sometimes associated with nonoral feeding tubes as well. I worked with an infant whose medical complications necessitated early feeding through an N-G tube. After this tube was removed, the child remained aphonic, apparently related to the trauma caused to the vocal mechanism by the tube passing behind it (through the child's esophagus). He produced both laughing and crying behaviors without voice. The aphonia was particularly unfortunate in his case because he was also blind. Thus, two peripheral communicative avenues were severely impaired. We had to work hard to find other ways to provide both receptive and expressive communication access for this infant, while still encouraging his attempts to produce noncry vocalizations.

Proctor (1989) reviewed recent research on normal noncry vocal development in infancy. She noted that different researchers use different theoretical models and measurement strategies to characterize those developments, ranging from articulatory and phonatory methods to phonetic and acoustic approaches. Proctor compiled the major markers from each of these approaches into the five stages of early vocal and phonological development listed in Box 7.5. She also provided an assessment protocol for establishing baseline infant vocal stages and suggested that it might be used in planning intervention and measuring progress. However, she noted that "There are no normative values for the amount, quality, or type of noncry vocalizations during the infant's first year" (p. 33) and suggested that speech–language pathologists must use clinical judgment to interpret the results of early stage vocal assessments. In addition, she noted that, "Depending on the child's other medical problems,

stimulation of vocalization may not be the highest priority for intervention, or perhaps intervention should not focus solely on vocal behavior" (p. 34). Instead, it may be more appropriate to target increases in the infant's vocal output in the context of more general communicative intervention strategies (Proctor, 1989).

It has long been recognized that stages like those outlined by Proctor (1989) in Box 7.5 are followed with relative uniformity across varied linguistic communities (Owens, 1988). No matter what language a child is exposed to, babies begin by cooing, then produce reduplicated consonant–vowel (CV) syllables, and finally produce "variegated" babbling that has sentence-like intonation patterns before producing words and word-like forms around the time of their first birthday (Oller, 1978, 1980). As children approach their first word productions, their babbling begins to sound more and more like the phonological patterns common to their own native languages—that is, if they can hear their native language adequately and can hear their own babbling.

Several studies have demonstrated more limited consonantal repertoires in the prespeech vocalizations of children with severe hearing impairments (R. Kent, Osberger, Netsell, & Hustedde, 1987; Oller, Eilers, Bull, & Carney, 1985). For example, Stoel-Gammon and Otomo (1986) and Stoel-Gammon (1988) analyzed a series of babbling samples gathered longitudinally over the 4- to 39-month age range from a group of infants and toddlers with normal hearing and with hearing impairments. Their results confirmed other indications that the babbling of children with hearing impairments differs, both quantitatively and qualitatively, from babbling by normal-hearing children. Consonantal inventories of normal-hearing children increased with age; inventories of hearing impaired children started smaller and decreased over the study period. The hearing impaired children also showed a tendency to produce (1) fewer multisyllabic utterances containing true consonants; (2) a higher proportion of vocalizations with glides or glottal stops; (3) a higher proportion of labial consonants; (4) a higher proportion of prolongable consonants like nasals, glides, fricatives, and syllabic consonants; (5) a lower proportion of alveolars; and (6) a lower proportion of stops and nonsyllabic affricates.

These data support the targeting of vocal and phonological development in the early stages of intervention, particularly for children with hearing impairments. Daniel Ling (1976) devised one of the most

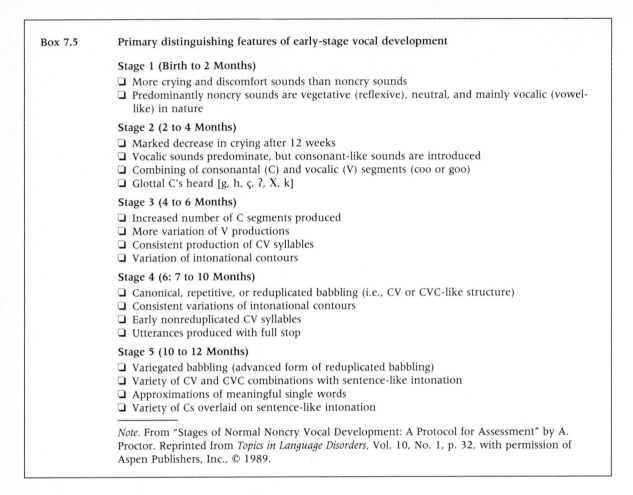

Box 7.5   **Primary distinguishing features of early-stage vocal development**

Stage 1 (Birth to 2 Months)
❏ More crying and discomfort sounds than noncry sounds
❏ Predominantly noncry sounds are vegetative (reflexive), neutral, and mainly vocalic (vowel-like) in nature

Stage 2 (2 to 4 Months)
❏ Marked decrease in crying after 12 weeks
❏ Vocalic sounds predominate, but consonant-like sounds are introduced
❏ Combining of consonantal (C) and vocalic (V) segments (coo or goo)
❏ Glottal C's heard [g, h, ç, ʔ, X, k]

Stage 3 (4 to 6 Months)
❏ Increased number of C segments produced
❏ More variation of V productions
❏ Consistent production of CV syllables
❏ Variation of intonational contours

Stage 4 (6: 7 to 10 Months)
❏ Canonical, repetitive, or reduplicated babbling (i.e., CV or CVC-like structure)
❏ Consistent variations of intonational contours
❏ Early nonreduplicated CV syllables
❏ Utterances produced with full stop

Stage 5 (10 to 12 Months)
❏ Variegated babbling (advanced form of reduplicated babbling)
❏ Variety of CV and CVC combinations with sentence-like intonation
❏ Approximations of meaningful single words
❏ Variety of Cs overlaid on sentence-like intonation

Note. From "Stages of Normal Noncry Vocal Development: A Protocol for Assessment" by A. Proctor. Reprinted from *Topics in Language Disorders*, Vol. 10, No. 1, p. 32, with permission of Aspen Publishers, Inc., © 1989.

widely used approaches for this purpose, based on a view of speech acquisition as an orderly and sequential process in which developmental advances occur on two developmental levels in parallel. On the phonetic level, children learn to produce and to perceive (differentiate) sounds to a precise level of accuracy and automaticity, but without assigning meaning to them. On the phonological level, children develop awareness of the meaningful use of speech sounds in their own speech and that of others.

This parallel organization is a departure from earlier programs designed on the basis of a progression from nonverbal to verbal stimuli. In Ling's (1976) approach, the seven stages of the phonetic level are (1) vocalization freely and on demand; (2) production of suprasegmental patterns (intonation and stress variations accomplished by shifting duration, intensity, and pitch relationships); (3) production of all vowels

and diphthongs with voice control; (4) differentiation of consonants by manner; (5) differentiation of consonants by manner and place; (6) differentiation of consonants by manner, place, and voicing; and (7) production of initial and final blends.

Judgments of adequacy at the phonetic level are based on automaticity and speed as well as accuracy to avoid the development of exaggerated, unnatural speech-production habits. Ling (1976) reported that failure to address both the phonetic and the phonological levels during early intervention can lead to less natural speech for hearing impaired children. Part of the process of encouraging this degree of naturalness and functionality of speech production and perception is for adults to avoid providing exaggerated visual models during phonetic level interactions.

As speech sounds become part of the child's seven-stage phonetic repertoire and the child begins to demonstrate communicative functions using other means, the seven parallel stages may be addressed on the phonological level. These stages include (1) using vocalization as a means of communication; (2) using different voice patterns meaningfully; (3) using different vowels to approximate words; (4) saying some words clearly and with good voice patterns; (5) saying more and more words clearly and with good voice patterns; (6) saying most words clearly and with good voice patterns; and (7) producing all speech intelligibly and with natural voice patterns.

Although Ling's (1976) procedures and targets were designed specifically for children with peripheral hearing impairments, they are based on normal developmental principles. Other children with early phonological processing problems in both perception and production may also need more deliberate attention to the development of their sound systems, as well as perception and control of paralinguistic vocal features.

Baltaxe and Simmons (1985) considered how prosodic development appears to differ for infants with autism. They observed that some children with autism demonstrate seemingly advanced musical abilities and exact echoing of prosody, both of which require precise auditory perception, but simultaneously appear unable to attach linguistic value to prosodic indicators. Baltaxe and Simmons hypothesized that some of the mixed picture for children with autism arises out of difficulty in hemispheric switching and integrating prosodic and linguistic functioning. They noted evidence that, in normal development, early use of prelinguistic prosody is reported to be exclusively affective in nature and that subsequent linguistic use evolves from this initial affective basis. This suggests that early prosodic processing may occur largely in the right hemisphere but that, as linguistic abilities begin to unfold, processing begins to interact with specifically linguistic function and to move increasingly to the left hemisphere. They hypothesized that "Autistic children may not be equipped to make an adequate switch, either because of deficits that directly or indirectly affect the dominant hemisphere or because of a possible maturational lag at the cortical level or both" (p. 117). Unfortunately, Baltaxe and Simmons did not offer clinical suggestions for encouraging more normal developmental patterns of prosodic development.

When making everyday clinical decisions for children with autism, I have sometimes faced the dilemma that these children seem to comprehend better when somewhat exaggerated prosody is used, but I wonder if I might have encouraged a maladaptive pattern when I hear my slightly exaggerated prosody echoed back stereotypically. I usually then vow to try to keep my own prosody more natural and to attempt to enhance comprehension and attention through other nonlinguistic contextual support.

For other children with autism whose speaking capabilities are extremely limited, intervention efforts often focus on training in the use of nonverbal communication methods, such as signing, rather than vocal development and speech. However, Koegel and Traphagen (1982) questioned the sometimes automatic assumption that these efforts might yield faster and better results than a more deliberate focus on phonological development with nonverbal autistic children. Their research showed that two nonspeaking autistic boys (ages 7:6 and 9:11) learned to say simple CV words (CVC combinations were more difficult) fairly readily when the initial target words were selected carefully from CV combinations of phonemes already in the boys' nonverbal self-stimulatory phonetic repertoires. Koegel and Traphagen hypothesized that, when vocal–verbal targets (i.e., spoken words) were selected in this way, learning might occur even more readily than when nonvocal–verbal targets (e.g., signs) were chosen.

Early Feeding Behaviors and Needs

Part of the potential for normal vocal communicative development comes from having a normally functioning biological mechanism that can support the development of speech. This may lead to suggestions to work on feeding behaviors in preparation for speech, but generalization from vegetative nonspeech functions to voluntary speech functions cannot be assumed. S. E. Morris (1981) commented that, "It is not uncommon to see children who have made excellent gains in developing oral-motor skills and sound play skills through preschool programs who do not translate these sensorimotor skills into speech production" (p. 217).

On the other hand, children who cannot use the oral-motor tract adequately for eating are unlikely to use it for talking. This suggests that adequate oral-motor foundation skills are necessary, but not sufficient, for the development of normal early speech. As mentioned, long-term mechanical disruptions may be particularly problematic. As Jaffe (1989) noted, "Infants who breathe through endotracheal tubes and eat nonorally via intravenous or gavage tubes for an extended period may eventually demonstrate decreased sucking and oral-motor function" (p. 18). When infants' oral-motor experiences are limited mechanically, they may be assisted nevertheless to associate oral movements with feeling full and contented by the care givers' inducing nonnutritive sucking on a pacifier, nipple, thumb, or finger during tube feedings. The encouragement of nonnutritive sucking at other times also may contribute to normalization of oral-motor behavior and oral sensation toleration.

The nurturing atmosphere generally associated with infant feeding is important to both mothers and children. When infants or children have feeding problems, their mothers' "feelings of concern, anxiety, frustration, resentment, anger, and failure are inevitable" (Jaffe, 1989, p. 13). For example, S. E. Morris (1981) described some characteristics of cerebral palsy likely to interfere with nonverbal communication signals during feeding and potentially resulting in misinterpretation of intentional communicative signals:

> Movement patterns of head extension, flexion or constant turning to one side may limit the child's ability to gain eye contact with the feeder. This, in turn, will make it difficult for the child to regulate the speed of feeding or the amount of food given. An abnormal tongue thrusting movement may push the food out of the mouth, whether or not the child wishes to eat it. A bite reflex on the spoon or nipple may be interpreted as teasing or misbehavior. The child may be unable to vocalize, reach, point, or in other ways indicate readiness to eat or cease eating. (p. 222)

For some mothers, especially when they are given limited support, such confusing biological signals may turn feeding sessions into negative experiences. When infants or children, in turn, sense their mothers' (or other care givers') negative responses to the feeding difficulties, the result may be even more physical problems, such as an increase in abnormal muscle tone, making eating yet more difficult.

Thus, the role of speech–language pathologists and other professionals when working with mothers and infants experiencing feeding difficulties is complex. In addition to assisting with techniques related directly to feeding, the professional "facilitates communication between parent and child and enhances the child's language development" in the context of feeding (Jaffe, 1989, p. 24). This may include helping care givers to recognize their children's subtle or overt cues that an approach is working (or not), which might be an important part of helping children develop feelings of competence and communicative control. It may also consist of giving care givers sup-

port so they can relax and simply enjoy their child, not be their child's primary therapist.

One supportive technique may be to assist care givers to identify the most facilitative feeding position for their child, encouraging efforts to hold their infants in a gently flexed position while feeding to enhance nurturing sensations for both. As the child grows, alternate positions may be explored in consultation with an occupational or physical therapist, and specialized techniques, such as jaw control, may be needed (e.g., see *The Carolina Curriculum for Handicapped Infants and Infants at Risk* by Johnson-Martin, Jens, & Attermeier, 1986).

Throughout the process, however, professionals and parents should avoid the trap of focusing on feeding difficulties to the exclusion of facilitating social and communicative growth at mealtimes. S. E. Morris (1981) discussed using mealtimes to encourage the development of communicative reciprocity, causality, or mean–ends behaviors, object permanence, and the communicative development of gaze behaviors. She also described mealtimes as a context for introducing early augmentative communication techniques. For older children in school programs who stay at earlier stages of eating skill (e.g., children with cerebral palsy), Morris suggested using a "Lunch Club" approach to keep them from being totally isolated during lunch but without exposing them to the potentially overstimulating school cafeteria. In a Lunch Club, all children in the child's regular education classroom take turns eating with one or more children with disabilities in a quiet and controlled environment that is positive and special. Romski, Sevcik, and Pate (1988) also used mealtimes to facilitate symbolic communication in adolescents with severe retardation. Mealtime was one of the contexts that Lucariello (1990) identified as providing the kind of familiar routine communicative event that can help children with higher cognitive abilities move beyond talk just about the here-and-now (see discussions later in this chapter).

When a child with severe impairments has feeding difficulties and needs to be fed by a variety of persons, problems may arise as each attempts to read the child's confusing communicative signals regarding the timing of bites, food choices, and facilitative techniques. The construction of a mealtime book, with personalized instructions and photographic illustrations, was suggested by S. E. Morris (1981). The following are entries drawn from the mealtime book of a 9-year-old boy with cerebral palsy:

I enjoy my meals and like to enjoy being with the person who feeds me. My mealtime book will help you know me better. It will help you know the best ways for us to be real partners when you feed me. That makes it easier for me and for you too. . . .

When I am ready for a bite of food, I will look at the food and open my mouth. I may also say "yeah" or "more" first. Please wait until I tell you with my open mouth and with my eyes that I am ready. . . .

When the spoon is in my mouth, please keep it there until I have gently bitten on the spoon. This keeps my jaw steady and lets me begin to use my lips. Then you can pull the spoon out. (p. 231)

Feeding assessment and intervention often involve complex decisions guided by fluoroscopic observation of swallowing to judge the safety of oral feeding. Table 7.3 is Jaffe's (1989) summary of normal, primitive, delayed, or abnormal feeding behaviors. Jaffe also provided specialized suggestions for children with neurological impairment, Down's syndrome, or cleft palates.

Some relatively formal assessment tools address feeding concerns. One is the Pre-Speech Assessment Scale (PSAS) (S. E. Morris, 1982), which facilitates observation of respiration, phonation, sound play, and meaningful speech behaviors that appear from birth through 2 years of age. Another is the Feeding Assessment by S. E. Morris and Klein (1987), which also includes a questionnaire (administered either in Spanish or in English) and yields an analysis of the physical and communicative environment and of normal and limiting oral-motor skills relative to various treatment options.

TABLE 7.3
Major movement patterns related to feeding

Primitive Patterns (Usually Seen During the First 6 Months of Infant Development)	Higher Developmental Patterns (Usually Seen Between 6 and 24 Months)	Abnormal and Compensatory Patterns
Suckling: The early infantile method of sucking that involves extension–retraction of the tongue, up-and-down jaw excursions, and loose approximations of the lips.	*Munching:* The earliest form of chewing that involves a flattening and spreading of the tongue combined with up-and-down jaw movement.	*Tongue Thrust:* An abnormally forceful protrusion of the tongue from the mouth.
Sucking: Characterized by negative pressure in the oral cavity, rhythmic up-and-down jaw movements, tongue tip elevation, firm approximation of the lips, and minimal jaw excursions.	*Chewing:* Characterized by spreading and rolling movements of the tongue propelling food between the teeth, tongue lateralization, and rotary jaw movements.	*Tongue retraction:* A strong pulling back of the tongue to the pharyngeal space.
Rooting reaction: Head turning in response to tactile stimulation applied to the lips or around the mouth.	*Tongue lateralization:* Movement of the tongue to the sides of the mouth to propel food between the teeth for chewing.	*Jaw thrust:* An abnormally forceful and tense downward extension of the mandible.
		Lip retraction: Drawing back of the lips so that they form a tight line over the mouth.
Phasic bite reflex: A rhythmic bite and release pattern, seen as a series of small jaw openings and closings when the teeth or gums are stimulated.	*Rotary jaw movements:* The smooth interaction and integration of vertical, lateral, diagonal, and eventually circular movements of the jaw used in chewing.	*Lip pursing:* A tight purse-string movement of the lips.
		Tonic bite reflex: An abnormally strong jaw closure when the teeth or gums are stimulated.
	Controlled, sustained bite: An easy, gradual closure of the teeth on the food, with an easy release of the food for chewing.	*Jaw clenching:* An abnormally tight closure of the mouth.

Note. From "Feeding At-Risk Infants and Toddlers" by M. B. Jaffe. Reprinted from *Topics in Language Disorders*, Vol. 10, No. 1, p. 15, with permission of Aspen Publishers, Inc. © 1989.

Early Comprehension of Routines and Making Sense of Events in the World

By the time normally developing children are 3 to 4 months old, they incorporate early communicative dialogues into familiar feeding routines and game routines, such as "peekaboo," "this little piggy," and "I'm gonna get you." These routines include all the aspects of conversational communicative events (although each exchange might not include all of the components). Because of their similarity to conversational interactions, Bateson (1975) called them "proto-conversations." Wells (1986) noted that, "By six months, then, a baby and his or her chief caregivers have established the basis for communication: a relationship of mutual attention" (p. 34). Encouraging parents to engage in these routines when their infants show appropriate levels of sensitivity can provide an important strategy for engaging hard-to-reach children and extending their attention in social contexts.

For example, "I'm gonna get you" and "knee-riding" routines allowed one mother I knew to communicate with her 7-year-old daughter, Cathy, who was deaf (or profoundly hearing impaired) and blind. Yet, Cathy clearly communicated anticipation of sequence in the context of these routines and eventually learned to give a primitive sign to request more tickling in the context of the "I'm gonna get you" game. Like Cathy, many deaf–blind children learn best through predictable routines involving movement. Box 7.6 is a summary (from N. W. Nelson, 1988) of five intervention levels in a "movement resonance," or "coactive movement" program based on a communication program developed originally by J. van Dijk (1965) for deaf–blind children in Europe. This particular summary includes adaptations developed for children with other severe and profound handicaps (L. Sternberg, 1982; L. Sternberg, Battle, & Hill, 1980; L. Sternberg, McNerney, & Pegnatore, 1985; L. Sternberg & Owens, 1984; L. Sternberg, Pegnatore, & Hill, 1983).

Siegel-Causey and Guess (1989) presented a comprehensive approach for enhancing nonsymbolic communication with individuals who have severe disabilities. It was based on five instructional guidelines related to the following:

1. Developing *nurturant* relationships
2. Enhancing *sensitivity* to nonsymbolic communication
3. Increasing *opportunities* for communication
4. *Sequencing* experiences in predictable order
5. Utilizing *movement* within natural interactions (p. 3)

Helping children organize their behavior into routines that involve increasingly conventional communicative exchanges rests on the implementation of these principles.

The following example shows how predictable sequencing can help children function as communicative members of a social group:

> The service provider places a cup on the learner's tray to communicate that it is snack time. The learner, as a result of similar previous experiences, recognizes that the cup means snack and pushes the cup to the service provider to communicate "wanting juice." The service provider pours the juice and holds the filled cup out to the learner to determine if the learner's communication (i.e., pushing the cup) actually meant, "want juice." The learner smiles and reaches for the cup. The service provider responds by assisting the learner to bring the cup to his or her mouth. (Siegel-Causey & Guess, 1989, p. 8)

K. Nelson (1986) proposed that early routines like these contribute to the development of *event knowledge*, which she viewed as a central feature of early cognitive development. Nelson defined an event as a dynamic incorporation of objects and relations into a larger whole that occurs over time. This view of cognitive development as shifting representation of events in the world departs from predominant views of cognitive development as changes in general processes, such as seriation, classification, inference, or inductive reasoning. It also differs from Piagetian views of cognitive development as shifts in schemas in which young children are thought to be incapable of accurately representing changes in the state of objects (Piaget & Inhelder, 1971). Rather, K. Nelson (1986) stressed that

> even very young children represent events as complex and dynamic, that is, as holistic structures involving internal change over time. Both of these characteristics—holistic structure and internal variation in structural relations over time—are important in considering the implications of the content and structure of children's event representations for theories of cognitive development. The representation of a holistic structure implies a strong proclivity for structural organization in the mind of the young child. (p. 3)

It is because the "young child's cognitive processing is contextualized in terms of everyday experience" (K. Nelson, 1986, p. 4) that children can exhibit greater cognitive competence in everyday activities than in artificial cognitive tasks. Nelson also noted that, whereas older children and adults may learn about the world through books and other media, such

Box 7.6   A summary of the five levels of early communicative interaction in a "movement resonance" or coactive movement program for children with severe and profound handicaps

1. Preresonance
   a. Receptive indices:
      (1) Moves, but not in response to stimulation
      (2) Changes behavior when stimulated (movement is encouraged in a same-plane, body-to-body motion of caretaker and child)
      (3) Repeats movement; focuses on own body
   b. Expressive indices:
      (1) Produces undifferentiated cry
      (2) Produces different movements/vocalizations for specific discomforts
2. Resonance:
   a. Receptive indices:
      (1) Responds to another's cues by participating in movement modification (moving in an opposition plane; facing the caretaker)
      (2) Produces repetitive behavior on objects; focuses on what happens to object
   b. Expressive indices:
      (1) Gives indication of recognition of familiar person/object
      (2) Participates in familiar motion after caretaker initiation; physical contact necessary
      (3) Signals caretaker to continue activity (such as pushing or pulling against a caretaker)
3. Coactive movement ("Movement Dialogue"):
   a. Receptive indices:
      (1) Responds to tactile signals for movement (when caretaker and child are separated in space but remain in close proximity)
      (2) Anticipates next movement in sequence
   b. Expressive indices:
      (1) Imitates movements after caretaker stops movement as long as cues are provided by caretaker's position
      (2) Uses multiple signals to continue activities
      (3) Duplicates different movements while caretaker is moving; no physical contact necessary
4. Deferred imitation:
   a. Receptive indices:
      (1) Responds to simple gestural commands; no physical cues necessary
      (2) Anticipates routine event from cues
      (3) Responds to gesture for object provided gesture focuses on use of object and object is present
   b. Expressive indices:
      (1) Imitates movements after caretaker finishes movement; no cues necessary
      (2) Uses gestures that are specific to certain situations; no generalization
      (3) Imitates new movements after caretaker finishes modeling movements
5. Natural gestures:
   a. Receptive indices:
      (1) Responds to gestures for objects provided gesture focuses on use; object need not be present
   b. Expressive indices:
      (1) Uses gestures for objects/activities across various situations; generalization
      (2) Uses gestures instead of whole-hand pointing

Sources: L. Sternberg, 1982; L. Sternberg et al., 1980, 1983, 1985; L. Sternberg & Owens, 1984; L. Sternberg, Ritchey, Pegnatore, Wills, & Hill, 1986; J. van Dijk, 1965.

indirect knowledge sources are unavailable to young children who do not yet have the language skills to take advantage of them. Rather, "what young children know comes primarily from the analysis of their own experience rather than from mediated sources" (p. 5).

This is not to suggest that experience comes to the child as "raw encounters with a neutral physical world. Rather, in some important sense, all knowledge of the world is social or cultural knowledge" (K. Nelson, 1986, p. 5). Social and cultural agents, such as parents and interventionists (for children with disabilities), set the context for children's learning. That does not imply, however, that adult agents determine the child's experiences. Children's experiences are influenced by the developmental state of their cognitive systems and current knowledge.

The interplay between current knowledge and new experience is often the focus of early-stage intervention. Professionals strive to maintain this transactional balance by using reciprocation, imitation, and scaffolding procedures.

Reciprocation, Imitation, and Scaffolding

Reciprocation suggests a balanced interaction; both children and adults bring something to the process, and each values something of the other's contributions. The early turn-taking and feeding exchanges between adults and children discussed previously help to establish this kind of reciprocation.

Reciprocal interactions can also give early communicators a powerful tool for learning more—*imitation*. If children can acquire what MacDonald (1989) called "the rule of natural social learning: 'Do as others do'" (p. 132), they have access to innumerable incidental learning opportunities.

Infants can show signs of imitation soon after birth, much earlier than originally credited by Piagetian models. By around 5 months, rather deliberate imitations of movements and vocalizations are possible, with a peak in frequency of imitation of hand and nonspeech imitation by around 6 to 8 months (Owens, 1988). Even later, however, some kinds of imitation are more accessible than others. For example, children between 9 and 12 months of age are not observed to imitate intonation patterns of their parents involving vocal pitch, amplitude, or duration shifts (Siegel, Cooper, Morgan, & Brenneise-Sarshad, 1990).

The results obtained by Siegel and his colleagues (1990) suggest a need to further consider the rela-

tionships between imitation and language acquisition. Children in the 9- to 12-month age range would be unlikely to understand that they were supposed to repeat their parents' surface-level intonation patterns; the child's natural tendency is to try to interpret the deeper communicative meaning of those patterns and to respond to them.

When questioning the evidence that children use imitation as a primary strategy for normal language acquisition, Wells (1986) commented that, "Children are not learning to talk in order to be able to behave like their parents for the sake of conformity, but rather to be able to communicate with them in collaborative activities in which the roles played are *reciprocal* rather than imitative" (p. 42). Wells characterized the linguistic theoretical position that, for the most part, rather than imitating whole chunks of linguistic input, normally developing children seem to analyze the utterances they hear into smaller units. As previously considered, Prizant (1983) suggested (see Chapter 4) that an exaggerated preference for gestalt processing strategies over analytic ones may be a central feature of autism.

Although intervention to improve imitative ability is not without caveats, children who cannot imitate, or who do so poorly, seem to be at a disadvantage in all aspects of learning. Again, normal development can serve as an intervention model. The evidence suggests that, in early stages of normal development, it is easier for children to imitate behaviors that are not new but that integrate components already in their spontaneous repertoires. Thus, it makes sense in intervention to encourage adults to imitate something that the child already does. This technique is especially useful for children who show little interest in the reciprocal turn-taking interactions that are critical to establishing early prelinguistic communication (Bullowa, 1979; MacDonald, 1989; Siegel-Causey, Ernst, & Guess, 1987). In addition, adult imitation of infant behaviors occurs naturally in early interactions. P. H. Wolff (1963) observed that from about the 6th week of normal development, by imitating their baby's sounds, parents can engage in exchanges of between 10 and 15 vocalizations. Adult imitation of children has also been shown to maintain infants' play and to contribute to their normal emotional development (Brazelton, Koslowski, & Main, 1974; Greenspan, 1985).

Adult imitation of children also is a technique that can be used to coax older children with severe impairments into the reciprocal turn-taking mode. Tiegerman (1989) reported a case study illustrating a procedure for encouraging children with autism to acquire imitation and turn-taking skills in the context of limited social interaction. A clinician sits across the table from the child with autism with a set of objects identical to those of the child. As the child selects and manipulates the objects, the adult selects the matching objects and imitates the child's behavior. Among the advantages that Tiegerman noted for this approach are its ability to establish a contingency relationship in which adult imitations are a function of the child's object manipulation, the fact that activities are child-initiated, and the provision of opportunities for the child to exert some control over another person's behavior. According to Tiegerman's case study description, the procedure may increase both gaze behavior and object manipulation among older children with severe impairments.

MacDonald (1989) took the imitation strategy one step further in his "matching" process, which is a central principle of the ECO model. In the following comments, MacDonald described matching for parents and related it to Bruner's (1983) explanation of matching as a scaffolding process in which adults fine tune their expectations to what the child can already do but also challenge the child slightly:

> Matching is perhaps the most effective strategy you can use with your child, regardless of his level. By matching we mean acting and communicating with your child in a way that he can do. Consider again the image of a staircase with your skills at the top and your child's at the bottom. To show him the next step, you must get to his step or a little step above his. There you do something that he can do and that he shows some interest in. What then? Wait. Think of MATCH AND WAIT as one extremely effective, natural teaching package for helping your child do more, stay with you, and become more like the people around him. (p. 126)

Although, in the earliest stages simple imitation of the child, no matter what the child does, may be necessary as a way of matching, gradual provision of a scaffold can help the child to imitate actions that have some conventional communicative value. For example, waving "goodbye" or "hi" in appropriate contexts might be appropriate either for infants or older children with severe handicaps. Pointing is another possibility. All three have communicative signal value as well as clear contextual cues for establishment and generalization.

Kaiser, Alpert, and Warren (1987) suggested three steps to increase functionality of early communicative behaviors: (1) Start by selecting forms that can be used frequently in contexts where the child already participates; (2) encourage functionality by training gestural, vocal, and other forms (e.g., by using imitation and shaping techniques) during opportunities to display particular intentions (e.g., greeting, making choices, requesting); and (3) attend to the child's forms and respond to them functionally as if they were intended to be communicative.

INTENTIONALITY AND EARLY COMMUNICATIVE FUNCTIONS

Effects of Context on Early Comments and Requests

Normally developing children are generally credited with true intentional communication when they enter the illocutionary stage at around 8 or 9 months of age (you may wish to review stages of intentional and linguistic communicative development in Table 7.1). During the illocutionary stage, although the gestural and nonverbal communication signals of normally developing children become increasingly conventional and clear to varied communicative partners (e.g., pointing and showing with communicative gaze and vocalizations), children do not yet use conventional symbols for communicating their intentions. By around 12 to 14 months, children who are developing normally begin to encode their intentions with words.

Care givers who interpret their children's actions as communicative even during the perlocutionary stage seem to play a critical role in helping children move from the perlocutionary into the illocutionary stage. Therefore, frequent targets of assessment and intervention for young children and those with severe impairments involve the transactional relationship between sensitivity exhibited by care givers and signal clarity exhibited by children. Direct intervention may be needed partially because some signals of intention are rendered less "readable" by children's impairments, such as cerebral palsy and autism, as discussed in the context of feeding events (S. E. Morris, 1981). Figure 7.5 is a list of some forms of nonsymbolic communications that older individuals with severe disabilities might produce in a variety of contexts (Siegel-Causey & Guess, 1989). These may be used as examples to help sensitize both consul-

FIGURE 7.5

Forms of learner nonsymbolic communications.

Generalized movements and changes in muscle tone

Excitement in response to stimulation or in anticipation of an event
Squirms and resists physical contact
Changes in muscle tone in response to soothing touch or voice, in reaction to sudden stimuli, or in preparation to act

Vocalizations

Calls to attract or direct another's attention
Laughs or coos in response to pleasurable stimulation
Cries in reaction to discomfort

Facial expressions

Smiles in response to familiar person, object, or event
Grimaces in reaction to unpleasant or unexpected sensation

Orientation

Looks toward or points to person or object to seek or direct attention
Looks away from person or object to indicate disinterest or refusal
Looks toward suddenly appearing familiar or novel person, object, or event

Pause

Ceases moving in anticipation of coming event
Pauses to await service provider's instruction or to allow service provider to take turn

Touching, manipulating, or moving with another person

Holds or grabs another for comfort
Takes or directs another's hand to something
Manipulates service provider into position to start an activity or interactive "game"
Touches or pulls service provider to gain attention
Pushes away or lets go to terminate an interaction
Moves with or follows the movements of another person

tants and care givers to behaviors that might be responded to as communicative. Over time, if care givers do not recognize the communicative messages of these behaviors, the danger is that both care givers and children may fall into a mode in which children are increasingly passive and neither partner has much sense of a particular child's potential for communicative control.

To prevent that problem, the specialist must carefully observe children's early forms of communication, perhaps using formal assessment procedures and adult-elicitation techniques (Linder, 1990; A. M. Wetherby & Prizant, 1990) as well as naturalistic contexts that are largely child initiated (Coggins, Olswang, & Guthrie, 1987; Lund & Duchan, 1988; Norris & Hoffman, 1990a, 1990b). Regardless of the assessment and intervention strategy chosen, it is important to consider how contextual variables and the child's stage of development might interact to influence children's expression of intentions.

Figure 7.6 outlines a set of observational criteria for identifying communicative intent in children at preverbal levels of communication. Coggins et al. (1987) developed this particular summary to study the effect of context on children's communicative functions. Coggins and his associates divided the intentions observed in early childhood communication into comments and requests and used both low-structured observations and more structured elicitation tasks to study the interactions among stages of development, contextual variables, and communicative intentions. In the area of comments, they examined how infants direct adult attention. In the area of requests, they examined how infants direct adult behavior.

Coggins and his associates (1987) found that different contexts tend to elicit different intentions. Structured tasks worked better to elicit requests from young children, and unstructured observations worked better to elicit comments. Age was also a factor in influencing the results, with 9-month-olds encoding

FIGURE 7.5
continued

Acting on objects and using objects to interact with others

Reaches toward, leans toward, touches, gets, picks up, activates, drops, or pushes away object to indicate interest or disinterest
Extends, touches, or places object to show to another or to request another's action
Holds out hands to prepare to receive object

Assuming positions and going to places

Holds up arms to be picked up, holds out hands to initiate "game," leans back on swing to be pushed
Stands by sink to request drink, goes to cabinet to request material stored there

Conventional gestures

Waves to greet
Nods to indicate assent or refusal

Depictive actions

Pantomimes throwing to indicate, "throw ball"
Sniffs to indicate smelling flowers
Makes sounds similar to those made by animals and objects to make reference to them
Draws picture to describe or request activity

Withdrawal

Pulls away or moves away to avoid interaction or activity
Curls up, lies on floor to avoid interaction or activity

Aggressive and self-injurious behavior

Hits, scratches, bites, or spits at service provider to protest action or in response to frustration
Throws or destroys objects to protest action or in response to frustration
Hits, bites, or otherwise harms self or threatens to harm self to protest action, in response to frustration, or in reaction to pain or discomfort

---

Note. From *Enhancing Nonsymbolic Communication Interactions Among Learners With Severe Disabilities* (p. 7) by E. Siegel-Causey and D. Guess, 1989, Baltimore, MD: Paul H. Brookes Publishing Co. Copyright 1989 by Paul H. Brookes Publishing Co. Reprinted by permission.

---

few intentions of either type in the clinical setting whether engaged in 30 minutes of unstructured free play with a parent or in relatively structured elicitation tasks with the examiner. It is particularly interesting that the 9-month-olds produced few requests, a finding consistent with Halliday's (1975a, 1975b) report that requests were rare in his son's early communicative attempts. Perhaps results such as these should lead clinicians to reconsider their usual tendencies to encourage "wants and needs" as the first intentions when augmentative communication systems are developed for nonspeaking children (although the advantage of natural reinforcement following requests might outweigh this slight developmental disadvantage). When Coggins et al. (1987), however, observed the same group of 9-month-olds longitudinally at 3-month intervals until they were 24 months old, intentional requests began to show up, particularly in structured elicitation contexts. By 15 months, two thirds of the children produced requests in structured

contexts with tangible rewards. In contrast, by 12 months, two thirds of the children used comments to establish joint reference and to direct their parents' attention to interesting sights and sounds. Not until 21 months, however, were elicitation tasks as effective in obtaining comments as were unstructured interactions.

Norris and Hoffman (1990a) conducted another study to assess the differential effects of more structured (adult-initiated) and less structured (child-initiated) sampling contexts. They studied intervention and assessment for children with severe multiple handicaps. The children, between the ages of 2:6 and 2:10 years, all functioned at prelinguistic levels. To measure results, Norris and Hoffman used their Infant Scale of Nonverbal Interactions (described earlier in this chapter in the section on informal assessment). They hypothesized, and their results supported, that "children would exhibit a higher frequency of communicative vocalizations, limb movements, and body postures when their spontaneously occurring behav-

FIGURE 7.6
General and operational definitions for comments and requests.

I. *Comments.* Intentional behaviors that direct the listener's attention to an object or the movement of an object.
   A. Extends arm to adult to show an object already in hand; may vocalize or verbalize (i.e., produce a single word or multiword utterance).
   B. Picks up an object and immediately shows it to an adult; may vocalize or verbalize.
   C. Points to, looks toward, or approaches on object; may vocalize or verbalize.

II. *Requests.* Intentional behaviors that direct the listener to act on some object in order to make it move or to retrieve an unobtainable object.
   A. Stretches hand toward an object; whines or fusses while leaning toward object; may vocalize or verbalize.
   B. Stretches hand toward an object with ritual gesture; may vocalize or verbalize.
   C. Looks at an object that has ceased moving or has the potential to move or be moved; reaches or leans toward object; may vocalize or verbalize.
   D. Looks toward an object that has ceased moving, has the potential to move or be moved, and makes a ritual gesture; may vocalize or verbalize.
   E. Looks at or touches an object; points to or reaches toward object and produces a single word or multiword utterance.
   F. Looks toward an object that has ceased moving, has the potential to move or be moved; may point toward the object or adult; may give the object to an adult and produce a single word or multiword utterance.

Note. From "Assessing Communicative Intents in Young Children: Low Structured or Observation Tasks?" by T. E. Coggins, L. B. Olswang, and J. Guthrie, 1987, *Journal of Speech and Hearing Disorders, 52*, p. 46. Copyright 1987 by American Speech-Language-Hearing Association. Reprinted by permission.

iors were treated as initiations than when attempts were made to elicit communicative behaviors" (p. 29). They also found that the child-initiated condition was associated with higher developmental levels than was the adult-initiated condition.

A third investigation of the role of context in encouraging differential communication of intention was conducted with children with more specific language disorders. S. F. Warren, McQuarter, and Rogers-Warren (1984) used variations of the incidental teaching approach (e.g., B. Hart & Risley, 1975, 1980) to guide interactions with three children. The children's ages were 2:11, 3:7, and 3:2 at initiation of the study, but all scored in the 1- to 2-year-old age range (with mean length of utterance, MLU, from 1.1 to 2.0) on various measures of language functioning. All three had intelligible speech and no evidence of hearing impairments, emotional disturbance, or mental retardation. Yet, all were of special concern because they were "low initiators" in that they "consistently displayed very low rates of productive verbal behavior prior to the study and typically remained socially isolated and withdrawn from both teachers and peers in free play situations" (p. 45). (In Fey's, 1986, terminology, these children would be called "inactive communicators.")

Warren and his colleagues (1984) studied the three children in a special preschool classroom, which included four additional children with severe language delays and three children developing language normally (along with four teachers). The researchers gathered multiple baseline data across the three subjects. They used a variation on other investigations in which less structured, child-initiated procedures were contrasted with more structured, adult-initiated procedures. Warren et al. modified the usual child-initiated version of the incidental teaching model into a more structured mand-model procedure (Rogers-Warren & Warren, 1980), making it more adult-initiated and direct, while maintaining the characteristic that the topic (reinforcer) was still determined by the child. In this revised approach, adults were encouraged to use mands, in the form of instructions to verbalize, or by asking *Wh-* questions, and models, in the form of imitative prompts to increase the frequency of communicative interactions. The results of the multiple-baseline design showed that low-initiating children verbalized more, produced longer utterances, and even produced more nonobligatory initiations, during mand-model sessions.

Dalton and Bedrosian (1989) studied the effect of context on communication board use by adolescents functioning at preoperational cognitive levels. Prior studies consistently showed that such youngsters occupy the respondent role far more frequently than the initiator role in transactions with adults (e.g.,

Calculator & Dollaghan, 1982; D. Harris, 1982; Light, Collier, & Parnes, 1985a, 1985b, 1985c). Dalton and Bedrosian found that partner roles influenced outcomes, with adolescents assuming the respondent role primarily with their teachers. With nonspeaking peers, however, requests predominated, and with speaking peers, a variety of communicative functions appeared.

The results of these varied studies also support the importance of context and the value of an eclectic model of language intervention (as advocated in Chapter 6). Children with varied problems at varied developmental stages benefit differently from similar treatment approaches.

Ranges of Communicative Functions Expected at Different Levels

The preceding discussion centered around a limited number of communicative functions and roles, primarily comments and requests. Surely, however, young children can be expected to produce a greater variety of functional communicative attempts.

Many categories of communicative intentions have been proposed by different authors (e.g., Bates, Camaioni, & Volterra, 1975; Coggins & Carpenter, 1981; Dale, 1980; Dore, 1974; Greenfield & Smith, 1976; Halliday, 1975a, 1975b). Roth and Spekman (1984) compiled them into three sets of categories for children at (1) preverbal levels, (2) the single-word level, and (3) the multiword stage of language development. The first two developmental levels are reprinted here (see Tables 7.4 and 7.5; the third level is shown in Table 8.3) because they pertain to the early stage of language acquisition.

Children whose communicative abilities include multiple communicative intentions are in a stronger position to continue their development than those who express a limited variety of intentions. Communicative intentions are valid targets of early intervention efforts, but they also offer contexts for encouraging the early development of additional forms and content. Requests for objects, actions, and information can provide both the motivation and the method for acquiring new vocabulary. Greetings and attention-seeking behaviors can keep children in social interaction contexts that are rich with language learning possibilities.

Aberrant Expression of Communicative Intention by Children With Profound Disabilities

The process, of course, is not the same for all children with language disorders and risks for language

TABLE 7.4

Preverbal communicative intentions

Intention	Descriptive Example
1. Attention seeking	
a. to self	Child tugs on mother's jeans to secure attention.
b. to events, objects, or other people	Child points to airplane to draw mother's attention to it.
2. Requesting	
a. objects	Child points to toy animal that he wants.
b. action	Child hands book to adult to have story read.
c. information	Child points to usual location of cookie jar (which is not there) and simultaneously secures eye contact with mother to determine its whereabouts.
3. Greetings	Child waves "hi" or "bye."
4. Transferring	Child gives mother the toy that he was playing with.
5. Protesting/Rejecting	Child cries when mother takes away toy.
	Child pushes away a dish of oatmeal.
6. Responding/Acknowledging	Child responds appropriately to simple directions/Child smiles when parent initiates a favorite game.
7. Informing	Child points to wheel on his toy truck to show mother that it is broken.

Note. From "Assessing the Pragmatic Abilities of Children. Part I: Organizational Framework and Assessment Parameters" by F. Roth and N. Spekman, 1984, *Journal of Speech and Hearing Disorders, 49,* p. 4. Copyright 1984 by American Speech-Language-Hearing Association. Reprinted by permission.

TABLE 7.5
Communicative intentions expressed at the single-word level

Intention	Definition	Example
1. Naming	Common and proper nouns that label people, objects, events, and locations.	"Dog," "Party," "Table"
2. Commenting	Words that describe physical attributes of objects, events,and people, including size, shape, and location; observable movements and actions of objects and people; and words that refer to attributes which are not immediately observable such as possession and usual location. These words are not contingent on prior utterances.	"Big," "Here," "Mine"
3. Requesting object		
a. present	Words that solicit an object that is present in the environment.	"Gimme," "Cookie" (accompanied by gesture and/or visual regard)
b. absent	Words that solicit an absent object.	"Ball" (child pulls mother to another room)
4. Requesting action	Words that solicit an action be initiated or continued.	"Up" (child wants to be picked up), "More"
5. Requesting information	Words that solicit information about an object, action, person, or location. Rising intonation is also included.	"Shoe?" (meaning "Is this a shoe?") "Wɑdæt?" (What's that?)
6. Responding	Words that directly complement preceding utterances.	"Crayon" (in response to "What's that?") "Yes" (in response to "Do you want to go outside?")
7. Protesting/Rejecting	Words that express objection to ongoing or impending action or event.	"No" (in response to being tickled), "Yuk" (child pushes away unwanted food)
8. Attention seeking	Words that solicit attention to the child or to aspects of the environment.	"Mommy!" "Watch!"
9. Greetings	Words that express salutations and other conventionalized rituals.	"Hi," "Bye," "Nite-nite"

Note. From "Assessing the Pragmatic Abilities of Children. Part I: Organizational Framework and Assessment Parameters" by F. Roth and N. Spekman, 1984, *Journal of Speech and Hearing Disorders*, 49, p. 4. Copyright 1984 by American Speech-Language-Hearing Association. Reprinted by permission.

delay. Although, as considered previously, it is impossible not to communicate (Watzlawick et al., 1967), some children have such profound developmental limitations that communicating with them in conventional ways is very difficult. When working with children with profound impairments, the general rule is that the more limited a child's abilities and the more unconventional the child's signals, the greater is the burden for communicative interpretation on adults in the child's environment.

For some children in this category, "challenging" aberrant behaviors seem to be far more prevalent than behaviors that resemble positive communicative attempts. In spite of severe limitations in their ability to learn, these children may appear to have learned well how to manipulate their environments and the

adults in them through aberrant and aggressive behaviors such as screaming, biting, and self-abuse. Unfortunately, such behaviors tend to be reinforced and maintained when other more positive behaviors are not. Perhaps this is because these behaviors remove children from situations in which they do not want to participate (this is the negative reinforcement process of escaping an undesirable situation), or perhaps because such behaviors bring social attention (even if it is negative).

Rather than using a purely behaviorist approach in analyzing and intervening in such situations, Donnellan et al. (1984) reported on a procedure for analyzing the communicative functions of aberrant behaviors and developing intervention tactics based on that analysis. These authors suggested that, rather than trying to extinguish aberrant behaviors (through nonreinforcement) or to punish them, greater success might come from "teaching new functional behaviors that result in reinforcing consequences similar to those available following the aberrant behaviors" (p. 201). They likened this process to a pragmatic approach in which all behavior, regardless of its topography, is responded to for its functional message value (Schuler & Goetz, 1981). Thus, communicative intent can be determined only by examining the relationship between behavior and context, not by examining the topography (surface form) of behavior in isolation.

Contextually based analyses may show that some children with severe impairments produce communicative means that are function specific—used to communicate only one message—whereas others may be observed to serve a variety of functions (Schuler & Goetz, 1981). For example, some individuals seem to use self-injurious behavior in different contexts to serve the varied functions of sensory stimulation, eliciting attention from others, and terminating undesirable situations. Donnellan and her colleagues (1984) analyzed these functions as having the respective pragmatic message values of: "I'm bored," "Pay attention to me," and "I don't want to do this anymore" (p. 202).

Intervention in aberrant behavior involves establishing goals to expand the individuals' limited response repertoires rather than eliminating their inappropriate behaviors. Donnellan et al. (1984) described three approach alternatives and gave clinical examples for each: (1) Teach alternative communicative behaviors to replace aberrant responses, (2) teach other functionally related behaviors to replace aberrant responses, and (3) manipulate antecedent contexts.

Teaching alternative communicative behaviors to replace aberrant responses. The specialist may teach communicative behaviors explicitly to reduce aberrant behaviors. An example is Don, an 18-year-old with severe mental retardation whose formal communicative abilities were limited to about 15 signs, which he rarely used spontaneously. Don also engaged in self-injurious behaviors of head-banging, head-punching, and face-slapping, which his teacher apparently reinforced by paying social attention to him whenever the behavior occurred. Thus, this behavior seemed to carry the message value, "Pay attention to me, I need help" (Donnellan et al., 1984, p. 203). Don's

intervention consisted of prompting–fading and modeling techniques to teach him more conventional means to ask for assistance in the three-part sequence: (1) Elicit the teacher's attention by visually scanning the room for him, going over, and tapping him on the shoulder. (2) Make the manual sign for "help" to request assistance. (3) Specify the kind of help needed by walking back to the work area and pointing to the task at hand. The authors reported that "within six weeks, Don regularly performed the request-for-assistance sequence whenever he encountered task difficulty, and the self-injurious behavior was virtually eliminated" (p. 203).

Teaching other functionally related behaviors to replace aberrant responses. The second approach differs from the first in that the alternative responses taught are not designed to be specifically communicative. Sam, a 12-year-old boy with autism and moderate retardation, had a fairly extensive sign repertoire, which he used spontaneously. When he was in crowded, noisy, or novel situations (e.g., shopping malls, stores, and recreational facilities), however, he engaged in several auditory self-stimulatory behaviors, such as finger snapping and loud repetitive vocalizations. These behaviors seemed to communicate the message, "I'm anxious/tense/excited/overwhelmed by the input available" (Donnellan et al., 1984, p. 204). Sam's treatment consisted of teaching an alternative, appropriate behavior that could serve the same function: Screen out high levels of sensory input from the environment. Donnellan et al. provided Sam with a portable cassette recorder with headphones and taught him in two phases: first, to operate the tape system and to listen to soothing music whenever overstimulated (this procedure took a few weeks and led to his being able to participate in community activities), and second, to remain for increasingly long periods of time in stimulating environments before using the tape system. Following the second phase, which took 3 months, "Sam was able to tolerate exposure to novel environments for up to one hour at a time before using the tape set for a 10-minute period" (p. 204).

Manipulating antecedent contexts. In the third approach, the specialist manipulates antecedent conditions to reduce aberrant behavior. This approach is most useful when the aberrant behavior's message seems to be, "I don't want to do this anymore" (Donnellan et al., 1984, p. 204). Donnellan and her colleagues (1984) noted that treatment of this behavior starts with acceptance of the message as valid, followed by questioning why someone would want to escape from the particular situation. For example, the aberrant behavior of Sarah, a 7-year-old girl with autism and severe retardation, consisted primarily of aggression to staff members and throwing objects in the classroom. For Sarah, Donnellan et al. devised a plan to assess her more carefully to determine her learning strengths, weaknesses, and modality preferences to more closely match learning tasks to her learning abilities. For Sarah, this meant reducing linguistic complexity and augmenting explanations with much nonverbal support and physical prompting while redesigning tasks to be more motivational and functional. The outcome was a program "designed to acknowledge the legitimacy of the communicative message of Sarah's behavior ('I don't understand'), and her aggression and tantrum behaviors decreased as they became unnecessary for terminating the activity" (p. 205).

Limited Expression of Communicative Functions by Persons With Profound Disabilities

Not all individuals with severe impairments exhibit aberrant behaviors; many are basically cooperative but highly passive communicators. As these individuals are taught linguistic symbols and structures in relatively deliberate ways, they have difficulty also learning how to use language to communicate. The unintended outcome may be that language seems to function for them more as an academic task than a means of communicating intentions to others. It is as if the only function of communication they have down pat is to respond when prompted.

Mirenda and Santogrossi (1985) described one such individual. Amy was an 8½-year-old-girl who was nonspeaking and who demonstrated severe retardation with autistic-like tendencies. Although Amy had learned to identify a fairly large number of symbols on her communication board in formal teaching contexts, she used them only when she was specifically prompted to do so (e.g., "Show me what you want"). For Amy, a revised primary treatment target was needed—*spontaneous functional communication*. It was defined as any communicative act not "performed in response to an instructional cue or prompt, such as 'What do you want?' or 'Show me what you want' presented by either an adult or a peer" (pp.

143–144). Teaching Amy the communicative value of her augmentative system involved returning to a level in which she had only one symbol available (a can of soda pop). Mirenda and Santogrossi used a prompt-free approach. Amy was first rewarded with a drink of the beverage whenever she accidentally touched the picture in the context of other learning activities. When she did so, the adult interactant poured Amy a drink and said something like, "Oh, you'd like a drink; Here." As Amy's touches became more frequent, and apparently intentional, the adult shaped them into even more deliberate communicative acts by honoring her "request" only when she searched for the symbol, located it, and looked at the teacher expectantly. This process included several stages in which the teacher replaced the original picture with a smaller, more symbolic drawing, which was gradually removed from her immediate range, covered with a translucent cover, and later placed in a notebook (see N. W. Nelson, 1988b, for a sequence of objectives related to this approach). Eventually, the teacher introduced more pictures, and Amy began to communicate intentions with novel pictures in novel environments. Her communication book was built back up until she had 120 symbols in the categories of food, drink, activity, and self-care–clothing. Perhaps the most exciting outcome was a generalization of her original request behavior to varied communicative intentions. For example, at one point in school, after using her symbol book to request paper, crayons, and scissors, she drew a picture and cut it out. What was particularly nice about this event was that, after requesting and being given the crayons, Amy pointed back to the crayon symbol, communicating an intentional comment to her communicative partner. (Remember that A. M. Wetherby et al., 1989, found that the production of comments by children with autism was extremely rare.)

Not all children who demonstrate severe restrictions of communicative intentions are passive communicators. Gallagher and Craig (1984) described a 4-year-old boy named Clark who met Stark and Tallal's (1981) criteria as a child with a severe language impairment (see Chapter 6). Initially, Clark produced the phrase "It's gone" 60 times within a 2-hour 10-minute videotaped sample. The phrase accounted for 17% of the utterances and seemed to serve varied communicative functions. Far from being passive, this child used the phrase, "It's gone," frequently during activity transitions to reestablish interaction with his partners in a game-like event similar to the nonexistence–disappearance ("all-gone") game played by infants and toddlers with their mothers. Gallagher and Craig noted that although Clark's repetitive phrase met criteria for syntactic productivity as a spontaneously rule-generated phrase, for him, it was best characterized as a memorized stereotypic phrase. They also noted that Clark's behavior illustrated the advisability of not discarding information about stereotypic, highly repetitive phrases from language samples, as often done, but of analyzing them carefully for their communicative intent. Gallagher and Craig recommended establishing an intervention target to assist Clark to acquire an expanded repertoire of socially acceptable and recognizable access behaviors for gaining social attention. (Clark also may have been demonstrating a need to acquire more elaborated play routines, discussed in a following section.)

This kind of careful analysis also might be necessary when children with autism use echolalia to perform varied communicative functions. Echolalia often has been regarded primarily as noncommunicative behavior representing signs of children's comprehension difficulties. Prizant (1987), however, pointed out that echolalic behaviors are best described along three continua regarding (1) exactness of the repetition, (2) degree of comprehension, and (3) underlying communicative intent. Prizant defined *immediate echolalia* as "utterances that are produced either following immediately or a brief time after the produc-

tion of the model utterance" (p. 66) and *delayed echolalia* as "utterances repeated at a significantly later time" (p. 67). Others have suggested that the two kinds of echolalia might involve differential activation of echoic short-term and long-term memory (Hermelin & O'Connor, 1970). By providing a rich, contextually based analysis of the communicative intent underlying both immediate and delayed echolalia, Prizant and his colleagues (Prizant & Duchan, 1981; Prizant & Rydell, 1984) led clinicians beyond traditional views of echolalia as aberrant behavior to be ignored or extinguished. Varied functions that may be served by either immediate or delayed echolalia appear in Tables 7.6 and 7.7. The clinical implications are that this kind of analysis should be used to identify functional distinctions for echolalia produced by individual children in different contexts rather than lumping all occurrences into one category and targeting it for extinction.

Prizant (1987) provided intervention guidelines for incorporating echolalia into individualized intervention programs. He recommended using strategies that would (1) simplify language input, (2) respond to the child's apparent communicative intent when echolalia is used, (3) relate echolalic utterances to actions and objects in the child's environment, (4) follow Fay's (1979) suggestions to deemphasize correct pronominal usage in early stages, and (5) never punish or ignore a child for echolalia if it is intentful or interactive or the only means of communication available.

TABLE 7.6
Functional categories of immediate echolalia

Category	Description
Interactive	
1. Turn-taking	1. Utterances used as turn fillers in an alternating verbal exchange.
2. Declaration	2. Utterances labeling objects, actions, or location (accompanied by demonstrative gestures).
3. "Yes" Answer	3. Utterances used to indicate affirmation of prior utterance.
4. Request	4. Utterances used to request objects or others' actions. Usually involves mitigated echolalia.
Non-interactive	
5. Non-focused	5. Utterances produced with no apparent intent, and often in states of high arousal (e.g. fear, pain).
6. Rehearsal	6. Utterances used as a processing aid, followed by utterance or action indicating comprehension of echoed utterance.
7. Self-regulatory	7. Utterances which serve to regulate one's own actions. Produced in synchrony with motor activity.

Note. From "Theoretical and Clinical Implications of Echolalic Behavior in Autism" by B. M. Prizant in *Language and Treatment of Autistic and Developmentally Disordered Children* (p. 72) edited by T. Layton, 1987, Springfield, IL: Charles C Thomas. Courtesy of Charles C Thomas, Publisher, Springfield, Illinois.

TABLE 7.7
Functional categories of delayed echolalia

Category	Description
Prizant and Rydell (1984)	
Interactive	
1. Turn-taking	1. Utterances used as turn fillers in alternating verbal exchange.
2. Verbal completion	2. Utterances which complete familiar verbal routines initiated by others.
3. Providing information	3. Utterances offering new information not apparent from situational context (may be initiated or respondent).
4. Labeling (interactive)	4. Utterances labeling objects or actions in environment.
5. Protest	5. Utterances protesting actions of others. May be used to prohibit others' actions.
6. Request	6. Utterances used to request objects.
7. Calling	7. Utterances used to call attention to oneself or to establish/maintain interaction.
8. Affirmation	8. Utterances used to indicate affirmation of previous utterances.
9. Directive	9. Utterances (often imperatives) used to direct others' actions.
Non-interactive	
10. Non-focused	10. Utterances with no apparent communicative intent or relevance to the situational context. May be self-stimulatory.
11. Situation association	11. Utterances with no apparent communicative intent which appear to be triggered by an object, person, situation, or activity.
12. Self-directive	12. Utterances which serve to regulate one's own actions. Produced in synchrony with motor activity.
13. Rehearsal	13. Utterances produced with low volume followed by louder interactive production. Appears to be practice for subsequent production.
14. Label (non-interactive)	14. Utterances labeling objects or actions in environment with no apparent communicative intent. May be a form of practice for learning language.

Note. From "Theoretical and Clinical Implications of Echolalic Behavior in Autism" by B. M. Prizant in *Language and Treatment of Autistic and Developmentally Disordered Children* (p. 73) edited by T. Layton, 1987, Springfield, IL: Charles C Thomas. Courtesy of Charles C Thomas, Publisher, Springfield, Illinois.

EARLY SYMBOLS

The preceding discussion concentrated mainly on social interactions and communicative functions in the early stages of language acquisition, along with some early aspects of learning to vocalize and to control the oral-motor mechanism. The social aspects of communicative development are highly pragmatic. They focus on language use more than its content and forms. For children to move beyond prelinguistic communicative stages, they must begin to acquire linguistic content and forms as well. Around the age of 1 year, normally developing children begin to combine varied components of prelinguistic behaviors into the production of true spoken words.

The appearance of a child's first true words has been considered a major developmental milestone, probably as long as people have thought about talking. You may recall the infamous experiment con-

ducted by Psammetichus I, an Egyptian Pharaoh of the 7th century B.C., who placed two children to be raised with sheep. They were cared for physically but were allowed to hear no human speech. The idea was to determine which words the children would utter first as a way of identifying Egyptian as the "natural" language of humans. Of course, without language models and communicative interactions, the children did not begin to speak Egyptian or anything approximating human language (Owens, 1988).

The point of retelling this story is that children need to hear words to learn them. Consideration of the word-learning difficulties experienced by children with severe hearing impairments emphasizes this point further. But children need to do more than hear words to learn them. They need to hear words in meaningful contexts. I have a friend whose daughter was born with a severe hearing loss following the rubella epidemic of the 1960s. When speaking to my classes, my friend used to tell the story of how her daughter learned her first word. Having been told that hearing impaired children needed to hear words hundreds of times before learning them, the family devised a plan to encourage learning of the word *ball*. They did this by hiding balls of various sizes and colors all around the house (including the refrigerator drawer). Then, they would feign surprise and make a production out of labeling the balls when any one of them was discovered. Although the child seemed to enjoy the fun, she did not learn the word. Instead, some weeks into the program, as the family pulled into the driveway in their car, my friend and her husband heard a small voice from the back seat say, "Home." Their daughter's first true word was heard, not in the contrived context of the teaching situation (even though it was spread throughout the day), but incidentally in the real-life meaningful event of "coming home."

How Children Appear to Learn Early Words

The preceding story illustrates several aspects that need to be kept in mind when assistance is needed to help children learn early words. Again, information from normal development can be instructive.

K. Nelson (1985) proposed that learning to talk involves entering into a system of shared meanings in which children learn to use words that have the power to evoke in others a conceptual representation that, ideally, matches the one children intend to express. This ability does not emerge suddenly but develops through stages to which several interrelated components contribute: (1) the communicative context, (2) the current status of the child's cognitive system, and (3) cognitive, linguistic, and social developments that change the parameters of the overall system over time. Efforts to encourage the development of a child's semantic system when it does not proceed normally must recognize these three elements as well.

In the earliest stages of linguistic learning, context is particularly important. As K. Nelson (1985) explained it, early words are often inseparable from the contexts in which they appear; they are embedded in particular contexts and are only understood or used within those activities. For example, a child might crawl to the high chair when his mother says, "Do you want lunch?" It is not the words that the child understands so much as the activity, partially because, at this point in development, "the child's representational system is largely organized around

events that are undifferentiated, unanalyzed schemas without separable elements of concepts" (p. 121). K. Nelson argued that children's first spoken words are also grounded in the actions of familiar routines and are thus "pure performatives." "Even when the parent and child are focused on an object, the protolanguage form seems to be *part* of the activity rather than *referring* to the object of the activity" (p. 121). At this transitional point, K. Nelson considered the child's use of words to be prelexical activity language and not yet reflective of activities.

Bruner (1977) offered a similar explanation for the transition from prelinguistic to linguistic communication in the context of joint action routines. Bruner, however, emphasizes the role played by the child's knowledge about social communication before language as the critical factor helping the child crack the linguistic code. "Communication is converted into speech through a series of behavioral advances that are achieved in highly familiar, well learned contexts that have already undergone conventionalization at the hands of the infant and his mother (or other caretaker)" (p. 274).

Bruner (1975) also identified joint reference as a critical aspect of early word learning, developing out of earlier stages when joint attention is established. In the earliest joint-attention exchanges, parents follow their infants' leads, using gaze cues, such as the child's line of regard, to identify objects of the child's attention so that parents may label, comment, or elaborate on those objects. Owens (1988) summarized the age-stage relationships in this process (see Box 7.7).

For infants at risk, intervention might encourage early communication along a similar sequence. Especially when motor problems preclude the production of clear gestural and vocal signals by children, parents need to learn to interpret their children's intentions through alternative indices. They also may need to be encouraged to stay with each stage of the process for longer periods than expected in normal development. In addition, they may want to be more deliberate in labeling the objects of their children's attentions. Even in normal development, labeling by parents, in addition to pointing, can sustain infants' attention to objects beyond the time when labeling occurs and may help children to learn mappings between words and objects (Baldwin & Markman, 1989). A final clinical implication is that early word learning should occur within meaningful contexts, in which words are associated with familiar routines.

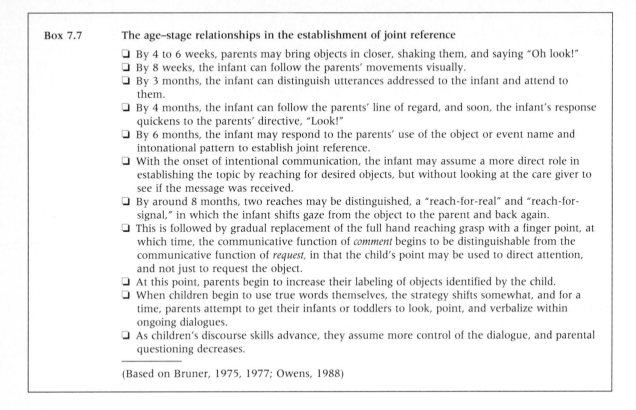

Box 7.7   The age–stage relationships in the establishment of joint reference

❏ By 4 to 6 weeks, parents may bring objects in closer, shaking them, and saying "Oh look!"
❏ By 8 weeks, the infant can follow the parents' movements visually.
❏ By 3 months, the infant can distinguish utterances addressed to the infant and attend to them.
❏ By 4 months, the infant can follow the parents' line of regard, and soon, the infant's response quickens to the parents' directive, "Look!"
❏ By 6 months, the infant may respond to the parents' use of the object or event name and intonational pattern to establish joint reference.
❏ With the onset of intentional communication, the infant may assume a more direct role in establishing the topic by reaching for desired objects, but without looking at the care giver to see if the message was received.
❏ By around 8 months, two reaches may be distinguished, a "reach-for-real" and "reach-for-signal," in which the infant shifts gaze from the object to the parent and back again.
❏ This is followed by gradual replacement of the full hand reaching grasp with a finger point, at which time, the communicative function of *comment* begins to be distinguishable from the communicative function of *request*, in that the child's point may be used to direct attention, and not just to request the object.
❏ At this point, parents begin to increase their labeling of objects identified by the child.
❏ When children begin to use true words themselves, the strategy shifts somewhat, and for a time, parents attempt to get their infants or toddlers to look, point, and verbalize within ongoing dialogues.
❏ As children's discourse skills advance, they assume more control of the dialogue, and parental questioning decreases.

(Based on Bruner, 1975, 1977; Owens, 1988)

Assessing Early Word Knowledge

Some formal assessment techniques have been devised to assess word knowledge for children at the single-word stage of expressive language development. A. M. Wetherby et al. (1989) reported on language-sampling techniques appropriate for this stage that are similar to those used in the CSBS (A. M. Wetherby & Prizant, 1990, described previously in this chapter). Language sampling is especially useful for attempting to elicit one-word or longer utterances in relatively structured communicative contexts.

Rescorla (1989) developed the Language Development Survey (LDS) as a screening tool to identify language delay in 2-year-old children. The survey, which can be completed by parents in about 10 minutes, is a vocabulary checklist that includes 242 words arranged in 17 semantic categories. Parents are asked to check off any words that their children say but are advised not to include any words that their children can understand but not say or say only in imitation. Rescorla found that the results of the LDS were highly correlated with the results of other

commonly used language assessment tools and that it showed both good sensitivity and good specificity (low false-negative and false-positive rates). The screening criteria that proved appropriate for defining language delay were fewer than 50 words or no word combinations at 2 years of age.

Words, Referents, and Meanings: Selecting Symbol Systems

Early semantic intervention requires an appreciation of the relationships among words, referents, and meanings. *Meaning* is inherent in people, not things or words.

> The word is a sign that signifies a referent, but the referent is not the meaning of the word. If, for example, you say to a child, "Look at the kitty," the actual cat is the referent but is not the meaning of *kitty*. If the cat ran away or were run over by a truck, the word would still have the same meaning because meaning is an act of cognition. (Pease, Gleason, & Pan, 1989, p. 102)

Words have arbitrary relationships to the things they represent, but some words are more arbitrary than others. This arbitrary relationship between signs (e.g., the word *kitty*) and their referents (e.g., the cat) is *symbolic*. Symbolic relationships may be represented by nonverbal signs (e.g., stop lights) as well as verbal signs, but not all signs are symbolic. Some do not have arbitrary relationships to the things they represent. A nonsymbolic sign that can be interpreted as having meaning is called an *index*. Examples are rain on the roof, footprints of animals, and cries of babies. They are less arbitrary, and are also not symbolic. When a sign has a strong physical relationship to the thing it represents and can be recognized on the basis of physical similarity alone, the sign is said to be *iconic*, or *transparent*.

It is not too surprising that, even in normal development, many of the early words or protowords learned by children are less arbitrary. For example, bumps on the knees may be called "owies," and clocks may be called "tick-tock." Parents provide some of these words, but others are children's own creations (Pease et al., 1989).

Older children who remain at early stages of language development may have particular difficulty learning arbitrary symbols. Some may never be able to say words and make them intelligible to others. What symbols, signs, and indexes should be used in trying to help such children acquire word knowledge? Miranda and Locke (1989) considered this issue systematically by studying 11 different symbol sets and nonsymbolic means of representing objects with 40 nonspeaking individuals who experienced varying degrees of intellectual disabilities. Their review of the literature in this area showed that "persons with intellectual handicaps can learn symbol–referent associations and that some types of symbols are more difficult to learn than are others" (p. 131). Miranda and Locke differentiated issues of symbol transparency (i.e., the degree to which a symbol looks like the thing it represents—its iconicity) from symbol learnability (i.e., how easy a symbol is to learn), although they recognized that the two are probably related. Miranda and Locke did not attempt to teach the meaning of the symbols and thus measured only transparency and not learnability. Because of differences among the capabilities of the individuals taking part in the study, the authors assessed 29 with a standard receptive language protocol (3 used eye gaze to select objects), 1 with a yes–no protocol, and 10 with a matching protocol. As expected, all of the symbols assessed were found to be less transparent

than were objects or pictures of objects. One of the most unexpected findings (although it had previously been hypothesized by Vanderheiden and Lloyd, 1986) was the low transparency of miniature objects. Apparently, miniature objects are not seen by some individuals with cognitive limitations as being representative of real objects. In fact, color photographs are more transparent than miniature objects. Miranda and Locke also noted that Blissymbols and written words were about equally transparent (although they may not necessarily be equally learnable).

Symbol Learning by Individuals With Profound Impairments

Because of their cognitive limitations, some individuals may never learn to communicate with symbols; however, this does not mean that they will never learn to communicate (Siegel-Causey & Guess, 1989). The most appropriate service-delivery model for these individuals may be collaborative consultation in which the specialist assists care givers to read communicative signs produced by the individuals and to teach them to make those signs in increasingly conventional ways so that they can be interpreted accurately by a wider range of partners. The long-term intervention process for receptive communication with these individuals may involve guiding them through stages in which they (1) recognize indexes provided by their care givers (see Table 7.8 for a list of possibilities provided by Siegel-Causey & Guess); (2) associate real objects with the sequence of the daily routine (e.g., a segmented wooden trough might be designed to hold objects that represent the major activities of the day in sequence); and (3) recognize photographs of objects to indicate where they are supposed to be and what they are supposed to be doing, and to represent available choices where appropriate.

Some individuals with profound disabilities also may be able to learn to recognize and use arbitrary symbols, especially when they are taught in deliberate ways over extended periods with careful attention to coordination of multiple components. Romski et al. (1988) described how three out of four adolescent and young adult women with severe retardation acquired a vocabulary of 20 lexigrams (arbitrary printed symbols composed of geometric forms) in this way and used them in meaningful ways. Romski and her colleagues initially taught the women to use symbols to request their favorite foods, and later objects. The women's requesting skills did not initially

TABLE 7.8
Forms of service providers' communicative expressions

Modality	Symbolic	Nonsymbolic
Auditory	Service provider speaks to learner	Service provider turns on music to indicate the start of physical therapy
		Service provider uses a nonspeech vocalization to attract the learner's attention
Visual	Service provider signs to learner	Service provider makes pointing movement to draw learner's attention to an object
		Service provider holds out spoon to see if learner is ready for a bit of food
		Service provider draws a picture with learner to indicate the next activity
		Service provider makes a twisting motion over the lid of a container to demonstrate to the learner how to open it
		Service provider makes an exaggerated movement to elicit learner's attention
Tactile	Service provider fingerspells in learner's hand	Service provider taps learner's hand to prompt the learner to pick up an object
		Service provider puts hands under the learner's arms and pauses to indicate that the learner is about to be picked up
		Service provider rubs learner's legs in a downward direction to request learner's assistance in pulling pants off
		Service provider ties bib on learner to indicate lunch
Kinesthetic	Service provider manipulates learner's hands through the "finish" sign to indicate that the activity is over	Service provider pauses while rocking with the learner to elicit a signal to continue
		Service provider manipulates the learner's hands through the start of pouring from a container to elicit the learner's participation
Olfactory		Service provider holds spoon near learner's nose to see if learner wants the particular food item

Note. From *Enhancing Nonsymbolic Communication Interactions Among Learners With Severe Disabilities* (p. 6) by E. Siegel-Causey and D. Guess, 1989, Baltimore, MD: Paul H. Brookes Publishing Co. Copyright 1989 by Paul H. Brookes Publishing Co. Reprinted by permission.

generalize to labeling and to comprehension tasks (the symbols were apparently used in ways that K. Nelson, 1985, called *activity language*—tied to specific events). Additional request experiences, however, resulted in improvements in the other functional areas. Romski et al. also observed that the participants later began to initiate lexigram communications spontaneously and that spoken language comprehension and production attempts were facilitated.

Selecting Words to Target in Intervention: The Meanings and Functions of First Words

An important issue for the specialist is selecting words to target early in the language process. Perhaps it is easier to select a lexicon for young chil-

dren than for children at later stages of language development, but in either case, it is an ominous task when one considers the rapidity of word acquisition in normal development and the huge number of possible choices. Crais (1990) noted that children between 1.5 and 6 years of age add an estimated five word roots daily and that the comprehension vocabulary of the average 6-year-old is around 14,000 words.

How then should we select among all of the possibilities to find the best target words for children—in order, from easiest to more difficult to learn? The best answer to this troublesome question probably is *let the context and the child be your guide.* When identifying target words in early language intervention, MacDonald (1989) suggested to parents that they should select (1) words to code their child's knowledge, (2) words to code their child's communication, (3) words to code their child's interests, (4) words with high communicative utility, and (5) "language for communication, not for storage" (p. 198). To reinforce these ideas, MacDonald told parents that the words should come from the adults' matched words, the child's communications without words, the child's current knowledge, and the child's own interests. For children who need AAC systems, Beukelman and Tice (1990) have been developing a software program for Macintosh computers, called the Vocabulary Tool Box. The program allows a professional to act as "editor" in consultation with one or more "informants," who select a customized lexicon for a particular child based on contextual observations with the assistance of lists of potential vocabulary sets that may be called up based on developmental and contextual criteria.

The first words of normally developing children generally have two types of meaning: (1) *Referential* meanings appear among words that stand for things such as objects ("milk"), events ("up"), and conditions ("hot"). (2) *Functional* meanings appear among words that accomplish things such as drawing attention ("hi") and rejecting undesirable actions ("no"). Intervention to assist children to acquire first words may be most successful if these dual levels of content and function are kept active and relevant to the child's needs. Box 7.8 is a summary of a first lexicon suggested by Lahey and Bloom (1977), based on a normal developmental model of language content, form, and use.

When encouraging early word learning, it is also important to remember the "linguistic universal"

(Ingram, 1974) that children generally comprehend words before they can produce them. Benedict (1979) confirmed this expectation when he analyzed the first words of eight normally developing children who comprehended 50 words before they produced 10. Box 7.9 is a list of the kinds of words Huttenlocher (1974) identified as comprehended by the four 10- to 18-month-old children she studied. She also noted that the phonological complexity of words that children comprehended often exceeded the phonological complexity of words they produced. Recognition of this discrepancy may be useful in intervention.

When K. Nelson (1973) inventoried the first 50 words produced by children, she noted that the highest proportion, 65%, was made up of names of either general or specific things. R. Schwartz and Leonard (1984) also found that the 12 toddlers they studied acquired object words and concepts more rapidly than action words and concepts. K. Nelson's (1973) findings for the expressive lexicons of the 18 children she studied showed the following proportions of early words:

1. *General nominals*, including objects (*ball*) 31%; animals and people (*doggie, girl*) 10%; substances (*milk*) 7%; and letters and numbers (*e, two*) 2%
2. *Specific nominals*, including people (*Mommy*) 12%; animals (*Fluffy*) 1%; and objects (*car*) 1%
3. *Action words*, including demand–descriptive (*up, bye-bye*) 11%; and notice (*look, hi*) 2%
4. *Modifiers*, including states (*hot, dirty, all gone*) 6%; locatives (*there, outside*) 2%; attributes (*big, pretty*) 1%; and possessives (*mine*) 1%
5. *Personal–social*, including assertions (*no, yes, want*) 4%; and social-express (*please, ouch*) 4%

Box 7.8	A first lexicon: Suggested content and forms (in parentheses) based on normal development (adapted from Lahey & Bloom, 1977)

  ❑ Rejection (*no*)
  ❑ Nonexistence or disappearance (*no, all gone, away*)
  ❑ Cessation of action (*stop, no*)
  ❑ Prohibition of action (*no,* or content word with negative head shake)
  ❑ Recurrence of objects and actions on objects (*more, again, another*)
  ❑ Noting the existence of objects, people, or animals (*it, this, that, there*)
  ❑ Identifying objects, people, or animals (*Mama, Daddy, doggie, baby, sock,* etc.)
  ❑ Actions on objects (*give, do, make, get, throw, eat, wash, kiss*)
  ❑ Attributes or descriptions of objects (*big, hot, dirty, heavy*)
  ❑ Persons and pets associated with objects (as in possession) (relevant proper names)

Box 7.9   Categories and examples of words comprehended by normally developing children between 10 and 18 months (based on Huttenlocher, 1974)

❑ Name of a family member or pet (*Mommy, fish*)
❑ Label for a game or social ritual (*bye-bye, peek-a-boo*)
❑ Manipulable object/toy (*blanket, telephone, shoe*)
❑ Body parts (*hair, nose, belly button*)
❑ Food related (*cookie, bottle*)

---

6. *Function words*, including questions (*what, where*) 2%; and miscellaneous (*is, to, for*) 2%.

When planning intervention programs (N. W. Nelson, 1988), the specialist might use this information to set up events that tend to encourage toddlers to interact in what R. A. Brown (1958) called "The Original Word Game." This is the normal developmental interaction in which an adult "tutor" supplies the label for an entity, and the child "player" then forms hypotheses about the named entity. The player tests these hypotheses by applying the label to other entities that appear to the child to be members of the same conceptual set. The tutor then evaluates the accuracy of the fit and provides evaluative feedback.

Potential Problems With Early Word Acquisition

Even when developing normally, children may differ in the things they like to talk about and the classes of words they seem to acquire most easily. K. Nelson (1973) described children who used substantive words primarily to talk about things as referential and children who used words and formulaic phrases primarily to direct social interactions as expressive. Horgan (1979) called such children "noun lovers" and "noun leavers."

This suggests that children can vary from the expected early semantic encoding proportions without those differences' necessarily representing pathological differences. When the specialist identifies individualized learning patterns in assessment, she may use them to advantage when selecting intervention content and contexts. On the other hand, when proportions are extremely out of balance—such as when a child seems to have no substantive words, except perhaps a few glued into stereotypic phrases—concern is appropriate. The specialist then should design some intervention strategies to help

children learn the symbolic value of words (Prizant, 1983). A little later in development (during what I call the *middle stage*), other children may begin to use multiple-word phrases but continue the telegraphic pattern of producing mostly content words without morphological inflections or function words. A different kind of concern then is justified; intervention is needed to help children with these specific impairments learn to use grammatical markers in their language.

Another area that is expected to vary normally, but in the extreme may represent pathology, is the difference in the size of receptive and expressive vocabularies. Both *overextensions* (i.e., applying a word to a category larger than the conventional one, such as calling horses *doggie*) and *underextensions* (i.e., applying a word to a category smaller than the conventional one, such as calling only Oreos, *cookie*) may occur in normal development either in comprehension or expression. These misapplications may be viewed as signs of developmental adjustments in semantic systems and not necessarily matters of concern, as long as they do not persist for extended periods of time even when new learning opportunities are presented.

Tager-Flusberg (1989) noted that numerous studies have shown that children can differentiate varied words in their receptive vocabularies (e.g., *motorcycle, bike, truck*), which they cannot yet use expressively (e.g., the same children who can point to pictures representing each kind of vehicle may call them all *car*). K. Nelson, Benedict, Gruendel, and Rescorla (1977) offered an explanation for this disparity, suggesting that early word-learning strategies differ during three different stages of early word development. (1) From 10 to 13 months, children seem to match adult words to preexisting concepts in comprehension. (2) From 11 to 15 months, they acquire a small number of words in production that are constrained in use only to a particular context or to the action-function component of the concept to which they are bonded. (3) From 16 to 20 months, they acquire new productive words for old concepts, form new concepts to match novel words, and begin to use words to categorize new instances. According to this theoretical position, comprehension and production involve different processes at different stages, and "errors," such as calling all vehicles *car*, may actually indicate more about a child's positive ability to draw inferences and to form categories than about limitations of expressive vocabulary.

For children who are nonspeaking and whose communication boards can hold only so many symbols, the ability to overextend a limited set of expressive symbols for wider uses may be critical to their ability to communicate. At the same time, their parents should be urged not to fall into the trap of limiting the vocabulary that such children hear. Parents may need to relate several different words for the child by pointing to the same symbol on the communication board. For example, parents may talk about *jets* and *helicopters* when the child notices them flying overhead, while pointing to the symbol for *airplane* on the child's board. When children can handle more arbitrary and less transparent symbol sets, Blissymbols may be preferred over more transparent or iconic symbol sets for their flexibility in communicating extended and more abstract meanings.

Parents of children with hearing impairments face a slightly different dilemma. These parents must strike a careful balance between keeping vocabulary to a level that will permit recognition and comprehension without overly limiting lexical input and preventing the child from learning a rich vocabulary. As Ling (1976) noted, parents must present natural speaking models to their children without exaggerating critical features if they want their children to have more natural speech. On the other hand, because of their reduced sensory input, children with severe hearing losses may have difficulty abstracting enough phonological information to segment words along their boundaries and to recognize the same words in different contexts. A variety of strategies has been suggested for helping children to compensate for this deficit. Besides total communication (Ling, 1984b)—the simultaneous use of multiple modalities including sign language symbols to communicate meaning—tactile stimulation devices (Lynch, Eilers, Oller, & Cobo-Lewis, 1989) may be

used to assist children to feel some characteristics of sound they cannot hear. Cued speech (Cornett, 1967, 1972) is another tool (proponents stress that it is not a method or a philosophy) that involves a set of four hand positions and eight hand shapes that can be used near the mouth to accompany spoken words and to supplement speech reading information already available to the "listener" (Ling & Clarke, 1975, 1976). However, the technique is not without controversy (Moores, 1969). In particular, Wilbur (1976) suggested that cued speech may be more appropriate for later stage speech instruction than for initial language learning.

Other children with central language processing problems, such as those with autism or with apparent word-retrieval deficits, may need programs that include specific attention to preventing their semantic systems from getting stuck in inflexible or weak processing patterns. Particularly, children with autism are likely to develop semantic underextension, insisting on using certain words to refer only to specific exemplars of a concept rather than to all exemplars.

Underextensions and overextensions that occur in autism also seem to arise out of cognitive and linguistic difficulties that these children have in isolating the set of features characterizing referents for one word and separating that semantic concept from others. "To produce a word in a variety of contexts, the child must first separate the word from the context to which it was first attached. Once this major feat is accomplished, the child can use the word as a symbol for, rather than a feature of, its referent" (Pease, Gleason, & Pan, 1989, p. 114).

I once worked with a 6-year-old boy with autism who had learned to use the word *in* to refer either to containment ("in") or support ("on") relationships with a particular kind of container and used *on* to refer either to containment or support relationships with a different kind of container. The critical feature that he had apparently abstracted for using *in* and *on* was nonconventional. He focused on the type of container rather than the discriminating feature of containment or support as the key to the meanings of those two words. He needed many examples of *in* and *on* with the same container (a clear plastic box) over many sessions before he could abstract the critical semantic features of containment and support and could separate them from association with the physical characteristics of particular containers (N. W. Nelson, 1988b).

ENCODING SEMANTIC RELATIONS AND COMBINING TWO WORDS TO DO MORE

First words are acquired in normal development as children become increasingly interested in what things are called and in the functional uses of words to communicate. At around 18 months, when single-word lexicons include a small core of words, normally developing children begin to combine words to communicate more elaborate meanings. However, children continue to mix two-word constructions with many single-word utterances throughout the latter half of the 2nd year (Owens, 1988). During R. A. Brown's (1973) first stage of language development, as MLU grows from 1.0 to 2.0, most of children's utterances are two words long, although a few may be as long as three or even four words.

Before the appearance of the first true two-word combinations, several transition behaviors may appear. These include combinations of nonmeaningful, "empty," CV and CVCV combinations with meaningful words (e.g., *ma baby*, *beda baby*); reduplication of single-word utterances (e.g., *doggie doggie*); and production of successive one-word utterances made up of two words, both produced with falling intonation (e.g., *mommy, laugh*) (Owens, 1988). Children may also appear to use generative rules to construct two-word utterances by imitating formulaic or gestalt units before they actually do so. Common examples listed by Owens that may occur in normal development include *all gone, go bye, so big, go potty* (p. 216).

Specialized Assessment Techniques for Early Multiword Utterances

Language comprehension abilities continue to develop while children move toward producing two-word combinations. Early language comprehension, however, may be based on situations as much as it is on relationships among words. Chapman and Miller (1980) described children's early nonverbal comprehension strategies, which toddlers use in the early stages to assist partially adequate verbal comprehension: (1) Locate the objects mentioned. (2) Give evidence of notice. (3) Do what you usually do (e.g., put objects in containers). (4) Act on objects in the way mentioned. (5) Perform as agent of action.

Because of the difficulty in determining the role of context in language comprehension by this age group under natural circumstances, specialized techniques have been developed to measure linguistic comprehension among 1- and 2-year-olds. One technique (designed by Golinkoff, Hirsh-Pasek, Cauley, & Gordon, 1987) involves positioning two video monitors so that very young children can see both monitors equally well while seated on their mother's laps. When using this technique, Golinkoff and colleagues showed that children as young as 17 months of age looked measurably longer at the appropriate video monitor when they heard the sentence "Cookie Monster is tickling Big Bird" than at the screen that displayed the relationship of Big Bird tickling Cookie Monster. The authors thus concluded that children can comprehend word order even before they begin using two-word utterances.

Another procedure for assessing comprehension of two-term semantic relations was devised by J. F. Miller et al. (1980). The examiner uses sets of objects to measure children's understandings of constructions involving the semantic relations of action, location, possession, and attribution. First, the examiner teaches the child (to 80% criterion) to show, demonstrate, look toward an object, or perform an action following the examiner's request. Then the examiner presents the child with four examples of each of the relational categories tested. For example, the action category might be tested with the four exemplars *throw block, open door, baby drink,* and *boy ride.* Results are expressed as the proportion of times comprehension (or production) was demonstrated out of four trials for each semantic category.

When children reach the stage of being able to scan pictures that represent various word combinations and to point (or to eye-point) to those being named, specialists may use other procedures to assess early-stage comprehension of semantic-grammatic relationships, as long as they keep in mind the limitations of formal testing. The Assessment of Children's Language Comprehension (Foster, Giddan, & Stark, 1973) presents sets of pictures representing single words that children select to demonstrate a basic one-word vocabulary level. Then the examiner asks the child to point to appropriate pictures (from contrasting foils) in other sets that represent two-word (e.g., *broken cup*), three-word (e.g., *cat under table*), and four-word (e.g., *happy little girl jumping*) combinations.

Special analytical techniques have also been recommended to assess whether children really are demonstrating creative, rule-based strategies in their production of two-word utterances (rather than just repeating language they have heard as unanalyzed chunks). Leonard, Steckol, and Panther (1983) suggested that two approaches could be used for this purpose. Using the *interpretive approach*, the specialist collects many spontaneous utterances over several sessions and then judges utterances as rule-based if they meet these criteria: (1) a high degree of positional consistency of elements and (2) some degree of creativity in word combinations. For example, the utterance, "hug mommy," would qualify as being based on the semantic–grammatic rule action plus object if *hug* and *mommy* both appeared also individually or combined with some other word and if other word combinations also representing action plus object relations appeared. Using the second method, the *relevant component approach*, the specialist constructs specific probes, attempting to elicit a wide variety and range of possible semantic segmentations, in which the child combines the same words in various ways. Although the relevant component approach requires more planning, it takes less time for data gathering and analysis.

Stockman and Vaughn-Cooke (1986) presented data supporting the use of early spontaneous language sampling with young children in working-class families who speak nonstandard dialects of English. They recommended gathering at least 50 to 100 utterances in natural interactions using a variety of stimulus materials. They then assigned the utterances to semantic categories to be compared with developmental data that they summarized from several sources, including their own research. As guidelines for identifying nonstandard speakers who may require clinical intervention, Stockman and Vaughn-Cooke recommended that by 30 months of age, working-class nonstandard speakers should "(a) use mainly two-word combinations, and (b) encode the following types of semantic categories: *existence, action, locative action, state, locative state, negation, possession, attribution, notice, intention, and recurrence*" (p. 23).

Targets and Methods of Intervention at the Two-Word Stage

The relevant component analysis procedures suggested by Leonard and his colleagues (1983) relate to the matrix training approach that has been suggested by many authors for helping children with disabilities acquire early two-word combinations (e.g., Bunce, Ruder, & Ruder, 1985; Stremel-Campbell & Campbell, 1985; B. Wetherby & Striefel, 1978). A matrix provides a system for pairing a variety of content words representing a targeted semantic role with another set of content words representing a related semantic role. The instructor combines a limited set of words in one semantic category with another set in a related semantic category to help children maximize their abilities to recombine lexical items in unique and communicative ways and to generalize those skills to new content and contexts. Figure 7.7 shows a set of stimuli for an agent–action matrix suggested by H. Goldstein (1985). Other matrices have been designed to teach productive action–object sequences (Stremel-Campbell & Campbell, 1985) and the comprehension of preposition–object phrases (Bunce et al., 1985). Ezell and Goldstein (1989) reported on a matrix training procedure that was designed to teach two moderately retarded children (a 6:1-year-old girl and a 9:11-year-old boy) to combine known and unknown words. When Ezell and Goldstein added imitation training to comprehension training, it not only facilitated comprehension learning but also helped the two students transfer the new constructions to expressive language.

Awareness of the most prevalent early semantic relations expected in normal development is helpful when selecting two-word combination targets. A fairly small set of rules has been observed consistently from culture to culture. L. Bloom's (1970) observations of semantic relations observed among the productions of three American children were similar to those that R. A. Brown (1973) reported among children learning Finnish, Swedish, Samoan, French, Russian, Korean, Japanese, and Hebrew. Stockman and Vaughn-Cooke (1986) also described similar semantic category acquisitions for African-American children in working-class families.

R. A. Brown (1973) suggested that this commonality in early semantic rules appears among toddlers worldwide because all toddlers appear to be preoccupied with objects, people, and actions at about the time they begin to combine words. Brown noted that these are the concepts that children have been developing during the immediately preceding Piagetian stages of sensorimotor development. When children talk about objects, they point out things (demonstrative) and name them (nominative), talk about where objects are (location), where they are not (nonexistence), what they are like (attributive), that they have disappeared (disappearance), who owns them (possession), who is acting on them (agent–object), and having more of them (recurrence). In talking about actions, children comment on the actions that people perform (agent–action), actions performed on objects (action–object), and actions oriented toward certain locations (action–location). Table 7.9 includes listings of the two-word semantic rules identified by R. A. Brown (1973) and L. Bloom (1970, 1973) as most common.

Noting the speculative nature of prior efforts by R. A. Brown (1973) and Edwards (1974) to connect Piagetian conceptual developments with semantic category acquisitions, Olswang and Carpenter (1982a, 1982b) designed research to look more deliberately at the process by which young children acquire the concept of a particular semantic category, the *concept of agent*. Based on observations of three children in their homes once per month from the time they were 11 months old until they were 22 months old, Olswang and Carpenter (1982a) described a five-level developmental sequence in acquiring the cognitive notion of agent. They characterized the first three levels as antecedents of the mature cognitive notion of agent: (1) in single-recipient acts, children might act

on an object *or* a person (e.g., when a wind-up toy runs down) but will not directly signal the adult to help with object; (2) in nondirective multiple-recipient acts, children might act on both objects and people in turn but do not direct the adult's attention to the need to fix the toy; (3) in directive multiple-recipient acts, children begin to direct the adult's attention to the toy but do not yet use the adult in unique ways, only in familiar helping roles. Olswang and Carpenter describe the last two levels as representing a mature cognitive notion of agent; (4) in new adult recipient acts, children request help efficiently and effectively from adults for roles that they have not previously seen the adults perform; and (5) in unobserved-adult recipient acts, they seem to realize that an adult agent must have been needed to activate a new toy that runs down even if the adult was not there when the original activation occurred.

In further analysis of the data gathered from the three children, Olswang and Carpenter (1982b) described the development of the corresponding linguistic expression of the concept of agent. At first, the children's vocalizations did not appear to be paired with any nonverbal indications of the awareness of the notion of agent. When the mature cognitive notion of agent did emerge, the children began to

FIGURE 7.7

An example of stimuli for an agent–action language matrix.

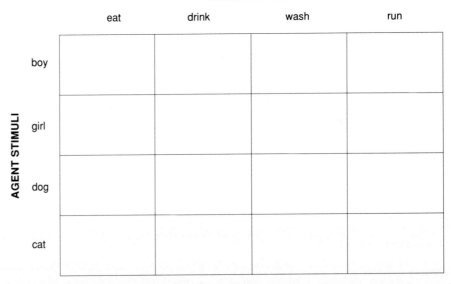

code the agent in agent–action–recipient events using single-word utterances. Eventually (before the age of 22 months), two of the children also began to use two-word utterances to code two of the elements in agent–action–recipient events.

The clinical implications of this research (Olswang & Carpenter, 1982a, 1982b) are that efforts to teach children to encode semantic relationships with one word or more can benefit from embedding the interventions in events designed to teach the concepts along with the words. It also suggests that familiarity may be an important component (in both people and objects used) in earlier sessions, but that variety should be introduced as children begin to demonstrate the targeted skills.

Clinical procedures for teaching two-word semantic relations have been described for working with young children with autism (Scherer & Olswang, 1989), with borderline to moderate retardation (S. F. Warren & Bambara, 1989), and with hearing impairments (Schirmer, 1989). In all three, the scaffolding behaviors of adults, including imitations, acknowledgements, modeling, and expansions, have seemed to play an important role in helping the children move forward in their word-combination production attempts.

In their study of children with autism, Scherer and Olswang (1989) allowed children to select objects for the intervention sessions from several boxes to provide the content for the constructions. The authors credited modeling and expansion procedures as being particularly instrumental, first in increasing spontaneous imitations of two-word utterances and, later, in increasing spontaneous productions of two-term utterances (with corresponding decreases in imitations).

S. F. Warren and Bambara (1989) embedded their training sessions with mentally retarded children in a *milieu approach*. They selected toys for each session according to a central play theme, and used teaching techniques combined from the mand-model and incidental teaching procedures (described previously in this chapter). Warren and Bambara also noted differences in the relative skills with which the different teachers of their three subjects engaged the children in conversations with opportunities to learn the new structures. One teacher (whose student showed the greatest improvement and generalization, even though she was the most developmentally delayed and had the fewest sessions) was particularly good at using scaffolding utterances to assist children to climb to the next step. She presented models for the child to imitate but within a natural turn-taking exchange. The teacher might say, "I'm pushing the car," and push the car toward the girl, who would then push the car back and say "push car" with appropriate intonation and apparent pragmatic intent (see Table 7.10 for other examples).

Schirmer (1989) also emphasized the importance of adult communicative partners who could provide appropriate interaction strategies and support with young hearing impaired children. She noted that "Hearing impaired children need the opportunity to interact linguistically in an environment structured to

TABLE 7.9

Commonly observed early two-word semantic–grammatic rules with examples

R. A. Brown (1973)	L. Bloom (1970, 1973)	Examples
Agent + action	Agent + action	Mommy come; Doggy sit
Action + object	Action + object	Drive car; Eat cereal
Agent + object	Agent + object	Daddy sock; Baby book
Entity + attribute	Attributive	Crayon dirty; Big doggy
Possessor + possession	Genitive	My bed; Mommy dress
Recurrence	Recurrence	More cookie
Nonexistence	Nonexistence	Allgone milk
Disappearance	Disappearance	Bye-bye car
	Rejection (of proposal)	No eat
	Denial (of statement)	No wet
Demonstrative + entity	Demonstrative + predicate nominative	There potty
Entity + locative	Noun + locative	Mommy stair
Action + locative	Verb + locative	Go pool; Sit chair
	Noticing + locative	Me here

TABLE 7.10

Examples of milieu prompting episodes using the mand-model and incidental teaching procedures

Mand-Model

Example 1

Context: Child is scooping beans with a ladle and pouring them into a pot.
  Trainer: "What are you doing?" (target probe question)
  Child: No response
  Trainer: "Tell me." (mand)
  Child: "Beans"
  Trainer: "Say, pour beans." (model)
  Child: "Pour beans."
  Trainer: "That's right, you're pouring beans into the pot." (verbal acknowledgment + expansion)

Example 2

Context: Trainer gives each child a turn to blow bubbles.
  Trainer: (holds the wand up to the child's mouth) "What do you want to do?" (target probe question)
  Child: "Bubbles"
  Trainer: "*Blow* bubbles" (model)
  Child: "Blow bubbles"
  Trainer: "OK, you want to blow bubbles. Here you go." (verbal acknowledgment + expansion + activity participation)

Incidental Teaching

Example 1

Context: Making pudding activity. Trainer gives peer a turn at stirring the pudding as the subject looks on.
  Child: "Me!" (Child initiates) and reaches for ladle.
  Trainer: "Stir pudding" (model)
  Child: "Stir pudding"
  Trainer: "Alright. You stir the pudding, too." (verbal acknowledgment + expansion + activity participation)

Example 2

Context: Trainer and subject are washing dishes together in a parallel fashion.
  Child: "Wash" (Child initiates with an action-verb, partial target response)
  Trainer: "Wash what?" (elaborative question)
  Child: "Wash" (incorrect response)
  Trainer: "Wash *what?*" (elaborative question)
  Child: "Wash cups"
  Trainer: "That's right. We're washing cups." (verbal acknowledgment + expansion)

Note. From "An Experimental Analysis of Milieu Language Intervention. Teaching the Action–Object Form" by S. Warren and L. Bambara, 1989, *Journal of Speech and Hearing Disorders*, 54, p. 461. Copyright 1989 by American Speech-Language-Hearing Association. Reprinted by permission.

maximize appropriate-level language input and the freedom to take risks in experimenting with new language meanings, forms, and uses" (p. 87). Schirmer's recommendations extended across R. A. Brown's (1973) five linguistic stages and did not relate only to the period of two-word utterances. In assisting children to move from one level to the next, she noted the importance of matching children's current linguistic levels and stretching them slightly through modeling and expansion.

PARENTAL ROLES IN HELPING CHILDREN GO BEYOND THE HERE-AND-NOW

At around 20 to 24 months of age, normally developing children begin to talk about objects and events from the past or in the future (Lucariello, 1990). This freeing of talk from the here-and-now is called *tempo-rally displaced* talk. Its appearance is associated with the development of increasingly mature event knowledge, but its emergence is facilitated through scaffolding by parents.

Event knowledge (as discussed earlier in this chapter) includes concepts about frequently experienced sequences of actions, goals organizing the actions, and the actors, roles, and props associated with them. When Lucariello (1990) observed children aged 2:0 to 2:5 in varied contexts with their mothers, temporally displaced talk occurred far more frequently in highly scripted contexts about aspects of the child's routines than in nonscripted contexts. Scripted contexts included routines for getting dressed in the morning, having lunch, and bathing and getting ready for bed. Nonscripted contexts included free play and interactions with novel toys.

The second key to children's transitions from talk only about the here-and-now to talk about there-and-then is the scaffolding that parents provide to make temporally remote (but familiar) topics accessible to their children (Lucariello, 1990). One kind of scaffolding is illustrated in the following exchange:

M: You did get a boo-boo.
Look at that foot.
How'd you do that?
C: Door.
M: On the door?
C: Yeah. (Lucariello, 1990, p. 20)

It is important to note that most parental scaffolding attempts in normal development aim to help children make sense using language (either receptively or expressively) not to elicit or teach particular vocabulary items or grammatical structures. Although many middle-class parents conduct fairly direct vocabulary teaching toward the end of their child's 2nd year, those efforts tend to be concentrated into a fairly short period of helping children learn the principle that everything has a name (Wells, 1986). As Gordon Wells noted, "Thereafter, only a minority of parents continue to teach vocabulary, and even then, this tends to be limited to common nouns and adjectives; verbs, adverbs, and other parts of speech are hardly ever explicitly taught at all" (p. 41). Furthermore, little evidence indicates that any parents engage directly in instruction of grammar. Yet children with normal developmental abilities continue to learn. Apparently, shared experiences, parental ability to mediate more difficult meanings, and positive social interaction elements all work together with increases in event knowledge to enable the cognitive and linguistic shift beyond the here-and-now.

For toddler-age children with disabilities, an important target of the intervention process may be assessment and enhancement of the facilitative characteristics of parental communicative interactions in naturally occurring contexts. Such efforts may need to occur in concert with efforts to change any maladaptive patterns that might have developed and to prevent development of any new maladaptive patterns. The evidence is not altogether clear in this area because it may not be possible to identify who is affecting whom.

Cross (1984) reviewed the literature on parent–child interaction in which interaction patterns of parents and their children with language impairments were compared with those of parents and their normally developing children. She noted many methodological problems with the studies but also summarized results that were fairly consistent across the studies in several areas. In the area of discourse contingencies, parents of children with language impairments (1) are less likely to use semantically or referentially contingent utterances; (2) are less likely to provide positive, accepting acknowledgments of their children's utterances; and (3) are more likely to produce exact repetitions of their own utterances. In the area of sentence types and associated functions, parents of children with language impairments (1) are more likely to use imperatives to control their children's verbal and nonverbal behaviors (a finding that correlates negatively with children's gains in syntactic development); (2) are more likely to use *wh-* questions, but less likely to use *yes–no* questions (parental recasts of children's utterances into *yes–no* questions have a high positive correlation with children's elaboration of the auxiliary verb system in normal development); and (3) are less likely to use declarative syntactic forms for the functions of commenting and stating. In the area of input parameters, parents of children with language impairments (1) are possibly less verbally assertive and/or responsive with their children (although results in this area are mixed); (2) are more likely to use less complex speech (perhaps the reduction in complexity acts as an appropriate adjustment to children's communicative problems, but parents may need assistance to keep their input complexity low enough to facilitate their children's comprehension while high enough to encourage new language learning); (3) possibly are more likely to speak rapidly to their children (although less evidence is available in this area, it may be appropriate to encourage parents to slow down); and (4) are more likely to be disfluent and unintelligible.

The irony of helping parents to appreciate the importance of their roles as primary language intervention agents with their young children at risk is that it may be counterproductive for them to feel this responsibility too keenly, because it may lead them to become tense and anxious about their language-teaching roles and to convey that anxiety to their children. This was one of the concerns expressed by S. J. White and White (1984) about interaction patterns of parents of children with hearing impairments. They cautioned that intervention efforts should aim not so much to encourage parents to bombard their children with talk, as to *interact with their children* in language.

Currently, more evidence describes what is typically observed than the efficacy of efforts to modify contextual variables in the form of parental interaction patterns in early development. Therefore, determining which parental interaction patterns aid children's language development is difficult. Based on her review, Cross (1984) recommended that practitioners employ procedures to

> (a) enhance the semantic contingency of parents' language on child's language; (b) reduce parents' directiveness; (c) increase their fluency, intelligibility, and tendency to question; and (d) generally encourage the parents of children with language impairments to talk with them more frequently than they do. (p. 12)

One intervention study (Tiegerman & Siperstein, 1984) aimed to modify parental styles of interaction by four mothers with their language-impaired children. The children ranged in age from 3 to 5 years, and had MLUs ranging from 1.0 to 2.0. None of the children had concomitant hearing, visual, or neurological problems. The procedure consisted of a series of pretraining videotapes, and 6 weeks of group and individualized weekly training sessions, in which parents were taught to become more child centered in their interactions and to focus on different aspects of semantic relatedness. They were also given "homework" assignments each week (e.g., transcribe a 5-minute sample of a father–child play session and identify features they had discussed). The results showed an increase in semantically related utterances and an expansion of communicative roles and behaviors used by the mothers, with more opportunities being given to their children to talk and to receive positive acknowledgments for that talk.

Moeller (1989) has also noted the specialized concerns that arise when assisting parents of children with hearing impairments to enhance their simultaneous signed and spoken communication with their children. Hearing parents of young children with profound hearing losses may be attempting to learn a new communication mode while they strive to provide facilitative linguistic input to their children and to deal with all of the other stresses of having a child with a severe disability. Moeller described efforts to determine the efficacy of designing individualized programs to teach hearing parents of children with profound losses the trilogy of signing skills, parenting skills, and language stimulation skills. Preliminary results suggest that parents can acquire the contexts as well as the content to modify their communication with their children in ways that are highly relevant to their everyday parenting needs.

EARLY LEARNING ABOUT LITERACY

Relatively direct but naturalistic teaching continues into the toddler and preschool years in homes where literacy is valued and books are available in the context of joint book reading activities (Heath, 1982; McGee & Richgels, 1990; Ninio, 1983; van Kleeck, 1990). These reading activities are useful not only for teaching new vocabulary but also for providing the context for conveying, either implicitly or explicitly, a variety of special rules for interacting with print.

Snow and Ninio (1986) gathered transcripts of parents interacting with their young children using books. They found evidence that parents use direct and indirect instruction to help children learn that (1) books are for reading, not manipulating; (2) books control the topic in book reading; (3) pictures are not things but represent things; (4) pictures are for naming (especially at the single and two-word utterance stage); (5) pictures can represent events even though they are static; (6) book events occur outside of real time; and (7) books represent an autonomous fictional world.

Early book experiences offer a rich context to assess and intervene in parent–child interactions (even children functioning at the 1- or 2-year-old level). By interviewing parents about this type of activity, professionals also may be able to encourage more of it. Simply suggesting more book reading is not enough, however. Particularly when children have language delays and related disabilities, parents may have become discouraged about their initial attempts to "read" books with their children. Parents may need to be shown techniques to pace the page turning, to establish joint attention and referencing (e.g., pointing and commenting on the pictures), and to take turns in a naming game before asking many questions and before trying to read the words printed on the pages. Remember also, that parents of children with disabilities may lead lives packed full of special meetings and appointments that make it difficult to spend time reading books with their children. Perhaps the best way to ensure that parents do find the time is to collaborate with parents to find literacy activities that will fit in with other activities (e.g., waiting in the physician's office) or as part of daily living (e.g., writing grocery lists, reading signs, taping notes to the refrigerator).

Most of this discussion of parental roles in early language and literacy learning has focused on generalized expectations about middle-class mainstream families (regardless of ethnicity). Not all families, however, are alike, even when they have similar cultural and sociolinguistic histories (Lieven, 1984). When families come from diverse cultural backgrounds, the culturally based differences in both beliefs about and expectations of children in the areas of preliteracy and other communicative interactions may be large (Heath, 1983; Snow, 1977b).

Focus on book reading may be primarily a middle- and upper-class phenomenon, but books are not the only way that children are introduced to print early in life (McGee & Richgels, 1990; D. Taylor, 1983; D. Taylor & Dorsey-Gaines, 1987). Van Kleeck (1990) reviewed many ethnographic studies with families in diverse geographic, cultural, ethnic, and socioeconomic situations. These studies "have found literacy artifacts and print-related events to be pervasive in all kinds of homes in literate societies" (p. 27). However, most print-related events in low-income families occur through activities of daily living, and not through books (D. Taylor & Dorsey-Gaines, 1987). Perhaps, intervention embedded in those naturally occurring practical activities is the best way to encourage early print experiences for young children with special needs in these homes.

When professional intervention teams work with families from cultures different from their own, the need for ethnographic sensitivity to different interaction styles and values also must be a part of the system. Prescriptive approaches that emphasize the "right" way to do things, only from the perspective of the professional, are doomed to failure. If parents and professionals work together to establish mutual goals and to develop interaction patterns that facilitate the child's development and are consistent with the family system, children may be able to consolidate gains in language and literacy and to continue to make new ones. Parents may also find that they like to learn new ways of interacting with their children if they can do so in a supportive and nonjudgmental context.

BUILDING MORE COMPLEX IDEAS THROUGH PLAY

Parental input and parent–child interactions contribute to the quality of children's early language and learning experiences, but they are not the only factors. The children themselves supply other factors. These relate to children's abilities to use their own current cognitive and linguistic abilities to help pull themselves up to the next step in the developmental process. (Linguist Steven Pinker, 1984, in arguing for the linguistic theory of language acquisition, called this process "bootstrapping." See Chapter 2 for a discussion of the linguistic theory.) Continued advances in children's abilities to represent events and meanings symbolically are demonstrated particularly in their increasingly sophisticated abilities to play. Current understanding of the relationships of language and play do not permit a strong conclusion that play is a prerequisite of language (or vice versa), but the two abilities do seem to develop hand in hand.

Several theoretical explanations have been offered for possible relationships between language and play. Both Piaget (1962) and Vygotsky (1967) linked the emergence of symbolic play to the development of representational skills, and the ability to represent one thing with another (e.g., pretending that beads are food) provides evidence that a child can function symbolically. Bates, Benigni, Bretherton, Camaioni, and Volterra (1979) found a correlation among symbolic play, vocal imitation, and language production in normally developing children. Casby and Ruder (1983) found that symbolic play also is a strong correlate of early language development in children with mental retardation. McCune-Nicholich (1981) found preliminary support for hypothesized correspondence between language and play in four areas: "(1) presymbolic behaviors in both domains [language and play], (2) initial pretending and first referential words, (3) the emergence of combinatorial behaviors in both domains, and (4) hierarchically organized language and symbolic play" (p. 795).

Kelly and Dale (1989) also found play skills to vary significantly among normally developing 1- and 2-year-old children, depending on whether their language was at the level of no words, single words, nonproductive syntax (defined as gestalt two-word phrases produced as formulaic routines or stereotyped units), or productive syntax (multiword utterances produced with evidence of rule-based creativity). In addition, however, they found evidence that the attainment of particular skills might be relatively more advanced or delayed either in language or in play.

Play-based assessments can be used to obtain information about children's internalized scripts and event knowledge. They also offer a context for naturalistic intervention (Norris & Hoffman, 1990b). In an ecological perspective, children's play may be viewed as an external context that the child creates, by bringing together certain objects and roles, thus making play an outward expression of the way that the child perceives the world (Bronfenbrenner, 1979), which can be quite useful in intervention.

Developments in Decentering, Object Symbolism, and Social Relations in Play

Developmentally, pretend play may appear in primitive form as early as 18 months and possibly earlier. It is found in most normally developing children by the age of 3 years, and it increases steadily into middle childhood before pretending begins to disappear (Chance, 1979).

During early-stage language development, assessment of and intervention in play might focus on three concerns (N. W. Nelson, 1988b). The first is the degree to which children can engage in pretend actions that are increasingly decentered from sensorimotor schemes (McCune-Nicholich, 1981). This includes evolution of play ability from a level of (1) presymbolic schemes (children can demonstrate function of real objects in real situations) through a level of (2) autosymbolic schemes (children can pretend by using objects in a nonliteral way but only for highly familiar schemes relating to the child's own body (e.g., "drinking" from a cup-like object), before reaching a level of (3) decentered symbolic games, marked by children's abilities to distance pretend actions from their own sensorimotor actions (e.g., using dolls for pretend).

A second assessment and intervention issue concerns the degree of similarity of pretend objects to the real objects they are supposed to represent. This focus is based on the work of Elder and Pederson (1978), who observed a developmental hierarchy in the following order: (1) similar substitute objects (e.g., a bristle block for a hairbrush), (2) dissimilar substitute objects (e.g., a plastic apple for a hammer), and (3) no object present. Elder and Pederson found that children under the age of 3 years were most dependent on the presence of similar substitute objects, but by the age of 3½, children could pretend equally well under all three conditions.

A third area of concern is the interaction of the development of social routines with the ability to pretend. Howes's (1985) research focused on this area and suggested that social play should be separated from social pretend play, which is more likely to appear after the child is around 23 months old. Howes suggested that substages for the development of social play might include (1) noninteractive parallel play, (2) simple social play with a turn-taking structure of at least three turns, and (3) complementary–reciprocal social play with reversal of play actions with another. Howes described three advancing types of social pretend play: (1) solitary pretend play, with a pretend action in the context of a social situation but not responded to by the partner; (2) simple social pretend play, in which both partners perform pretend actions that may be related temporally or using the same objects but not engaging in complementary roles; and (3) cooperative social pretend play, in which both partners engage in ongoing play with complementary pretend roles (e.g., mother and baby; daddy and mommy).

Targeting Play Skills in Intervention

Many relatively formal assessment instruments, scales, and strategies have been constructed to take advantage of play as an indicator of early development in a variety of areas, including language (e.g. McConkey, 1984; McCune-Nicholich & Fenson, 1984; Norris & Hoffman, 1990b; Westby, 1980, 1988). One, TPBA (Linder, 1990) was reviewed earlier in this chapter.

Using these tools and informal techniques the specialist can assess play skills to demonstrate varying patterns of sensorimotor, cognitive, linguistic, and social development among children with different disabilities. These patterns may suggest specific intervention target areas (Linder, 1990). Particularly young children with specific language delays may demonstrate play skills slightly below age level but relatively less impaired than their language skills (B. Y. Terrell, Schwartz, Prelock, & Messick, 1984). This finding suggests that play contexts might be used in intervention to target "verbal expressions of the meanings and relations already evidenced in play" (B. Y. Terrell et al., 1984, p. 428). When children make doll figures, cook food, or drive a tractor, they demonstrate knowledge of the coordination of the concepts of agent, action, and object. The next step might be to help them to encode those relationships linguistically. Westby (1980, 1988), in her Symbolic Play Scale, showed how cognitive and linguistic elements may correspond in the context of play. The first five stages in her scale are represented as Table 7.11. A set of expectations for kinds of play and strategies for engaging others in play that are appropriate at the toddler level appear in Box 7.10.

TABLE 7.11
Symbolic Play Scale—the first five stages (pp. 319–320).

DECONTEXTUALIZATION: What Props Are Used in Pretend Play?	THEMATIC CONTENT: What Schemas/Scripts Does the Child Represent?	ORGANIZATION: How Coherent and Logical Are the Child's Schemas/Scripts?	SELF/OTHER RELATIONS: What Roles Does Child Take and Give to Toys and Other People?	LANGUAGE: Function	LANGUAGE: Forms and Meaning
0–Stage 1: 17 to 19 months					
Tool-use (uses stick to reach toy) Finds toy invisibly hidden (when placed in box and box emptied under scarf) Uses common objects and toys appropriately in real and pretend activities; requires life-like props to pretend	Familiar, everyday activities (eating, sleeping) in which child has been active participant	Short, isolated schemas (single pretend action)	Self as agent (autosymbolic or self-representational play, i.e., child pretends to go to sleep, to eat from spoon, or to drink from cup)	Directing Requesting Commanding Interactional Self-maintaining Protesting Protecting self and self-interests Commenting Labeling (object or activity) Indicating personal feeling	Beginning of true verbal communication. Words have following functional and semantic relations: Recurrence Existence Nonexistence Rejection Denial Agent Object Action or state Location Object or person associated with object or person
Stage II: 19 to 22 months					
		Short, isolated schema combinations (child combines two actions or toys in pretend, e.g., rocking doll and putting it to bed, pouring from pitcher into cup, or feeding doll from plate with spoon)	Child acts on doll (doll is passive recipient of action): brushes doll's hair, feeds doll, covers doll with blanket Child performs pretend actions on more than one object or person, e.g., feeds self, a doll, mother, and another child	Refers to objects and persons not present	Beginning of word combinations with following semantic relations: Agent–action Action–object Agent–object Attributive Dative Action–locative Object–locative Possessive
Stage III: 2 years					
		Elaborated single schemas (represents daily experiences with details, e.g., puts lid on pan, puts pan on stove, turns on stove; or collects items associated with cooking/eating such as dishes, pans, silverware, glasses, highchair)			Uses phrases and short sentences Appearance of morphological markers Present progressive (ing) on verbs Plurals Possessives

TABLE 7.11
continued

DECONTEXTUALIZATION	THEMATIC CONTENT	ORGANIZATION	SELF/OTHER RELATIONS	LANGUAGE	
What Props Are Used in Pretend Play?	What Schemas/Scripts Does the Child Represent?	How Coherent and Logical Are the Child's Schemas/Scripts?	What Roles Does Child Take and Give to Toys and Other People?	Function	Forms and Meaning
Stage IV 2 ½ years					
	Less frequently personally experienced events, particularly those that are memorable because they are pleasurable or traumatic Store shopping Doctor-nurse-sick child				Responds appropriately to the following WH questions in context: What Whose Where What . . . . do Asks WH questions (generally puts WH at beginning of sentence) Responses to why questions inappropriate except for well-known routines
					Asks why, but often inappropriate except for well-known routines Asks why, but often inappropriate and does not attend to answer
Stage V: 3 years					
	Re-enactment of experienced events, but modifies original outcome	Evolving schema sequences, e.g., child mixes cake, bakes it, serves it, washes dishes; or doctor checks patient, calls ambulance, takes patient to hospital (sequence is not planned)		Reporting Predicting Narrating or story-telling	Uses past tense, such as, "I ate the cake," "I walked" Uses future aspects (particularly "gonna") forms, such as, "I'm gonna wash dishes."

Note. From Westby, C., Children's Play: Reflections of Social Competence, in *Seminars in Speech and Language*, Volume 9, Number 1, New York, 1988, Thieme Medical Publishers, Inc. Reprinted by permission.

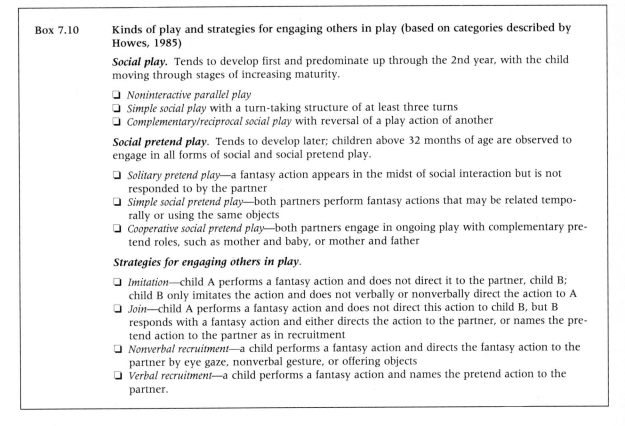

Box 7.10   **Kinds of play and strategies for engaging others in play (based on categories described by Howes, 1985)**

Social play. Tends to develop first and predominate up through the 2nd year, with the child moving through stages of increasing maturity.

❑ *Noninteractive parallel play*
❑ *Simple social play* with a turn-taking structure of at least three turns
❑ *Complementary/reciprocal social play* with reversal of a play action of another

Social pretend play. Tends to develop later; children above 32 months of age are observed to engage in all forms of social and social pretend play.

❑ *Solitary pretend play*—a fantasy action appears in the midst of social interaction but is not responded to by the partner
❑ *Simple social pretend play*—both partners perform fantasy actions that may be related temporally or using the same objects
❑ *Cooperative social pretend play*—both partners engage in ongoing play with complementary pretend roles, such as mother and baby, or mother and father

Strategies for engaging others in play.

❑ *Imitation*—child A performs a fantasy action and does not direct it to the partner, child B; child B only imitates the action and does not verbally or nonverbally direct the action to A
❑ *Join*—child A performs a fantasy action and does not direct this action to child B, but B responds with a fantasy action and either directs the action to the partner, or names the pretend action to the partner as in recruitment
❑ *Nonverbal recruitment*—a child performs a fantasy action and directs the fantasy action to the partner by eye gaze, nonverbal gesture, or offering objects
❑ *Verbal recruitment*—a child performs a fantasy action and names the pretend action to the partner.

When older children stay at early stages or have severe physical disabilities, how might play be used in intervention? Success may depend on staying within the limits of individuals' cognitive and physical abilities while not violating their needs for age-appropriate materials and experiences. Carlson (1982) provided a resource book for adapting toys for children with motoric handicaps and Musselwhite (1986) discussed broader aspects of encouraging these children to play.

One approach that I found helpful for a group of nonspeaking teenage boys with limited expressive language and cognitive abilities, along with profound motor impairments, was to collude with them in playing practical jokes on each other and the staff members in their school. For example, eye pointing and joint referencing were never so motivated as when these adolescents did things such as directing the teacher to put a plastic spider in her hair (or on the shirt of one of the boys) until other unsuspecting staff members arrived on the scene and were directed to

notice it. Their eyes danced (and their minds were active) at those times.

When play is used to encourage language and cognitive development, it is essential to remember that *play is supposed to be fun.* Play is "what children do when they are *not* involved in activities that meet biological needs or that are required by adults" (Singer, quoted by Chance, 1979, p. 1). Therefore, to make play into a work session would be counterproductive. When adults do take part in play with children, it is important that they engage as "partners" (MacDonald, 1989), not just talk about playing (Chance, 1979). Although some evidence suggests that modeling of pretend play by adults may be an effective intervention strategy (S. Singer & Singer, 1977), it is probably most effective for adults to respond to children-initiated actions so as not to dominate the play with adults' ideas (this is the scaffolding strategy discussed previously). For children whose symbolic representational skills are just emerging, it may also be helpful to use real objects to set a meaningful context in which substitute objects can then be introduced for pretending (G. Fein, 1975). The most important thing is to keep play fun.

MAKING SPEECH MORE CLEAR

Children will not benefit much from having more ideas to communicate, or attempting to engage their peers in social pretend play, if they lack the means to articulate messages clearly enough to be understood by unfamiliar listeners. Stoel-Gammon (1987) pointed out that the normative information available for making judgments of children's phonological development at 2 years of age typically is based on extremely limited samples. For example, only about half of 21 subjects at this age studied by Prather, Hedrick, and Kern (1975) could respond to direct metalinguistic prompts, such as "Say *fish*," used to gather normative data in that study. It also may be more useful to analyze children's speech patterns independently from adult models rather than to focus on "mastery" of adult speech pronunciation patterns, as done traditionally.

To add prior information and to correct earlier methodological problems, Stoel-Gammon (1987) conducted an analysis of the word and syllable shapes in conversational speech samples produced by 33 two-year-olds. She also inventoried the initial and final consonantal phones produced and the percentage of consonants correct in those samples. The results of these analyses are summarized in Box 7.11. Essentially, they show that normally developing 2-year-olds can produce a range of sounds and structures and show evidence of synchrony in the developing sound system; children with larger initial inventories in earlier samples also tended to have larger inventories in later samples. Stoel-Gammon also found synchrony (in the form of a positive correlation) between the

total inventory size for individual children and the percentage of consonants correct and interpreted this as evidence "that phonetic abilities (as measured by the number of different consonants produced) and phonological abilities (as measured by appropriate use of consonantal phones in matching the segments of the adult model) go hand in hand" (p. 326). The profile represented in Box 7.11 is also consistent with earlier research that has shown a preponderance of stops, nasals, and glides in early meaningful speech, as well as simple monosyllabic and disyllabic words, such as CV, CVC, and CVCV shapes, before 2 years of age.

These findings have implications for the kinds of words selected for early productive lexicon training with children who have severe phonological production deficits. The first priority in lexical selection for these children should be selecting words to map onto concepts that are already relevant and important. The child may also benefit if words are selected to approximate the phonological patterns prevalent in early normal development and/or in the children's existing phonetic repertoires (Koegel & Traphagen, 1982).

Some attempts have been made to tie early phonological ability to imitation skill and other cognitive developments. R. Schwartz and Leonard (1982) studied the imitations of 12 normally developing children who were single-word users. They found that the children were better able to imitate words with characteristics already evident in their spontaneous phonological production systems than words with characteristics outside of those systems. The majority of this group had also not yet attained the means–end skills of Piaget's (1962) sensorimotor stage VI. This was in contrast to vocal imitation results obtained by Leonard, Schwartz, Folger, and Wilcox (1978) for slightly older children, all of whom had at least a 50-

---

Box 7.11	Phonological abilities demonstrated by the "typical" child by age 2-years (based on Stoel-Gammon, 1987)

  ❏ Produces words of the form CV, CVC, CVCV and CVCVC.
  ❏ Produces a few consonant clusters in initial position and maybe one or two in final position.
  ❏ Produces 9 to 10 different consonantal phones in initial position, including exemplars from the classes of stops (b/t/d/k/g), nasals (m/n), fricatives (f/s), and glides (w/h).
  ❏ Produces 5 to 6 different consonantal phones in the final position, mostly stops, but also a representative from the nasal, fricative, and liquid sound classes.
  ❏ Matches the consonant phonemes of adult words with at least 70% correctness.

word vocabulary and most of whom had begun using two-word utterances. Most of the children in the older group demonstrated stage VI means–end ability. They also showed a tendency to imitate words whether or not the imitated consonants or syllabic shapes were part of their existing phonological systems.

More research is needed to guide decisions about selecting intervention targets and strategies for children who have specific speech and language impairments. As you may recall from Chapter 4, scatter among cognitive and linguistic indicators often is an identifying factor in diagnosing specific language and learning disabilities. Clearly, however, assessment and intervention of phonological skills should be incorporated into comprehensive programming for many young children with language and speech delays.

SUMMARY

This chapter considered the expectations of normal development during the first 3 years or so of life. During this time, children and their care givers exploit children's natural desires to communicate and to learn about their world and how it works. In the transactions of early-stage development, the seeds of language begin to grow in contexts that have shape, meaning, and purpose. Although the discussion did not dwell on the differences associated with various causative conditions, the chapter stressed that not all children learn in exactly the same ways (even in normal development) and that the same children may need different approaches at different stages of development. In particular, when older children have early-stage language abilities, they are still older children, and their needs differ from those of infants and toddlers.

Normally developing children smoothly and rapidly accomplish the transitions from the earliest stages of almost complete dependence on their care givers' understanding, through emerging stages of expressing their own intentions, to using language symbols to create and communicate their own unique messages. However, it is easy to lose sight of how complex the navigation is until a child has difficulties. When children and their care givers need assistance to move through the tiny steps and major stages of language acquisition, the process is no less marvelous if they pass the landmarks at slower rates. Accountability practices do more than prove to agencies who provide funds for services that their money is well spent. They also provide occasions to survey a child's progress and to appreciate the value of the journey.

8

Middle Stages

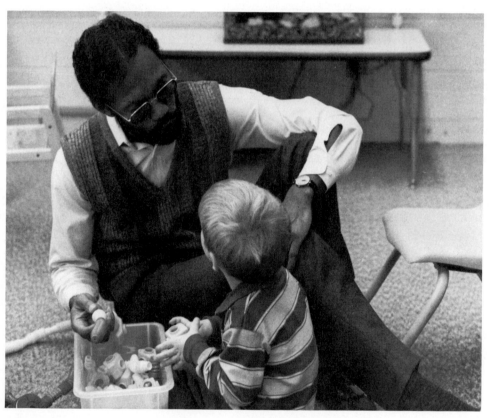

Children Needing
Intervention Aimed at
Middle-Stage
Developments

Measurement of
Middle-Stage
Abilities, Needs, and
Accomplishments

Methods and Targets
of Middle-Stage
Intervention

❏ Who may need treatment for middle-stage problems?
❏ What tools can be used for measuring middle-stage needs and abilities?
❏ What kinds of intervention targets and methods are appropriate?

The middle stage of language acquisition occurs quite early in normal development. It starts during the transition from toddlerhood to preschool age (at approximately 3 years of age)—when children begin to increase the number of multiple-word utterances in their expressive language—and it extends through ages 7 or 8 years (with no clear dividing line) into the threshold of preadolescence. Looking at the developmental process in this way, when children are in the middle stages, one observes that the primary feat is the acquisition of the grammatical code. Although, as considered in Chapter 9, much more recognition is now given to the developmental enrichments of the later stages of language development (those that normally occur during preadolescence and adolescence), the preschool and early elementary years still take the prize for dramatic language acquisition accomplishments, particularly in the area of grammatical development (language *form*) but also in expansion of concepts that children can talk about (language *content*) and in their resources for modifying their communications to be appropriate in particular contexts (language *use*).

The purpose of this chapter is to provide information on developmental expectations and potential intervention targets that can be used with children in the middle stages of language acquisition, whether they are in this age range or are older but still have middle-stage language needs in addition to age-related needs. As in the early stages, the focus for children who can "almost but not quite" (ABNQ) keep up with their same-age peers with language learning and use is more likely to remain on *prevention* and on *intervention* than on *remediation*. For these children, intervention involves an intensified, deliberate process, primarily of fostering normal development. When children are markedly behind their same-age peers in language acquisition, the focus may include efforts aimed toward *remediation and compensation* for communicative needs that are clearly out of the ordinary (e.g. by providing augmentative communication devices and techniques, encouraging compensatory learning strategies, and modifying information to be received in different modalities).

In practice, intervention and remediation processes are not necessarily distinguished. In many discussions, the terms are treated as synonymous, although *intervention* is used by some as a broader, more all-encompassing term, and *remediation* is reserved for the provision of specific assistance to children with identified delays or disabilities to bring them closer to their age-level peers (Sameroff & Fiese, 1990). *Remediation* implies "fixing," whereas *intervention* may apply to any type of deliberate attempt to influence a system (including both child and contextual factors) to make it work better. *Intervention* does not necessarily imply a particular approach, or one focused exclusively on the child with the problem, but this term is used more frequently by professionals who adopt a sociolinguistic view of language acquisition in which children are seen as active participants in their own development and the context is viewed as an integral component of the developmental (and intervention) process.

Two of the early-stage intervention approaches discussed in Chapter 7, redefinition and reeducation (Sameroff & Fiese, 1990), are still appropriate in the middle stages of language acquisition. The target audience for redefinition and reeducation, however, may expand at this level to include teachers in addition to parents. Both care givers and teachers may need assistance to redefine their perceptions of children's abilities by receiving help in reevaluating those children's strengths and weaknesses. Both may also need reeducation regarding better ways to communicate with and to teach children who have difficulty learning language and using language to learn. The language specialist may wish to use collaborative techniques, which generally work better than directive ones to encourage change among colleagues.

All children have individualized needs. Nevertheless, as a general rule, when children exhibit relatively severe disabilities, focusing on their abilities is particularly important. Conversely, when children exhibit more specific and apparently "mild" disabilities, it may be more efficient and effective for some intervention activities to focus directly on those disabilities, not forgetting the need to use the children's greater areas of strength to build success and confi-

Personal Reflection 8.1   "I am told that some remarkably high percentage of a child's learning — in language and other things — happens before the age of five. (I never can remember the percentage here, only that it is big). I have never understood how one could possibly give particular weights to particular learnings. How does one weigh the child's early acquisition of "shoe," "hat," "key," and "mommy" against the child's later development of complex relational notions and the forms that express them: "if–then," "although," "because," "unless"? How does one weigh the child's earlier interaction through talk, with her later development of ways of interacting through writing? How does one weigh the earlier simple, direct requests ("want juice") with her later development of more subtle and various ways of requesting — ways that take different partners and situations into account ("I just love orange juice" or "I'll trade you my juice for your crackers")? I just don't know how anyone decides what each chunk of learning is worth I (or even what a chunk is), and without knowing this, how does one total up the chunks and decide what proportion happened before age five and what proportion happened after that age? For me, this way of thinking about children's development doesn't make sense."

From Judith Wells Lindfors, *Children's Language and Learning,* Second Edition (p. 217). Copyright © 1987. Reprinted with permission of Allyn and Bacon.

dence in language-related activities (and almost all activities are language-related).

As an example of a child with severe disabilities, consider the needs of an 8-year-old nonspeaking girl with cerebral palsy and moderate mental retardation. This girl uses a communication board to produce simple sentences and loves to hear books read aloud as a way to vicariously experience broader aspects of the world. Testing has revealed that she has a specific disability in perceiving and naming shapes and quantities which exceeds her other areas of difficulty. However, rather than hours of weekly drill of those items, a more productive intervention approach might be to focus on this child's interest and ability in learning about people's motivations and interactions and about how the world works. Conversational skill and problem solving may evolve best for her when the vocabulary added to her communication board is the vocabulary she needs to discuss the problems and possibilities facing the characters in the stories she hears (perhaps the same stories as those being studied by grade-level classmates). This may enhance her emerging abilities for analyzing social interactions, may foster her linguistic development for combining basic sentence constituents, and she will be less likely to develop a self-image as a person who has difficulty learning.

As an example of a child with mild disabilities, consider the needs of a first-grade girl with a specific language-learning disability whose vocabulary is strong and whose social skills are among the best in the class, but who exhibits a specific disability in analyzing sound–symbol relationships and detecting the sound sequences within words and sometimes transposes words in sentences. This student is at high risk for reading disability. She needs an intensive program aimed directly at the area of disability, not ignoring her strengths in understanding linguistic and text-level meaning, but focusing on teaching her to recognize sound–symbol and syllable–morpheme associations. This child might benefit from an approach that would help her to analyze associated auditory–print sequences in reading and spelling tasks while using her more intact discourse abilities to assist her to comprehend written language. A direct intervention approach with intensive practice of graphophonemic decoding and encoding during the early grades may enable this child to spend much less time out of class in later grades learning skills that the other children in the class have acquired with little direct instruction. She will also be more likely to practice communicating through reading and writing. Such a program may also prevent years of failure and "faking it" later on. Those are the kinds of mistakes that this chapter is designed to help you avoid.

CHILDREN NEEDING INTERVENTION AIMED AT MIDDLE-STAGE DEVELOPMENTS

This chapter focuses primarily on children with language disorders functioning at the middle stage of development but with the caveat that, although developmental level may provide the best blueprint for selecting an intervention procedure, chronological age cannot be ignored. Children who are ABNQ on a level with their same-age peers are most likely to be found participating in the same activities with those peers. Children who have more severe impairments associated with any of the conditions discussed in Chapter 4 are more likely to be school-age but functioning at a preschool level or to qualify for special education classroom services during the middle stages of language acquisition. Some persons with severe disabilities may never leave the middle stages linguistically and may never enter the later stages involving greater abstract language use and reliance on nonliteral meanings. Nevertheless, their communicative needs are likely to change as they grow older. Many of the concerns discussed throughout this book—about communicative opportunity, special education placement, and possibilities for regular education integration with same-age peers—apply to these individuals.

IDENTIFYING LANGUAGE DISORDERS IN THE MIDDLE STAGES

Child-Find Efforts and Preschool Screening

Children who need speech and language intervention services during the preschool years from 3 to 5 may be identified in several ways. The Child-Find efforts discussed in Chapter 7 are pertinent. Medical referral is also common during this period, particularly resulting from well-child clinics and follow-up monitoring of children who have had difficult births. Recently, pediatricians and family practitioners in many communities seem to have become increasingly appreciative of the importance of early communication development and its relationship to later school success and depend on local communication professionals to collaborate with them. As they become better informed, fewer adopt the well-known "Don't worry, she'll outgrow it" posture.

At the same time, more parents are aware of early developmental expectations, and they are not afraid of asserting their own concerns about their children's developmental needs without apologizing for those concerns. Thus, parental referral continues to be a common source of identification of children with speech and language delays throughout the preschool years. Preschool teachers also may refer children during this stage. If children have not been identified by the time they enter school, early elementary school teachers may be more likely to refer them for speech–language evaluation than their parents. In some school districts with highly conservative qualification criteria, however, concerned parents may seek out private speech–language intervention services for their children during the early elementary school years when their children do not qualify for school services. Other public sector programs, such as Head Start, provide intervention.

Regardless of who makes the referral and where services are provided, the national priority of Child Find and PL 94–142 and 99–457 is that any child who needs special services should receive them. Thus, it is important that all potential referral sources be informed about danger signs that may indicate that language and communication development are not proceeding as they should. A listing of some of the danger signs that may signal the need for referral of 3- to 5-year-olds for speech–language evaluation appears in Box 8.1.

Different sets of factors predict a child's later need for special services better than others at certain developmental stages. In the early years from birth to 3, parental traits, such as maternal education levels, are better predictors of disabilities in adolescence than children's own behavior. In the middle stage years, from ages 4 to 7, however, child-centered skills are better predictors of later status than maternal educational attainment (Kochanek, Kabacoff, & Lipsitt, 1990).

This suggests that screening tools that focus on children's developing speech–language, communicative, and cognitive abilities may be used appropriately during the middle-stage years. Many are available; some broad, comprehensive screening tools, and some are aimed more exclusively at speech and language development (N. W. Nelson, 1981b). Many commonly used screening and assessment tools appropriate for this developmental level are listed in Appendix A.

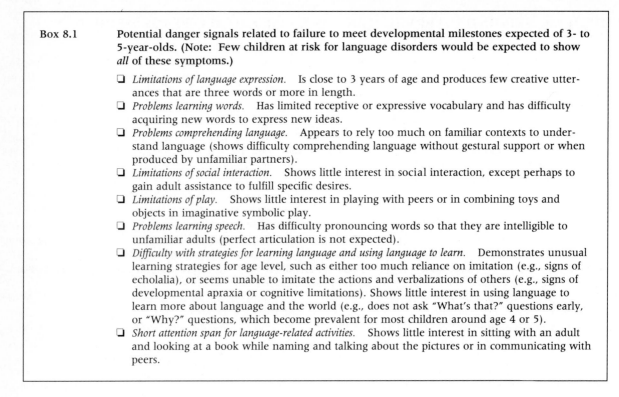

Box 8.1   Potential danger signals related to failure to meet developmental milestones expected of 3- to 5-year-olds. (Note: Few children at risk for language disorders would be expected to show *all* of these symptoms.)

❑ *Limitations of language expression.*   Is close to 3 years of age and produces few creative utterances that are three words or more in length.
❑ *Problems learning words.*   Has limited receptive or expressive vocabulary and has difficulty acquiring new words to express new ideas.
❑ *Problems comprehending language.*   Appears to rely too much on familiar contexts to understand language (shows difficulty comprehending language without gestural support or when produced by unfamiliar partners).
❑ *Limitations of social interaction.*   Shows little interest in social interaction, except perhaps to gain adult assistance to fulfill specific desires.
❑ *Limitations of play.*   Shows little interest in playing with peers or in combining toys and objects in imaginative symbolic play.
❑ *Problems learning speech.*   Has difficulty pronouncing words so that they are intelligible to unfamiliar adults (perfect articulation is not expected).
❑ *Difficulty with strategies for learning language and using language to learn.*   Demonstrates unusual learning strategies for age level, such as either too much reliance on imitation (e.g., signs of echolalia), or seems unable to imitate the actions and verbalizations of others (e.g., signs of developmental apraxia or cognitive limitations). Shows little interest in using language to learn more about language and the world (e.g., does not ask "What's that?" questions early, or "Why?" questions, which become prevalent for most children around age 4 or 5).
❑ *Short attention span for language-related activities.*   Shows little interest in sitting with an adult and looking at a book while naming and talking about the pictures or in communicating with peers.

Professionals are urged to be careful when selecting and interpreting screening and assessment tools. For example, Bailey and Brochin (1989) pointed out that the inclusion of items on a screening measure does not mean that they are necessarily important in a particular context or that they have been encouraged within a particular child's cultural experiences. In addition, different test makers may use different standards for assigning age levels to items. Although a common procedure is to decide where to place assessment items by selecting items passed by 50% of the children at a given age level, not all tests use this criterion. For example, the Battelle Developmental Inventory (Newborg, Stock, Wnek, Guidubaldi, & Svinicki, 1984) used the criterion of the age at which 75% of the normative sample audience passed an item. It is important to be aware of these varying standards when interpreting screening test results and deciding which children should be given more comprehensive assessments.

An even more serious problem is that some instruments allow the generation of developmental age scores even though they were never normed themselves (Bailey & Brochin, 1989). Examples are the Early Learning Accomplishment Profile (Glover, Preminger, & Stanford, 1978; Sanford & Zelman, 1981), the Hawaii Early Learning Profile (Furuno, O'Reilly, Hosaka, Inatsuka, Allman, & Zeisloft, 1979), and the Early Intervention Developmental Profile (Rogers, D'Eugenio, Brown, Dononvan, & Lynch, 1981). These tests assign developmental ages based on reference to such standardized sources as the Bayley Scales of Infant Development (Bayley, 1969), the Denver Developmental Screening Test (Frankenburg, Dodds, & Fandal, 1969–1970), or the Manual of Developmental Diagnosis (i.e., the Gesell Development Schedules; Knobloch, Stevens, & Malone, 1980). The problem with this approach is that the equivalence of measures gathered in different years and on different populations is uncertain, particularly because norms established on more recent populations tend to show developmental milestones being reached at younger ages than those reported on older measures (Bailey & Brochin, 1989).

A third concern is the degree to which a screening test is based on a normative group that can be considered representative of the population as a whole.

Bailey and Brochin (1989) recommended that, "Ideally, the sample should be stratified, with proportionate representation of various racial groups, geographic regions, sex, income levels, and urban/rural distribution" (p. 28). The Developmental Indicators of the Assessment of Learning (DIAL) is an example of a comprehensive screening instrument that was originally standardized only in Illinois on a sample of just 320 children (Mardell & Goldenberg, 1975). However, the restandardization of the DIAL-R involved 2,447 children from geographical proportionate regions of the United States, with approximately equal numbers of boys and girls, and with a minority population of 44.5% of the group (Mardell-Czudnowski & Goldenberg, 1984, 1990). It can be used with children ages 2 to 6 years and provides statistical data based on three norming groups; 1990 census, white, and minority. The DIAL-R provides standardization data for the three screening cutoff points: ±1, ±1.5, ±2 standard deviations. The DIAL has also been shown to correlate highly with the Boehm Test of Basic Concepts (Boehm, 1971) as a quick screening instrument to detect potential difficulties with basic language concepts in a young kindergarten population (Sarachan-Deily, Hopkins, & DeVivo, 1983). In its newest version (Mardell-Czudnowski & Goldenberg, 1990), the language items include (1) articulation, (2) giving personal data, (3) remembering, (4) naming nouns, (5) naming verbs, (6) classifying foods, (7) problem solving, and (8) sentence length. Before selecting any screening test, the specialist should carefully examine the methods used for standardizing it and the validity of the constructs on which it is based.

Prekindergarten Screening

Although screening may be conducted at any point throughout childhood, the practice of screening children before they enter kindergarten, for example, by using the Manual of Developmental Diagnosis (Gesell, Knobloch et al., 1980) or DIAL-R (Mardell-Czudnowski & Goldenberg, 1990), is particularly widespread. The usual purpose of this practice by school districts is to identify children who may not yet be ready to enter the regular school curriculum at the kindergarten level so that assistance may be provided if needed. The outcome of the screening process may be a recommendation to wait another year before starting a child in school, to refer the child for special education assessment, or to place the child in a developmental kindergarten program, with the intention that the child will participate in regular kindergarten the following year. Speech–language pathologists often participate in this screening activity and use it to identify prekindergarten-level children with communicative disorders in the schools they serve.

The use of prekindergarten screening, however, is not without controversy. Some see it as leading to an early form of ability tracking that may carry many of the detrimental effects associated with tracking throughout the grades, including (1) weaker learning environments, (2) lowered expectations, (3) cumulative losses compared to same-age peers, and (4) resegregation of children in minority groups (when busing and other methods have been used to achieve racial balance), particularly for children of lower socioeconomic status (Braddock & McPartland, 1990). On the other hand, when children have wobbly language and communicative skills and have had little exposure to preliteracy experiences, a strongly language-based developmental kindergarten experience may provide the boost they need to begin school successfully and avoid a later need for special education services. More research is clearly needed in this area, as we attempt to understand what is best for children.

Early Elementary School Referral Criteria

When children are in the early elementary school years, teachers serve critical roles as referral sources. Because whole-grade screening by speech–language pathologists is now less common than before the implementation of PL 94–142, it is particularly important that specialists assist teachers to identify children at risk for language disorders and related learning impairments. One problem in eliciting appropriate referrals from teachers results from the fact that some language-based, debilitating school problems are not necessarily obvious to teachers. Like all of us, teachers tend to be tuned to hear errors rather than to notice the absence of developmentally appropriate features. It is easier to pick up the existence of negative symptoms, such as misarticulations, pronoun substitutions, and morphological immaturities, than to notice the lack of important positive developments such as later developing logicogrammatical structures or adequate language comprehension ability.

Part of the problem is that most screening and referral criteria are based on expressive language and speech criteria alone. Exclusively expressive criteria present problems for identifying children with language disorders in their school-age years for several related reasons. When individuals spontaneously express their own ideas, they can select lexicon and syntax from items and structures they know well. Therefore, children may choose to express messages with primarily simple structures and concrete vocabulary, and no one may notice that their linguistic formulations are not complex or abstract because they make few or no errors. On the other hand, the same kind of luxury does not accompany language comprehension activities. It is well documented that children spend much more time in school settings listening than talking (e.g., Cazden, 1988; N. W. Nelson, 1985; Sturm, 1990; Wells, 1986). When children listen to others speak, or read what others have written, they have no choice except to try to understand that language. When they do have opportunities to speak in classrooms within the teachers' hearing, it is often as members of large groups, and their utterances are generally expected to be short answers to their teachers' questions. When a child fails to volunteer in class, he or she may not be noticed. When a child is called on and has difficulty answering, teachers might assume many explanations, aside from linguistic impairment, for not answering the teacher's ques-

tions (e.g., being inattentive, not listening, not trying, or being a slow learner). Language impairment is not usually one of the first explanations that occurs to teachers unless they are given specific guidance in identifying the danger signs.

Damico and Oller (1980) studied varied kinds of referral criteria to discover which work best for children in the elementary grades. They provided inservice to two groups of teachers (54 teachers in grades kindergarten through fifth). Group S (surface-oriented) teachers were taught to use "traditional," superficial morphological and syntactic criteria, such as noun–verb agreement, possessive inflections, tense marking, auxiliary verbs, irregular verbs, irregular plurals, pronoun case or gender, reflexive pronouns, and syntactic transpositions as the basis for making referrals. Group P (pragmatically oriented) teachers were taught to use the criteria shown in Box 8.2. Following the inservice, a panel of judges reevaluated the referrals from both sets of teachers, using statewide criteria for determining speech–language impairment. The results showed that the teachers in Group P identified significantly more children and were more frequently correct in their identification than those in Group S. Both groups identified significantly fewer children as grade level increased.

| Box 8.2 | Pragmatically oriented referral criteria for elementary education teachers suggested by Damico and Oller (1980). |

❏ *Linguistic nonfluency.*   Disruption of speech production by a disproportionately high number of repetitions, unusual pauses, and excessive use of hesitation forms.

❏ *Revisions.*   Breakup of speech production by numerous false starts or self-interruptions; multiple revisions are made as if the child keeps coming to a dead end in a maze.

❏ *Delays before responding.*   Pauses of inordinate length following communication attempts initiated by others.

❏ *Nonspecific vocabulary.*   The use of expressions such as *this, that, then, he,* or *over there* without making the referents clear to the listener; also, the overuse of all-purpose words such as *thing, stuff, these,* and *those.*

❏ *Inappropriate responses.*   The child's utterances appear to indicate that the child is operating on an independent discourse agenda — not attending to the prompts or probes of the adult or others.

❏ *Poor topic maintenance.*   Rapid and inappropriate changes in the topic without providing transitional clues to the listener.

❏ *Need for repetition.*   Requests for multiple repetitions of an utterance without any indication of improvement in comprehension.

Note. From "Pragmatic vs. Morphological/Syntactic Criteria for Language Referrals" by J. S. Damico and J. W. Oller, Jr., 1980, *Language, Speech and Hearing Services in Schools, II,* p. 88. Copyright 1980 by American-Speech-Language-Hearing Association. Adapted by permission.

Although whole-grade screening is much less common following the implementation of PL 94–142 (because of the law's requirement that no child be placed in a special education program on the basis of screening results alone), speech–language pathologists still may find widespread, whole-grade screening activities to be appropriate particularly in the early elementary years. A story-retelling procedure (see Box 8.3) was devised by Culatta, Page, and Ellis (1983) to perform this function. When Culatta and her colleagues compared this measure of integrated communicative performance with performance on two standardized screening tools that tested knowledge of discrete language rules, they found that the story-retelling measure was more stringent than the standardized discrete item tasks for kindergarten, readiness (a transitional level between kindergarten and first grade), and first-grade children. Although some of the children who scored adequately on the standardized measures — the Screening Test of Auditory Comprehension of Language (STACL; Carrow, 1973a) and the Evaluation of Language Scale (ELS; Vane, 1975) — were unable to relate events conveyed in a story, all children who performed poorly on the story-retelling task also had difficulty on the standardized measures. Because more children were identified at the kindergarten level than at the transitional first-grade or first-grade levels using this procedure, the authors suggested that perhaps graded stories and sets of comprehension questions should be devised in the future. To my knowledge, no standardization of this kind of task has yet been accomplished.

Considering the Middle-Stage Needs of Individuals With Multiple and Severe Disabilities

Most children with multiple impairments, including hearing loss, mental retardation, autism, and physical impairment, are identified during their preschool years as needing special help, and they often continue to receive help over the years as they mature. Other children with multiple impairments may receive language intervention services during their preschool years but fail to meet eligibility criteria for specialized speech–language services as they advance in age, even though their language abilities continue to lag considerably behind those of their same-age peers. What criteria should be used for deciding which children need speech and language intervention services when speech and language delays are integral parts

of other handicapping conditions? Should all children like this qualify because their communicative abilities are inconsistent with their chronological ages? Should none of them qualify because other conditions are primary? In some school service-delivery systems, either of these extremes may be evident. Either approach may lead to inappropriate decisions about children when their needs as individuals are not considered.

One way to decide when to refer children with other disabilities for speech–language services is to look for mismatches between communicative skills and other developmental abilities, particularly cognitive ones. This is the kind of language age–mental age mismatch criterion discussed in Chapter 6. A communication processes assessment model, such as that exemplified by the Michigan Decision-Making Model (N. W. Nelson, 1989a; N. W. Nelson, Silbar & Lockwood, 1981) discussed in Chapter 7, can assist in the process of identifying children whose communicative skills are not commensurate with their cognitive and social interaction skills. Such a procedure, however, can have all of the pitfalls discussed previously regarding the difficulty of obtaining uncontaminated estimates of cognitive abilities when children have communicative impairments.

A possible solution to this dilemma is to solicit referrals not only for children who demonstrate uneven developmental patterns but also for children who are unable to meet the communicative demands of the important contexts of their lives. Professionals should remember to ask questions not only about what is wrong with children's communicative skills but also about what children need to be able to do in certain contexts and what opportunities they have to participate in contexts that parents, teachers, and children identify as important. Regional rules should be written so that all children who need special education services are eligible to receive them in a way that does not limit their participation with same-age peers.

The challenge to professionals when working with older individuals with middle-stage communicative abilities is to offer services appropriate to their individual developmental levels without relying on activities and materials that are either irrelevant or inappropriate to their age levels. A particular danger with older students who have not yet acquired skills that are common targets of preschool curricula (e.g., independent dressing, shape recognition, color naming, or number identification) is that their programs will become mired in a focus on those developmental

Box 8.3   **Story retelling as a screening tool in the early elementary grades**

Administration

☐ Introduce the story-retelling task by saying, "I'm going to tell you a story. You listen and when I'm finished you tell me the same story."

☐ Read the story to the child.

☐ Say, "Now you tell me the story."

☐ If the child does not begin, say, "Can you tell me the name of the little boy in the story?" Provide additional open-ended prompts if necessary, such as: "That's OK, what's the rest of the story?" "What did Tommy want?" "Really — what else happened?"

☐ Present the 10 comprehension questions.

Make One of Three Disposition Decisions

1. *To enroll the child for language intervention.*   Legally, under PL 94–142, a comprehensive multi-disciplinary evaluation should be conducted at this point — children cannot be determined to have a handicapping condition on the basis of a single procedure administered by a single professional. The story retelling activity is judged to support a diagnosis of language impairment if the child is unable to relate the story or if the child's version deviates significantly from the original version in either sequencing or content.

2. *To re-evaluate the child's language.*   Children who seem to be "on-the-borderline" may be observed carefully in the regular education context or rescreened before receiving a comprehensive multidisciplinary evaluation if that seems more appropriate. This decision is made if the child tells a story that is sketchy but relevant and properly sequenced.

3. *To terminate contact.*   Children whose integrated language skills are clearly adequate may be considered to have passed the screening. This decision is made if the child tells a detailed version of the story that is properly sequenced.

Stimulus Story With Number of Events

                           1   2   3

Tommy was five years old, but his birthday was coming soon. He wanted a puppy for his

      4   5

birthday, but his mother said he was too little to take care of it. Tommy didn't think he

            6   7 8

was too little. When his birthday came Tommy had a party. Five of his friends came to his

      9   10   11   12

house. They played games, ate animal crackers and cokes, and Tommy opened his pres-

   13   14   15   16   17

ents. He got a GI Joe, a fire truck, some comic books, and a baseball bat. He liked the

     18   19

presents, but he was disappointed because he didn't get a puppy. All of Tommy's friends

         20

were getting ready to go home when his daddy brought out another present for him to

   21   22   23

open. Inside was a little black puppy. Tommy was really happy because he got the present

   24

he wanted.

academic and self-help objectives to such an extent that their other needs (e.g., for social interaction and even emergent literacy) will be ignored. Contrary to popular opinion, self-dressing, color identification, and shape naming are not necessarily prerequisites for learning to read (Vellutino & Shub, 1982).

Students who have cognitive impairments, in par-ticular, need periodic review of programs to ensure that they are given opportunities to acquire skills that will enable them to function as independently as possible while in school and as they mature into adults. Their communicative needs should be reassessed periodically in contexts appropriate to their chronological age needs, because changing contexts may sig-

Box 8.3   *Continued*

Comprehension Questions

1. Who was the boy in the story?
2. How old was he?
3. Who said he was too little for something?
4. What was he too little for?
5. How many friends came to Tommy's house?

6. Why did the friends come over?
7. Name two presents Tommy got.
8. What did they eat at the party?
9. Who gave Tommy the puppy?
10. What color was the puppy?

Note: This is a nonstandardized procedure whose interpretation rests largely on clinical judgment. When the procedure is used within a particular school district, local norms might be established by quantifying some of the observations and performing statistical analyses to compute cutoff scores for children who fall more than 1 or 1.5 standard deviations below the mean for children when judged within the context of the normative group in their own linguistic and sociocultural community (see Saber & Hutchinson, 1990).

Note. From "Story Retelling as a Communative Performance Screening Tool" by B. Culatta, J. L. Page, and J. Ellis, 1983, *Language, Speech and Hearing Services in Schools, 14,* pp. 68, 73. Copyright 1983 by American Speech-Language-Hearing Association. Reprinted by permission from p. 73; adapted by permission from p. 68.

nal changes in their abilities to meet communicative demands of the new contexts. Special education and language intervention programs often focus on helping these individuals develop functional abilities (rather than focusing on meeting adult standards of correctness) for participating with as much independence as possible in school, community, and job settings, and in **activities of daily living (ADL)**. This focus on functionality is appropriate, but the professional should not overlook the possibility that functional literacy skills and other middle-stage language developments might be needed to support such activities. As functional goals are pursued, speech–language pathologists can collaborate with others to foster a better match, both by stretching individuals' communicative abilities beyond their current limits and by increasing these youngsters' opportunities to participate in activities from which they might acquire additional middle-stage communicative skills. For example, some older children and adolescents with moderate-to-severe cognitive disabilities may benefit from a team approach that considers how their oral speech and language limitations and abilities might influence their potential to learn to read and write. Programs to identify this potential might involve the solicitation of referrals. Then, dynamic assessment and diagnostic teaching activities might be designed to see whether further advances might

be possible for these youngsters if a team approach targets new skill acquisition.

Summary

This section considered a variety of methods for identifying the presence of language and other communicative disorders among middle-stage children and older individuals who are still in the middle stages of development. Both formal and informal methods were reviewed. Whereas large-scale screening programs using standardized instruments may be appropriate before kindergarten, the pitfalls of such programs should not be ignored, particularly for children from diverse cultural backgrounds. When children are in their early and middle elementary school years, a strong information dissemination program should be designed to solicit appropriate referrals based on observation of communication abilities in naturalistic and classroom settings. When children at middle-stage chronological ages stay at early-stage developmental levels, or when older children and adolescents stay at middle-stage developmental levels, other considerations become important. Then, a more individualized approach, involving consultation, referral, dynamic assessment, and diagnostic teaching may be needed to identify those individuals who both need, and can be expected to benefit from, language intervention services.

MEASUREMENT OF MIDDLE-STAGE ABILITIES, NEEDS, AND ACCOMPLISHMENTS

CONTEXTS FOR MIDDLE-STAGE ASSESSMENT AND INTERVENTION

The Continuing Importance of the Family and the Child's Primary Culture

Parents continue to play a primary role in the development of communicative ability throughout the preschool and early elementary years. It is largely through interactive experiences in the home that children come to understand their world and to have the language for mapping onto and extending concepts and to gain access to additional learning experiences.

By the time children leave toddlerhood, if their language and speech skills are noticeably limited, most parents begin to attempt to "do something" about what they increasingly perceive as a problem. Depending on their own resources and community education efforts, parents may or may not be aware of the availability of professional help, but evidence shows that they modify their interactions with their children, consciously or subconsciously (e.g., Cross, 1984; Lasky & Klopp, 1982). To summarize previous discussion of research on parental interaction styles with children with and without language disorders (discussed at several points throughout this book), most evidence seems to indicate that parental interaction styles with children with language delays are more direct (sometimes even corrective) and are less semantically contingent on the child's interests than are parental interactions with normally developing children. Some parents appear to adopt strategies of asking too many test-like questions and making informal learning opportunities too much like school, and others go to the opposite extreme, rarely asking questions (Cross, 1984). In either case, opportunities for experiencing the naturally rewarding consequences of meaningful interactions may suffer.

The evidence does not lead to the conclusion, however, that parents are to blame for their children's language delays. Both Cross (1984) and Leonard (1987) urged caution in concluding such a causative role. A better explanation seems to be one of interactive causative patterns (as described in the system theory discussion of Chapter 1), in which children's communicative delays influence parental interaction strategies and vice versa. Acceptance of this explanation not only removes the need for blame, it also sug-

gests some possibilities for designing assessment and intervention activities to escape from maladaptive downward spirals. Assessment within the family involves collaborating with parents to help them to identify strategies for fostering development while communicating parental affection and disciplinary expectations in culturally consistent ways.

Sensitivity to cultural differences continues to be an important feature of contextually based assessment activities in the preschool years. When a young child's communication is inconsistent with mainstream norms, professionals should never fail to consider whether the difference may be consistent with expectations in the child's nonmainstream culture rather than impaired performance. For example, Shirley Brice Heath (1983) described differences in adult expectations and interactions with young children in the African-American working class community she called "Trackton." In this community, where Heath spent a considerable amount of time as a participant observer, babies and young children were constantly part of the adult communication scene, but except when boys were coached in public "stage" presentations, children were not particularly encouraged to join in the conversations with adults. Unlike the parents in mainstream middle-class cultures, the adults in this community did not interpret babies' prelinguistic babbling noises as having meaning. Nor did they address much of their talk directly to infants. As Heath put it, "Everyone talks *about* the baby, but rarely *to* the baby" (p. 75). Differences in adult–child communication actions and interpretations were also found by Philips (1983) in the Warm Springs Indian Community in Oregon, where greater attention is given to the comprehension of language evidenced by young children than its expression. "Children are given many directions and then watched closely to see if they do what they are told. If they do what they are told, it is taken as evidence of comprehension" (p. 64).

Because professionals cannot possibly know all culturally based communication rules in our pluralistic society, they must often act as their own ethnographers, carefully observing children who seem to be developing normally in the same contexts as the children who are at risk. They may also find that interviewing participants in the culture can yield a critical perspective in helping to sort out whether a linguistic–cultural difference or a language disorder accounts for the behaviors they observe.

Increased Interactions With Peers

Children have varying opportunities to interact with other children during the preschool years from age 3 to 5. For many, their first opportunities are interactions with their own siblings. Efforts to make sense of the influences of sibling order and other factors on language development have met with limited success. Wells (1986) followed 32 children through the final year of their elementary education in his longitudinal study of language development in Bristol, England. He found great variability among the developmental rates of siblings in the same families but no particular pattern regarding whether parents described their older or younger children as relatively more advanced or delayed. Wells reported that interpretation of results was further complicated by varied age gaps between siblings and their differential preferences for interacting with younger or older siblings. The only generalization that seemed justified was that "there was a slight tendency for only children or those without a sibling close in age to develop more rapidly, due most probably to the more frequent opportunities these children had for interaction with their parents on a one-to-one basis" (p. 132).

In what context besides interactions with siblings at home do preschool children communicate with other children? One of the most important peer-interaction contexts is social play. Howes (1985) found that social play tended to precede social pretend play in normal development, but that both were established in normal development by 3 years of age. Westby (1988) outlined the interwoven developmental pathways of play and language (development of play behaviors is discussed later in this chapter; see Table 8.5). Children's interactions with peers are an important context for conducting language assessment and intervention activities. However, most of the normative or descriptive data about children's language acquisition come from interactions of children with adults. Because of the lack of data about child–child interactions, this is clearly an area where the standard for assessment, at least for now, must be criterion referenced to the standard of communicative competence, which might be defined as the ability to express and receive messages effectively and appropriately. In other words, it must be based on the question of "Does this child have the skills he or she needs to participate successfully in the important contexts involving communication with peers?" rather than being based on the norm-referenced assessment question "Does this child have skills that are within normal limits when conversing with peers?" Reliable normative data are simply not available.

Making the Shift From Home to School in the Preschool Years and Kindergarten

Although families continue to serve a primary role in children's development throughout childhood, when children reach the age of 3 years or so, their worlds begin to expand. Many enter a preschool setting, either Head Start or a private preschool or a combined day-care–preschool setting, and some may enter a public school-sponsored special classroom for children with identified communicative disorders or a generic preschool special education classroom. Others may not be exposed to the relatively more formal communication interactions of classrooms until kindergarten. In classrooms, children are on their own as communicators as never before. For the first time, they may be expected to be able to communicate with an adult in authority without a parent, grandparent, or familiar child-care worker to mediate the exchange. They also may be brought into large groups of peers for the first time. All such changes necessitate the acquisition of new communicative strategies.

Children's readiness to assume this relative independence as communicators follows on the heels of early-stage developments that rely on much more dependent relationships with primary care givers. When describing an early-stage child named Mark, for example, Wells (1986) noted that, "when he is talking with someone who knows him well and who is able to interpret his intention from the combination of his utterance and its context, he is successfully able to mean more than he can say" (p. 23). Wells likened the developmental accomplishments for Mark and his peers over the next few years of middle-stage development as an almost sheer climb up the face of a cliff, after which the rest of the mountain remains, but the pathway is less clearly defined, many routes are possible, and the going, in general, is somewhat easier.

Having acknowledged the importance of shifts in communicative expectations from home to school, Wells (1986) noted the continuity in the shift from one context to the other as well, particularly for children whose home experiences have helped them get ready. He commented:

> As far as learning is concerned, therefore, entry into school should not be thought of as a beginning, but as a transition to a more broadly based community and to a wider range of opportunities for meaning-making and mastery. *Every* child has competencies, and these provide a positive base from which to start. The teacher's responsibility is to discover what they are and to help each child to extend and develop them. (p. 69)

The problem is that, all too often, the language of the school setting does not particularly facilitate further language learning. Wells (1986) noted the lack of reciprocity in traditional classroom interactions. In his comparison of home and school interactions with young children, Wells found that teachers were twice as likely as parents to develop meanings that they themselves had introduced into the conversation rather than following the child's lead. He commented, "Small wonder that some children have little to say or even appear to be lacking in conversational skills altogether" (p. 87).

Wells (1986) also provided an example from the transcripts of a child called Rosie, whom he presented as possibly learning disabled. Rosie was the youngest in a low-income family with five children. Her mother stayed home, and her father was unemployed and usually at home. Although, in comparison to the other children studied, when she entered school at age 5, Rosie was a "slow developer" both socially and linguistically, she was far from being nonverbal. Furthermore, Rosie's mother demonstrated many of the same kinds of facilitative strategies in her interactions with Rosie at home as did mothers of children of middle-class socioeconomic status, and Rosie capably conversed with her mother. Nevertheless, in a transcript gathered in interaction with one of her teachers, Rosie was completely lost. Even though they were talking about a picture that Rosie had just pasted on a calendar she had made, she seemed to have no comprehension of the teacher's questions and was unable to answer coherently, possibly because Rosie had no experience with snow skiing, which the picture illustrated. The teacher also provided little scaffolding, placing Rosie at an added disadvantage. Yet in another interaction on that same morning with another teacher in a seemingly more complex early reading task, Rosie was allowed to take the leading role in a conversation about chimneys and heating stoves. In this case, she appeared much more competent as a communicator. She contrib-

uted to this topic from her own experience. *Problems are not just within children, and neither are their solutions.*

The Elementary School Classroom as a Context for Language Learning and Use

Classrooms play such an important role for school-age children that they warrant special consideration as assessment and intervention contexts. The formal interactions of classrooms have some unique features that differ considerably from the informal interactions of dyadic communication as it occurs most often in homes and individual adult–child conversations. In classroom discussions, the power differential between teachers and students is usually obvious (Cazden, 1988; Lindfors, 1987). In fact, McDermott (1977) argued that "teaching is invariably a form of coercion" (p. 204). That is, teachers almost always fill the role of authority in the classroom, controlling topics and the allotment of turns, asking test-like questions to which they already know the answers, and establishing a variety of special communication rules (such as flipping the light switch to signal that children should stop talking).

Contrast this style with interaction in homes, where children more often are given the opportunity to establish topics and to guide the evolution of conversations with their own interests. J. N. Britton (1979) contrasted the kind of discourse occurring in true conversation, where both partners play an equal role in negotiating its transitions, which he called the *participant* mode, as with a different style, which he called the *spectator* mode. In the spectator mode, one partner takes the lead in maintaining the unity and coherence of the total representation of experiences. Britton commented, "As participants, we use language to shape experience in order to handle it; as spectators, we use language to digest experience" (1979, p. 192). The spectator role is assumed much more often in classrooms.

As Cazden (1988) pointed out, teachers often guide discourse in the classroom, not only when they are in expressive control themselves, but when their students are presumably in control of extended expressive turns, as in sharing time. When teachers perceive that their students have begun to stray too far from announced topics, teachers say things like:

> OK I'm going to stop you // I want you to talk about things that are really very important // that's important to you but can you tell us things that are sort of different // can you do that? // (p. 13)

Problems arise for students when cultural differences in discourse styles learned at home do not match the expectations of their teachers. For example, Cazden (1988) pointed out that children from African-American homes are more likely to use a narrative style involving an episodic structure; one event is tied sequentially to the next but no overall theme is maintained. Such narratives might be evaluated as the norm by adults in the child's culture and are likely to have served as primary models that the child heard during preschool, but they are likely to be evaluated as inferior narratives by white mainstream teachers whose experiences with narration are limited to their own culture.

Beyond issues of power, control, and cultural variation, school–home expectations differ in presupposition, or the degree of knowledge shared by adult and child partners, and the opportunity for repair. Parents of young children generally know so much about their children's experiences, language, and world knowledge that they can easily provide scaffolding to help their children be competent in discussions that include vocabulary and concepts their children do not yet know. For example, when my own children were young, I remember many times in the pediatrician's office having to bite my tongue, knowing that my children had been asked a question in a way that would not make sense to them but knowing also that I should allow the physician the opportunity to do his own repair work and my children a chance to experience communicative independence from their very language-oriented mother.

When children begin acquiring word and world knowledge from sources beyond the home, many parents at first are surprised and even ask metacognitive questions that are probably beyond their children's comprehension. When I asked one of my children as a preschooler where he had learned something that surprised me, I remember relishing his reply, "I just knowed it." But I delighted in knowing that he was beginning to take advantage of experiences beyond those we shared to acquire new words and concepts.

The debate about the degree of distinction between language in the home and language in school has been going on for some time and in several disciplines (N. W. Nelson, 1988a). It is echoed in the debate about the degree of distinction between oral language and written language, which has been used as a forum for discussing whether persons in societies that are not literate are as capable of complex thought as those in which literacy is formally taught (Scribner & Cole, 1978) and whether cultures that have not developed literacy teaching and interaction methods can ever have access to world power without them (Whiteman, 1981). Even those who choose not to emphasize the distinctions between oral and literate communication point out that varied sets of linguistic and communicative rules are associated not so much with different communication modalities (i.e., reading–writing versus listening–speaking) as with the degree of formality of the communicative context (Blank, 1982; M. M. Cooper, 1982; Tannen, 1982).

Whether the distinctions between school and home language and oral and written language represent truly separate systems or merely different points on a continuum, professionals should appreciate them when evaluating young children in early elementary classrooms. Differences in lexical choices (more varied and abstract), sentence structure (more complex), and discourse organization strategies (more preplanned and cohesive) are associated both with written language and with formal spoken language, such as that used in classrooms. The differences in all of these linguistic dimensions generally can be traced to the influences of one key factor—the degree of contextualization.

When people communicate, at least three sources contribute meaning to the message; (1) Both partners bring with them some internalized meaning that may be more or less shared, depending on their common experiences and culture. (2) Some nonlinguistic meaning may be available in the immediate context, possibly through gestures, actions, and objects. (3) Speakers or writers encode some linguistic meaning in the words and phrasing of the discourse. As children shift roles as comprehenders from home to school, and from oral to written modalities, increasing decontextualization occurs. Less meaning is available in the situation, and more must be gleaned from words. This shift has been termed one of movement from situated meaning to lexicalized meaning by Cook-Gumperz (1977) (see Box 8.4 for a list of other terms that have been used by different authors for these shifts). When contextualization shifts occur, children whose linguistic comprehension skills are weaker than their nonlinguistic skills are at increasing risk for language disability.

For these children, several different consequences are possible. One is that no one will recognize the problem as involving a language disorder. Children then may

Box 8.4   Home language and school language — Oral language and written language

Home Language and Oral Language	Source	School Language and Written Language
Heavy reliance on non-linguistic context		Heavy reliance on linguistically encoded meaning
Situated meaning	(Cook-Gumperz, 1977)	Lexicalized meaning
Restricted code	(B. B. Bernstein, 1972)	Elaborated code
Particularistic meanings implicit in text		Universalistic meaning explicit in text
Exophoric meaning	(Gregory & Carroll, 1978)	Endophoric meaning

Note. From "The Nature of Literacy" by N. W. Nelson in *Later Language Development: Ages Nine Through Nineteen* (p. 17) edited by M. A. Nippold, 1988, Austin, TX; Pro-Ed. Copyright 1988 by Pro-Ed. Adapted by permission.

be called lazy and may be accused of not trying because no one recognizes that understanding the language and communicative expectations of classrooms is not automatic for them. Going unrecognized and untreated for what they are, the language-related problems of these children may mount as they experience increasing failure within the advancing language demands of classrooms, and they may be at risk for problems of other types as well, particularly those involving self-image. Another possibility is that the problem may be recognized as one involving language disorder, with the result that the child is removed from the mainstream to a special education context to address the problem.

Although the first outcome clearly should be avoided, the second is more difficult to evaluate. The determination of least restrictive environment (LRE) is relative to the child's needs (see discussions in Chapter 5). When problems are severe enough, placement in self-contained language intervention classrooms for a year or more may, in fact, be the preferred solution. The teacher (who may be a speech–language pathologist in some states) then can carefully control language input and provide linguistic and nonlinguistic scaffolding to improve the child's access to the curriculum (as long as special educators and speech–language pathologists keep an eye on the regular curriculum to prevent gaps from widening between children in regular and special education contexts). However, when children are closer to being able to comprehend in regular classrooms (those I call ABNQ children), keeping them in their regular classrooms and in the regular curriculum often is preferred.

Complexity of teacher language is not necessarily a negative factor. Gradual exposure to increasingly complex language helps children grow, as long as they can make sense of it. When children need help to make sense of instructional language, the best solutions may involve collaborative consultation with the teacher to modify language expectations slightly (e.g., by adding redundancy or slowing speaking rate), while at the same time helping children acquire stronger skills for processing increasingly complex language. Many teachers are willing to monitor a child's comprehension more closely and to engage in individualized communicative repair when they recognize that a child has failed to understand, not because of lack of trying or inattention, but because the child did not understand the language. As I have written before (N. W. Nelson, 1989b), it is far more likely that *children would (do their work) if they could, than that they could (do their work) if they would (only try).*

Just what kinds of communicative events and expectations happen in early elementary school classrooms? Language permeates all aspects of teaching and learning. "Language" is not something that happens from 9:00 to 10:00 on Monday, Wednesday, and Friday morning. It happens all the time. It happens when teachers and children study math or science. It also happens when children learn the new rules of a game on the playground. Language plays a role whether the children listen, speak, read, write or think.

As mentioned previously, language expectations become increasingly complex as children move from home to school and from oral to written contexts. What else do we need to know to evaluate children's abilities to process the language of classrooms? For the most part, the language of classrooms is used (1) for instruction in how to read and write language (fostering the acquisition of literacy is a critical function of school language); (2) to talk about language (much of school language is metalinguistic, from talking about words and sounds in kindergarten to talking about metaphor and simile in the later grades); (3) to use language to learn how to do other things (much of school language is used to convey procedure); and (4) to use language to learn about other things (in other cases, school language is used to convey content).

When Janet Sturm and I recorded and analyzed the language in first-, third-, and fifth-grade classrooms (five classrooms at each level), we coded the speech acts produced by both teachers and students in 9 minutes of group instruction and discussion discourse for three consecutive school days (Sturm, 1990). We gave every utterance at least one code, but some received more than one code. This occurred particularly for teachers when they used such linguistic devices as "Now . . ." or "OK . . ." to mark content (MC) for their students or to signal a shift in topic. Children were more often coded as producing a single speech act at a time. The results of that speech act analysis are presented in Table 8.1.

Table 8.1 shows that the speech acts that teachers used most often in formal classroom discourse were questions to "solicit information" (SI). Correspondingly, the speech acts children used most often were "supply solicited information" (SSI). Children showed extremely small proportions of any other kind of speech act in this type of interaction. Other speech acts that teachers frequently used were to convey content (CC) and to convey procedure (CP), each of which account for approximately 15% of speech acts across grade levels. These kinds of language require different kinds of linguistic abilities of children attempting to make sense of them.

Language that is used to convey procedure typically places greater demands on auditory memory and the ability to process language in sequence. Children often must reauditorize (D. J. Johnson & Mykle-

bust, 1967) procedural language as they seek to carry out the teacher's instructions. The following is an excerpt from a sample recorded by Sturm (1990) in a first-grade classroom, coded for the variables represented in Table 8.1 and coded for analysis with the Systematic Analysis of Language Transcripts (SALT) program (J. F. Miller & Chapman, 1986) (including bound morphemes marked with a slash, e.g., "trade/ed"). The teacher is conveying a procedure about the transitions in a cooperative learning task involving process writing. Notice the high demand on the ability to decode complex logicogrammatical (if–then) structures involving negative and temporal concepts and to remember the teacher's instructions (perhaps by reconstructing them) long enough to carry them out:

T OK, if you have not trade/ed job/s, it is now time for the listener to become the reader and the reader become the listener [MC][CP].
T If you have both had time to finish what you/'re do/ing, you/'ve read your story all the way, it is time to go back to your seat and make any correction/s that you need to make [CP].
S XXX [SI?] [A question asked by a student was unintelligible on the tape].
T Then she can read it as far as she is [SSI].
T (People who are not done. . .) OK, then you can go back to your seat and work [MC][CP].
T None of you need to be up here [CP][CA].

Teachers also use language to tell children about the content of the curriculum. The referents are often abstract and metalinguistic. An example is the following sequence, recorded in a first-grade classroom, where a teacher and students are editing the punctuation on a letter. She has just called on an individual student, coded as "solicit other" (SO):

T Chantel, what else should we do to our letter [SO][SI]?
= room silent waiting for an answer 00:10 seconds
S Put a comma after "love" [SSI].
T Alright a comma after "love" [MC][AE+].
T We call that our close/ing don/'t we [CC][SI]?
T We/'d always put a comma whether it/'s "yours truly," or "love," or "sincerely" [CC][CP].

Personal Reflection 8.2	"Where children and teachers are doing real work, there is no way to separate out 'language' and what is sometimes called 'content.'"
	Judith Wells Lindfors (1987), writing about the language of classrooms.

TABLE 8.1
Classroom speech acts

Communication Act Variables	Grade-Level Student Means			Grade-Level Teacher Means		
	1st	3rd	5th	1st	3rd	5th
1. To convey content (CC)	0.6%	1.4%	2.0%	12.3%	14.3%	15.9%
2. To mark content (MC)	0.1	0.2	0.4	11.9	12.3	16.3
3. To call on specific child, "solicit other"(SO)	0.0	0.2	0.0	9.8	6.0	5.3
4. To convey procedure (CP)	0.0	0.0	0.2	14.7	13.5	13.8
5. To convey attitude (CA)	0.1	0.2	0.3	2.7	3.4	3.5
6. To acknowledge evaluate (AE)	0.2	0.1	0.2	5.2	4.0	3.3
7. To acknowledge modify (AM)	0.0	0.0	0.1	6.4	6.5	4.5
8. To ask questions or "solicit information or action" (SI)(SA)	0.7	1.8	2.4	22.1	17.0	17.6
9. To answer questions/read aloud "supply solicited info" (SSI)	10.1	13.0	10.0	0.8	1.0	1.7
10. Performatives (P)	0.1	0.2	0.2	0.8	0.8	0.5
11. Free responses (FR)	1.4	4.1	1.8	0.0	0.0	0.0
Totals	13.3%	21.2%	17.6%	86.7%	78.8%	82.4%

CC, convey content; CP, convey procedure; MC, mark content; SI, solicit information; SSI, supply solicited information.

Note. Mean proportions of total speech acts produced at a grade level over the 3-day period in instruction–discussion discourse involving the class as a whole (total, 15 classes, based on data from Sturm, 1990).

To successfully process language conveying the curriculum content (in this case, rules of punctuation and capitalization), children often must understand multiple-meaning words (e.g., *letter* in this context does not refer to a letter of the alphabet, and *closing* is used as a noun, rather than as a verb as in "closing a door"). If children can immediately recognize that the referent for *closing* in this case is the word, *love*, but that the teacher is offering other exemplars from the same category in the listing, "yours truly," or "love," or "sincerely," they will have simplified the task of remembering the rule for when to use a comma. When children have trouble with the concrete vocabulary of everyday interactions, such abstract discussions often make no sense.

The language processing demands of classrooms are varied and complex. Often, within a single communicative event, children must apply a set of coordinated strategies for using oral and written language to (1) comprehend, (2) remember, (3) recall, and (4) express. For a language assessment to be fully relevant to the needs of children with suspected language disorders who spend much of their day in elementary school classrooms, assessment activities must address the interactions between the demands of those contexts and children's abilities. Although formal tests can contribute to understanding children's problems in the classroom, they are not enough.

TOOLS AND STRATEGIES FOR MIDDLE-STAGE ASSESSMENT

Gathering Background Information for Contextually Based Assessment

Having reviewed the contexts that are likely to be important for children in the middle stages of language acquisition, you should be wondering how a clinician might use that information in assessing a child's needs. Strategy adoption should be guided by the information gathered through observation and interview. As discussed in Chapter 6, strategies also differ with the varying purposes of assessment. When the purpose is to determine whether a child meets entry or exit criteria for receiving special education services (this is the basic question about impairment), the question of whether the child has lower language abilities than those expected for same-age peers is a primary one. It is answered most readily by administering relatively formal tests standardized on an appropriate reference group.

Norm-referenced assessment activities are inadequate by themselves, however, for meeting other assessment purposes. Another aspect of meeting entry–exit criteria involves determining whether a child needs special education services (this is the basic question about disability). The only way to answer this question adequately is to observe the child's ability to meet the linguistic demands of key contexts in the child's life. Those contexts can be identified only by collaborating with others who are concerned and knowledgeable about the child's communicative life. A sequence that might be followed in gathering this essential background information appears in Box 8.5.

Language Sampling and Other Informal Assessment Techniques

The *pièce de résistance* of most speech–language evaluations of children in the middle stages of language development is the spontaneous language sample. Although the professional may use formal language assessment tools to quantify various aspects of a child's language and speech abilities, the spontaneous language sample affords the richest opportunity to observe a child's integrated communicative abilities.

Language-sampling techniques can be used to gather quantitative data to support a diagnosis of language disorder (Lee, 1974; J. F. Miller, 1981; Roberts & Crais, 1989), or they can serve as a source of qualitative data for the intervention-planning process (Fey, 1986; Lahey, 1988; Lund & Duchan, 1988; J. F. Miller, 1981; Roberts & Crais, 1989). Both purposes are important, and both can be approached in a variety of ways.

Language sample analysis is not new. It has been used as a diagnostic and research technique at least since McCarthy (1930) reported that 50 utterances of spontaneous speech "would give a fairly representative sample of the child's linguistic development in a relatively short period of time, without tiring the child with a prolonged observation" (p. 32). Many versions of language-sampling and analysis strategies have been published since the early 1970s, including several

---

Box 8.5   **Procedures for gathering background information essential to the assessment of children in the middle stages of language acquisition**

1. Determine the **reason for referral** by interviewing the person who made the referral (or suggested that it be made). The fact that someone was concerned enough about the child's communicative development to make a referral is significant. If the child was identified through screening instead of referral, interview those who might have made a referral (but did not) to determine whether they have ever felt any concern about the child's communicative development.

2. Gather **history information** about the nature of the problem using the parents as informants, but also interview other informants who are significant in the child's life. Include questions about (a) the family and any communicative problems or disorders family members might exhibit (or may have exhibited as children); (b) the child's medical history and any significant injuries or illnesses; (c) the child's developmental history, especially related to major developmental milestones; (d) the child's educational history (if there is one), including any previous referral and/or enrollment in special services; and (e) the child's social history, including information about the child's interactions with peers and effects on those interactions from the child's communicative behaviors.

3. Collaborate with other important adults to **identify contexts** where it is important that the child meet communicative expectations. Include questions about (a) places (e.g., home, school, day-care center); (b) people (e.g., parents, siblings, day-care playmates or friends); (c) communicative events (e.g., show-and-tell, understanding parental requests, free-play time at preschool).

4. Use multiple strategies to **identify aspects of communicative competence in each of these important contexts**. Include both (a) observational strategies and (b) interview strategies. When using observational strategies, attempt to use strategies of both onlooker observation (the mouse-in-the-corner strategy) and participation observation (to explore the child's ability to be more effective when contextual conditions are modified somewhat). When using interview strategies, ask informants to list and prioritize areas of greatest strength and concern, and ask other questions that ask informants to give examples of what they mean by the way they choose to label behaviors.

5. Based on this initial compilation of background information, **form additional hypotheses about the child's relative areas of strength and difficulty** that can be tested in the remainder of the assessment process using both informal and formal assessment techniques.

computer software programs designed to make various aspects of the task easier. These are listed and described in Box 8.6. Unfortunately, however, no one has developed a way to avoid human transcription of the recordings. For most experienced clinicians, that remains the most time-consuming part of the process. Following is a description of transcription and other aspects of the language-sampling process: (1) gathering the sample, (2) transcribing it, (3) analyzing language form variables, (4) analyzing language content variables, and (5) analyzing language use variables. This discussion is an overview of generic concerns. For more detailed descriptions of methods described briefly in Box 8.6, readers are referred to the original sources.

| Box 8.6 | Language sampling and analysis strategies |

Crystal, D., Fletcher, P., & Garman, M. (1976). *The grammatical analysis of language disability*. London: Edward Arnold. Describes their Language Assessment, Remediation, and Screening Procedure (LARSP): Both morphological and syntactic developments are tallied on a LARSP chart, arranged in order from earlier to later developing forms, which can be used to plan intervention.

Lee, L. L. (1974). *Developmental sentence analysis*. Evanston, IL: Northwestern University Press. Describes Developmental Sentence Types analysis for children not producing at least 50% complete sentences (defined as including a subject and verb) and Developmental Sentence Scoring (DSS) for those who are. DSS is based on grammatical analysis of eight categories for a 50-utterance sample, which yields a score that can be compared with normative data for 3- to 7-year olds.

Long, S. H., & Fey, M. E. (1991). *Computerized profiling* [computer program; Version 7.1]. Ithaca, NY: Computerized Profiling. Provides computer assistance for several other analysis systems, including LARSP.

Lund, N. J., & Duchan, J. F. (1988). *Assessing children's language in naturalistic contexts* (2nd ed.). Englewood Cliffs, NJ: Prentice-Hall. Serves as a reference text, summarizing multiple language sampling and analysis strategies.

Miller, J. (1981). *Assessing language production in children: Experimental procedures*. Baltimore, MD: University Park Press. Serves as a reference text, summarizing multiple language sampling and analysis strategies.

Miller, J., & Chapman, R. (1986). *Systematic analysis of language transcripts (SALT)* [Computer program; A. Nockers, Programmer]. Madison, WI: Language Analysis Laboratory, Waisman Center on Mental Retardation and Human Development. Available in both Apple and IBM versions, this computerized analysis system can accommodate more than one speaker. Samples are entered using slashes to indicate bound morphemes and using customized codes. Offers standard analyses (e.g., MLU, type–token ratios, word counts) and customized analysis.

Palin, M. W., Mordecai, D. R., & Palmer, C. B. (1985). *Lingquest 1: Language sample analysis software* [Computer Program]. San Antonio, TX: Psychological Corporation. Available in both Apple and IBM versions, this software package yields type–token analysis, form analysis of eight grammatical categories, an error profile, structure analysis of 7 basic sentence types, 10 question types, and 12 complex sentence types. At least 50 utterance samples are typed in with glosses.

Stickler, K. R. (1987). *Guide to analysis of language transcripts*. Eau Claire, WI: Thinking Publications. A transcript guides readers through varied procedures for analysis of semantic, syntactic, and pragmatic features. Procedures are most useful with young children with language disorders, but many are also applicable with older students.

Tyack, D. L., & Gottsleben, R. H. (1977). *Language sampling, analysis, and training: A handbook for teachers and clinicians*. Palo Alto, CA: Consulting Psychologists Press. A sample of approximately 100 sentences is transcribed on a form. The professional counts words and morphemes, computes a word–morpheme mean to assign the child to one of five linguistic levels, compares the child's language forms to a developmental chart of those expected for the child's level, and uses these results to make clinical decisions.

Gathering the sample. When gathering a language sample, the specialist's question is whether uniform control of contextual variables or more spontaneous natural samples are preferred. For example, should the professional gather samples entirely through conversation or ask children to retell a story or give instructions for playing a game? Should pictures or toys be used? Should the language specialist gather the samples or record children in interactions with other adults or peers?

These questions have no one best answer. The best answer to all of them is, it depends. It depends on the purposes of the assessment and on whether the clinician plans to apply an established set of analysis criteria that are at least partially quantitative. When quantitative comparisons are desired, the specialist should gather the sample using methods consistent with those recommended by the author of the analysis procedure. A caveat is in order, however. What looks like a standard procedure to the adult controlling the sequence of an interaction may actually be experienced in unequivalent ways by different children. Depending on past experiences with certain kinds of interactions and people, what may be easy for child A may be hard for child B; whereas in a different cultural milieu, child A may be disadvantaged. If clinicians are not careful, they may draw conclusions about a general lack of communicative competence when the child is demonstrating reduced communicative competence *in a particular context*. For example, telling a story about a picture may be a task that is highly familiar and comfortable to one child but totally foreign to another. In such cases, cultural factors may play a major role in how children have learned to interact with adults. Remember Crago's (1990) report in Chapter 2 of her surprise when an Inuk teacher she consulted about a highly verbal child Crago had judged as linguistically advanced was perceived by the teacher as having a possible learning problem because, in the teacher's cultural experience, "children who don't have such high intelligence have trouble stopping themselves" (p. 80).

When doubts are raised about a child's communicative competence in a sample gathered in one context, particularly when the child's culture and ethnicity differ from that of the person interacting with the child, the professional should seek other interaction contexts (both people and places) and should build an awareness of the communicative expectations of the child's culture into the process. Although practical concerns may limit the number of observational opportunities for clinicians with large caseloads, failure to observe the child's communicative abilities within his or her own language community may lead to biased assessment results, which must be avoided.

The usual goal of language sampling is to create an optimal language interaction context in which children can demonstrate their best language capabilities. Occasionally, sampling a child's ability to communicate in contexts identified as problematic may be desired.

The materials and discourse tasks best suited for gathering language samples will likely vary based on children's ages and language levels as well as assessment purposes. As a general rule, the younger the child, or the more limited the child's language abilities, the more toys and other props are helpful in the language sampling interaction. Older children who have higher level language skills can interact more when the context is established through linguistic rather than nonlinguistic means. Conversational interaction, in which children are allowed to set the topics, may also be particularly desirable for young children. Yes–no questions and questions that can be answered elliptically should be avoided. When children are particularly reticent, it is generally helpful to avoid questions altogether, engaging instead in joint focus or parallel play activity, gradually commenting on aspects of the environment to which the child is attending. This usually takes the pressure off talking and leads to more natural interactions. As Lund and Duchan (1988) commented, when clinicians insert their own opinions or comments occasionally, a more natural and less "testing" atmosphere may be created. Manipulable materials like play dough and puzzles are not particularly effective for gathering rich language samples. Many children with language impairments become so preoccupied with the motor activity, that they say little when their hands are busy.

Some conversational strategies that work better with more talkative children include asking the usual questions about brothers and sisters and then asking whether the child's siblings ever bother the child's "stuff." This almost invariably elicits a spontaneous response that has an emotional flavor and can lead to more natural interactions. Children love emotionally based topics. That may be why Grimm's Fairy Tales have held children's attention for centuries. Children also enjoy pretend play with adults using toy figures.

Remember (from Chapter 6) that Hubbell's (1988) review of the literature showed that children are likely to talk more (1) when they have equal or greater power in a relationship, (2) when there are fewer constraints on them, and (3) when the topic is of immediate interest to them.

Narrative discourse should also be probed for most middle-stage children. The appropriateness of probing the narrative genre, even for 3-year-olds, is supported by K. Nelson's (1989) report of "narratives from the crib" (see discussion in Chapter 7). These were amazingly complex private stories produced by a young child between the ages of 21 and 36 months. Interestingly, during this time, her spontaneous bedtime conversations with her parents were much more linguistically limited. For example, Emily's monologues had a mean length of utterance (MLU) of 5.40 morphemes, whereas her dialogues had an MLU of 3.61 morphemes. Either MLU is advanced from that usually expected of 2-year-olds, which is predicted to be closer to 2.0 to 3.0 morphemes (J. F. Miller, 1981). Even very young children, when conditions are right, can use connected discourse without heavy support from an adult. The probing of narrative discourse is useful because attempts at story telling are generally associated with the production of longer and more complex utterances, the use of cohesive devices, and the opportunity to observe whether the child has a sense of story grammar.

Because story telling from memory may be highly variable depending on the familiarity of a particular event being retold, some have suggested using story retelling. The clinician first tells the story, and then the child retells it (see the screening technique reported earlier and in Box 8.3). During story retelling, the presence of pictures will affect memory cueing and sequencing of events in the retelling. The strength of the story's script and the child's familiarity with the type of script may also influence performance. Recognizing the variability inherent in such task, Dollaghan, Campbell, and Tomlin (1990) recommended using narration of videotaped cartoons to provide a relatively standard context for sampling "spontaneous expressive language" that would depend less on memory and recall strategies. They found this sampling context to be particularly useful for individuals who had experienced head injuries.

When one considers all of the variables that may influence the quality of language in a particular sample, it may seem inappropriate to compare children's language characteristics to those of a set of standard samples. Yet, J. F. Miller (1981) and J. F. Miller and Chapman (1981) reported research for children between the ages of 17 and 59 months from middle- and upper-middle class homes in Madison, Wisconsin, that demonstrated a fairly predictable and linear relationship between MLU and chronological age (see Table 8.2). This relationship was later confirmed by Klee, Schaffer, May, Membrio, and Mougey (1989) for 24 normally developing children from lower-middle-class homes in Nashville, Tennessee, whose MLU scores compared favorably with the earlier MLU scores from the J. F. Miller and Chapman (1981) study. Klee and his colleagues also analyzed the relationship between MLU and chronological age for an additional 24 children with specific language impairments. They found that MLUs for children with specific language impairments were consistently lower, as might be expected, but that MLU for the children with language impairments changed at a rate similar to that observed for normally developing children, suggesting that slower rate of development may not be the best way to explain the variation in their language acquisition processes.

Although quantified norm-referenced data are often important when making decisions about impairment, they are not sufficient for making decisions about disability. For that purpose, criterion-referenced standards are necessary. Then, the question becomes, "Is this child's language adequate to meet the communicative demands of important contexts?" rather than, "Is this child's language at age level?"

Recording the sample.   For very young or physically impaired children, videotaping is essential to capture the nonlinguistic as well as the linguistic context, but when children enter middle-stage language acquisition, audiotaping may suffice for most clinical purposes. When children produce mostly utterances of three words or more in length, enough of the context is usually encoded in language to enable judgment of their linguistic and communicative abilities from the language sample itself. In these instances, the clinician should transcribe the audiotape as soon as possible, so that contextual notes may be added.

Whenever professionals document clinical activities, it is important that they keep in mind the absent audience for the written report of each activity, the purpose of the report, and alternative purposes to which the report might be put. In this case, the audience is most

TABLE 8.2
Predicted MLUs and MLU ranges within 1 *SD* of predicted mean for each age group

Age ±1 Month	Predicted MLU[a]	Predicted SD[b]	Predicted MLU ±1 *SD* (middle 68%)
18	1.31	0.325	0.99–1.64
21	1.62	0.386	1.23–2.01
24	1.92	0.448	1.47–2.37
30	2.54	0.571	1.97–3.11
33	2.85	0.633	2.22–3.48
36	3.16	0.694	2.47–3.85
39	3.47	0.756	2.71–4.23
42	3.78	0.817	2.96–4.60
45	4.09	0.879	3.21–4.97
48	4.40	0.940	3.46–5.34
51	4.71	1.002	3.71–5.71
54	5.02	1.064	3.96–6.08
57	5.32	1.125	4.20–6.45
60	5.63	1.187	4.44–6.82

[a] MLU is predicted from the equation MLU = $-0.548 + 0.103$ (age).
[b] SD is predicted from the equation $SD_{MLU} = -0.0446 + 0.0205$ (age).

Note. From Jon F. Miller, *Assessing Language Production in Children: Experimental Procedures* (p. 27). Copyright © 1981. Reprinted with permission of Allyn and Bacon.

likely other professionals, and its primary purposes may be (1) to capture the essential qualities of the child's linguistic and communicative abilities, (2) to make quantitative judgments about normalcy and/or progress in comparison with dimensions of earlier samples, and (3) to select target goal areas for special attention in the intervention process. When others also review the report (e.g., parents, teachers, or auditors), they should be kept in mind as potential audience while the tape is being transcribed and contextual notes are being included. Particular concerns are provision of sufficient contextual information so that someone who was not there can understand the transcript, and protection of the child's and family's right to privacy.

Transcribing the sample. Aside from the time transcription takes, most problems in transcription arise around decisions for segmenting utterances. Segmentation decisions are particularly important because they influence measurements such as MLU that depend on the size of sentence-like utterance units. Different authors recommend different strategies, which may be more or less appropriate depending on the child's linguistic and developmental level. J.F. Miller (1981) recommended that "Utterance segmentation should be based on terminal intonation contour, rising or falling" (p. 14). This strategy may be especially appropriate when transcribing samples of children in the early stages of language acquisition. For children at middle stages of language development however, who are learning to elaborate and combine sentences, it must be augmented by other syntax-based segmentation rules. Then, the problem may become how to give credit for compound sentence constructions without inflating the child's MLU from multiple run-on clauses, such as those conjoined with "and then" starters. Lee (1974) suggested a way to satisfy these concerns, restated and elaborated on by Lund and Duchan (1988) (summarized in Box 8.7).

An alternative strategy for dividing utterances might be more appropriate for children who are beyond Brown's Post Stage V (MLU = 4.50+). According to J.F. Miller's (1981) normative projections (see Table 8.2), the predicted mean for the age 60 months (5 years) ±1 month is 5.63 (±1 *SD* for MLU at this age is represented by the range 4.44 to 6.82). Traditionally, the MLU has been assumed to become less meaningful as a measure of children's development beyond the age of 5 years. At that point, advancing maturity begins to be marked by children's ability to say more in fewer words (Hunt, 1965), and a different criterion for dividing utterances for analysis then becomes appropriate. Kellogg Hunt (1965) therefore proposed the T-unit as "one main clause with all the subordinate clauses attached to it" (p. 20). As Hunt pointed out, the advantage is that this method preserves all of the youngster's subordination and all of the coordination between words and phrases and subordinate clauses, but does not overcredit the less mature strategy of coordinating main clauses.

Box 8.8 illustrates how the same sample might be divided using the two different strategies proposed by Hunt (1965) and Lund and Duchan (1988). It is the attempt of a child with a language-learning disability to retell the story of "Dumbo." This sample also illustrates how to handle linguistic nonfluencies when transcribing language samples by placing in parentheses such devices as initial conjunctions, pause fillers (um, ah, er, OK), part-word or whole-word repetitions not intended for emphasis, and revisions. Revisions sometimes look like linguistic dead-ends and were labeled *mazes* by Loban (1963). (Hunt, 1965, called them *garbles*.) Linguistic nonfluencies, although they might appear extraneous to the message being conveyed, provide important information about internalized processing efforts and should be maintained in language sample transcripts. However, they should not be included when counting morphemes to determine utterance length or when assigning credit for grammatical features (e.g., when performing Laura Lee's, 1974, developmental sentence analysis).

Analyzing language form variables.   The clinician's analysis of the language sample depends on the questions raised during the observations and interviews when gathering background information. Questions about **language form** may be divided into three types: (1) questions about inflectional morphology, (2) questions about syntactic construction and comprehension, (3) and questions about contextually-based variation of language form.

First, **questions about language morphology** are usually guided by reference to information about the acquisition of the 14 morphemes studied by Roger Brown (1973) and by Jill and Peter de Villiers (1973). These are summarized in Box 8.9.

When analyzing morphological development, the clinician generally starts by computing MLU for a sample of at least 50 utterances. This MLU is used to assign the child to a developmental level (usually corresponding to one of R.A. Brown's, 1973, stages). Then the clinician seeks from the target child's language sample that morphological developments expected for the child's age and MLU are occurring. J.F. Miller (1981) referred to the analysis of simple sentences as Assigning Structural Stage (ASS). His procedure compares the evidence from a child's language sample to a series of charts summarizing developmental expectations. In a similar procedure,

---

Box 8.7	Guidelines for segmenting utterances

Judgment of utterance boundaries must be made at the time of transcription, using contextual and intonation cues. Once the words are written down, the information is lost. Indicate pauses with a slash (/).

1. The end of an utterance is indicated by a definite pause preceded by a drop in pitch or rise in pitch.
2. The end of a sentence is the end of the utterance. Two or more sentences may be said in one breath without a pause, but each one will be treated as a separate utterance for syntax analysis.
3. A group of words, such as a noun phrase, that can't be further divided without losing the essential meaning is an utterance, even though it may not be a sentence.
4. A sentence with two independent clauses joined by a coordinating conjunction is counted as one utterance. If the sentence contains more than two independent compound clauses, it is segmented so that the third clause, beginning with the conjunction, is a separate utterance.
5. Sentences with subordinate or relative clauses are always counted as single utterances.

Note. From *Assessing Children's Language in Naturalistic Contexts* (p. 209) by N. J. Lund and J. F. Duchan, 1988, Englewood Cliffs, NJ: Prentice-Hall. Copyright 1988 by Prentice-Hall. Reprinted by permission.

Box 8.8   Two methods of utterance segmentation

Excerpt from a language sample produced by a 9-year-old with a language-learning disability who is retelling the story of "Dumbo" (slashes indicate pauses).

so a circus was there and they had these other hands/he had these other people in it/so he first got in a train/and so he didn't get in the train cause he could fly/so he/Mr. Tyler wasn't/he was happy/he didn't care if the train was broke down/and so this little guy, Timothy, a little mouse, he gets on and they found a boat/so they sailed on the boat/and so hippopotamus/no/the elephant had to go up in a tiny bed/so the bed broke down and they try to XXX hippopotamus up there . . .

METHOD I.   Segmentation keeping the first two main clauses in coordinated compound sentences together (Lee, 1974; Lund & Duchan, 1988):

1. (so) a circus was there and they had these other hands/
2. he had these other people in it/
3. (so) he first got in a train/
4. (and so) he didn't get in the train cause he could fly/
5. (so he/Mr. Tyler wasn't/) he was happy/
6. he didn't care if the train was broke down/
7. (and so) this little guy, Timothy, a little mouse, he gets on and they found a boat/
8. (so) they sailed on the boat/
9. (and so hippopotamus/no/) the elephant had to go up in a tiny bed/
10. (so) the bed broke down and they try to XXX hippopotamus up there . . .

METHOD II.   Segmentation into T-units of one main clause with all subordinate clauses attached to it (Hunt, 1965):

1. (so) a circus was there
2. (and) they had these other hands/
3. he had these other people in it/
4. (so) he first got in the train/
5. (and so) he didn't get in the train cause he could fly/
6. (so he/Mr. Tyler wasn't) he was happy/
7. he didn't care if the train was broken down/
8. (and so) this little guy, Timothy, a little mouse, he gets on
9. (and) they found a boat/
10. (so) they sailed on the boat/
11. (and so hippopotamus/no/) the elephant had to go up in a tiny bed/
12. (so) the bed broke down
13. (and) they try to XXX hippopotamus up there . . .

Tyack and Gottsleben (1977) defined mastery of a particular structure as correct adult usage in 90% or more in obligatory contexts. Tyack and Gottsleben's system consists of constructing an outline of baseline forms (morphological developments) and constructions (syntactic developments) that have been mastered (1) at and below the assigned level or (2) above the assigned level. The specialist then can propose intervention goals based on evidence about forms and constructions that are at or below the assigned level and either (1) do not appear or (2) appear inconsistently (i.e., in less than 90% of obligatory contexts).

Another similar approach, called language assessment, remediation, and screening procedure (LARSP), was described by Crystal, Fletcher, and Garman (1976). Using the LARSP, the specialist summarizes evidence of both morphological and syntactic developments on a tally sheet, based on a 30-minute language sample. Crystal and his colleagues emphasized that positive evidence about the forms and constructions a child uses in spontaneous language is always more directly useful and reliable in defining a pattern than the negative evidence is. "The presence of a score is a positive indication of ability, whereas the absence of a score may mean only that the sample is biased" (p. 113). Once a child's sample is outlined on the summary chart, Crystal et al. defined the purpose of intervention as assisting the child to move "down the LARSP chart [from earlier to later developments] in as controlled a way as possible" (p. 117).

Perhaps the most complex aspect of morphological development in English is the acquisition of rules related to auxiliary verb construction. Auxiliary verbs are particularly important syntactic elements for their contributions to conveying, for example, questions (e.g., "He found it ⟶ Did he find it?"); negation (e.g., "He found it ⟶ He didn't find it"); tense (e.g., "He finds it ⟶ He will find it ⟶ He has found it"); and mood (e.g., "He can find it ⟶ He could find it"). Lee (1974) used Chomsky's (1957) auxiliary verb construction schema (see Figure 8.1) to design verb scoring for the Developmental Sentence Scoring (DSS) system (assigning credit ranging from 1 to 8) in the area of main verbs. Lee's procedure can give clinicians an internalized system for helping children to acquire more flexible strategies for conveying meanings using auxiliary verbs.

Other important aspects of morphological development include personal pronouns and articles. Recall from Chapter 4 that persistence in pronoun case problems is one area where the performance of children with specific language impairments has been discriminated from that of children with normally developing language skills (Leonard, 1980). When children have trouble including appropriate articles in their expressive language, they may have difficulty learning to recognize similar elements in written language and those opportunities may need to be probed as well.

Second, **questions about syntactic construction and comprehension** play an important role in language form analysis. When the analytical focus shifts from the level of inflectional morphology and function words to the level of sentence construction, the clinician should ask questions about children's abilities to construct well-formed simple sentences that include all essential elements in an acceptable sequence. A particular concern may be whether sentence subjects are included when obligated by the linguistic context. This is because, as noted in Chapter 4, the omission

---

Box 8.9	Development of 14 morphemes	

Brown's Order		De Villiers & De Villiers's Order	
-ing (no auxiliary verb)	(STAGE II)	*-ing* (no auxiliary verb)	(STAGE II)
in		regular plural, *-s*	
on		*in*	
regular plural, *-s*		*on*	(STAGE III)
irregular past (imitated)		possessive, *-'s*	
possessive, *-'s*		regular past, *-ed*	(STAGE V)
uncontractible copula, *be*	(STAGE III)	irregular past (imitated)	
articles, *a the*		regular third-person sing, *-s*	
regular past, *-ed*		articles, *a the*	
regular third-person sing, *-s*	(STAGE V)	contractible copula, *be*	
irregular third-person sing. (*does, has*)		contractible auxiliary, *be*	(STAGE V+)
uncontractible auxiliary, *be*		uncontractible copula, *be*	
contractible copula, *be*		uncontractible auxiliary, *be*	
contractible auxiliary, *be*		irregular third-person singular (*does, has*)	

Note. Although the sequences of morphological development reported by R.A. Brown (1973) and De Villiers and De Villiers (1973) are quite similar, some differences are evident, especially in the order of contractible and uncontractible verb forms. (Brown also found some variation in order and stage of acquisition for his three famous subjects, Adam, Eve, and Sarah.) All 14 regular morphemes are acquired by Stage V+ (MLU 4.5+) by children acquiring standard English normally, but most children continue to sort out irregular forms into their school-age years. Children learning dialectal variants of English such as Black English-Vernacular or Spanish-influenced English follow a different developmental pattern.

FIGURE 8.1

Chomsky's (1957) auxiliary verb construction rule. C + (Modal) + (have + en) + (be + ing) + MV

Score	Developmental Verb Forms	Chomsky's schema: C(M) (have + en) (be + ing) V	Transformations and Colloquial Forms
1 0	I *play*. It *is* good. It's good. He *play*. She *play*. It *play*.	V	
0	I *playing*. He *playing*.	ing V	
0 1	I *is playing*. You *is playing*. He *is playing*.	is + ing V	
2 2 2	He *plays*. He *played*. I *am playing*. He *was playing*. We *are* good. They *were* good.	C pres. past (be + ing) V -s -ed am, are was, were	
4 4 4 4	I *can play*. He *will play*. Transformations: I *don't* play. They *don't* play. *Do* you *play*? Do they *play*? They *do play*.	C (M) V pres. can, will, may	Transformations: Obligatory *do* + negative + question Emphasis
6 6 6 6 6	He *could play*. He *would play*. He *might play*. He *should play*. Transformations: He *doesn't* play. He *didn't* play. *Does* he *play*? *Did* he *play*? He *does play*. He *did play*.	C (M) V past could, would might, should	Transformations: Obligatory *does, did*: + negative + question Emphasis
7 7 7 7 7	I *must play*. I *shall play*. (rare) I *have eaten*. I *had eaten*. Colloquial form: I*'ve got* to play. The music *was being played*. The music *could have been played*.	C (M) V pres. must, shall C (have + en) V pres. past. Passives of all tenses are scored the same.	Colloquial form: *have got* Transformation: Passive
8 8 8 8	I *have been playing*. I *may have eaten*. I *might be playing*. I *might have been playing*. Etc.	C (M) (have + en) (be + ing) V pres. past	

C, an abstract symbol for markers indicating person (first, second, or third), tense, and number; MV, main verb.

Note. From *Developmental Sentence Analysis* (p. 13) by L. L. Lee, 1974, Evanston, IL: Northwestern University Press. Copyright 1974 by Northwestern University Press. Reprinted by permission.

of sentence subjects may be a danger sign that a young child's language development is not proceeding normally. Development of question and negative forms have also been studied extensively, and data from that research may be used to analyze the target child's constructions as well (e.g., Crystal et al. 1976; Lee, 1974; J.F. Miller, 1981; Tyack and Gottsleben, 1977).

Beyond the simple sentence level, it is important to ask about children's abilities to construct and comprehend complex sentences. Rhea Paul (1981) suggested some strategies for analyzing complex sentence development to accompany J. F. Miller's (1981) ASS procedure. To perform this analysis, it may be helpful to make a listing transcript, in which all of the sentences of a particular type are pulled out from the overall sample and listed. A set of criteria for analyzing complex constructions is summarized in

Box 8.10. Some information about complex sentence development also may be obtained from the J.F. Miller and Chapman (1986) SALT program for computer analysis of language samples by asking the software program to list the number of different conjunctions and the number of times each conjunction appears in the sample.

Third, **questions about contextually based variation related to language content and use** are used to guide assessment of the child's ability to adjust lan-

---

Box 8.10   The development of compound and complex sentences

Developmental stage information is based on suggestions by R. Paul (1981) for the point at which 50% to 90% of children exhibit a structure and by Lee (1974) for assigning Developmental Sentence Scores (DSS). As a rule of thumb, whenever a sentence contains two verbs that are not related as auxiliary and main verb, a compound or complex sentence form is evident.

Catenative (semiauxiliary) forms *gonna* **(in Black English Vernacular, children may use** /fɪn tə/ **"fixin' to"),** *wanna, hafta.*   These forms appear early, and rather than representing infinitival embeddings, probably function more as auxiliaries in simple sentences.
(Stage II; scores 2 as secondary verb in DSS.)
     "I'm gonna make some."
Early forms *let's, let me.*   These forms also act similar to unanalyzed catenatives. Note that they involve obligatory deletion of the infinitival *to.*
(Early Stage IV; scores 2 as secondary verb in DSS.)
     "Let me do it."
Simple infinitives with equivalent subjects in both clauses.
(Early Stage IV; scores 3 as secondary verb in DSS.)
     "I have to see."
     "He wants to come."
Compound sentences conjoined by *and.*   These are sentences in which two independent clauses are joined.
(Early Stage IV; the conjunction *and* scores 3 in DSS.)
     "He looked out the door and he saw a big dog."
Full propositional complements.   Full propositional complements occur when a complete sentence is used as the object of another sentence, usually following verbs such as *know, wonder, guess, think, pretend, hope, show,* and *forget,* which name an action that brings something into existence. The clause may or may not start with *that,* but does not begin with a *wh-* word.
(Early Stage IV; if used, *that* scores 8 as a conjunction in DSS.)
     "I know (that) he did it."
     "I think (that) that's right."
     "He said (that) he might come."
Simple noninfinitive *wh-* **clauses.**   Other early subordinate clauses are introduced by the subordinating conjunctions *what, where, why,* or *how* (these were called *indirect or embedded questions* by R. A. Brown, 1973).
(Early Stage IV; some *wh-* words score 6 as relative pronouns, and others score 8 as conjunctions in DSS.)
     "That's why it happened."
     "That's what I thought."
     "She knows how it works."

guage form to covary appropriately with language con-tent and use. Children must know how to use rules for expressing language content–form interactions to make sense to their communicative partners and to express their ideas effectively (Lahey, 1988). A vari-ety of assessment questions can be asked about these abilities. For example, one might ask whether a child in the latter part of the middle stages has the syntactic flexibility to emphasize the importance of an event affecting the object of a sentence by using a complex passive construction to move the object to the initial position (e.g., "After she fell, the girl was chased across the parking lot"). Additionally, can the child understand passive-construction sentences encountered in teacher talk or in books? Can the child paraphrase individual or multiple sentences that encode multiple semantic relations in complex or embedded sentences? Can the child understand and use productively rules of complex pronominal refer-ence that contribute to discourse cohesion?

Box 8.10   *continued*

Double embeddings.   These forms are credited when one clause is embedded within another (one of which might include a catenative).

(Late Stage IV – Early V; all primary and secondary verbs score in DSS.)
  "I'm gonna think about how to do it."
  "You hafta let me come."

Infinitive clauses with differing subjects.   In these sentences, the subject of the embedded sentence differs from that of the main sentence.

(Late Stage V; score 5 as secondary verbs in DSS.)
  "I want you to be my friend."
  "How do you get this to work?"

Subordinating conjunction *if* is used.

(Late Stage V; *if* scores 5 in DSS.)
  "I can come if you invite me."

Relative clauses.   These modify noun constituents of main sentences. They are introduced by one of the relative pronouns *which, who, that,* or *what.*

(Late Stage V; relative pronouns score 6 in DSS.)
  "It's the one that I want."
  "That's the dog who bit me."

Unmarked infinitive clauses.   These are embedded infinitive clauses that do not contain *to* in the surface sentence, and usually follow verbs like *let, make, watch,* or *help.*

(Stage V+; score 5 as secondary verbs in DSS.)
  "He made her fall down."
  "She'll let me go."

***Wh-* infinitive clauses.**   These clauses are introduced by a *wh-* word and include the infinitival *to.*

(Stage V+; score 5 as secondary verbs in DSS.)
  "Do you know how to do it?"
  "Show me what to do."

Coordinating conjunction *because* is used.

(Stage V+; *because* scores 6 in DSS.)
  "The boy fell because his bike hit a rock."

Gerund clauses.   Gerunds are verbs with *-ing* endings that are used as part of a noun clause.

(Stage V+; gerunds score 8 as secondary verbs in DSS)
  "I like making noise."
  "He hurt me by pushing me down."

Subordinating conjunctions *when* and *so* are used.

(Stage V++; *so* scores 5, and *when* scores 8 in DSS.)
  "Tell me when it's time."
  "He whispered so she wouldn't hear him."

What about language form–use interactions? For example, what happens when an adult or child conversational partner fails to understand something that the child has tried to communicate? What are the target child's syntactic resources for rephrasing the utterance and repairing the communication? Can anything be learned from the child's linguistic nonfluencies, such as revision and maze behaviors, about potential problems in language formulation? Do contextual variables (linguistic, situational, or emotional) appear to co-occur with difficulty in formulating language? What are the child's syntactic resources for making polite, indirect requests (and understanding them)? Does the child use different syntactic style appropriately when communicating with different kinds of partners in different kinds of settings? Does the child have syntactic resources for expressing and understanding deictic relationships of person, place, and time? (*Deixis* is reference to relationships that vary with the speaker's perspective, e.g., *your book* becomes *my book* when the person speaking changes; *here* becomes *there* when the speaker's relative position to an object changes; "We are going to the zoo *tomorrow*" becomes "We went to the zoo *yesterday*" when the relative temporal relationship to the event changes.)

An additional set of questions that should be asked, particularly when analyzing contextually based language form interactions is whether any variations noted might represent the influence of a set of linguistic rules differing from the standard English rules on which most analysis systems are based. For example, if the child hears a mixture of Spanish and English spoken at home, or is learning English from parents who themselves learned English as a second language, it is highly likely that morphological development (particularly) will not follow the expected developmental pattern for middle-socioeconomic-class native standard English speakers. Children whose primary home language is Black English Vernacular (BEV) also will learn different language rules as part of the normal developmental process. When professionals assess the language of these children, they must consider which features represent developmental delays or abnormalities and which represent legitimate rules of other linguistic systems. This requires knowledge of more than one linguistic system and the ability to apply contrastive linguistic analysis techniques to identify features representing language difference.

Appendix C demonstrates one system for differentiating language difference from disorder, called Black English Sentence Scoring (BESS). I have developed this technique over several years, most recently in collaboration with Yvette Hyter (N.W. Nelson & Hyter, 1990a, 1990b), and with consultation from Walt Wolfram of the Center for Applied Linguistics. BESS is not an independent assessment system. It is an analysis procedure that uses the techniques of Lee's (1974) Developmental Sentence Scoring (DSS). Children who use features of BEV also use features predicted by rules of standard English. Therefore, when a child's language sample is analyzed using BESS, the child is given credit for all structures that score in eight grammatical categories analyzed with DSS (indefinite pronouns and noun modifiers, personal pronouns, main verbs, secondary verbs, negatives, conjunctions, auxiliary inversion in questions, and Wh- questions). In addition, the child receives credit for structures that are acceptable according to the rules of adult BEV as represented in the scoring standards of BESS. By adding up the points awarded according to DSS and BESS standards (including sentence points given differentially according to DSS and BESS standards) and dividing by 50, a mean BESS is computed that can be compared to a set of preliminary normative data gathered based on samples from 64 normally developing children of African-American descent (most were from Kansas and Michigan, but a few were from Florida, Texas, Chicago, and Washington, DC) between the ages of 3:0 and 7:0 who were all learning BEV as a primary linguistic system. Nonbiased evidence about the development of language form can be added to other pieces of information about the child and his or her language to make quantitative as well as qualitative decisions about the child's need for special services and potential areas to be targeted by short-term objectives.

Analyzing language content variables. Analysis of middle-stage language content should include description of (1) the child's lexicon at the word level; (2) semantic roles the child uses and understands at the sentence level; (3) topics and topic organization strategies available to the child at the discourse level; and (4) the child's ability to linguistically encode and decode information representing world knowledge at broader cognitive processing levels.

First, the clinician should attempt to **characterize the lexicon in the spontaneous language sample**.

Lexical quantification for children beyond the stage of early vocabulary acquisition is difficult. Most language samples tap only a small portion of the total lexicon a child might be able to use. When a child does not use certain words in a spontaneous sampling context, it is difficult to know whether the child's lexicon is limited or whether the sampling context was limited. This problem may be particularly acute when children and clinicians come from different cultural backgrounds and world experiences.

A quantitative technique sometimes recommended for measuring vocabulary diversity is the type/token ratio (TTR). Type/token ratios are computed by dividing the total number of different words (types) in a speaker's sample by the total number of all words produced (tokens) by the speaker in the sample. The SALT program (J.F. Miller & Chapman, 1986) computes the TTR automatically, making it a fairly easy measure to obtain. The question is, what does the measure mean? A problem with the TTR is that it tends to be negatively related to increasing sample lengths, because, as sentence length increases, grammatical function words tend to make up a greater proportion of the total sample. Therefore, older children, who generally produce longer samples and use more complex grammatical constructions (with a higher proportion of function words), may in fact have relatively lower TTRs. If the sample length is not controlled, TTR comparisons may be meaningless, or even deceptive. However, as Loban (1963) commented, the TTR measure "can disclose important distinctions *when the size of the language sample is kept uniform*" (p. 22). It is also helpful to be aware of the general rule of thumb suggested by J.F. Miller (1981) based on the data Mildred Templin (1957) gathered for 480 3:0- to 8:0-year-old children. Across this age range, across both genders, and regardless of socioeconomic status, Templin found TTRs of approximately 1:2, or 0.50. Miller suggested, if a normal hearing child's TTR is significantly below 0.50 we can be reasonably certain the sparseness of vocabulary use is *not* an artifact of SES but is probably indicative of a language-specific deficiency" (1981, p. 41).

Because of problems with the TTR, Bennett (1989) developed another analysis technique, which he called Referential Semantic Analysis (RSA), as an alternative method to measure expressive vocabulary diversity. Rather than using a ratio that varies little with increasing age and vocabulary development,

Bennett and Alter (1985) gathered normative data on the means for the total words and number of different words produced in 50 utterance samples by youngsters between the ages of 2 and 15 years. These data provide evidence of developmental advances. Bennett's original samples included 20 middle-class normally developing children (rural and urban Virginians) at each age level. The children were grouped into 6-month intervals from ages 2 to 5 years, into 1-year intervals from 5 to 12 years, and into 2-year intervals for the age range of 13 to 15 years. In a follow-up study, Olson and Bennett (1987a, 1987b) studied test–retest reliability and possible geographic differences for a group of 24 children (6- and 7-years-olds) by comparing 12 children from Virginia with 12 children from North Dakota. Their findings showed no significant geographic differences and significant test–retest reliability coefficients of .68 for number of different words and .88 for number of total words. A computer software program (Bennett, 1989) facilitates the computation of RSA data and generates separate counts for the number of different words and total words coded as nouns, verbs, adjectives, adverbs, pronouns, conjunctions, prepositions, articles, and "other." The program can also generate the derived ages, as well as the overall number of different and total words for the complete sample, along with derived ages (age-equivalency scores).

Bennett's (1989) RSA probably still should be considered preliminary for several reasons. The normative sample was somewhat limited in size and in geographic, socioeconomic, and cultural representativeness. Questions, such as those discussed in Chapter 6, also might arise about the decision to use age-equivalency scores rather than other kinds of standard measurements (e.g., those using standard deviations) to judge developmental adequacy. The decision to code words by parts of speech rather than by more semantically representative categories might also be questioned. Nevertheless, this is an interesting new approach that holds promise for making quantitative comparisons to normative data and for making qualitative decisions about areas to target in intervention. For example, Bennett and James (1990) presented several guidelines for interpreting RSA results, noting that maximum growth patterns for an individual child's total lexicon should be considered as well as patterns based on different rates in normal development. However, when children's RSA data show patterns (based on derived age scores) such as low use of verbs, low use of conjunctions, or a high use of pronouns combined with a relatively low use of nouns, language intervention may need to specifically target corresponding aspects of their lexical systems.

Many other questions might be asked about the child's lexicon based on evidence from spontaneous language samples. For example, does the child have a variety of words to indicate fine shades of meaning or seem to have to make do with a limited set of nonspecific "all-purpose" words such as *stuff* and *thing?* Does the child create any new words using derivational morphemes that seem generative rather than merely imitative (e.g., "destoppable tank")? By the middle grades in elementary school, does the child understand many multiple-meaning words and figurative meanings? Does the child use appropriate memory and recall strategies to acquire the lexicon appropriate to key contexts of the child's life, such as preschool and early elementary school classrooms?

Second, questioning about language content might address **semantic roles the child uses and understands at the sentence level**. For example, does the child use words that fill a variety of semantic roles (e.g., actor, action, state, location, time), or does the child encode only a limited variety of semantic relations? A summary of four studies of the development of semantic relationships (Stockman & Vaughn-Cooke, 1986) showed that 11 major and 12 minor semantic categories were all represented in the language samples of children in Post Stage II (MLU > 4.0) by the age of 53 to 54 months. Even more important, these findings were consistent across the three subject populations, working class black children, working class white children, and middle-class white children. The 11 major categories were *existence, action, locative action, state, locative state, negation, possession, attribution, notice, intention,* and *recurrence*. The 12 minor categories were *Wh- question, place, action + place, dative, instrument, quantity, time, mood, coordination, causality, epistemic,* and *antithesis*.

A third level of analysis might address **topics and topic organization strategies available to the child at the discourse level.** Brinton and Fujiki (1989) described this area as encompassing both what speakers talk *about* and how speakers *manage* what they talk about. In asking what children talk about, the clinician might ask whether particular categories or topics appear frequently and might ask questions about the nature of the topics. For example, does the child talk mostly about concrete things or also some abstract topics? By the time children enter the middle stages of language acquisition, they should be able to talk about remote topics as well as the here-and-now (review discussion in Chapter 7). For children in elementary school the specialist may use language sampling to probe their understanding and ability to talk about curricular content.

Questions might also address topic organization and manipulation strategies. Brinton and Fujiki (1989) included questions about how topics are introduced, continued, changed, and recycled. They noted that topic manipulation strategies change with increasing age and linguistic maturity. Roots of topic management are found in the interactions of care givers and infants with the establishment of joint reference (discussed in Chapter 7). Growth in topic management involves a reduction in the child's dependence on adults to construct and change topic sequences and a reduction in the number of different topics introduced in a particular time period. Five-year-olds are more likely to recycle previous topics in conversations than 9-year-olds are, but research has also shown considerable variability in several areas across different age groups (Brinton & Fujiki, 1984). The development of independent strategies to manipulate topics is observed well into middle childhood (Brinton & Fujiki, 1989). Many questions might be asked in this area. For example, can the child organize topics logically and follow topic shading strategies to connect one with another? Are there any unusual delays in responding or perseverative topics that might suggest emotional impairment or other processing difficulties? Does the child focus on tangential aspects of topics and seem unable to grasp the big picture?

A final level of analysis regarding language content might address the child's ability to **linguistically encode and decode information representing world knowledge at broader cognitive processing levels.** At the information processing level, what can be hypothesized about the child's developing perceptual and cognitive abilities based on topics the child talks about? Are the child's word memory and recall strategies adequate?

How do higher levels of language comprehension relate to broader understanding of the world? Milosky (1990) reviewed alternative language comprehension models. According to the traditional decoding model of language comprehension, listeners start by using semantic and syntactic decoding strategies to generate a small number of possible meanings for individual sentences, after which, as necessary, they disambiguate the limited number of possible meanings by using available contextual information. The alternative model suggests that almost every word has many possible meanings, and that, to understand, listeners must *start* the language comprehension process by drawing on existing world knowledge. Then they activate only relevant senses of words and information and attempt to make incoming information relevant to what they already know. Milosky described this more efficient process as follows:

> The relevant information, or world knowledge, that is accessed and activated is, in part, determined by what knowledge is relevant given the speaker, the physical environment, the social occasion, the goals of the interaction, the affective variables, and the prior discussion. These all enable a listener to determine rapidly and selectively what a speaker is saying. (1990, p. 3)

The implications of this alternative view are significant for guiding language assessment and intervention. Assessment and intervention goals shift from learning a set of words or structures to learning how "to call up relevant knowledge and to use language in order to interact and add to that knowledge in some coherent fashion" (Milosky, 1990, p. 4).

Analyzing language use variables. Analysis of middle-stage language use might include description of (1) the child's ability to use language to communicate a variety of intentions and to perform a variety of pragmatic functions; (2) the child's ability to organize discourse of several types; and (3) the child's ability to use and understand contextually based variations in linguistic, paralinguistic, and nonlinguistic communicative features.

Questions about the adequacy of children's language use relate ultimately to definitions of communicative competence. The classic definition of communicative competence was provided by sociolinguist Dell Hymes (1972b), who defined it as a language user's

> . . . knowledge of sentences, not only as grammatical but also as appropriate. He or she acquires competence as to when to speak, when not, and as to what to talk about with whom, when, where, in what manner. In short, a child becomes able to accomplish a repertoire

of speech acts, to take part in speech events, and to evaluate their accomplishments by others. (p. 277)

When assessing communicative competence, the first level of analysis might address the child's **use of varied pragmatic functions and expression of intention.** This aspects relates to the first of three clusters identified by Dollaghan and Miller (1986) to guide observations of communicative competence. They identified it as the set of "communicative intents, communicative functions, or speech acts: the reasons for which speakers communicate" (p. 116).

This analysis is based on the question "What purposes do the child's utterances seem to serve?" It may be difficult to decide how to categorize the speech acts of a particular child. As noted in Chapter 7, taxonomies of communicative intentions have been proposed by a variety of authors (e.g., Bates et al., 1975; Dale, 1980; Dore, 1974; Halliday, 1975a, 1975b), some of whom argue that no one taxonomy should be applied to all children because one set of categories may characterize the language of a given normally developing child better at one point than another (Halliday, 1975; Lund & Duchan, 1988). Dollaghan and Miller (1986) also noted that taxonomies based only on normal development may "fail to capture numerous aspects of the performance of the disordered subjects" (p. 109). The need to consider how variations of communicative intention may be expressed by children with language disorders was illustrated by the work of Prizant and his colleagues (Prizant, 1987; Prizant & Duchan, 1981; Prizant & Rydell, 1984) when they analyzed the echolalic utterances of children with autism into different categories based on the varied functions they served.

Taxonomies for organizing pragmatic functions into categories for children functioning at the preverbal and single-word levels were presented in Chapter 7 (see Tables 7.4 and 7.5), based on summarizes by Roth and Spekman (1984). Here, Roth and Spekman's third level, which summarizes categories appropriate to middle-stage multiword levels of production, is reprinted (see Table 8.3). The inclusion of this particular taxonomical set should not suggest, however, that these are the only, or even the most important, categories to consider.

To be useful in intervention, speech-act analysis should surpass merely coding and counting pragmatic intentions. Fey (1986) proposed a decision-making matrix based on the relative use of assertive and

TABLE 8.3

Communicative intentions expressed at the multiword stage of development

Intention	Definition	Example
1. Requesting information	Utterances that solicit information, permission, confirmation, or repetition.	"Where's Mary?" "Can I come?"
2. Requesting action	Utterances that solicit action or cessation of action.	"Give me the doll." "Stop it." "Don't do that."
3. Responding to requests	Utterances that supply solicited information or acknowledge preceding messages.	"Okay." "Mary is over there." "No, you can't come." "It's blue."
4. Stating or commenting	Utterances that state facts or rules, express beliefs, attitudes, or emotions, or describe environmental aspects.	"This a bird." "You have to throw the dice, first." "I don't like dogs." "I'm happy today." "My school is two blocks away." "He can't do that."
5. Regulating conversational behavior	Utterances that monitor and regulate interpersonal contact.	"Hey, Marvin!" "Hi," "Bye," "Please." "Here you are."
6. Other performatives	Utterances that tease, warn, claim, exclaim, or convey humor.	"Know what I did?" "You can't catch me." "Watch out." "It's my turn." "The dog said 'moo.'"

Note. From "Assessing the Pragmatic Abilities of Children: Part 1. Organizational Framework and Assessment Parameters" by F. P. Roth and N. J. Spekman, 1984, *Journal of Speech and Hearing Disorders, 49,* p. 5. Copyright 1984 by American Speech-Language-Hearing Association. Reprinted by permission.

responsive conversational acts by young children that can contribute to goal setting. In Fey's system, *assertive acts* include requestives of four types (for information, action, clarification, and attention); *assertives* of three types (comments, statements, and disagreements); and performatives (e.g., claims, jokes, teasing, protests, and warnings). *Responsive acts* include responses to requests of four types (for information, action, clarification, and attention), and responses to assertives and performatives. Fey uses two other categories to classify individual utterances as imitations or as other (when they do not fit well into any of the other three categories). Beyond the utterance level, conversational acts are also coded at the discourse level, depending on whether they serve to initiate, maintain, or extend topics, or to extend topics tangentially (not adequately). Children who show a high rate of both assertive and responsive conversational acts are *active conversationalists.* Children who show a high rate of assertive acts but a

low rate of responsive ones are *verbal noncommunicators.* Children who show a low rate of assertive acts but a high rate of responsive ones are *passive conversationalists.* Children who are low in use of either assertive or responsive acts are *inactive communicators* (see Figure 4.1). Children with these varied patterns of conversational speech acts are considered to have different intervention needs (see Box 8.13, later in chapter, for potential goals).

Another system for coding spontaneous social interactions among preschoolers was devised by Rice, Sell, and Hadley (1990). Called the Social Interactive Coding System (SICS), this is an observational tool that can be used "on-line" (i.e., while the events are occurring) to code behaviors in a variety of categories related to social interaction in free play. These include the start time (5-minute blocks are observed), play activity, addressee, verbal interactive status, script code (type of play area), play level (solitary, adjacent, or social interactive), and language used (the approach may be used with bilingual children). The verbal interactive behaviors that are coded include initiation (coded as repetition if repeated after the first initiation fails), response (coded as one-word verbal R-V-1, multiword verbal R-V, or nonverbal R-NV), and ignore.

After gathering information about speech act behavior the specialist might address a second level of analysis, the child's **ability to organize and participate in the production of discourse of several types.** This cluster was identified by Dollaghan and Miller (1986) as the cluster of pragmatic phenomena related to "rules for sequencing communicative acts, or for constructing and managing discourse" (p. 116). The major types of organization to be probed include free conversation, narrative, and expository discourse.

The usual discourse context for gathering language samples is free conversation with an adult. This is the genre of participant discourse (J. N. Britton, 1979), discussed previously. As examples of the kinds of rules used in structuring conversational discourse, Dollaghan and Miller (1986) listed (1) initiating and terminating conversational sequences, (2) exchanging speaker turns, (3) introducing and maintaining topics, and (4) identifying and repairing conversational breakdowns. A variety of potential problems have been identified in this area among children with specific language impairments. For example, Brinton and Fujiki (1982) found that children with specific language impairments who were between ages 5:6 and 6:0 years frequently ignored or responded inappropriately to conversational requests. However, some of their problems seemed to be related more to difficulty in managing language content than in managing language use. Some of the children showed skill in using strategies that facilitated the flow of conversations but showed no understanding of the content.

In their book on conversational management with language-impaired children, Brinton and Fujiki (1989) suggested a variety of questions to ask when screening conversational samples of children with potential language disorders, including the following: Does the child initiate topics or mostly respond to questions asked by the conversational partner? Does the child seem to stay on topic or make frequent switches without preparing the listener? (Questions of this sort also relate to language content.) Does the child have presupposition skills to judge how much information should be shared with the listener? Does the child have strategies to repair communication when it breaks down?

Although conversational discourse provides an important context for judging communicative competence, it is not the only discourse style to probe. As illustrated by K. Nelson's (1989) bedtime transcripts of 2-year-old Emily, not unusually, rather young children produce monologues that approximate the structure of narratives. By probing narrative discourse contexts, professionals can determine whether a child has internalized rules related to the genre of spectator discourse (J. N. Britton, 1979) involving longer turns, more organized structures, and domination by a single speaker. (See further discussion of the narrative genre and criteria for assessing six levels of narrative organization, suggested by Applebee, 1978, in Chapter 9.)

When observing narrative development, the clinician can also ask questions about the child's apparent internalization of a narrative schema, sometimes referred to as "story grammar." Several variations of story grammar schemata have been proposed (e.g., N. S. Johnson & Mandler, 1980; Rumelhart, 1975; Stein & Glenn, 1979; Thorndyke, 1977). Most describe a discourse schema that includes one or more episodes with information about setting (e.g., person, place, and time), a problem, some action aimed at alleviating the problem (more complex story grammar schemas include a plan by the protagonist before taking action), an outcome, and an ending, which completes the story by relating logically to issues raised in the beginning. A description of feelings, personality traits, and motives of main characters are also observed in more mature narratives (Westby, 1984, 1985, 1991).

Telling and comprehending narratives requires more than a knowledge of story grammar. Judith Johnston (1982) suggested that professionals analyze narrative ability by looking for evidence that children use story grammar (including both a setting and a coherent episode structure); use mature organization; use knowledge of common event scripts and sequences in constructing a plot; operationalize linguistic textual cohesion devices (e.g., pronoun reference and complex sentences); and demonstrate sensitivity to the needs of the listener. The ultimate test is whether the story was communicated clearly.

The third discourse type that the specialist might probe through spontaneous sampling is **expository.** Because of its importance in later stages of language acquisition, expository discourse is discussed more fully and illustrated in Chapter 9. Expository discourse may be defined simply as discourse that conveys factual or technical information. This discourse is demanded when a child is asked to explain the rules of a game, how to make something, the characteristics of an object, or to engage in "show-and-tell." Some expository discourse, such as that used to explain the making of a peanut butter sandwich, is ordered by temporal sequence. Other expository discourse, such as a discussion of pets, may be organized as a series of hierarchically or horizontally related categories, with definitions and examples of each. Most academic discourse produced by teachers and in textbooks is expository.

Questions to ask about expository discourse include the following: Does the child have enough cognitive control of the topic to organize an explanation logically? Does the child use linguistic cohesion devices, such as complex sentences and logical connectors? Does the child demonstrate excessive linguistic nonfluencies (e.g., mazes, tangles, and revisions) that suggest internalized processing and text formulation difficulties? Does the child show evidence of comprehending expository discourse produced by others orally or in textbooks?

The third level analysis of pragmatic aspects of language development asks about the child's **ability to use and understand contextually based variations in linguistic, paralinguistic, and nonlinguistic form and content.** This cluster of behaviors was identified by Dollaghan and Miller (1986) as "the ways in which speakers and listeners integrate linguistic and nonlinguistic information and includes rules for presupposing and foregrounding information" (p. 116). Dollaghan and Miller also included rules for selecting and maintaining speech register and for using cohesion devices and deixis (considered previously under issues of language form). Children with language impairments, especially those with specific language impairments, may not always show delays relative to their normally developing peers in these areas. When Fey and Leonard (1984) investigated discourse adaptation skills of 4:6-to 6-year-old children, based on whether they were talking to adults, age-peers, or toddlers, they found that children with specific language impairments performed at least as well as normally developing younger-age language-matched peers and below the levels of same-age peers in only a few areas (related to form variables such as MLU and the ability to ask internal state questions).

Many questions might be used to focus language sample analysis on pragmatic adaptation, including the following: Does the child seem to have ways of altering the delivery style to achieve a certain effect (e.g., teasing, polite forms)? Does the child seem to understand such variations? Does the child have any strategies for helping out if the listener fails to understand something the child said? Can this child participate appropriately in classroom discussions?

Formal Assessment

Although informal assessment of spontaneous language samples provides some of the most useful information about the nature of children's language abilities and disabilities, it is not sufficient for all assessment purposes. Formal assessment with standardized instruments may be essential to identify children as having a language disorder, for example. It may also help a professional to check clinical impressions of relative strengths and weaknesses against the performance of normative groups.

Unfortunately, many formal standardized tests seem to promise more than they can deliver. McCauley and Swisher (1984) applied 10 psychometric criteria for norm-referenced tests to a review of 30 language and articulation tests designed to be used with preschool children: (1) description of the normative sample, (2) adequate sample size, (3) item analysis used to promote test reliability and validity, (4) report of measures of central tendency and variability for relevant subgroups, (5) evidence of concurrent validity, (6) evidence of predictive validity, (7) estimate of test–retest reliability, (9) detailed description of administration and scoring procedures, and (10) specification of qualifications required of test administrators or scorers. They found that half of the tests met no more than two of the criteria (most often, numbers 9 and 10). Most frequently *unmet* criteria were those requiring empirical evidence of test validity and reliability. Table 8.4 summarizes the results for the 30 instruments McCauley and Swisher reviewed. The full identification of these instruments appears in Appendix A with the summary of test instruments designed for the middle stages of language acquisition.

McCauley and Swisher (1984) noted the possibility that psychometric test-evaluation may discourage the use of standardized tests. Rather than avoiding formal test use entirely, however, they recommended that potential test users should become more sophisticated in recognizing psychometric flaws and should consider these limitations when interpreting test results and making clinical decisions. They also pointed out that "clinical decisions are never properly based on test results alone" (p. 41). Furthermore, they noted that, by being selective consumers, those who purchase standardized tests may influence premarketing development of these instruments.

Standardized tests are most useful when professionals select them to test diagnostic hypotheses. The first hypothesis tested may be rather broad. It may simply be that the child will score below normal limits on a broad comprehensive test of language abilities. For this purpose, tests that include a variety of sub-tests, such as the Clinical Evaluation of Language Fundamentals — Revised (CELF-R) (Semel et al., 1987) or the Test of Language Development – 2 Primary

(TOLD-2 P) (Newcomer & Hammill, 1988), may be used with children in middle stages of language acquisition. The best way to learn about the strengths and foibles of a particular instrument is to administer it to many children. No test is without its limitations, and it is important to remember that any standardized test may be either useless or harmful for children whose backgrounds differ from those of the normative group. Nevertheless, standardized batteries like the CELF-R and the TOLD-2 P provide a profile of relative strengths and weaknesses for many children. Directions for giving a standardized test must be followed explicitly. Some adjustments, however, may be made when interpreting results of subtests that may be biased for particular children.

In addition to results of broad comprehensive tests, participant interviews and spontaneous com-

TABLE 8.4
Tests meeting psychometric criteria established by McCauley & Swisher (1984)

Criterion	Number of tests	Tests
1. Description of normative sample	3	ITPA, PPVT-R, TOLD
2. Sample size	6	BTBC, ITPA, PPVT-R, STACL, SOLST, TOLD
3. Item analysis	9	BTBC, EOWPVT, ITPA, PPVT, PPVT-R, QT, SICD, T-D, TOLD
4. Means and standard deviations	7	ICLAT, PAT, PPVT, T-D, TACL, TOLD, TTC
5. Concurrent validity	5	CELI, PLAI, PLST, TOLD, VLDS
6. Predictive validity	0	—
7. Test–retest reliability	1	TOLD
8. Interexaminer reliability	0	—
9. Description of test procedures	25	ACLC, BLST, BTBC, CELI, DASE, EOWPVT, ICLAT, ITPA, LAS, NSST, PAT, PLAI, PPVT, PPVT-R, REEL-scale, STACL, SICD, SOLST, T-D, TACL, TOLD, TTC, UTLD, VANE-L, VLDS
10. Description of tester qualifications	14	BLST, ICLAT, ITPA, PLAI, PPVT, PPVT-R, QT, SICD, STACL, SOLST, TACL, TOLD, UTLD, VANE-L

ACLC, Assessment of Children's Language Comprehension; BLST, Bankson Language Screening Test; BTBC, Boehm Test of Basic Concepts; CELI, Carrow Elicited Language Inventory; DASE, The Denver Articulation Screening Examination; EOWPVT, Expressive One Word Picture Vocabulary Test; ICLAT, Illinois Children's Language Assessment Test; ITPA, Illinois Test of Psycholinguistic Abilities; LAS, Laradon Articulation Scale; NSST, Northwestern Syntax Screening Test; PAT, Photo Articulation Test; PLAI, Preschool Language Assessment Instrument; PLST, Preschool Language Screening Test; PPVT, Peabody Picture Vocabulary Test; PPVT-R, Peabody Picture Vocabulary Test—Revised; QT, The Quick Test; REEL, The Receptive Expressive Emergent Language Scale; SICD, Sequenced Inventory of Communication Development; SOLST, Stephens Oral Language Screening Test; STACL, The Screening Test of Auditory Comprehension of Language; T-D, Templin-Darley Tests of Articulation; TACL, The Test of Auditory Comprehension of Language; TOLD, Test of Language Development; TTC, The Token Test for Children; UTLD, Utah Test of Language Development; VANE, Vane Evaluation of Language Scale; VLDS, Verbal Language Development Scale.

Note. From "Psychometric Review of Language and Articulation Tests for Preschool Children" by R. J. McCauley and L. Swisher, 1984, *Journal of Speech and Hearing Disorders, 49*, p. 40. Copyright 1984 by American Speech-Language-Hearing Association. Reprinted by permission.

munication samples can be used to refine hypotheses about probable areas of greater strength and difficulty for a particular child. Then, deeper tests of more narrow areas may be selected to evaluate those hypotheses. I usually select at least one more specific assessment device in an area I hypothesize to be an area of relative strength as well as one of relative weakness. For example, if I am testing a kindergarten child whose primary difficulty seems to be in the area of language form, with relatively higher skills in the area of language content and use, I might use the Structured Photographic Expressive Language Test–II (SPELT-II) (Werner & Kresheck, 1983) to confirm and to round out the data from spontaneous sampling about expressive syntax. I might also administer the Boehm Test of Basic Concepts—Revised (BTBC-R) (Boehm, 1986) or the Bracken Basic Concept Scale (BBCS) (Bracken, 1984) to test my impression that this child can handle key relational concepts and

vocabulary important for understanding school discourse in kindergarten and first grade. If I am evaluating a slightly older child, I might use The Word Test—R (Huisingh, Barrett, Zachman, Blagden, & Orman, 1990) and informal strategies of curriculum-based language assessment (discussed in Chapter 9) to identify problems related to difficulty in understanding written and oral instructions and stories.

A difficult but important decision to be made during the comprehensive initial assessment of a middle-stage child is just how much standardized testing to do. This is always something of a value judgment involving cost–benefit analysis. By constantly asking oneself whether the benefit of additional information outweighs the cost of time borrowed from other activities the child (and professional) might engage in, professionals can avoid the trap of continued assessment that delays getting to the meat of intervention.

METHODS AND TARGETS OF MIDDLE-STAGE INTERVENTION

The methods and targets of intervention for the middle stages of language acquisition are designed to build on the linguistic and nonlinguistic abilities the child has already acquired and to extend the child's development in areas not proceeding normally. Like those in Chapter 7, the following discussions are intended not to constitute a "curriculum," or a set of program objectives appropriate for all children with middle-stage needs (sets of goals and short-term objectives are available in N. W. Nelson, 1988b, and, in computerized version, N. W. Nelson & Snyder, 1990). Rather, the following sections are intended to highlight some areas that pose problems for many children with middle-stage language acquisition needs and to suggest some ways that language specialists and others might assist children through a more normal development course. Although the discussion is organized more by behavioral description than causative concerns, the latter often play a role in clinical decision making (in some cases more than others, e.g., when a child cannot hear). Therefore, special issues related to cause and to circumstances that differ when older children stay at middle stages are discussed where appropriate, as illustrative, but not exhaustive, cases.

ROLES OF ADULT PARTNERS AND CONTEXTS IN LANGUAGE INTERVENTION

Although children in the middle stages of development are less tied to the home and to primary care givers than are infants and toddlers in the early stages, they nevertheless continue to learn much about language and communication through their interactions with adults. Therefore, part of the intervention process should continue to focus on adults' roles in encouraging more normal development.

Modifying Parent Discourse as Part of Intervention

In discussing language intervention with young children, Fey (1986) noted that "needs to use language arise much more frequently at home and at school than in any clinical setting" (p. 291) and that some of the best opportunities for language learning seem to occur when children are the most motivated to communicate. Conditions under which these needs arise are often difficult to simulate in the clinic, and learning new skills in context can increase the likelihood that they will generalize. Therefore, Fey proposed that

Personal Reflection 8.3

"It is a simple fact that the language impaired child spends much more time at home with family members and friends than she could ever spend at the clinic."

Marc Fey (1986, p. 291) writing about the practical need to include family in the intervention process, regardless of one's theoretical orientation.

intervention with young children is most effective when it involves family members.

As discussed in Chapter 5, however, not all parents are equally prepared to assume intervention roles with their young children. Many need considerable preparation before they can act as language intervention aides or primary intervention agents for their children, and they may not always recognize opportunities to serve as incidental intervention agents (roles discussed in Chapter 5). Although the research reviewed in Chapter 5 suggests mixed results of formal efforts to involve parents in intervention, their role in helping their children learn to communicate and to know more about the world is critical. This should involve helping parents focus on their children's abilities as well as disabilities and helping them encourage the delight of informal discovery rather than formal teaching. Parents may also need assistance in focusing on areas presenting difficulties to their children. They may need some guidance in helping to build linguistic and nonlinguistic scaffolds, to intensify experience, to help frame and focus their children's attention (as exemplified in Personal Reflection 8.4).

When we developed a preschool language intervention program for children in Berrien County Intermediate School District, one of the devices we used to increase immediate contact with the children's parents was to send notebooks back and forth each day in the children's pouches. Each child had a colored symbol that identified his or her notebook, carrying pouch, storage "cubby," placemat, and other items at school. Each also had a carpet square of the same color to define where the child was supposed to sit during "circle time." (These strategies helped the children learn the concept of abstract symbols representing a person's belongings, built meaningfulness into abstract colors and shapes, and made it possible to talk about such concepts as "Who is *not* here today?" based on empty carpet squares). Not all parents were immediately anxious to write in the notebooks each night, however, and the usual problems with getting the books returned each day were apparent in the early days of the program. The collaborating professionals soon discovered and modified a strategy that made all the difference. Each night, they asked parents to sit down with their children to sketch an event that had happened that day (profes-

Personal Reflection 8.4

When asked where the childlike expectation in her creativity came from, Jeannette Haien, concert pianist and novelist, responded:

"I credit my parents. One begins, or doesn't, with that. One of my first memories is of my father calling excitedly to say. 'Look.' He was looking up at the sky. I couldn't see what I was to look at. Then he said, 'Listen,' and I heard this peculiar sort of sound, very distant. He kept saying, 'Look higher, look higher,' and I did. Then I saw my first skein of geese and heard their call. He took my hand and said to me, 'Those are the whales of the sky.' I have never forgotten it. And I never look up at a sky without the expectation of some extraordinary thing coming — airplane, owls at night. I'm a great looker up to the sky."

Jeannette Haien, when interviewed by *Bill Moyers*, journalist, during his PBS series (quoted in Tucher, 1990, p. 53)

sionals modeled extremely primitive stick figure draw-ings to reduce parental anxiety about drawing). They also instructed parents to write down what their child said about the event in the child's exact words. The parents learned to take mini-language samples of their child's words, to transcribe them exactly, to become sensitive to limitations of form, but also to tune into their children's interests and understand-ings. The professionals instructed parents *not* to cor-rect their children's grammatical formulation errors but encouraged parents to show interest in their child's ideas and to model other ways to talk about the same topic and to extend it. Topics ranged from exciting visits to Grandmother's house to mundane teeth brushing. Soon, the children themselves (many with severe language limitations) were reminding their parents about their language books, because each child who brought the notebook spent some individual time talking about the picture with the speech–language clinician or the teacher during small-group time. During this time, the adult redrew the original sketch on larger paper and invited the child to fill in details and to recall and to talk about the event (a similar strategy could be used in pull-out ses-sions). When the group came back together in a cir-cle, children with story pictures talked about them with their peers. The instructor also encouraged peers to ask questions of each other (something they rarely did spontaneously). This all made it highly desir-able to take notebooks home and bring them back. It also gave the professionals an opportunity to inform parents of the "concepts of the week" (we usually used three contrasting pairs) and to suggest some enrichment activities at home to reinforce those con-cepts during family routines (e.g., "accidentally" putting on both a long and short sock during dressing and waiting for the child to comment on it).

Exactly *how* parents communicate with their chil-dren with language impairments may not be as important as *that* they communicate with them. However, a key seems to be that language input be appropriately complex. Geers and Shick (1988) stud-ied the language abilities of 5- to 8-year-old children who had either hearing parents or hearing impaired parents. The authors hypothesized that the better language skills demonstrated by children of hearing impaired parents were related to the signing ability of their parents, which allowed the parents to provide consistent language stimulation, of appropriate advancing complexity, throughout the elementary

school years. P. J. Yoder (1989) found that children with specific language impairments made greater improvement in mastering auxiliary verb use when their mothers used higher rates of information-seek-ing questions. Conti-Ramsden (1990) found that mothers of language-impaired children tend not to use verbal recasts and other contingent replies to seek clarification of their children's messages. Perhaps some specific instruction in how to do so would have a positive effect on their children's lan-guage acquisition. Clearly more research is needed in this area.

Modifying Teacher Discourse as Part of Intervention

As children enter school programs, adults other than their parents become significant interactants. As a result of PL 99–457, children likely will be identified at earlier ages, and more of these children may find their ways into specialized intervention programs. In such programs, teacher–child discourse interactions provide another potential source for influencing lan-guage development. Although the quality of adult–child discourse receives infrequent attention by researchers, it may have untapped potential for encouraging child development.

Chapter 6 introduced the principles of incidental teaching. B. Hart and Risley defined this approach as the "interactions between an adult and a child that arise naturally in an unstructured situation, such as free play, and that are used systematically by the adult to transmit new information or give the child practice in developing a communication skill" (1975, p. 411). Some evidence supports the effectiveness of these strategies, which tend to be "brief, positive, and oriented toward communication rather than lan-guage teaching per se" (S. F. Warren & Kaiser, 1986, p. 291). For example, during free play in a preschool classroom, a child may point to a ball on a shelf, per-haps even saying the word *ball*. The teacher will fol-low this initiation by using a mand-model, saying, "Tell me, 'want ball.'" After the child does so, the ball is handed to the child (a natural reinforcer), and the classroom routine continues. Another possible use of the procedure would be for a teacher to approach a child engaged in an activity and to ask, with interest, "What are you doing?" (a mand). If the child re-sponds verbally, the teacher says something like, "That's neat," or "Right." If the child fails to respond, the teacher produces a model for the child, such as,

"Say, I'm coloring." If the child does so, social reinforcement is provided; if not, the interaction continues.

The effectiveness of incidental teaching was investigated by S. F. Warren, McQuarter, and Rogers-Warren (1984) when they used it in a university preschool for language-delayed children. Their results showed increased rates of total verbalizations, including both responses to questions and nonobligatory speech initiations. They also found some evidence of increase in MLU and generalization to other free-play situations.

The descriptions of milieu teaching or incidental intervention rely heavily on the terminology and technology of behaviorism (Kirchner, 1991). Relying more on a sociolinguistic theoretical perspective, Norris and Hoffman (1990b) described a set of naturalistic strategies for providing interaction-based language interventions for middle-stage children. They emphasized that even when language intervention is provided within naturalistic environments (in which language is treated more as a medium of communication than a system of rules to be learned), it must be organized. The naturalistic intervention steps suggested by Norris and Hoffman included the following: (1) organize the environment so that appropriate information is available and the child has opportunity to interact; (2) initiate and refine communication, encouraging the child to initiate, responding to the child's behaviors as if they are communicative, elaborating and expanding the child's topics, and using scaffolding to help the child reach the next level of complexity; and (3) provide consequences that are natural to the communicative event, emphasizing the criterion of communicative effectiveness, using clarification or repair strategies as necessary.

In describing a dialogue approach to intervention, Marion Blank (1973) emphasized that the quality of adult–child interactive discourse depends on the degree to which it might encourage development of the "abstract attitude." Blank argued that, despite the fuzziness of the concept and breadth of phenomena subsumed under the rubric *abstract attitude*, advantages accrue from targeting its development rather than targeting the development of specific skills among children with developmental risks. Furthermore, Blank argued that the abstract attitude could best be developed in the context of extended, connected one-on-one dialogues between a child and an intentioned adult (not in discrete single-unit exchanges or group lessons). She emphasized the need for children to participate in contextually grounded sequences of discourse interactions, noting that, "The opportunity for the sustained pursuit of an idea is acquired" (p. 22). The notion that ideas can "attain their full potential only when embedded in context" (p. 22) is easier to understand when one considers that a sentence such as "The car is red" takes on entirely different meanings if it follows a question such as "How did he recognize the car?" or "How is the car different from the other car?" Consider how this kind of discourse interaction differs from common clinical discourse exchanges when clinicians ask a series of unrelated parallel questions such as "What color is the ___?" Such a series does not require children to make any cognitive connections beyond the surface ones. An example of the kind of "tutorial" discourse advocated by Blank appears in Box 8.11.

For children at the school-age level, N. W. Nelson (1984, 1985, 1989b) also suggested that "teacher talk" be considered a legitimate focus of intervention. At least, the specialist should ask questions about how the demands of classroom discourse intersect with the child's language abilities and disabilities. It might be appropriate to consider teacher discourse styles, speaking rate, and other variables that may facilitate or impede children's language processing in regular education classrooms. Choices about the best classrooms for children might be made on these bases. Or the specialist might encourage teachers, through collaborative consultation, to be aware of ways they might enhance the comprehension of children with wobbly language competencies by their own discourse strategies, such as using more frequent comprehension checks and giving explicit directions.

Enhance the Auditory Language-Learning Context

Amplifying the volume of adult speech is another way to modify the environment to encourage communicative development among middle-stage children. Recently, a few investigators have reported the use of sound field amplification in classrooms to enhance the signal-noise ratio of teachers' language to background noise, even for children who have normal peripheral hearing (Flexer, 1989; Flexer, Millin, & Brown, 1990; Ray, Sarff, & Glassford, 1984; Sarff, Ray, & Bagwell, 1981). Sometimes teachers' speech has been amplified (using a standard portable public address system or a personal FM auditory trainer) in

Box 8.11   The pattern of tutorial discourse (illustrating scaffolding) used in storytelling in which a bit of content is read and is then used as a takeoff point for posing a series of relevant cognitive questions

Dialogue	Interpretation
Teacher — Where is this nest?	
Child — On a tree.	This sounds correct but the child has still not shown
Teacher — And where is the nest in the tree?	that she has grasped the concept of height.
Child — (No response.)	
Teacher — Near the ground?	
Child — High up in the tree?	The posing of an incorrect alternative led in this case
Teacher — That's right! And if he just walks out high up in the tree what will happen to him?	to the correct elaboration of the response.
Child — He'll fall out.	
Teacher — That's right. I guess he thinks he can fly. But why can't he fly? His mother can fly!	
Child — He and the bird can fly.	The pictorial information told her that the bird would fall; her verbal associations to birds are that they fly. This is an illustration of how the child holds two opposing views without any awareness of their conflict.
Teacher — You think he can fly? Let's see (turns the page).	
Child — He fell.	
Teacher — Why did he fall? Why didn't he just fly?	
Child — Cause, cause he took one foot off the nest!	A good use of memory, but still an incomplete answer to the question "why didn't he fly?"
Teacher — Yeah. But his mother took one foot off of the nest and what did she do?	This question is to help the child realize that her initial response is obviously not correct.
Child — She didn't fall out.	
Teacher — Why not?	
Child — (Shrugs shoulders.)	
Teacher — Who's bigger and stronger? The mommy bird or the baby bird?	While this question poses an alternative which may cause difficulty, the child's strong verbal associations make this a reasonable option to chance.
Child — The mommy.	
Teacher — And who can fly?	
Child — The mommy.	The teacher concludes the sequence since it would
Teacher — That's right. But the bird cannot fly yet because he is not strong. His wings are not strong enough to help him fly. What could happen?	probably be too difficult for the child to do it, especially at the end of a lesson. Nevertheless, a question is left for the child to answer in order to make her use some of the information she has been given.

Note. From *Teaching Learning in the Preschool: A Dialogue Approach* (pp. 190–191) by M. Blank, 1973, Columbus, OH: Merrill/Macmillan. Copyright by M. Blank. Reprinted by permission.

regular education mainstream environments (Ray et al., 1984; Sarff et al., 1981). In one case, the use of amplification was explored in a special education context. Children with developmental disabilities attending a primary-level special education class made significantly fewer errors on a word identification task with amplification than without (Flexer et al., 1990).

The provision of amplification to children with language disorders but normal hearing is still in an experimental stage. In addition to sound field amplification, the use of amplification devices such as FM systems, auditory trainers, personal amplification devices, and other assistive listening devices has been reported with normal hearing children. When they reviewed these studies, the American Speech-Language-Hearing Association (ASHA) Committee on Amplification for the Hearing Impaired (1991) cautioned that the work is preliminary and that more information is needed in the areas of efficacy, consumer safety, and professional liability before the procedures are considered a standard element in language treatment.

The provision of amplification for children with hearing impairments is, of course, another matter. The multiple considerations involved in making these decisions exceed the boundaries of this text. They involve the professional contributions of audiologists and other hearing health-care specialists. However, speech–language pathologists and other special and regular education professionals cannot afford to ignore those needs, or others that extend beyond amplification. "While the appropriate and effective use of FM units is essential for the classroom management of hearing impaired children, equipment use alone may not be sufficient for successful mainstreaming" (Flexer, Wray, & Ireland, 1989, p. 17). Other programming components that these children may need include specific training for using auditory skills in functional contexts, helping teachers and students maximize the auditory information available in educational activities, and providing intervention specifically related to understanding the language of the curriculum.

DEVELOPING SKILLS IN SYMBOLIC PLAY

In the middle stages of language acquisition, play, especially role play, remains a valuable context for developing multiple aspects of language. By its nature, play offers particularly rich opportunities for encouraging children to develop the symbolic function of language. Other developments may come in the area of language content as it is embedded within the context of varied schemas and scripts, language forms as they are needed to express relatively complex meanings across integrated events, and social uses as they are required for setting up play with peers and acting out scripted roles.

Questions about the relationships of thought and language come to the fore in the context of child's play. Both Piaget (1962) and Vygotsky (1967) linked the emergence of symbolic play to the development of representational skills. Bates and her colleagues (1979) found early correlations among symbolic play, vocal imitation, and language production in normally developing children during infancy. But the relationships are far from clear.

In at least one study, some aspects of language development preceded some aspects of play development among children with "specific" language impairments. Roth and Clark (1987) compared the symbolic play and social participation of six children with language impairments with eight children who were learning normally. Those authors found that the language-impaired children demonstrated "deficits" in symbolic play compared to younger language-matched normally developing children. For example, more than half of the language-impaired children failed to perform play behaviors such as putting a doll to bed or placing a toy figure in a tractor, items from the Symbolic Play Test (Lowe & Costello, 1976). They also demonstrated social participation difficulties when rated on a continuum of levels ranging from nonplay to cooperative play with role differentiation. Roth and Clark noted that the social interaction results may have been influenced by pairing the normally developing children together and the language impaired children together as play partners. (Perhaps these findings have some further implications for integrating children with and without disabilities.) They also emphasized the heterogeneity among the group of children with language impairments in their play interaction styles.

Roth and Clark's (1987) results, when compared with the studies on younger children, show that children with language disorders change over time. Chronological age does make a difference; 7-year-olds with language impairments are not the same as 3-year-olds with language impairments, even when the same child is compared across the two ages. Yet, because longitudinal data are lacking, we can only surmise that what happens in the years between toddlerhood and early elementary years may be critical in determining how children with language problems relate to others and entertain themselves during play.

Ignoring the possibility that 7-year-olds may be less interested in engaging in doll play in the presence of strangers with video equipment than 3-year-olds, how might language interventionists encourage children to develop the rich imaginative and communicative skills needed to play with peers in the preschool and early elementary years? Opportunity seems to be one key to the process. Children need to be placed in situations where they can feel included in their peers' games. The kinds of "Let's pretend" that come only when a group of children decides to play "restaurant," "shoestore," "horses," or "jungle" (all fondly remembered from my own childhood) are hard to orchestrate. But enlisting the aid of an older child to help figure out an appropriate role for the child in the wheelchair or one who can walk and run but cannot talk so well is a possibility.

Part of the problem may be that children with language problems simply do not know how to make appropriate social overtures to potential play partners. Some of this may be modeled for them, and in some cases, older siblings or other interested peers can help instruct target children in how to join play groups. This differs from forcing the participation, and it takes quite a bit of ground work by adults. Expectations for the play and communicative behaviors appropriate to middle stages of development are summarized by Westby (1988) in the last three stages of her Symbolic Play Scale, which appears in

Table 8.5 (the earlier stages were summarized in Chapter 7).

USING LANGUAGE TO ACCOMPLISH EXPANDED CONVERSATIONAL PURPOSES

Goals Related to Individual Patterns of Communication

In their preschool and early elementary years, children continue to expand the pragmatic functions they are able to accomplish with language. Children with language disorders, however, may be more limited in their communicative interaction patterns than their normal language-learning peers. Previously in this chapter, patterns of communicative assertiveness or responsiveness were described (Fey, 1986; see also Figure 4.1). Different communicative function patterns justify different intervention goals. The intervention goals Fey suggested for children exhibiting particular communicative patterns are summarized in Box 8.12.

Making Requests

It would be a mistake to think of intervention to expand communicative functions as affecting or targeting only single dimensions of communicative behavior. For example, one cannot simply target a function such as "making requests" without recognizing all of the kinds of knowledge and skills that must be integrated before a child can effectively do so. For example, Ervin-Trip and Gordon (1986) noted that a speaker must solve five different problems to make requests effectively: (1) get attention, (2) be clear, (3) maintain desired social relations, (4) be persuasive, and (5) make repairs. Some developmental

| Personal Reflection 8.5 | Play often provides wonderful opportunities for intersections of cognitive and linguistic development. My own family enjoys retelling the story of when, as a child, I was sent down the block during a cowboy game to bring back 100 head of cattle and returned lugging a heavy imaginary "bag" full of those 100 heads I had just lopped off with an imaginary sword. Besides being an embarrassing moment, this is an example of how play can be rich in idiomatic language use and how it is a normal part of childhood for younger children to learn from older, more advanced peers. |

TABLE 8.5
Symbolic Play Scale—the last three stages

DECONTEXTUALIZATION	THEMATIC CONTENT	ORGANIZATION	SELF/OTHER RELATIONS	LANGUAGE	
What Props Are Used in Pretend Play?	What Schemas/Scripts Does the Child Represent?	How Coherent and Logical Are the Child's Schemas/Scripts?	What Roles Does Child Take and Give to Toys and Other People?	Function	Forms and Meaning
Stage VI: 3 to 3½ years					
Carries out pretend activities with replica toys (Fisher-Price/Playmobile doll house, barn, garage, airport, village). Uses one object to represent another (stick can be a comb, chair can be a car). Uses blocks and sandbox for imaginative play. Blocks used as enclosures (fences, houses) for animals and dolls	Observed events, i.e., events in which child was not an active participant (policemen, firemen, schemas/scripts from familiar TV shows—Superman, Wonder Woman)		Uses doll or puppet as participant in play Child talks for doll Reciprocal role taking—child talks for doll and as parent to doll	Projecting: Gives desires, thoughts, feelings to doll or puppet Uses indirect requests, e.g., "mommy lets me have cookies for breakfast." Changes speech depending on listener Reasoning (integrates reporting, predicting, projecting information)	Descriptive vocabulary expands as child becomes more aware of perceptual attributes. Uses terms for following concepts (not always correctly): shapes sizes colors textures spatial relations Uses metalinguistic and metacognitive language, e.g., "He said . . .", "I know. . . ."
Stage VII: 3½ to 4 years					
Uses language to invent props and set scene Builds 3-dimensional structures with blocks		Schemas/scripts are planned Child hypothesizes, "What would happen if . . ."	Uses dolls and puppets to act out schemas/scripts Child or doll has multi-roles (e.g., mother and wife; fireman, husband, and father)	Uses language to take roles of character in the play, stage manager for the props, or as author of the play story	Uses modals (can, may, might, will, would, could) Uses conjunctions (and, but, so, if, because) Note: Full competence for modals and conjunctions does not develop until 10–12 years of age. Begins to respond appropriately to why and how questions which require reasoning
Stage VIII: 5 years					
Can use language totally to set the scene, actions, and roles in the play	Highly imaginative activities that integrate parts of known schemas/scripts and develop new novel schemas/scripts for events child has never participated in or observed (e.g., astronaut builds ship, flies to strange planet, explores, eats unusual foods, talks with creatures on planet)	Plans several sequences of pretend events. Organizes what is needed—both objects and other children. Coordinates several scripts occurring simultaneously			Uses relational terms (then, when, first, next, last, while, before, after) Note: Full competence does not develop until 10–12 years of age

Note. From Westby, C., Children's Play: Reflections of Social Competence, in *Seminars in Speech and Language,* Volume 9, Number 1, p. 13, New York, 1988, Thieme Medical Publishers, Inc. Reprinted by permission

Box 8.12   Suggested intervention goals based on conversational speech-act analysis

Goals for active conversationalists

1. Train [the child in] new content–form interactions to perform available conversational acts.
2. Facilitate the use of old forms to fulfill alternative conversational acts.

Goals for passive conversationalists

1. Increase the frequency of use of available assertive conversational acts in a variety of social contexts.
2. Increase the child's repertoire of assertive conversational acts, using existing forms when possible.
3. Train new linguistic forms that are useful in performing available assertive acts.

Goals for inactive communicators

1. Increase the child's rate of positive social bids (verbal and nonverbal) in a variety of social contexts.
2. When the child becomes more responsive and begins to initiate communication more frequently, goals for passive conversationalists probably will be appropriate.

Goals for verbal noncommunicators

1. Increase the relatedness of the child's responses to the assertive acts (e.g., requestives, assertives, performatives) of the partner.
2. Facilitate the child's production of sequences of utterances that are topically related to one another.

Note. From Mark E. Fey, *Language Intervention With Young Children* (pp. 80–98). Copyright © 1986. Reprinted with permission of Allyn and Bacon.

---

expectations in this area are summarized in Box 8.13. These expectations may be used to guide intervention goals in the middle stages of development.

Being Polite

Most normally developing children in mainstream Western cultures begin to be held accountable for politeness by their parents during the preschool years. Being polite is more than a matter of being able to say *please* and *thank you* (as evident in the review by Ervin-Tripp and Gordon, 1986, summarized in Box 8.13). Nippold, Leonard, and Anatopoulos (1982) characterized development in production and understanding of polite forms as sensitivity to the function of these forms in an increasing number of sentence types related to increasing ability to assume perspectives of listeners. Intervention strategies might focus on the development of this perspective-taking ability by modeling and reinforcing it as well as by directly modeling polite conversational behaviors and linguistic markers.

Taking Turns, Managing Topics, and Making Repairs

John Dore (1986) described growth in the development of conversational competence as being context dependent. He also tied it to growth of cohesion (making sensible connections) and coherence (relating to a topic). During the one-word stage, according to Dore, children begin to develop cohesion by choosing one word as a single option among several to fit the circumstances. This kind of cohesion is primarily lexically determined. Discourse cohesion across turns develops more slowly. At preschool level, Dore pointed out that children begin to work out new relationships with peers, school authorities, and others. While doing so, "the child explores the options for getting and constructing his turns at talk and for exploiting the conversational subsystems in negotiating his social power and solidarity" (p. 36). When children enter grade school, significant shifts in conversational influences are observed again:

Box 8.13   Developmental advances from ages 2 to 8 years in skills needed for making requests (based on Ervin-Trip & Gordon, 1986)

Getting Attention

Ages 2 to 4: Children tend to make requests without first attempting to gain attention. By age 3, they improve in this regard, but tend to call "Hey" rather than the more specific, "Hey, Joe."
Ages 4 to 8: Children increase the specificity and effectiveness of attention forms.

Clarity

Ages 2 to 4: Children learn a full array of basic forms for making instrumental moves, and clarity ceases to be their major problem. During this time, they learn to be specific about the agent, action, and goal in their requests.
Ages 4 to 8: Whereas young children are not good at attending to the cognitive needs of their listeners, this awareness increases in the early elementary years. During these years, interviewing shows that children are more explicit in their requests when they think the listener does not expect a request.

Social Distinctions

Ages 2 to 4: By age 2, children already show some distinctions in their speech for different listeners (e.g., on the basis of age, familiarity, and role). By age 2:6, they begin using auxiliaries that give them the possibility of adding polite questions to mark social contrasts, often combining requests with the word "Please." They also begin to use forms like "Can you," and "D'you wanna" when compliance cannot be assumed.
Ages 4 to 8: Children seem to become more sensitive to the effects of interruption on the listener. When they expect listeners to be compliant, children tend not to use imperatives. Polite forms are used more frequently when children interrupt their listeners. By age 8, children tend to be better at perspective taking.

Persuasion

Ages 2 to 4: Spontaneous explanations or justifications for requests are rarely provided by 2- and 3-year-olds.
Ages 4 to 8: By age 4 or 5, children often supply reasons or check willingness when making requests of their peers. Older speakers eventually use the justification statements or reasons alone as indirect requests.

Repairs

Ages 2 to 4: Younger children are likely to attempt to make repairs by increasing their requests over and over with increasing urgency. By age 2:6, children who have developed politeness strategies will use them on second attempts if first attempts are unsuccessful.
Ages 4 to 8: When older children fail to have their requests met, they are more likely to use tactics of conveying obligation, justification, or bribery in addition to increased aggravation or urgency (as younger children tend to do).

The child's initiation into studenthood involves him with a much wider social milieu, a more structured authority system, an expansion of his relationship to others from peer to educational collaborator and a sense of being one-among-many, perhaps even of being an interchangeable member of a vast institution. Student membership brings with it many new responsibilities for "behaving like a good pupil." (Dore, 1986, p. 55).

These efforts involve not only cooperation strategies but also competition strategies, such as in classroom attempts to get and to avoid turns to speak and read. Much of the research on the conversational strategies of children with language learning disabilities has been done with children in the later grades. However, in her research review, T. Bryan (1986) noted that some of the learning disabled children studied were as young as first graders. Although the learning disabled children were not inferior to their language-normal peers in all areas of conversational interaction studied, they were found to have difficulties in many areas. They had difficulties delivering bad news to peers tactfully, their messages were less informative, and they had difficulty asking clarification questions when given ambiguous messages. On the playground, they were less likely to give positive, encouraging remarks to their peers, such as "Good catch," and more likely to make negative, discouraging comments, e.g., "Look, he can't even get up there" (p. 239).

Responses to requests for clarification by children ages 4:10 to 9:10 were studied by Brinton, Fujiki, Winkler, and Loeb (1986). They used a series of stacked responses from children with specific language impairments and children with normal language skills at three age levels. Their findings showed that all children demonstrated the willingness and ability to respond to these neutral clarification requests. However, the quality of the responses differed. The language-impaired children produced more inappropriate responses than did the normally developing children across age groups and clarification request types. The children with language impairments showed particular difficulty repairing multiple times in stacked sequences, perhaps because they had less linguistic flexibility, were less aware of their listener's needs, or interpreted the repeated requests for clarification as disapproval of the form or content of their messages.

Pragmatic Functions

Most clinicians agree that pragmatic functions can be targeted effectively only within the contexts of naturalistic communicative interactions. To some extent, such opportunities may be contrived, or enhanced with techniques of focusing and modeling, but the essential intervention strategy is to help children move through developmental sequences by giving them opportunities to practice their advancing skills in meaningful contexts.

In discussing intervention for problems related to conversational management, Brinton and Fujiki (1989) commented that clinical procedures must be devised to fit the child, the clinician, and the target. For example, children with more severe impairments are likely to need more highly structured conversational contexts, whereas children with less severe impairments may benefit more from naturalistic exchanges. In either case, however, the final goal should be a set of integrated communicative abilities, "not to teach turn taking or topic mechanics per se but rather to facilitate the conversational management skills that enhance effective communication" (p. 142). Intervention objectives should be written to be consistent with this goal. Box 8.14 includes two kinds of objectives, one written in a way that Brinton and Fujiki considered to be less effective than the other.

Conversational contexts not only provide rich opportunities to observe and foster integrated language, speech, and communicative abilities, they also may be used to gain insights into possible factors contributing to communicative problems. Effective assessment during intervention involves identification of contributing factors to be addressed along with primary symptoms. For example, Brinton and Fujiki (1989) listed 10 related problems that might undermine smooth turn exchange and successful topic manipulation: (1) peripheral hearing loss, (2) selective attending difficulty, (3) language comprehension difficulty, (4) language production deficits, (5) problems with immediate memory span, (6) stuttering behaviors, (7) difficulty with relevance constraints, (8) being oblivious to the needs of other speakers, (9) being too easily intimidated, and (10) psychological disturbance.

Intervention strategies aimed directly at conversational interaction are implemented by first engaging children in conversations with enough environmental support to ensure success, starting with nonverbal exchanges or games if necessary. The support should be based on the child's needs. The strategy might include the use of such suprasegmentals as pause and stress to encourage children to notice cues for initiating turns, providing repair, or asking for clarification. Other strategies might involve direct or indirect modeling. Gradually, the clinician should reduce the environmental support to allow more equal responsibility for managing conversations (Brinton & Fujiki, 1989).

Intervention of this type may be delivered using a variety of service models. Conversational interaction strategies may be targeted in dyadic clinician–child conversations or in the contexts of small groups or special or regular education classrooms. A key to

Box 8.14	Less and more effective ways of designing intervention objectives for topic maintenance.

Less effective objective: Teach the child to talk about any given topic for 30 seconds.
More effective objective: Facilitate the child's participation in topical sequences to share information when interacting in a dyad.
_____

(From Brinton & Fujiki, 1989, p. 142). |

remember is that the outcome of intervention contexts should be legitimate conversation that is communicative and not distorted by intervention. For example, it would be a disservice to teach children to make multiple clarification requests when teachers find that behavior inappropriate without also teaching the children to recognize cues regarding appropriate timing of questions to the teacher. Teachers may also need to be assisted to appreciate the need for children to ask clarification questions through mutual goal setting and collaborative consultation.

PRODUCING AND COMPREHENDING MORE COMPLEX CONTENT–FORM CONSTRUCTIONS

Part of the process of gaining communicative competence involves making advances in producing and understanding more complex content-form constructions. Although superficially these developments may appear to be simply a matter of learning aspects of language form, meaningful uses of content–form constructions require sensitivity to semantic and pragmatic constraints as well. This section considers production aspects of syntactic and morphological rule usage separately from those related to comprehension. In actual communicative events, the two modalities are probably closely related but not necessarily mirror images of each other because of the different processing demands associated with each.

Producing More Complex Content–Form Constructions

When children reach the beginning of the middle stages of language development, if they are learning language normally, they can combine such basic sentence constituents as agents, actions, and objects. In the middle stage, they acquire additional rules for elaborating the detail of those basic constituents, for making them agree with each other in number and tense, and for formulating variants of basic sentences, such as negatives and questions.

Subjecthood. Learning some of the formal grammatical properties of subjecthood and subject–verb

Personal Reflection 8.6	The following sample was reported by *Bonnie Brinton* and *Martin Fujiki* (1989) in their book *Conversational Management With Language-Impaired Children*.

Child: What do you do at work anyway?
Clinician: Well, I help kids who have trouble talking.
Child: What happens to them?
Clinician: Sometimes they don't understand people, and sometimes people don't understand them.
Child: So how do you help them?
Clinician: Oh, we do a lot of things. We help them to say things clearly. We help them to learn new words, and we help them to make sentences.
Child: But how do they learn to talk to people?
Clinician: We work on that too.
Child: Oh. (looks thoughtful) You gotta talk to people, you know.
Clinician: I know. (pp. 214–215) |

agreement appears to give many children with language disorders particular difficulty (Connell, 1986b), perhaps because the properties are not directly tied to meaning (Johnston & Kamhi, 1984). Properties to be learned relating to subjecthood include subject–verb agreement, the copula and auxiliary *be*, the third-person singular present-tense marker, the nominative case of pronouns, and the auxiliary inversion of questions.

An intervention strategy to teach multiple subject properties using a single procedure was devised by Connell (1986b). He tested the strategy with four children ranging from 3:4 to 4:2 who were diagnosed as having language disorders. The children were taught individually in ½-hour sessions 3 to 4 times per week. When the intervention procedure began, the children with language disorders were producing structures such as "Him walking," "Him walk," "Him big," or "Him a man." Connell described these as early topic-comment forms, which did not, in the child's system, require subject–verb agreement or subjective (nominative) case on pronouns because they were used simply to name a topic and then comment on it. Connell designed the intervention procedure to move the children forward toward subject–predicate structures by "dislocating the topic." He modeled sentences with an accusative (objective case) pronoun placed before the nominative pronoun and the rest of the sentence. For example, children heard models like, "Him, he is walking," which used the accusative pronoun *him* to serve the topic function, followed by the nominative pronoun *he* to serve the subject function, and the auxiliary *is* to agree with the subject. The children were taught to give this response when shown two contrasting pictures and asked, "Which one is walking?" Alternatively, the model "He is walking" was used with the question "What is the man doing?" presented with other pictures. By alternating the types of models and questions (with their corresponding stimulus pictures), Connell found that the strategy could help the children acquire the various aspects of subjecthood using a single set of varied models and questions.

Modal auxiliaries. Elaborating the verb phrase depends heavily on the acquisition of rules for using the modal auxiliaries *can, will, shall, may, must* (with corresponding past-tense forms *could, would, should, might,* and *must*). These forms have strong semantic, pragmatic, and syntactic implications. (Bliss, 1987). Syntactically, the modal auxiliaries play important roles in forming negative and interrogative constructions, such as "May I have some?" and "I can't reach it." Semantically, they convey varied meanings: ability (*can*), intention (*will*), permission (*may, can*), obligation/necessity (*should*), probability/possibility (*may, might*), and certainty (*will*). Pragmatically, modals serve varied functions, such as making requests, especially polite, indirect requests, and performing other social interactive functions.

As discussed earlier in this chapter, problems with modal auxiliaries may be identified through language sample analysis. For example, Lee's (1974) DSS requires fairly elaborate analysis of modal auxiliaries and their contribution to forming negatives and interrogatives. The normal development of modal auxiliaries occurs over several years (Bliss, 1987), extending from the 2nd year, when modals begin to emerge, until at least the age of 8. Bliss (1987) suggested intervention guidelines for working on modal auxiliaries that were based on the normal developmental sequence and included the following:

1. Focus on [the semantic roles] ability and intention early, as these are frequent and early acquired concepts [ability is expressed by the modals *can* or *can't*; intention is expressed by the modal *will* —"I'll show you how"].
2. Begin with *can* versus *can't*. Once these are mastered, wait several weeks to begin *will* and *won't*. The contrast eases learning. An interval is necessary to prevent confusion by the child.
3. Use self-reference early (first person pronouns or the child's name), as this form is the first to be associated with modals (Fletcher, 1979).
4. Link the modals with actions. Modals are initially used with an activity (Fletcher, 1979). An associated activity should facilitate learning. For example, "I *can* reach (it)." vs. "I *can't*."
5. Initially, use short sentences with the modal occurring at the end of an utterance (Stimulus: :Can you reach the star?" Response: "Yes, I *can*" or "No, I *can't*"). This procedure increases the saliency of the form.
6. Make the words critical to a situation. Provide meaningful situations in which concepts are linked to the modals that have been targeted.
7. Generalization of modal usage to speakers other than the clinician is crucial for adequate carryover. Parents and teachers need to be involved in a successful intervention program.

Note. From "'I Can't Talk Anymore; My Mouth Doesn't Want To.' The Development and Clinical Applications of Modal Auxiliaries" by L. S. Bliss, 1987, *Language, Speech, and Hearing Services in Schools, 18,* p. 77.

Other complex verb forms.   Acquiring rules for modal auxiliaries is only one way that children learn to elaborate verb phrases. Even before children's earliest uses of *can't* and *don't,* auxiliary forms of *be* may begin to show up in children's present progressive (*is* + V*ing*) constructions. The auxiliary *is* appears as one of R. A. Brown's (1973) first 14 morphemes (see Box 8.9). Yet, perhaps because it carries such a light semantic and pragmatic load, and perhaps because its acoustic qualities are often light as well, many children with form-based specific language impairments seem to need direct attention to acquire the grammatical rule for *is* + V*ing.*

Recall Chomsky's (1957) auxiliary construction rule (see Figure 8.1):

C + (modal) + (*have* + *en*) + (*be* + *ing*) + MV

In this rule, the C is an abstract symbol standing for the obligatory inclusion of markers indicating person (first, second, third), tense (present, past), and number (singular, plural) expressed on the first item in the verb string, which must agree with the subject of the sentence. The preceding discussion of *subjecthood* considered how intervention might help children acquire some of the subtleties of subject–verb agreement.

Except for the main verb (MV), all of the other items of Chomsky's (1957) verb construction rule, which appear in parentheses, are optional, depending on the linguistic context. As mentioned previously, modals may be used to shade meaning and to convey intention. The *be* + *ing* option of the rule is used to convey progressive action. When the auxiliary *be* is used in a present tense form (remember that syntactic tense can only be marked as present or past), such as "The boy is yelling," the semantic tense is present progressive, indicating ongoing action. When the auxiliary *be* is used in a past-tense form, such as "The boy was yelling," the semantic tense is past progressive, indicating action that was ongoing during some past moment. When the *have* + *en* option is selected, the semantic tense of the verb changes to the "perfect" tense. When the auxiliary *have* is used in present tense, such as "She has arrived," it merely conveys that some action has been completed. This is called *present perfect tense.* When the auxiliary *have* is used in the past tense, such as "She had arrived by the time we got there," it conveys the past

perfect semantic tense, meaning that the action was completed in the past.

Setting up situations that help children notice meaning contrasts like these may encourage them to use syntactic forms to convey similar shades of meaning in their own constructions. For example, Fey (1986) noted that children are more likely to understand the use of perfective verb forms if children are placed in a context requiring their use, rather than if children simply form isolated sentence pairs primarily to please the clinician. Two of the sample discourse contexts he suggested for eliciting perfective verb forms appear in Box 8.15.

Children learning BEV have more options for forming semantic tenses than children learning standard English (SE) alone. According to the rules of the BEV linguistic system, including third-person singular present-tense markers and forms of the auxiliary and copular *be* is optional. When evaluating samples of spontaneous language or responses to test items, clinicians must be extremely careful not to penalize the use of such "zero copula" and "zero auxiliary" forms by BEV speakers (Black English Sentence Scoring [BESS], N. W. Nelson & Hyter, 1990a, was designed for this purpose; see Appendix C). Such forms should never be described as "incorrect" for BEV speakers. Children learning BEV also may use two later developing verb tenses that exist in BEV but not in SE: (1) the invariant *be* and (2) the remote time aspect with *been.*

The invariant *be* in BEV may be further subdivided into two uses: (1) as the uninflected main verb, or (2) as the distributive or nontense *be.* In BEV, unlike SE, in which forms of *be* must be inflected differently depending on the subject of the sentence (e.g., *is, are, am; was, were*), "the form *be* can be used as the main verb, regardless of the subject of the sentence" (Fasold & Wolfram, 1970, p. 66). In one variation of this occurrence, phonological deletion rules make *be* appear to occur alone although the contracted auxiliary has simply been deleted phonologically (e.g., "He['ll] be here pretty soon" and "If you gave him a present he['d] be happy"). The other invariant *be* expresses a unique temporal meaning. The "distributive or nontense *be*" is used to indicate when an exact time cannot be clearly specified because the event is distributed intermittently in time (Fasold & Wolfram, 1970). Examples from a connected discourse sample spoken by a normally developing girl [age 6:3] illustrate this feature:

Box 8.15   Discourse contexts used to evoke past perfect verb constructions

Clinician:	Suzy liked to bake chocolate chip cookies. One day, she decided to make some. She mixed the batter and spread the cookies on the sheet. Then she put them in the oven and turned on the timer. When the timer went off, Suzy got a big surprise. There was smoke everywhere and the cookies were black! What had happened?
Child (or model):	She had set the timer wrong. She had left the cookies in too long. They had burned.
Clinician:	Basil, the dog, loved children. One day Karen decided that she would surprise the family with fried chicken for dinner. She laid the chicken on the table. Then, she remembered that she had no flour. She rushed to the store in her car. When she returned, she was surprised to find that her chicken was gone. Can you guess what had happened?
Child (or model):	Basil had been hungry. He had jumped on the table and had eaten all of the chicken.

Note. From Mark E. Fey, *Language Intervention With Young Children* (p. 188). Copyright © 1986. Reprinted with permission of Allyn and Bacon.

My mama don't like it neither. She be sayin' it stinks. My brothers be gettin' me in trouble. They be tellin' lies on me. [girl, 6:3]

The remote time aspect with *been* is used in BEV to indicate that a "speaker conceives of the action as having taken place in the distant past" (Fasold & Wolfram, 1970, p. 62). For example, a boy [age 5:3] established his prior right to play with a toy airplane by saying "I been wanted this."

Intervention should never be designed to eliminate culturally acceptable forms from a child's communicative interactions. They represent rich and meaningful expressions. As children learning different dialects or languages encounter SE forms through literacy activities and oral interactions in school, they may be more likely to acquire varied forms for varied contexts and purposes if all of their communicative attempts are accepted and encouraged and if they are allowed to try out different forms in speech and in writing as they develop (see the following section on emergent literacy). When children whose first language experiences differ from SE demonstrate language impairments within their native systems, the collaborative planning process may be used to decide whether SE forms should be encouraged along with acceptance of the forms of the child's first dialect or language. When making these decisions, the specialist should consider the language skills the child will need to participate in the important contexts of the child's life.

Complex sentence development. Previously in this chapter, a listing of expectations for complex sentence development was included in the discussion of language sample analysis (see Box 8.10). The acquisition of these forms may be an appropriate target when planning intervention for children who use complex forms rarely or incorrectly. Yet, such problems tend to be overlooked because it is easier to recognize misuse of a particular construction than to notice its absence. For example, when a kindergarten teacher hears a child produce sentences like "Me want to do it," or "Him coming to my house," the teacher is more likely to be alerted to the possibility that a language disorder might be present than when the child use only simple forms for expressing ideas but makes few alerting "errors." Besides, short, simple utterances may be the expected norm in classroom group instruction (Sturm, 1990). On the other hand, the language of the curriculum itself is often filled with many complex sentence demands, and these show up from the earliest grades (N. W. Nelson, 1984). Children who have not learned to produce and comprehend such sentences in other contexts are then increasingly disadvantaged as grade level and linguistic demands increase.

Intervention plans targeting the acquisition of rules for forming complex sentences consider many variables. These were summarized by N. W. Nelson (1988b) as including developmental ordering and timing, relationships between comprehension and production, and recognition of the semantic and cognitive demands on speakers, listeners, readers, and writers. Infinitive embeddings are often the first complex forms to appear (Tyack & Gottsleben, 1986), and "at very young ages, as early as 2:6, children begin combining sentences to express complex or compound propositions" (Tager-Flusberg, 1985, p. 161). The first conjunction to emerge, *and,* appears even before children have mastered the grammatical morphemes (Laughton & Hasenstab, 1986; Tager-Flusbert, 1985). Other meanings of *and* are not acquired until much later. In one study, L. Bloom, Lahey, Hood, Lifter, and Fiess (1980) found that the meanings of the word *and* emerged in the following order (presented with the authors' examples):

1. Additive —"Maybe you can carry this and I can carry that."
2. Temporal —"Jocelyn's going home and take her sweater off."
3. Causal —"She put a bandage on her shoe and maked it feel better."
4. Adversative —"Cause I was tired and now I'm not tired."
5. Objective specification —"It looks like a fishing thing and you fish with it." (pp. 243–245)

Other conjunctions that can express varied conceptual relationships were summarized by N. W. Nelson (1988b) to include the following types:

1. Causal (*because, so, therefore*)
2. Coincidental (*while, during*)
3. Comparative (*as . . . as, . . . than*)
4. Consequential (*since, therefore, so*)
5. Conditional (*if, if . . . then*)
6. Disjunctive (*but, or, although, however*)
7. Temporal (*when, before, after, then*) (p. 171)

When teaching rules for combining and embedding sentences, it is important for the clinician to ensure that children comprehend the conceptual relationships occasioning the use of these varied conjunctions. N. W. Nelson (1988b) suggested a sequence of objectives to target increasing independence from nonlinguistic context and linguistic modeling as children advance in their ability to understand and produce complex sentence forms. Kamhi's (1982) research with normally developing 3:0- to 5:2-year-old children also supported that children best acquire complex linguistic forms in contexts that encourage their own actions to represent compound and complex relationships in the presence of linguistic models.

Metalinguistic monitoring.   Intervention approaches for young children of preschool and early elementary school age typically do not rely heavily on metalinguistic awareness. However, whenever a child is asked to imitate a comment rather than respond to it, a certain amount of metalinguistic expectation is evident.

Metalinguistic awareness is also needed when children are asked to monitor their speech for grammaticality of their utterances. The research on syntactic awareness reviewed by Sutter and Johnson (1990) suggested that the identification of grammatical errors is most closely correlated to advancing chronological age; that it is not noticeably exhibited until around the age of 6 or 7 years; but that considerable variablilty is evident that can usually be attributed to contextual factors. Sutter and Johnson noted that focus on the early elementary schoolchild suggests that "a relation may exist between tacit knowledge of grammatical rules and the ability to contemplate syntactic form" (p. 85). If this is the case, one wonders about the advisability of asking children with delayed acquisition of grammatical rules to perform an intervention step that requires them to recognize the presence of grammatical errors in their own language or the language of others, perhaps by raising their hands or performing some other action to indicate notice.

The linguistic and cognitive processing demands of surrounding context also seem to influence children's ability to focus on surface-level features such as grammatical correctness. In their study of 6-, 7-, and 8-year-olds, Sutter and Johnson (1990) found that school-age children were less able to spot grammatical errors when the sentences with errors were embedded in a story than when the errors occurred in isolation. The authors hypothesized that this result might reflect children's efforts to focus their energy on getting the message of the story. They also found that children were more likely to spot errors involving auxiliaries and suffixes than adverbial constructions and that the normally developing 8-year-olds in their study were substantially better at identifying ungrammatical forms than their younger schoolmates.

At present, little research evidence guides decisions about the wisdom of requiring specific focus on monitoring of grammatical errors in intervention with middle-stage children. The research evidence available for normally developing children suggests that intervention time may be better spent on other avenues to build intrinsic linguistic proficiency, at least until the middle grades, when children begin to monitor for grammaticality in their written work as well as their oral language.

Comprehending More Complex Content–Form Constructions

Although it might be assumed that once a child begins to produce a particular grammatical form, the child should also be able to comprehend it, that is not necessarily the case (Guess & Baer, 1973). Conversely, comprehension of language forms is usually assumed to precede production of language forms in normal development. Yet that also is not necessarily the case, as exemplified by children's use of forms such as *because* clauses before they can fully comprehend causal relationships (L. Bloom & Lahey, 1978; R. S. Chapman, 1978). Comprehension and production, although related, do not seem to be fully reciprocal processes. The cognitive demands of recognition are not the same as those of recall, making comprehension a somewhat less demanding process in many respects, especially when other contextual variables support the child's ability to comprehend. Yet, the complexity of receptive processes needed to sort out the varied elements of content and form in compound and complex sentences results in production skills preceding comprehension skills for some structures at some intervals (Bates, 1976; Hood & Bloom, 1979), especially when the nonlinguistic context does not support listening comprehension. In comparison, even without external contextual support, middle-stage speakers may choose to talk about things they know (in essence, bringing their own context to the task), and production may be relatively easier than listening to someone else who controls the topic and the linguistic complexity.

It is interesting to track development of a linguistic form in different modalities. For example, in a series of studies, D. L. Johnson (1985) noted that the sense of past time is understood at around 4 to 5 years of age, that production of these same forms is not fully mastered by 6 years of age (Sutter & Johnson, 1988), and that the ability to monitor metalinguistically for errors in these verb forms is not very solid until around age 8 (Sutter & Johnson, 1990). Given this evidence, it may be inappropriate to expect children with language impairments to exhibit evidence of similar forms of processing all in the same semester or year.

Some language intervention programs have been designed on the premise that teaching children to focus on a new form without necessarily requiring production at the same time may be the most effective approach to language acquisition. Based on some of these procedures, some workers reported that successful teaching of language forms in comprehension resulted in improved production (Leonard et al., 1982; Winitz, 1973). However, when Connell (1986a) tried to teach six 3-year-olds with language disorders both to produce and to comprehend semantic role distinctions, even though all of the children learned to produce constructions using correct word-order relationships, none of them learned word order through comprehension training alone. Furthermore, learning to produce word order appropriately in spontaneous speech did not help children learn to use word-order cues to decode semantically reversible sentences on comprehension tasks.

Results of comprehension training on expression capabilities may be rather confusing partly because linguistic comprehension is often thoroughly confounded with world knowledge (R. Paul, 1990). It is also important to recognize that children use different comprehension strategies at different ages and stages of development (R. S. Chapman, 1978; R. Paul, 1990; Wallach, 1984). Box 8.16 presents a summary of some of the changes that can be expected over the years from 4 to 10.

Separate studies, reviewed by R. Paul (1990), showed that children with autism, specific language impairments, and hearing impairments use comprehension strategies similar to each other but different from those used by younger, language-matched normally developing preschoolers. Children in all of the disorder groups relied more heavily on canonical word-order strategies than on strategies based on world knowledge or later developing syntactic strategies (a finding supported by van der Lely & Harris, 1990). All of the children with impairments, however, even those with autism, used some knowledge of event probabilities and scripts to guide their responses.

R. Paul (1990) emphasized the need to evaluate both contextualized and decontextualized language comprehension for all children referred for language problems, even if their parents report comprehension to be unaffected. She was less firm about a recommendation to help children acquire comprehension strategies when they have not learned them on their

---

Box 8.16   Changes in comprehension strategies over the ages 4 to 10 years

1. Children move from almost exclusive reliance on *canonical order* (SUBJECT–VERB–OBJECT) strategies prior to age 4 [as infants and toddlers, their comprehension is largely context-determined], through *semantic constraints* and *probable event* strategies at age 4, to the ability to use *syntactic strategies,* at around age 5, for reversible passive sentences, in which the canonical order is violated (*The giraffe is kicked by the elephant*).
2. They also develop more mature strategies for comprehending *clause relationships* as they advance in age beyond 5, after which they learn to go beyond the *order-of-mention* and *pay-attention-to-the-main-clause* strategies that they have used earlier for processing clauses, and the *minimal-distance-principle* and *pronominalization* strategies that they have used earlier for determining reference.
3. Children also advance in their abilities to use cognitive *constructive* strategies to comprehend complex meanings between the ages of 4 and 10. As early as age 4, children can demonstrate *integration* strategies by distinguishing semantically consistent pictures that belong in a sequence from those that are semantically inconsistent and do not belong. But not until between the ages of 7 and 10 do children develop *inferencing* strategies for reading beyond the words to fill in information that makes sense even though it was not explicitly stated. For example, after age 7, the word *broom* can cue memory of the sentence, *Her friend swept the kitchen floor,* even though *broom* was never explicitly stated in the sentence.

Note. From *Planning Individualized Speech and Language Intervention Programs*—Revised and Expanded, by Nickola Wolf Nelson, copyright 1988 by Communication Skill Builders, Inc., PO Box 42050, Tucson, AZ 85733. Reprinted with permission.

---

own. She suggested using highly repetitive, highly ordered contexts, such as nursery rhymes and songs to use the word-order strategies common among many children with language impairments. She also recommended stretching children's comprehension capabilities by providing "opportunities for the child to process sentences slightly above the current level of functioning" (p. 72). Most important, Paul noted, was to encourage children with language disorders to take risks in their attempts to comprehend to prevent the later development of maladaptive patterns of nonresponsiveness.

When children have difficulty comprehending the language of others, their problems are often exacerbated because they do not realize that they did not understand, and they fail to ask for clarification. Skarakis-Doyle and Mullin (1990) noted a symbiotic relationship between primary linguistic comprehension and comprehension monitoring, blending reliance on both communicative and cognitive factors for efficient operation. Although children with language disorders may have difficulty with both factors, research by Skarakis-Doyle and Mullin supported a

greater influence of communicative than cognitive factors in reducing comprehension monitoring by children with specific language disorders between the ages of 3:6 and 8:4 years. In a related study, language-impaired children distinguished ambiguous from unambiguous messages but did not always clearly signal that detection (Skarakis-Doyle, MacLellan, & Mullin, 1990). Alternatively, children with weak language skills may assume that everyone else understands everything they hear all of the time, and that they are the only ones who do not. Or children with communicative deficits may feel too intimidated to ask for clarification or lack the linguistic prowess to do so. When any of these conditions is present, the clinician may facilitate language-related performance by directly teaching children to monitor their comprehension and to use strategies to request clarification when they have not understood.

Dollaghan and Kaston (1986) taught four children with language impairments (ages 5:10 to 8:2 years) to recognize inadequate tape-recorded messages and to ask for appropriate modifications. The intervention was designed in stages so that children first learned to recognize, label, and demonstrate an active orientation to listening, including sitting still, looking at the speaker, and thinking about what the speaker is saying. Second, they learned to detect and to react to messages that had "signal inadequacies," such as insufficient loudness or excessive rate that obscured the message by saying, for example, "I can't hear you," or "Slow down." Third, they learned to evaluate and react to messages containing inadequate content, by saying, for example, "What do you mean?" or "Which one?" Finally, they learned to respond to messages that exceeded their comprehension owing to the presence of unfamiliar lexical items, excessive length, or excessive syntactic complexity by saying things such as "Say those one at a time" or "Can you show me?" Following the implementation of intervention techniques that included direct instruction, modeling, role playing, and guided discussions, these early elementary schoolchildren demonstrated rapid increases in queries about inadequate messages and they maintained high-level monitoring skills following a nontreatment interval of 3 to 6 weeks.

Content, Contexts, and Strategies for Content–Form Intervention

The strategies used to select target structures and to conduct intervention depend in part on the underlying theoretical position one adopts. Approaches driven by linguistic rule induction or behaviorist theories tend to involve careful specification of target structures and sequences of intervention steps. Interestingly, many of the approaches aimed at helping children acquire rules for producing and comprehending content–form constructions were first introduced in the 1970s when the psycholinguistic focus on grammatical rule acquisition was at its height, but the main strategies being implemented by speech–language pathologists and special educators were behavioristic. Hence, in the 1970s, many of the intervention approaches designed to teach language forms used the high structure that Fey (1986) labeled "trainer-oriented" programs: Clinicians select particular target structures; control stimuli and reinforcers (e.g., tokens to be turned in for small toys); and use strategies requiring children to make many responses of similar types (massed trials) in a short amount of time. The intended result is that children will induce rules under these focused conditions that they have not been able to induce from more random evidence in natural communicative interactions.

Gray and Ryan (1973) designed a structured, highly controlled intervention program that gradually moved children from heavy dependence on imitative modeling and 100% reinforcement schedules, to more indirect modeling, and then no modeling. Sometimes known as the *Monterey language program,* it included several subprograms for different grammatical structures with similar series of steps in which children learned first to imitate particular pieces of sentence forms and then learned to respond in the same way to questions after the imitative prompts were removed. In the early stages of the program, the context and content for the practice sentences came from sets of pictures illustrating various situations (often cut from magazine advertisements), which sometimes led to the use of an interesting and varied lexicon. In the later stages of each subprogram, parents were taught to administer similar prompts and reinforcers to those used earlier by the clinician in contexts that at first were semistructured (looking at storybooks) and later unstructured.

As sensitivity to pragmatic features such as functionality and context-dependence became more common in the 1980s, programs such as Connell's (1986b) approach (described previously in this section) were designed to teach more multidimensional aspects of language forms and to be sensitive to context and to conversational partners. However, even those approaches tended to remain highly structured and strongly dependent on operant methods, including such features as massed trials, gradually faded imitative models, and extrinsic reinforcers delivered on a preplanned schedule.

Contrast such structured, trainer-oriented approaches with those called "child oriented" (Fey, 1986) or "naturalistic" (Norris & Hoffman, 1990b). In less structured approaches, intervention is less focused on one target structure at a time. Although objectives may still be written that target the acquisition of particular structures, multiple structures may be targeted at once. The actual amount of the child's practice on each target structure is determined more by the occasions that necessitate its use, based on the child's choices of context and topic, than on the basis of some predetermined sequence and number of productions. This approach is guided more by social interaction theory than by linguistic rule-induction theory. It is consistent with the argument that children will be more likely to acquire a particular structure and to generalize it to everyday use when they need to use it during real communication for real purposes (rather than a contrived set of parallel sentences).

Research is needed to compare the results of the two kinds of approaches for acquiring the rules of content–form constructions. Different children may benefit differentially from the two types of approaches. In my personal experience, children who are active conversationalists (using Fey's, 1986, terminology, see Figure 4.1) with relatively specific deficits of language form, may benefit from an efficient, structured, trainer-oriented approach; however, children who are passive conversationalists, inactive conversationalists, or verbal noncommunicators are more likely to benefit from a more child-oriented naturalistic approach that uses classroom contexts as well as direct one-to-one intervention.

CONTINUED PHONOLOGICAL DEVELOPMENT

Phonology is one of the five rule systems (including morphology, syntax, semantics, and pragmatics) that children must acquire to become competent communicators. Consistent with system theory advocated throughout this book, it is impossible to consider other aspects of language development apart from acquisition of the phonological system. The influence of phonological complexity on syntactic performance by children with language disorders has also been noted (Panagos & Prelock, 1982).

The problem in designing intervention programs is in knowing how much time to devote to activities primarily aimed at reducing phonological impairment and how much time to devote to other aspects of language acquisition. Fey (1986) suggested that, as a rule of thumb, increasing intelligibility should be targeted as a basic goal within more comprehensive programs for children with language impairments in cases where two conditions hold: (1) Speech sound production deficits are a significant component of the child's communication problem, and (2) the child has at least a 50- to 100-word expressive vocabulary. Fey also noted that children in any of his four categories might require direct attention to phonological development.

In their three-part review of factors related to the classification, management, and severity of phonological disorders in children, Shriberg and Kwiatkowski (1982a, 1982b, 1982c) emphasized the role of individ-

ual differences among children with developmental phonological disorders. They suggested that children's intervention needs might be better met if professionals considered those individual differences when planning intervention. For example, some children might benefit most from a program with mechanism emphasis, which focuses on surface forms and speech motor control, using drill and drill-play modes early in treatment and structured play and free-play modes later for transfer. Other children might need a more cognitive-linguistic emphasis, which focuses on underlying forms and phonological rules, using drill-play and structured play early for acquisition and the free-play mode later for transfer. A third group of children might benefit most from programs using a psychosocial emphasis, in which sociolinguistic forms become the primary phonological targets; the play mode is used early for "acclimation," drill play and structured play modes are used later for acquisition, and play modes are used still later for transfer. This strategy is consistent with the eclectic approach advocated throughout this book.

ACQUIRING AND RECALLING WORDS AND CONCEPTS

Building a Lexicon: Fast Mapping and Other Processes

It is artificial to separate word meaning from the acquisition of the ability to produce and comprehend language constructions. Yet, it is sometimes helpful to focus relatively more on one domain or the other in intervention.

When children reach the middle stages of language acquisition, they already have a substantial vocabulary. From 18 months to 6 years of age, they can be expected to add words at a rate unsurpassed at other stages of development. Crais (1990) summarized research showing that children add approximately five word roots per day during this time and comprehend around 14,000 words by the time they are 6 years old.

How do children accomplish such an amazing feat normally, and what differences might be expected for children with language disorders? As we considered in Chapter 7, infants and toddlers are heavily dependent on context and event-based strategies for learning word meanings. Part of the process of developing more mature lexical acquisition strategies involves changing from solely event-based processing to multiple processing strategies. However, this does not mean that event-based strategies are abandoned entirely. Even adults use event-based strategies to comprehend unfamiliar words and to recall less familiar words at times (Crais, 1990).

Establishing meaningful contexts that encourage children to add new words to their lexicons is one intervention strategy that can be used with children of all ages. This strategy draws on children's abilities to "map" information about words into memory. Carey (1978) described the mapping process as having two phases. In the first, called *fast mapping,* children map only a small portion of the available information into semantic memory by using episodic and contextual cues to form preliminary associations. The second phase is more gradual, involving subsequent encounters with the word, when additional information is mapped.

Fast mapping has been demonstrated for preschool-age children. Carey and Bartlett (1978) used the naturalistic context of snack time in a preschool to show that 3- and 4-year-olds could fast map a meaning of *chromium* when exposed only once in the context, "See those two trays? Bring me the chromium one, not the red one." A week later, more than half of those children demonstrated partial knowledge of the word *chromium* in comprehension and production tasks. As might be expected, however, the children's word concepts at that point were highly varied, supporting the idea of a second (perhaps indefinite) stage of mapping, in which word meanings continue to be clarified and amplified. This study also illustrates "the-rich-get-richer" phenomenon: children who already had solid control of the meaning of the word *red* and the syntactic construction conveying contrast were much more likely to have the tools needed to fast map.

Dollaghan (1985) designed a similar task. She asked 2- to 5-year-old children to hide three familiar objects and then to hide a "koob" (a novel plastic object). Later, a majority of the children comprehended the word sufficiently to select a "koob" from a set of five objects (two familiar and three unfamiliar) and feed it to a puppet. During a production task, when Dollaghan asked children to perform a phonetic reproduction of the word, more problems arose. Indeed, the production task in the "koob" procedure was the only one that discriminated performance of a group of 4- and 5-year-old normally developing children from a matched group with language impair-

ments (Dollaghan, 1987a). Dollaghan was unsure whether the difficulty experienced by the language-impaired subjects (who were equally able to choose a referent, to comprehend the word, and to store nonlinguistic information about it) was due to storage or retrieval difficulties. She suggested, however, that breakdown more likely occurred during retrieval, because four of the five children who did not name the object recognized "koob" when given "soob" and "teed" as foils.

Rice, Buhr, and Nemeth (1990) identified several points in the fast-mapping process that might be vulnerable to the negative effects of language impairment: (1) attention to the stream of words presented, (2) identification of a novel item, (3) a quick assessment of the linguistic and nonlinguistic context for probable meaning, (4) entering the probable meaning into the appropriate slot in the available lexicon, and (5) storage for immediate or later use. In a study that showed fast mapping by 5-year-olds with language impairments to be significantly poorer than fast mapping by MLU-matched and chronological age-matched peers, Rice et al. found that the most striking difference between the groups was the rate of fast mapping. Also, object words were the most discriminating between the groups, perhaps because the normally developing children fast mapped them so readily, making the children with language impairments comparatively much poorer; and the children with language impairments performed more poorly on comprehension as well as recall tasks. Based on their analysis, Rice et al. concluded little support for attention deficits, limitations of lexical and grammatical knowledge, or the ability to store new lexical items in memory as primary explanations for the deficit.

Perhaps the strongest implication of these studies is that children with language disorders need more time, more repetitions, and heightened focus on new words and concepts to acquire new meanings. They may also may need more deliberate productive practice of novel words before making them their own, and they may be less apt to acquire new words effectively in the context of completely naturalistic experiences. The intervention techniques best suited for this kind of problem are scaffolding and mediation, including Blank's (1973) dialogue approach, in which adults interact with children in meaningful contexts, framing and focusing the children's attention on key relationships and highlighting contrastive details within existing knowledge, and giving them opportunities to use the words many times in appropriately varied ways.

Intervention for Word-Finding Impairments

The relationships among processes of word comprehension, short- and long-term memory storage, retrieval, and production are difficult to sort out. Researchers have observed, however, that some children with language impairments and learning disabilities have difficulty "finding" the words they want to use in specific contexts, particularly under stressful conditions, even when they appear to "know" those words under other conditions and at different times (Denckla & Rudel, 1976; German, 1979; D. W. Johnson & Myklebust, 1967; Wiig & Semel, 1980). Stated most simply, word-finding difficulties (also called *dysnomia*) involve problems in generating appropriate words to use in particular contexts (Kail & Leonard, 1986). In some cases, children with these problems may also substitute unintended for intended words (German, 1982, 1983; see Personal Reflection 8.7), much like the paraphasic errors produced by adults with acquired aphasia. German described other secondary characteristics that might be observed for children with word-finding problems as follows: (1) talking around the word they are trying to retrieve (circumlocutions), providing a description or function "you cut with it" instead of the word (*knife*); (2) using time fillers during long pauses (*um, er, ah*); (3) using empty words (*stuff*); (4) substituting indefinite pronouns (*thing*); (5) producing attempts at self-correction ("fork, no, I mean knife"); (6) using gestures; and (7) producing extra verbalizations ("it's a, oh, I know it . . ."). Alternate explanations have been proposed for these phenomena.

Following a series of experiments with school-age children between the ages of 7 and 14 years, Kail and Leonard (1986) concluded that retrieval problems experienced by children with language disorders were mainly a result of limits of semantic elaboration.

They cautioned against the use of intervention approaches designed to teach children processing strategies for word retrieval without providing information about the meaning, use, and syntactic privileges of occurrence of words to be retrieved.

German (1989; D. German, personal communication, April 17, 1990) presented a slightly different explanation for the occurrence of word finding problems, at least in some children. She suggested that three groups of children with word-finding problems can be differentiated: (1) individuals with specific language impairments who meet the classic definition of retrieval difficulty in the presence of good comprehension; (2) individuals with specific language impairments who have related receptive language problems and difficulty retrieving because their word images are unstable (this describes the group studied by Kail & Leonard, 1986); and (3) individuals who have multiple disabilities that affect both their acquisition of words in comprehension and their ability to retrieve words they know. German's analysis suggested that some children are more likely to experience breakdowns of lexical representation in memory at the semantic level, and others at the phonological level. As German has refined the Test of Word Finding (1989, see also annotated bibliography in Appendix A), she has added tasks that can help sort out different levels of processing breakdown and has developed procedures to analyze children's word-finding skills in more informal discourse contexts (German, 1991).

German (1983) noted that teachers can be the best sources of referral of children with word-finding difficulties. A word-finding survey designed to be completed by teachers to aid in referral appears in Box 8.17.

Intervention for word-finding difficulties may differ somewhat, depending on whether one views the primary problem to stem from lack of semantic elaboration, impaired phonological representation, or a

Personal Reflection 8.7	"Mary is seven and in the second grade. In her attempts to give specific responses to a set of picture cards, she made the following errors: 'question mark' for 'check mark,' 'head cover' for 'crown,' 'checkers' for 'jacks,' 'It's the thing you make a hole with' for 'drill,' and 'stool' for 'spool.'"
	Description of a child with word-finding problems by *Diane German* (1983, p. 539).

Box 8.17   German's (1983) Word-Finding Survey for use by teachers

Teacher's Name _____   Child's Name_____

Does the child frequently (+ = yes, − = no)

1. Know the word he wants to retrieve, but can't think of it?
2. Show a delayed response time when he is trying to think of a word?
3. Talk around the word he wants to use?
4. Give word substitutions that have the same meaning as the word he wants to use?
5. Give the function of the word he wants to use?
6. Give a description of the word he wants to use?
7. Give a substitution that sounds like the word he wants to use?
8. Have difficulty finding the word he wants to use when he is trying to relate an experience to you?
9. Use such vague words as they, stuff, you know, in place of words he wants to retrieve?
10. Use filler words such as um, er, ah, when he is trying to retrieve a word?
11. Have difficulty retrieving a specific word, object name or fact?
12. Use gestures to pantomime the word he wants to retrieve?
13. State: "I know that word, but I can't think of it"?
14. Use incomplete phrases and self corrections when describing an experience or event?
15. Have good understanding of oral language used in class?

_____

Note. From "I Know It but I Can't Think of It: Word Retrieval Difficulties" by D. J. German, 1983, *Academic Therapy, 18,* pp. 542. Copyright 1983 by Pro-Ed. Reprinted by permission.

retrieval processing deficit in the presence of adequate internalized word concepts. In any of these cases, however, part of the process must be assisting the child to gain practice in making rich associations and to develop multiple strategies for building stable semantic categories and associations of words (in their auditory, oral, read, and written forms).

PARTICIPATING IN STORYTELLING: EMERGING LITERACY

The previous discussion of language sample analysis for middle-stage children mentioned the need to consider varied modes of discourse, not only conversational interaction. As noted, even 2-year-olds may use some of the features of organized narrative discourse, such as longer turns, more organized structures, and domination by a single speaker, when they produce bedtime monologues (K. Nelson, 1989). A review of the literature on emerging literacy (Norris & Bruning 1988) suggested that "the development of literate-style language begins as early as 2 years of age for children who have opportunities to engage in story-book reading and storytelling" (p. 416).

The importance of positive early literacy experiences on later language learning can hardly be overstated. Cullinan (1989) reviewed a series of studies, all of which supported the conclusion that children who have heard written language read aloud as preschoolers have dramatic advantages later in learning to read and in understanding the world at large. For example, in Gordon Wells's (1986) longitudinal study (discussed earlier in this chapter) one child had never heard a story read aloud before entering school and continued to lag behind the other students at the end of elementary school. Meanwhile a child who had heard more than 5,000 stories during same time was at the top of the class in literacy-related activities. Although simple cause–effect relationships cannot be assumed, the need to experience good children's literature (see Cullinan, 1989, or Westby, 1985/1991, for selection suggestions) in positive social interactions with parents should never be ignored when programming for middle-stage children with language disorders.

The need for literary experiences may be particularly acute when children's other life experiences are limited. In Chapter 4, we considered possible limita-

Personal Reflection 8.8 "The Garcia family also has found a special way of sharing books. Books are read in both English and Spanish. Raphael, age six, listens to the stories with his little sister, Maria, age two. When their mother, Carmen, begins reading the story of *Hester the Jester* by Ben Schecter, she starts in English. Raphael and Maria listen, and ask questions about the story. Carmen answers them, and then she gives a Spanish translation of the story. It is a family time, and the children enjoy listening to their mother as she reads and talks to them in the English and Spanish of their bilingual home."

Family literacy experiences described by *Dorothy Strickland* and *Denny Taylor* (1989, p. 31).

tions in language development related to physical impairment. One example of the value of early literacy experiences for those children was reported by Butler (1980), who described the importance of books in the early development of Cushla, a girl with severe physical impairments. Cushla's parents used stories to calm her through long hospital stays and sleepless nights as she struggled with her disabilities. Because she was unable to hold objects, crawl, sit up, or watch what happened around her, books became Cushla's chief means of learning, as well as her chief source of delight. Although Cushla's parents had been told to expect her to be mentally retarded, her intelligence was assessed as being well above average when she was tested at age 3:8.

Providing opportunity to participate in varied literacy activities, such as hearing written language read aloud, looking at books, participating in storytelling, writing notes, and drawing pictures about stories, all may be part of reducing disabilities and handicaps of children with language impairments and middle-stage needs. Not all children with disabilities have parents like Cushla's, however (Butler, 1980). Far too often, delayed language skills and associated attention and cognitive deficits result in children with language disorders receiving fewer opportunities to engage in positive narrative discourse activities with their parents and other adults than are received by their siblings and peers. The professional may need to design direct intervention strategies to assist parents to acquire skills that will make reading to their children enjoyable for all.

To tell and to understand stories, children need at least two kinds of experience. First, they need to understand enough about how the world and people work in their culture to construct scripts or schemas

for common interactions and events. Second, they need to have heard enough stories that they can begin to construct internalized schemas for story structures, which are ways of reorganizing and reconstructing reality. When literacy activities work best, the two kinds of experience are likely to be thoroughly intertwined. Indeed, as Cushla's experience suggests (Butler, 1980), books may provide the opportunity for vicarious experiences that can at least partially compensate for unavoidable limitations in real-life experiences.

Narrative constructions do not spring forth fully formed from most children. Rather, they undergo gradual development, when children learn to create logical chains of events and to maintain consistent motivations and personality characteristics of main characters before learning to combine both features (Applebee, 1978; Westby, 1984). Many examples of children's literature parallel this developmental sequence and it may be helpful for the professional to match literature selections fairly closely to children's own expressive storytelling in the early stages. As noted previously in this chapter (Cazden, 1988), cultural differences also should be honored.

Scott (1988a) emphasized the need to recognize the influence of different stories and storytelling contexts when analyzing stories told by children with language disorders. She noted that the same child may tell stories with different qualities, depending on the surrounding events and degree of prompting the child receives before beginning the narration. The three types of narratives that have received the most attention in prior research include (1) personal narratives; (2) TV program, film, or book summaries; and (3) fictional tales. For stories retold from TV programs or books, Scott's review suggested that the medium in which children originally experience narratives might influence their later ability to retell them. Children's retellings of TV dramas and cartoons tend to lack explicit references to character's goals and discernible endings, perhaps because TV characters' motivations tend to be nonexplicit, and even normally developing 9-year-old children have difficulty answering inference questions about TV narratives (Collins, Wellman, Keniston, & Westby, 1978). Books that discuss characters' motivations and feelings explicitly may be better suited for modeling such considerations, particularly for children with language disorders. Their stories tend to include less information in the story grammar categories of internal response (Ripich & Griffith, 1985) and protagonist attempt (Roth & Spekman, 1986) than their peers who are learning language normally. In my experience, when asked to tell or write personal narratives from their own experiences, many children use more story grammar categories when prompted to talk about some problem and how they solved it. If they are asked only to tell or write about something interesting that happened to them, the "narrative" that results is far more likely to be a sequenced chain of events experienced on a vacation trip to an amusement park. Hearing examples of mature personal narratives modeled by adults may also help some children to incorporate more organized and thematically connected details in their stories. Telling stories with "sparkle" (Peterson & McCabe, 1983) may also be more likely to occur when children have some commitment (Perera, 1984) to the topic of the narration, as they do in a personal narrative involving themselves.

Assisting children to organize their narratives in mature ways may involve direct targeting of the inclusion of the key components of "story grammar" (N. W. Nelson, 1988b, Westby, 1984, 1985/1991). Research evidence suggests that children can learn to include more of the macrostructure elements as a result of training (Carnine & Kinder, 1985; Gordon & Braun, 1983). However, children need to be guided to do more than to make sure that they have something in each slot in the organizational schema. Westby (1984) emphasized the need for specific and sustained social interaction dialogue to support early narrative development, including discussions leading to knowledge of cause and effect and motives. Children with weak language skills, including poor readers, may be less likely to exhibit logical cohesion in their narratives (Norris & Bruning, 1988), and helping them

to achieve better organization may depend as much on encouraging the development of complex ideas as the development of complex sentence structures. Indeed, mediated discussions about interesting stories may be the best way to target the acquisition of complex linguistic structures by children with wobbly language competencies.

Westby (1985/1991) described a scaffolding strategy in which a teacher led a discussion about a picture showing two children injured in an accident. The teacher guided the interaction by asking a series of focusing questions that led the children to describe a possible setting, initiating event, internal response, internal plan, attempts, consequence, and ending. These responses were outlined in separate columns on the chalkboard. Then the children constructed their story:

> Angel and Michael got hurt in a car accident. An ambulance came real fast and took them to the hospital. Dr. David and Nurse Michelle washed their cuts. Then they put bandages on them. Officer Joe called Mrs. Chavez on the phone. He said, "Your children were hurt in a car accident. They are at the hospital. I'll pick you up in my police car." Mrs. Chavez was worried and scared. She asked Dr. David if she could take her children home. He said, "You may take them home. Give them soup and put them to bed." Angel and Michael got well and lived happily ever after. (reported by Costlow, 1983, in personal communication to Westby, 1985/1991, p. 200)

Although learning to understand and to tell stories seems to be critical to the emergence of literate language during the preschool years, the importance of encouraging narrative discourse does not stop when children begin to learn to read. Narrative skills continue to develop into adulthood (N. W. Nelson, 1988c). Indeed, the best storytellers are rewarded handsomely for their novels and screenplays. Targeting narrative language skills for intervention in the later stages of language development may be as appropriate as in the middle stages. However, because of wide variations in narrative discourse among individual samples produced by the same children in different contexts, the specialist may not always be able to separate issues of the need for normal development (language arts) from the need for special services (language intervention). Clearly, in this area, speech–language pathologists need to work closely with regular and special educators to conduct ongoing criterion-referenced assessments, such as by comparing writing samples across portfolios in all of the children in a second-grade classroom. Even if a child with a language impairment seems not to have a disability in constructing narratives relative to contextual demands, a finding of relative strength in discourse processing may be useful in designing intervention approaches. For such children, emphasizing top-down processing can help them compensate for weaknesses in surface-level processing needed in, for example, written language decoding. Encouraging children to use their grasp of deeper text-level meanings may help them predict words in listening or written language, provided they are also taught to use perceptual level cues to check the accuracy of their predictions. Otherwise, some bright children with specific language-learning disabilities may tend to construct marvelous stories as they attempt to read, but stories that diverge further and further from the text on the page (see Personal Reflection 8.9).

BEGINNING SCHOOL

The Early Stages of Learning to Read

In the minds of children, parents, and teachers, learning to read is perhaps the most important hallmark of the middle stages of language acquisition. If learning to talk did not occur so seemingly automatically, the oral language accomplishments of the preschool years might appear far more dazzling than early elementary school accomplishments of learning to read. Learning to talk, however, usually occurs without direct instruction, but learning to read is what children and parents in literate cultures talk about and look forward to as a primary motivation for going to school.

Learning to process written language is not equally accessible to all children. Even in kindergarten, some children become so discouraged with themselves in school that they start each day with a headache or stomachache, and children with a history of language acquisition difficulties are particularly at risk. Preventing such misery involves concentrated collaborative efforts of special and regular educators and speech–language pathologists as all seek ways to help children with language-learning difficulties crack the written language code and make sense of written words.

To understand how to help these children, one must first understand the process of mature reading. Reading is more than pronouncing words on a page. Although acquisition of strategies for transforming text to speech certainly plays a role in obtaining meaning from print, reading involves much more than sounding out words. Mature readers focus their primary attention on decoding strategies only when they come to unusual or difficult words. Even then, they tend to sound out words syllable-by-syllable rather than sound-by-sound. Whether readers use phonemic, syllabic, or whole-word units to connect print with auditory and spoken word images, they use graphophonemic cues, which involve associations of graphemes to phonemes but not necessarily one-to-one correspondences between single graphemes and phonemes. Rather, they often require associating irregular patterns such as *cough* and *through* with two- or three-phoneme sequences or directly with morphemic meanings, or they may involve associating irregularly spelled morphemes like *-tion* with other sound sequences and meanings.

Mature readers use two or three additional cuing systems, all based on knowledge of language and discourse, to form hypotheses about the messages they are attempting to get through print. K. S. Goodman (1969, 1973a, 1973b) proposed that mature readers use the three linguistic cuing systems (1) graphophonemic, (2) syntactic, and (3) semantic to form and test predictions as they read. In addition, it may be equally important to use (4) text and discourse knowledge and understanding of scripts to make sense of

---

Personal Reflection 8.9   "Some readers of low skill appear to compensate for ineffective word-level processes by relying more on discourse-level information to identify words. Compared with skilled readers, such low-skill readers identify words much more quickly in context as long as the context is helpful. However, when context is misleading, such readers are slowed down more than skilled readers."

Steven Roth and *Charles Perfetti* (1980 p. 26).

written language texts and to ensure that later and earlier parts of texts are integrated and connected (a more complex model of written language processing is presented in Chapter 9). In fact, mature readers rely heavily on their knowledge of language and the world to form hypotheses and to make predictions about the words on the page. They sample only enough perceptual data from the printed text to confirm that their predictions are accurate. If something does not make sense, they may backtrack to gather further perceptual data and relate it to what they know about how words sound and what words and sentence constructions mean but only to the degree necessary to obtain meaning and for the text to make sense.

The assumptions cannot necessarily be made about beginning readers. Chall (1983) proposed a developmental model of the stages of reading acquisition. She called the initial prereading period, stage 0, the stage from birth to 5 or 6 years of age, when children pretend to "read" familiar stories that they have heard read aloud many times. She noted that it was followed by stage 1, an initial reading or decoding stage, when children are "glued to print." During stage 1, occurring in 5- to 7-year-olds, Chall proposed that children devote a great deal of attention to the process of learning phoneme–grapheme correspondence rules. During stage 2, in 7- to 9-year-olds, children undergo the subsequent process of ungluing from print. They begin to rely more heavily on the redundancies of language and their knowledge of scripts and story structure to derive meaning more easily and fluently from text.

Other theorists would disagree that Chall's (1983) model is truly developmental and would argue that it only appears to be developmental because it is the way that adults have organized the curriculum for teaching children to read traditionally (K. S. Goodman,

1986; D. F. King & Goodman, 1990; Norris & Damico, 1990; Schory, 1990). Instead, this second group of theorists, who advocate keeping language whole in early literacy instruction, argue that a better developmental explanation for early reading acquisition emphasizes children's motivations and abilities to make sense of their world as the driving force that leads children to begin to derive meaning from print (see Personal Reflection 8.10). They argue that the parts of language are processed most effectively when encountered in whole-language contexts, and that fragmenting language to teach it is unnatural and counterproductive (Norris & Damico, 1990).

A similar philosophy has guided language and reading instruction in the culturally diverse island nation of New Zealand for more than 20 years, and the program is reported to have met with considerable success with all kinds of children (Mabbett, 1990). Mabbett articulated some of the principles of that approach:

❏ Reading, talking, and writing are inseparably interrelated;
❏ The foundations of literacy are laid in the early years;
❏ Reading for meaning is paramount;
❏ Books for children learning to read should use natural idiomatic language that is appropriate to the subject;
❏ There is no one way in which people learn to read. A combination of approaches is needed. (1990, p. 60)

When children with language-learning impairments have difficulty learning to read, speech–language pathologists may identify weak language skills that contribute to the difficulty. Phonological processing limitations may be involved. Kamhi and Catts's (1989) review of the literature showed that children with reading difficulties often have deficits in encoding, retrieving, and using phonological memory codes. These problems tend to show up as deficits in performing metalinguistic tasks, such as rhyming and

---

Personal Reflection 8.10   "The term [*whole language*] originated in response to methods used in schools that fragment and tear language asunder. The subsystems of language are often the focus of useless, time-wasting, and confusing instruction. Speaking, listening, reading, and writing are often taught as if they were separable pieces of language, each composed of separable smaller units. We have had, in fact, a 'part-language' curriculum. The 'whole' in whole language emphasizes the integrity of language and the language process."

Dorothy King and *Kenneth Goodman* (1990, p. 222) writing about whole language as a philosophy about learners.

recognizing sound families. However, that does not necessarily mean that teaching children to rhyme isolated words is a particularly good intervention approach. Another common recommendation is that children who have trouble with phonological skills such as word pronunciation and sequencing complex sound sequences should be taught to read by methods emphasizing visual patterns and whole-word recognition and avoiding attention to phonics. In my experience, these approaches often fail to meet children's needs. Memorizing individual words places an immense load on memory and makes it difficult for children to decode words they have never seen. On the other hand, children with weak phonological processing skills may learn to make sound–symbol associations and to sequence them when reading and writing if deliberately assisted in making the associations.

Many children automatically make such associations in whole-language contexts as they learn to read. The same may not be true, however, of children with language-learning difficulties who find it more difficult to induce such connections. They may need more "code emphasis" (I. Y. Liberman & Liberman, 1990) to become aware of the segments of language and the alphabetic principle by which artifacts of alphabet are associated with natural units of language. Although deliberate instruction may need special prominence, it should not be isolated completely from the top-down processes of obtaining meaning from text. In my experience, children with language-learning difficulties benefit from a combination of bottom-up teaching strategies that focus on decoding sound patterns in combination with activities designed to teach children to focus on the construction of meaning. For example, in classroom programs for children with severe language impairments, my colleagues and I used an eclectic model of language intervention. We instructed children in phonological analysis and synthesis skills, focusing on form, during part of the day, and helped them to construct and "read" their own personal news journals, focusing on meaning, during another part of the day (N. W. Nelson, 1981a). As children become stronger in both skills, they can integrate multiple components of the reading and writing process.

The Early Stages of Learning to Write

An integral part of the philosophy that views literacy development as language learning is that reading, writing, and talking are not separate but are integrated processes. This suggests that, rather than waiting to teach children to write until after they have gained facility with reading and speaking skills, the best strategy might be to teach writing in tandem with the other skills, using it to facilitate reading and even speaking and auditory sequencing.

Learning to produce written language is a complex process involving the coordination of language formulation, phonological processing, graphomotor, and cognitive monitoring skills. Effective writers also use pragmatic knowledge to consider the needs of their imagined audience. One way that teachers encourage children to write is to serve as a real and interested audience for their messages (Calkins, 1983; Graves, 1983).

Written language, like spoken language, may serve varied sociolinguistic functions. In one classroom, students might use written language to label, to remember, to entertain, and to learn academic content (McGee & Richgels, 1990). Children who have difficulty grasping the abstract nature of the writing process may need illumination of the communicative function of writing by conversing with a real audience, such as the teacher, through written notes. Parents who exchange notes with their children also find that they can communicate some things better in writing than orally. Teachers should be encouraged to allow children to write surreptitious social notes without appearing to sanction the process. This kind of spontaneous conversational writing is mapped onto early discourse functions, and the recipient almost always accepts and never criticizes it. Children who do not have access to the usual modes of writing because of motor deficits need augmentative systems that can support social and academic writing.

In the early stages of learning to write, children may lack sufficient knowledge to spell words they want to write. Box 8.18 lists some strategies that children adopt as they learn to spell. Recognizing the normal variation that can occur in word-production strategies may prevent specialists in language and learning disabilities from becoming overly critical of the normal "errors" that children make when learning to produce words in writing.

As children develop more mature written language abilities, other discourse functions also may be encouraged. Children who have encountered written language in shared reading experiences may have more conceptual support for constructing stories of their own. In the early stages, a combination of printed words and drawings might be particularly

Box 8.18   A description of developmental word-creation strategies

Physical Relationship.   Child tries to relate the number or the appearance of marks to some physical aspect of the object or person represented. The child might use three marks, for example, to write her name if she is three years old.

Visual Design.   Child accepts the arbitrary nature of words—that they do not resemble their referents physically. The child tries to recreate some designs. The first design attempted is often the child's name. Placeholders—others letters, circles, solid dots, or vertical lines—often are used in the place of those letters that the child cannot form.

Syllabic Hypothesis.   Child realizes there is a relationship between the oral and written version of words and also that spoken words can be segmented into "beats" or syllables. The child codes words syllabically, using one mark for each of a word's syllables.

Letter Strings (visual rules).   Children create words by stringing letters together so that they look like words. They use several rules. (1) Don't use too many letters. (2) Don't use too few letters. (3) Use a variety of letters, with not more than two of the same letter in succession. (4) Rearrange the same letters to make different words. Children ask, "What word is this?"

Authority Based.   This strategy often follows on the heels of the letter string strategy, apparently because children decide that it is more efficient to ask for spellings, since so many of their letter strings yield nonwords. Children ask for spellings of whole words, or they copy known words from environmental print or books.

Early Phonemic.   Children begin to generate their own words by coding sounds they hear—an idea they might get as adults provide spellings and make letter–sound associations explicit when giving spellings during the time that children are using the Authority Based strategy. Independent spelling may be delayed in children who receive complex answers to their spelling questions during the early part of this stage. No known disadvantage is associated with delay of this kind.

Transitional Phonemic.   Children begin to realize that their sound based spellings do not look quite like words they see in the environment and that specific spellings they generate are not always identical to ones they see elsewhere. Children often become dissatisfied with their own spellings and begin to ask again for whole word spellings, or they generate a spelling on their own and ask, "Is that right?" This strategy is not common among preschoolers, although children who read early often use it, presumably because they have more visual information about words than do typical preschoolers.

Note. The order of use for the strategies typically follows the order of this list, although different environments provide different information to children, which can result in variations in children's word creation strategy development.

Note. From "The Place of Specific Skills in Preschool and Kindergarten" by J. A. Schickedanz, in *Emerging Literacy: Young Children Learn to Read and Write* (p. 103) edited by D. S. Strickland and L. M. Morrow, 1989, Newark, DE: International Reading Association. Copyright 1989 by International Reading Association. Reprinted with permission of Judith A. Schickedanz and the International Reading Association.

effective for children who can more easily represent meanings in nonprint modes. In our Berrien County, Michigan, classrooms for children with severe language impairments, students either wrote or dictated personal narrative "news" each day in special booklets. They also illustrated their news and read it aloud for their classmates in the whole-group context later in the day. During the full-group interaction, the class decided together what news to record on the 4 × 6-inch cards that were later stapled to the bulletin board for each day of the month as a calendar. One child was selected to illustrate each bit of group news. At the end of the month, the daily cards were taken down and tied together with yarn to make a familiar book that any of these students with dyslexia could read. For older children with multiple impairments who remain at middle language stages of written language development, special devices such as computer software programs (Beukelman, Tice, Garrett, & Lange, 1989) may be used to assist children to learn to spell, and story frames (Stewart, 1985) may be used to assist children to see the structure of texts.

Other Uses of Language in Classrooms

The uses of language for learning to read and write and for communicating in written language are highly visible in early elementary classrooms, but they are certainly not the only uses of languages. As mentioned previously in this chapter, language plays many roles in classrooms.

Some of the language used to teach reading and writing is language used to talk about language, or *metalinguistic* language. One function that traditional speech therapy has sometimes served for children with articulation disorders is that they acquire concepts for metalinguistic terms such as *sound, letter, syllable, word,* and *sentence* before other children do. When children have difficulty functioning in early elementary classrooms, their ability to use language to talk about language may be one area that could benefit from intervention. The focus of the intervention might be to help the children acquire the meanings of such terms in contexts meaningful to the child and relevant to classroom interactions.

A similar use of language in classrooms might be called *metapragmatic*. This is the language and non-verbal communication used by teachers to convey the rules for communicating in the classroom. For example, children need to learn to recognize when they must raise their hands to talk and when talking is permitted.

A variety of other specialized uses of language occur in particular aspects of the curriculum. When teachers, parents, and students prioritize areas of the curriculum that present the most difficulty for a student, those areas should be the focus of investigation when performing curriculum-based language assessment activities (as described in Chapter 9).

Different parts of the curriculum make different kinds of language demands on the learner. For example, mathematics uses its own nonlinguistic symbol system. Some famous individuals, best exemplified by Albert Einstein, have shown great difficulty learning to talk and read but genius when manipulating mathematical symbols. In the elementary classroom, however, children who are good at understanding language concepts, such as *many, each, all* and so forth, have a distinct advantage. So do children who are good at using their verbal memories to remember teachers' instructions and to verbally recall and paraphrase instructions to direct their own thinking. When children have difficulty using any of these language functions, they may find themselves in serious difficulty in classrooms without knowing exactly why.

What can be done about it? Different problems justify different intervention strategies. Verbal mediation can assist in many areas. For example, when a child in first or second grade seems unable to remember whether to add or subtract when completing worksheets of mixed addition and subtraction problems, one possibility is that the student is not using verbal mediation strategies to label each problem before attempting to solve it. Some metacognitive modeling of how to use "thinking language" to talk to oneself while working and some practice in using the strategy might help these students. When verbal mediation techniques are taught, it is best for language specialists and classroom teachers to collaborate in selecting labels for the desired behavior so that they may prompt the child in similar ways to use the strategy in everyday activities. For example, if the speech–language pathologist uses the term *thinking language* to prompt the behavior in small-group settings, the special or regular education teacher should prompt with the same label. However, teachers might want to move the child toward using "whisper thinking" as the new strategy becomes established.

When the problem is identified as limited conceptual development for instruction vocabulary, the language specialist may assist the child best by targeting unfamiliar or misunderstood vocabulary within regular classroom curricular materials. A three-part sequence might be used to structure this kind of curriculum-based language intervention. In the first step, the language specialist sits side-by-side with the student as the student attempts to complete a curricular assignment. The professional acts as onlooker-observer and analyzes the language demands of the activity and the student's language skills and strategies without attempting to influence him. In the second stage, the professional begins to mediate the interaction between the demands of the task and the student's address to the task and asks questions designed to help the student to focus on key elements of the activity ("what are we supposed to do here?"); sometimes asks the child to paraphrase the instructional language ("what do you think that means?"); sometimes asks the child to identify the referent for a particular pronoun ("I wonder who the 'he' is in this problem?"); or asks the child to sketch the elements represented by the language of a story problem ("let's sketch what we think that means"). The attitude to convey is one of co-conspirator in unlocking the mysteries of the problem, not one of teacher who knows it all and is just testing whether the student does too. This is not to suggest that the adult should play dumb, but it does allow the adult to participate with the student in the problem-solving activity, interjecting scaffolding comments when appropriate, but primarily, facilitating the child's making discoveries independently. When the child makes an "error," rather than correcting the child or simply indicating that an error has occurred, the interventionist shows the child how the child's response is inconsistent with the data of the problem ("When you call that word *saw* [the word is *was*], I expect it to start with the /s/ sound," or "'The box *saw* full,' does that make sense?"). In the third step, the interventionist attempts to perform the "question transplant" operation introduced in Chapter 1. In this step, the adult encourages the child to internalize the strategies and to become more independent in problem solving. At this point, labels such as "thinking language" for the new strategies are helpful, because adults in multiple settings can all give the child the same prompt to implement the newly acquired strategy.

Increasingly, as children advance through the early grades, they are expected to use nonliteral language to think and to discuss abstract concepts. A review of almost any textbook or literature selection intended for the first few years of elementary school yields examples where children must draw inferences,

understand idioms and metaphors, and use analogical reasoning. One of the dangers of placing children with language-learning difficulties in special curricula is that they will have less exposure to such rich language uses. That is unfortunate for children who can ABNQ handle the language demands of the regular curriculum. Although early elementary school children with language impairments have significantly more difficulty with analogical reasoning than their normal learning peers (Kamhi, Gentry, Mauer, & Gholson, 1990; Nippold, Erskine, & Freed, 1988) some evidence suggests that they can learn to use analogical language when assisted (Kamhi et al., 1990; N. W. Nelson & Gillespie, 1991).

The communication needs model advocated in this book suggests that professionals should use assessment to identify intervention targets based on what children need to do to function successfully in key contexts. This differs from the more traditional approach of the communication processes model—basing target selection on areas of weakness identified on formal tests. When the communication needs model guides assessment, the professional is less likely to underestimate both the communicative demands of contexts and children's potential to acquire new abilities to meet those demands.

FUNCTIONAL GOALS FOR OLDER STUDENTS AT MIDDLE STAGES

Much of the research about disordered language development in the middle stages has been conducted with children who have specific language impairments. Although the category of children with learning disabilities is the largest federally reported special education category in the United States, many children with other problems require language intervention services for middle-stage problems as well.

As noted throughout this book, professionals should consider children's needs from multiple per-

Personal Reflection 8.11	"Each year I come closer to understanding how logical thinking and precise speech can be taught in the classroom. . . . The teacher must help the child see how one thing he knows relates to other things he knows."
	Vivian Paley (1981, p. 213), kindergarten teacher and researcher, describing how she encourages children to learn and to think, using their fantasies and stories.

spectives and should be aware that children's disabilities are relative to the demands of contexts. As these demands become more complex, children whose communicative abilities cannot keep up are likely to be at an increasing disadvantage. Any contributing factors, such as mental retardation, hearing loss, autism, or psychiatric disorder can further negatively influence the child's communication system.

Children with middle-stage language development needs may be adolescents or young adults in transition from school to work settings. The intervention team's job then is to juggle concerns related to the young person's pattern of developmental levels with needs related to chronological age and stage of life expectations. Recall the general purpose of language intervention introduced earlier in this book: to make changes relevant to persons' needs in the domains of (1) social appropriateness, acceptance, and closeness; (2) formal and informal learning; and (3) gainful occupation (paid or unpaid). Keeping these broader purposes in mind will help professionals avoid missing the forest for the trees, which sometimes happens when people work for years on the same discrete skills.

What role should the communicative specialist play when it appears unlikely that young people will ever master the fine points of linguistic use usually acquired during the middle stages of language acquisition? In many U.S. school districts and community service plans, far too many of these individuals receive no services aimed specifically at their communicative needs because they do not show discrepancy between their cognitive and language levels using formal standardized tests. Yet, as noted in Personal Reflection 8.12 when their contextually based needs are considered, many appropriate goals emerge.

Most goals appropriate for older individuals with middle-stage developmental needs are related to functional outcome, and they are often expressed in situation-specific terms. Professionals then plan sequences of subobjectives based on task analysis. For example, Mire and Chisholm (1990) listed seven different goal areas, each of which related to a specific functional context: The client will independently (1) place an order in a fast-food restaurant, (2) use a telephone, (3) shop, (4) communicate needs and comments during leisure time, (5) communicate needs while traveling, (6) communicate while banking, and (7) communicate at the post office. The authors reported an increase in motivation among staff and clients as they worked toward skills that clients were eager to learn and that were clearly relevant.

Persons with developmental disabilities are particularly at risk for being socially disvalued (handicapped) because of inadequate communication abilities (see Personal Reflection 8.13). Part of the communication disorders specialist's role is to minimize the negative effects of external evaluations of their capabilities. Duchan (1986) suggested that clinicians can do this, and can be more relevant to the needs of persons with multiple disabilities by using principles of sense making and fine tuning to guide language intervention. By *sense making,* Duchan referred to "what the participants in the interaction think is going on and what ideas structure that thinking" (p. 188). By *fine tuning,* she meant "the various ways partners adjust their part of the interactions to be in accord with their model of the person they are interacting with" (p. 188). To use sense making in intervention, Duchan suggested that clinicians learn to focus on how children or young people make sense of events as whole processes. Some of the sense of events is based on the scripts that characterize them, and some events and aspects of events have stronger scripts than others. For example, ordering a Big Mac at McDonald's has a standard script, but deciding what to do if the sandwich falls on the floor is an unforeseen part of the script. Both may be legitimate intervention tar-

gets. The structure of some events may also influence clients' agendas regarding their participation. The agenda may be getting the sandwich or getting some tokens and pleasing the clinician. In the first case, the agenda is more clearly the client's, and the clinician can fine tune the interaction to be consistent with that agenda. In the second, the locus of communicative control has shifted to the clinician, and opportunities for client-based fine tuning are diminished. Duchan summarized the advantages of sense making and fine tuning over either traditional "pragmatics intervention" or "behavioral intervention" approaches:

> Clinicians can do more than model and expand on what they take the child to mean; they can be responsive to the child's intent, agenda, and overall sense of the event. They can do more than positively reinforce the child; they can also match the reinforcement to each act and to what the child wants to accomplish with it. (1986, p. 209)

SUMMARY

This chapter considered the communicative contexts, abilities, and needs of children at middle stages of language development. During this period, children advance beyond one- and two-word utterances to formulating and comprehending complex sentences, weaving them into discourse events of many types, and accomplishing varied communicative purposes.

For middle-stage children, the spontaneous communicative sample is an essential assessment context, and methods were suggested for analyzing language form, content, and use in conversational contexts. Other types of discourse were also identified as important, including narrative and expository discourse in both informal and academic contexts.

Intervention targets and strategies related to problems of middle-stage development were discussed as they relate to interactions with adults, play activities, conversational management, developing knowledge of content–form constructions, phonological production and processing capabilities (including those

related to early reading instruction), lexical development and recall strategies, learning to read and write, learning the language of school, and acquiring skills related to functional outcomes appropriate to later stages.

No one intervention approach was advocated as best for all abilities and all children. Some skills (e.g., phonological, morphological, and syntactic rule development) may be more amenable to direct, structured intervention approaches; whereas others (e.g., conceptual knowledge, pragmatic appropriateness, and contextually sensitive linguistic variations) may only be encouraged in meaningful, more naturalistic contexts. Finally, the underlying message throughout Chapter 8 (and the book) advocates identifying the child's current functioning levels in relationship to the communicative demands of important contexts of the child's life and then designing plans to help narrow the gap.

9

Later Stages

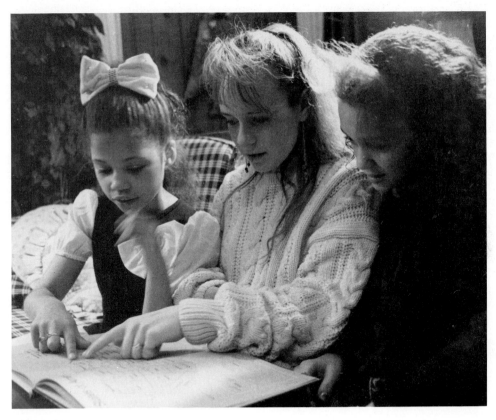

Children Needing
Intervention Aimed at
Later Stage
Developments

Measuring Later Stage
Needs and Abilities

Methods and Targets
of Later Stage
Intervention

❏ Who may need treatment for later stage problems?

❏ What tools can be used to measure later stage needs and abilities?

❏ What kinds of intervention targets and methods are appropriate?

The era called here the *later stages of language acquisition* covers the preadolescent period of later childhood (ages 8–9 to 10–12) through adolescence and the transition to adulthood (ages 10–12 to 21). This period of development was largely ignored in the early years of the psycholinguistic movement. In fact, publication of Carol Chomsky's book, *The Acquisition of Syntax in Children From 5 to 10,* drew so much attention in 1969 partially because it was unusual to think that much language acquisition of any consequence happened beyond age 5. The possibility that age-related changes in language use might extend even into the geriatric years had barely been considered. As recently as 1986, Reed wrote that "there is no cohesive, integrated body of knowledge regarding normal language development during adolescence" (p. 229).

Now a considerable body of literature is available regarding development of language in the later childhood years, and to a certain extent, across the age span. Nevertheless, the territory encompassing the later stages of childhood and adolescence is still less charted than that for early and middle stages of language development. The shape of the developmental landscape also differs from that of earlier language acquisition. In the introduction to *Later Language Development: Ages Nine Through Nineteen,* Nippold (1988b) identified eight points of contrast that can be observed between earlier and later stages of language learning (see Table 9.1 for a summary).

Many of these factors make identification of clear indicators for normal language development more difficult in the later stages of childhood and adolescence than in the earlier stages. The gradual incline of the language learning curve, magnified individual variability, and increasing contributions of formal education and sociocultural-linguistic variation all make it particularly difficult for specialists in language disorders to be clear about who should qualify for service in this age range. In addition, few formal assessment instruments have been designed to reflect the more subtle, abstract, and discourse-related nature of later stage language acquisition (Nippold, 1988b; Stephens & Montgomery, 1985). The available tests tend to reflect exclusively a mainstream cultural and linguistic orientation. This factor, in the face of sociolinguistic variability that influences written as well as oral language acquisition, means that it is quite difficult to know who among the "almost but not quite" (ABNQ) group should be identified as having a language disability and who should be considered "at risk" for school failure or dropping out for other reasons.

The purposes of this chapter are to outline developmental expectations and potential intervention targets for children and adolescents in the later stages of language development, to discuss assessment and intervention methods for the language problems associated with this developmental stage, and to continue to foster the systems perspective that problems are not just within children and neither are the solutions. Cultural and linguistic variations are considered important contextual variables, and their potential influence is highlighted through the chapter. Another

---

Personal Reflection 9.1

"When the apostle Paul said, 'I put away childish things,' he reduced to five words a period of growth that psychologists and pediatricians eagerly study, parents anxiously anticipate, and children inevitably undergo. This is the period called adolescence. Although Paul's description is admirably succinct, it hardly does justice to the process that begins with the early, subtle, biological stirrings of the 10- or 11-year-old and does not end until mature independence is achieved in the mid-20s. The course of adolescence can be orderly and serene, or it can be turbulent and unpredictable. So can the experience of working with adolescents."

Harry E. Hartzell (1984, p. 1), Clinical Professor in the Department of Pediatrics at Stanford Medical School, writing on "the challenge of adolescence."

TABLE 9.1

Contrasts between earlier and later stages of language development

Characteristic	Earlier Development (Ages 0–9)	Later Development (Ages 9–19)
1. Speed of acquisition	Rapid change, with highly salient changes occurring year-to-year and even month-to-month in the earliest years.	Gradual change, with subtle changes noted only when sophisticated linguistic phenomena are analyzed in nonadjacent age groups.
2. Emphasis in growth	Acquisition of spoken language skills.	Acquisition of written language skills.
3. Primary sources of input	Spoken communication.	Both spoken and written forms.
4. Degree of linguistic and cognitive freedom	Relative uniformity of developmental advances enable provision of reliable normative data.	Greater individualism and personal choice make it difficult to establish linguistic and cognitive norms.
5. Nature of settings and instructions	Most language learning occurs in nondirected informal settings.	Some language is learned in informal settings, but much language is acquired through formal instruction in grammar, spelling, etymology, literature, and composition.
6. The use of metalinguistics	Few requirements for metalinguistic focus on language as an object are made before school-age years.	Metalinguistic knowledge is required to learn to read and write, perform complex word analysis, and interpret figurative language.
7. The level of abstraction	Vocabulary and language interpretation are literal and concrete.	Newly learned words often represent abstract notions; nonliteral meanings are appreciated increasingly.
8. Social ability	Immaturity makes it difficult to take the perspective of another.	Increased perspective taking enables individual to adjust the content and style of language to an audience for conversation, story telling, and writing.

Note. Summary of "Introduction" by M. A. Nippold in *Later Language Development: Ages Nine Through Nineteen* (pp. 1–10) edited by M. A. Nippold, 1988, Austin, TX: Pro-Ed. Copyright 1988 by Pro-Ed.

undercurrent of the discussions is the need to provide attention to individuals' linguistic and nonlinguistic abilities in addition to their disabilities.

Because the expression of language disorders may change over time (Bashir, 1989; S. E. Maxwell & Wallach, 1984), the same individual may need different services at different stages of development. Although prevention may seem to be most appropriately associated with prenatal care and the earliest stages of development, it continues to be an important consideration of later stage development. Recall (from the end of Chapter 4) that there are three kinds of prevention. *Primary prevention* fosters conditions to keep problems from appearing; *secondary prevention* uses early identification and intervention to minimize long-term handicaps; and *tertiary prevention*

remediates current problems and limits further ones, once they have appeared (S. E. Gerber, 1990).

In later childhood and adolescence, primary prevention tends to involve public information programs. Older children and adolescents are not particularly susceptible to most of the conditions that cause language disorders in adulthood (e.g., atherosclerosis and heart disease), but they are establishing eating and health-care habits that remain with them throughout their lives. Adolescents can have strokes, can experience near-drowning accidents, can be exposed to infectious diseases that affect the brain, or may experiment with brain-damaging drugs or alcohol. Adolescents and young adults are particularly susceptible to traumatic brain injury, with young men between the ages of 15 and 24 years among those at greatest risk (Beukelman & Yorkston, 1991). One third of all permanent disabilities among children are caused by accidents; motor vehicular accidents are the leading cause of death and disability for persons between the ages of 1 and 45, and bicycle accidents, many involving teenagers, injure almost a half-million young people in the United States annually (S. E. Gerber, 1990). The use of seat belts and helmets may diminish the incidence of head injury and its long-term consequences for many young people, and these are forms of primary prevention that should be encouraged universally.

Secondary prevention in the later stages of language development aims primarily to identify and minimize societal, environmental, familial, and personal factors that limit the ultimate achievement of communicative, social, vocational, and economic independence. Encouraging desirable communicative contexts and encouraging the development of mature abilities and healthy attitudes and strategies for meeting needs associated with those contexts are aspects of secondary prevention. With the implementation of Public Law 100–476—the Individuals With Disabilities Education Act (IDEA; described in Chapter 6 as amendments that renamed the Education for All Handicapped Children Act, PL 94–142)—Individualized Educational Plans (IEPs) for individuals age 16 or older must include transition plans to prepare the individual for postschool employment or postsecondary education. These plans constitute another form of secondary prevention.

Because tertiary prevention involves remediating existing problems and limiting the development of further ones, it is particularly appropriate in the later stages of child development. Here, as in the early and middle stages, redefinition and reeducation may be combined with more direct intervention and remediation goals to target a whole system and not just an individual with a problem.

During adolescence, young people with and without disabilities often redefine themselves. Parents, teachers, and other professionals may attempt to influence the redefinition process in positive directions. Particularly, youngsters who previously have been defined primarily as "special education students" may search out new peer groups (not always healthy ones) or jobs as they move toward adulthood. In interviews, Hartzell (1984) noted that adolescents with learning disabilities "frequently said that their first feelings of self-confidence came from a work

experience. School may have been frustrating, an experience in failure; but in a job, they perceive the possibility of a useful role for them in society" (p. 5).

Because in many adolescents, metacognitive and metalinguistic awareness increase and they can focus more consciously on their own abilities, adolescents may also be able to more actively plan their own programs. They may exhibit a new readiness to respond to reeducation intervention techniques that take advantage of their increased capabilities to reflect on their own behavior and to adopt conscious strategies to reduce impairment or compensate for disabilities. Approaches that involve modification of problem-solving strategies are often called *strategy-based intervention*. This differentiates them from *skill-based intervention* approaches, which are more typical of earlier stage programs that target basic abilities and naturalistic communication. Such changes may also influence roles played by interventionists (e.g., speech–language pathologists and special educators), who may begin to function more as facilitators and less as direct instructors (Hoskins, 1990).

Facilitation sometimes involves deliberate efforts to encourage the use of compensatory strategies to perform tasks that would be impossible otherwise. Compensatory strategies also may be discovered independently, as young people attempt to cope with their disabilities. Not all compensatory techniques discovered by adolescents on their own are healthy, however. Therefore, the intervention program must offer remediation for problematic behaviors developed inadvertently. Remedial activities replace current ineffectual patterns with new, more appropriate, and effective ones.

Consider the example of a bright junior high student with dyslexia who fooled me at first by "reading" from a page of notes he had copied and mostly memorized. Probing further, I soon discovered that this young man had few decoding skills for reading these words or others in novel contexts. He had a history of early language delay and severe speech impairment. Although years of articulation therapy had enabled him to speak without overt errors, he still sounded as if he had learned English as a second language. His program had successfully focused on one area of specific disability (articulation) but had missed another related area entirely (graphophonemic analysis and written language decoding). His intervention team had missed the opportunity to use oral and written language skills for mutual facilitation. As an older junior high school student, this boy was unhappy and anxious about this "faking it" strategy but needed deliberate intervention to decode written language before he could abandon the unhealthy strategy.

CHILDREN NEEDING INTERVENTION AIMED AT LATER STAGE DEVELOPMENTS

Communication, learning, and social problems exhibited by adolescents with disabilities vary with related factors that determine whether or not they can acquire age-appropriate skills. For the most part, any young person who reaches the later states of language development in spite of having a language disorder can be expected to be in the ABNQ group. Generally, these are individuals with relatively normal cognitive ability but specific language-learning disabilities. Some individuals with emotional impairments and concomitant communication disorders, often involving pragmatics, also may fall into this category.

The heterogeneous group of older children and adolescents with language disorders and moderate-to-severe cognitive limitations related to mental retardation or autism clearly does not fit into the ABNQ category. For these more severely impaired individuals, language skills may remain commensurate with earlier stages of development as socioemotional needs advance. Language **content** and **form abilities** may stay at early- or middle-stage levels, while life circumstances necessitate later stage **functional capabilities** for relatively independent adult living and work arrangements. For example, adolescents with moderate-to-severe impairments might need to use early- or middle-stage language skills for later stage activities such as interviewing for and keeping jobs; becoming socially independent from parents; living in semisupported group homes; and engaging in increased social interactions with peers, perhaps even dating.

Yet another heterogeneous group of older children and adolescents has peripheral physical or sensory impairments that interfere with acquisition of language and social interaction skills, but their cognitive skills are basically intact. Impairments that involve selective deficits of peripheral auditory, visual, or motor systems may not interfere with the potential for language acquisition per se, but they often influence opportunities to participate fully and to benefit as much as possible from available opportunities. Sensory or motor impairments mixed with other disabling conditions further complicate the picture.

In summary, individuals who make up the population of adolescents with language disorders constitute three fairly distinct groups, each with somewhat unique needs. Using the system proposed by Beukelman and Mirenda (1992) for rating participation expectations as competitive, active, or included, the ABNQ group includes primarily individuals with diagnoses of speech–language disability, learning disability, and/or emotional or behavioral impairments who may be at least somewhat competitive in participation with same-age peers. The second group includes individuals with severe or multiple impairments that probably always will necessitate somewhat protected environments, but who may be able to be active or included (if not competitive) in some environments. The third group is rather diverse and includes individuals with a variety of peripheral impairments, both sensory and motor, that impair their acquisition of language and communication although their central language processing systems are presumed to be largely intact. Some of these individuals may be fully competitive with their same-age peers in regular academic, social, and work settings when aided by compensatory technology and only intermittent consultation from a language specialist. Others may require extensive environmental and therapeutic support and augmentation. A comprehensive assessment and intervention model for individuals in any of these groups should consider their communicative processes (for reducing impairment), their communicative needs (for reducing disability), and their communicative participation (for reducing handicap) (see previous discussions of these concepts in Chapters 1 and 3, based on Beukelman & Mirenda, 1992).

IDENTIFYING LANGUAGE DISORDERS IN THE LATER STAGES

School or health-care systems rarely implement extensive screening programs to identify the presence of communicative disorders in the later stages of childhood. The majority of individuals who need services for language, speech, and other communicative disorders at this stage will have been enrolled in programs steadily since preschool. By the later elementary and secondary school years, it may not be in the students' best interests for specialists to look for problems in the general population. Screening certain high-risk populations, however, may be entirely appropriate to identify whether previously unrecognized language disorders might explain clearly evident and negative aspects of academic, social, or behavioral problems.

In designing identification programs, the language specialist would be aided by information about the prevalence of communicative disorders among children and adolescents. However, because of limitations in special education services data-gathering requirements in the United States, the prevalence of communication disorders is impossible to determine: PL 94–142 requires each person with a disability to be counted only once. This "unduplicated count" means that many individuals with communicative disorders are not counted as having speech and language disorders but are counted in the categories associated with their other related disorders, such as learning disabilities or mental retardation. Prevalence figures also vary widely across regions, depending on philosophies about the need for services for older children and adolescents. The problem of identifying who qualifies for services therefore is circular; in some areas, children are not identified because no one provides services, and no one provides services because the need has not been identified.

Gillespie and Cooper (1973) estimated the prevalence of speech problems in junior and senior high schools in the United States to be around 5.5%. That figure is somewhat high compared to other estimates, which run closer to 1% to 2% (D. Fein, 1983); 3% to 5% is probably a fairly accurate prediction of

the prevalence of language or speech disorders in the general population (Reed, 1986). In certain specialized settings, the prevalence may be considerably higher. For example, in 1969, Taylor (cited in Larson & McKinley, 1987) found that 84% of youth incarcerated in juvenile detention centers in Missouri had communicative disorders. A study reviewed by Ehren and Lenz (1989) found evidence of language disorders among 73% of a group of high-risk middle school students, including students in compensatory education and special education, with the figure jumping to 80% for students with learning disabilities.

Individuals may be at risk for learning and language disorders for a wide variety of reasons (see Personal Reflection 9.2). Frymier and Gansneder (1989) identified at least 46 different factors that can contribute to risk for educational dysfunction. Larson and McKinley (1987) described one portion of the at-risk population as including adolescents who

> are not deviant enough for criminal justice services, not deprived enough for social service programs, and not disabled enough for special educational services. These students are described as having a high incidence of problems related to reasoning and communication skills, yet they may be receiving no help from established systems, including no speech-language services in the schools. (p. 8)

Screening

School-based screening programs at this age level are usually holdovers from earlier days when caseloads were reestablished following mass screenings each fall. With the implementation of PL 94–142 and ongoing IEPs, that approach became inappropriate and, in many cases, impossible because current IEPs had to be implemented continuously, eliminating the time to conduct annual massive screening. Some practitioners continue to recommend testing all students at

---

Personal Reflection 9.2

"The term high risk in the educational literature is no longer confined to the consideration of preschoolers who may encounter language or learning difficulties on entering school. With the growing interest and concern for the adolescent who has a language learning handicap, we have come to examine more closely those children and youth in the middle and high school populations across the country."

Katherine G. Butler (1984a, p. iv), editor of the journal *Topics in Language Disorders*, in her introduction to an issue on "Adolescent Language Learning Disorders."

least once during their secondary education years, perhaps during their English classes in 7th, 9th or 10th grades because their problems may be overlooked (O'Connor & Eldridge, 1981; Tibbits, 1982). I agree with Larson and McKinley (1987), however, that more efficient alternatives to mass screening may identify individuals needing service at these levels.

Most alternative approaches involve efforts to encourage referrals by informing primary referral sources—including teachers, parents, social workers, physicians, and students themselves—about the signs of a language disorder or other communicative impairment. A more efficient approach may also include selective screening among high-risk groups. Larson and McKinley (1987) recommended that groups screened routinely include (1) adolescents in special programs, such as programs for students with emotional impairment or mental retardation; (2) all seventh- and eighth-graders still receiving remedial reading services; (3) individuals about to drop out of high school; and (4) adolescents with academic difficulties not related primarily to attitudinal or motivational factors. Larson and McKinley also recommended selective screening programs as part of routine intake activities in juvenile detention centers and adolescent psychiatric assessment and treatment institutions.

A few instruments have been designed to screen adolescents' language skills. The following individually administered instruments all measure language comprehension and production and recommend pass–fail decisions based on comparison with established norms: Adolescent Language Screening Test (ALST; Morgan & Guilford, 1984); Screening Tests of Adolescent Language (STAL; Prather, Beecher, Stafford, & Wallace, 1980), and Clinical Evaluation of Language Functions: Advanced Level Screening (CELF; Semel & Wiig, 1980).

Caution should be exercised when interpreting the results of formal screening measures such as these. Some reflect earlier developing language skills and may not be sensitive to later language problems that can have significant negative influences on "real-life" functioning. For example, the ALST (Morgan & Guilford, 1984) evaluates earlier developing skills and ignores later developing skills (Nippold, 1988b). The STAL (Prather et al., 1980) is too easy for students in middle-class suburban areas, so it does not identify problems among them; practitioners in lower socio-

economic districts, however, have found it useful (Stephens & Montgomery, 1985). Whenever students from racially or culturally diverse communities are assessed (e.g. from inner cities or isolated rural areas, e.g., Appalachia or Indian reservations), standardized screening instruments are probably inappropriate. They do not adequately allow for influences of nonstandard English dialects or foreign languages.

Referral

Informed referrals from those in close contact with older children and adolescents may be the most productive and efficient identification method. Referrals may come from parents, medical personnel, counselors, employers, or other adults. Teacher referrals, however, are particularly important because of teachers' extensive opportunities to observe higher order language and thinking skills, where later language problems often appear. Older children and adolescents also may refer themselves.

Accurate referrals generally result from strong information dissemination programs about the nature of communicative disorders. In the later stages particularly, teachers need instruction to recognize communicative disorders when no overt speech impairments or obvious errors of grammatical formulation are evident. They also need to consider whether problems such as academic and social difficulties might signal the presence of previously untreated (or undertreated) communicative difficulties. The secondary-level referral form developed by Larson and McKinley (1987), includes observational signs of communicating disorders in the domains of thinking, listening, speaking, nonverbal communication, and survival language.

To keep making referrals, teachers need clear evidence that their students benefit from the time spent outside class for language assessment and intervention. Success stories provide the best stimulus for more requests for assistance. Magnotta (1991, p. 150) called it "invitation-by-success." On the other hand, if teachers refer students who they suspect of having language-based classroom problems only to be told that the students do not qualify for services, they likely will not refer more students or work to build collaborative relationships with speech–language pathologists. Disappointing outcomes are more likely when assessment involves only a limited set of standardized tests. Then it is difficult to be relevant to teacher and student needs. Constable (1987) described one teacher who commented on frustrating

Personal Reflection 9.3   "I do not have the training that you people [speech–language pathologists] have. However, I've been in the business for a long time, and I think I know when I see a child with a language problem. So I make all the referrals. Now I don't know what happens in the 1:1 session, or what kinds of tests you give the kids, but my speech person keeps sending these children back to me saying they don't have a language problem. Finally I just said to her, 'then you get in the classroom and see what is wrong'."

Frustrated teacher, whose comments were reported by Catherine Constable (1987, pp. 347–348).

experiences with such an approach (see Personal Reflection 9.3)

As children reach adolescence, they are more likely to refer themselves, especially if they have been provided adequate education about communicative disorders and are in the later stages of adolescence (Larson & McKinley, 1987). Self-referral is especially powerful because the student is motivated to change. Some individuals who refer themselves when provided a nonthreatening avenue to do so may have received speech–language intervention services in earlier grades several years previously. In the later grades, they may gain new appreciation of the value of strong communication skills and new insights into their own problems. They also may have increased access to professionals who understand the nature of later stage communicative difficulties and how to work with them.

Considering the Later Stage Needs of Individuals With Multiple and Severe Disabilities

As noted in Chapters 7 and 8, when individuals have severe or multiple disabilities, perhaps the greatest challenge in intervention is to offer services that are appropriate for their developmental stage levels without relying on activities and materials that are either irrelevant or inappropriate for their chronological age levels. For each individual, communicative needs should be reassessed periodically in age-appropriate contexts of home, school, community, and work, with a focus on activities of daily living (ADL).

Referral may be the best method for identifying these individuals, but referral criteria must be tailored to the purpose. Referral criteria based on discrete language abilities probably will not work, because most individuals with cognitive limitations have communicative skills considerably below those expected for their chronological ages. Shifting experiences in adolescence and adulthood may also bring new contextually based communicative demands for which they are inadequately prepared. Box 9.1 offers a set of potential referral criteria to assist professionals such as employment counselors and special educators to know when a communicative specialist might help to solve functional communication problems for older individuals with middle-stage (or even earlier) language abilities.

MEASURING LATER STAGE NEEDS AND ABILITIES

CONTEXTS FOR LATER STAGE ASSESSMENT AND INTERVENTION

The division of childhood into early, middle, and later stages in this text is intended to organize expectations for increasing developmental and chronological levels. Although developmental expectations have provided the primary framework, I have repeatedly noted that some individuals may remain at earlier developmental levels in terms of many cognitive and linguistic abilities yet may have communicative, social, and emotional needs associated with older chronological ages.

To understand the specialized needs of adolescents with developmental language disorders and related disabilities, professionals should consider that many of them have struggled for years to achieve the language and educational levels of their same-age

---

Box 9.1 **Suggestions for recognizing the need for consultation with a communicative specialist for older children and adolescents with moderate-to-severe multiple disabilities**

❏ **Failure to understand instructions.** When a person has difficulty performing essential job or daily living tasks, consider the possibility that the person may not understand the language of instructions and may not have sufficient communicative skill to ask for repetition or clarification.

❏ **Inability to use language to meet daily living needs.** When individuals can produce enough words to formulate a variety of utterances, including questions, then they can travel independently, shop independently, use the telephone when they need to, and ask for assistance in getting out of problem situations when they arise. If persons cannot function in a variety of working, shopping, and social contexts, consider that communicative impairments may be limiting their independence.

❏ **Violation of rules of politeness and other rules of social transaction.** The ability to function well in a variety of contexts with friends, acquaintances, and one-time contacts depends on sensitivity to the unspoken rules of social interaction. One of the most frequently cited reasons for failure of workers with disabilities to "fit in" with fellow workers is their inability to engage in small-talk during work breaks. Examples that might cause difficulty are failure to take communicative turns when offered, or conversely, interrupting the turns of others; saying things that are irrelevant to the topic; not using politeness markers or showing interest in what the other person says; making blunt requests owing to lack of linguistic skill for softening them; failing to shift style of communication for different audiences (e.g., talking the same way to the boss as to co-workers); and any other communicative behavior that is perceived as odd or bizarre. If people seem to avoid interacting with the target person, referral may be justified.

❏ **Lack of functional ability to read signs and other symbols and to perform functional writing tasks.** The ability to recognize the communicative symbols of the culture enables people to know how to use public transportation, to find their way around buildings, to comply with legal and safety expectations, and to fill out forms or use bank accounts. Communicative specialists may be able to assist in identifying the best strategies for teaching functional reading and writing skills and encouraging the development of other symbol-recognition and -use skills.

❏ **Problems articulating speech clearly enough to be understood, stuttering, or using an inaudible or inappropriate voice.** Other speech and voice disorders may interfere with the person's ability to communicate. When such problems are noted, refer the individual to a speech–language pathologist.

---

peers but continue to fall further behind. Later stage child development then may become increasingly complicated by self-image, identity, and motivational issues that are exaggerated in all adolescents, but perhaps excessively so in this group. Specialists, as well as these youngsters, sometimes have difficulty differentiating problems associated with the special experience of growing up with a disability from those associated with simply growing up. As an aid, Box 9.2 outlines expectations for normal social-emotional development in early, middle, and later stages of adolescence.

Because adolescence may be confusing to teachers, clinicians, and parents, and to adolescents themselves, knowing that the period of maximum turmoil smooths out with time and maturity may be comfort-ing to families. It is inappropriate to conclude, however, that just because some adolescents are rebellious, inconsistent, impulsive, or moody, that most of them are. As Larson and McKinley (1987) pointed out, "the vast majority of adolescents are thriving, healthy beings who feel confident, happy, and self-satisfied" (p. 1) (see Personal Reflection 9.4).

This section addresses the multiple contexts in which later stage children and adolescents participate. Of continued importance is the individual's family and primary culture, but the expanding world of adolescents beyond family also should be considered. Other important contexts for adolescents with language disorders include increased interactions with peers; participation in a variety of educational contexts that

Box 9.2   General expectations for change occurring within the early, middle, and later stages of adolescence

Early Adolescence	Middle Adolescence	Later Adolescence
Period of rapid physical growth that precedes sexual maturity (ages 10–13 for girls and up to 2 years later for boys).	Period that begins after the physical changes of maturity are complete (ages 13–16 in girls and 14–17 in boys).	Period by which full adult growth and strength are reached (begins about age 16–17 and may extend into the mid-20s).
Gangly and awkward period; both boys and girls are uncomfortble with their new body images.	Boys show great interest in their bodies; girls diet and exercise to lose weight; both show dissatisfaction with their bodies and worry that they may not be normal.	Comfort with body maturity increases.
Problem solving is egocentric and concrete.		Period of partial dependence on parents is often extended, compared to previous generations, owing to longer career preparations and postsecondary education.
Self-consciousness leads to the formation of intense relationships with peers based on similarities (e.g., in dress), but home and family remain the most important emotional and social factors.	Psychosomatic complaints may appear, and some need reassurance that stress and worry can cause physical symptoms like headaches and stomachaches.	Personal identity is developed with greater reliance on friends than family for social contact.
Approval of peers is important, with a strong yearning to be normal and average. Those in special education become strongly sensitive to its symbols (e.g., riding a different schoolbus, being called out of class, or working in a resource room).	Thinking is more abstract, theoretical, and idealistic. Interest in outside world and introspection both increase.	Sexual intimacy increases, as does ability to deal with interpersonal complexities.
Emotional lability may appear in the form of wide mood swings from depression to elation.	Beliefs persist in simple solutions for complex problems (from world hunger to fad diets and cures for acne).	Personal value systems are adopted, leading to the ability to make mature, independent judgments (in spite of earlier rebelliousness, most older adolescents adopt value systems similar to those of their parents).
Moral outlook for most is at the conventional level (individual conforms to authority and obeys laws and social rules).	Feelings of rebellion may be exhibited in dress styles, hair styles, adolescent slang, and fascination with rock music and rock stars. Extreme forms may involve drugs, alcohol, vandalism, and early pregnancy.	
	Social life is primarily with peers; dating becomes more common.	
	First jobs and participation in sports may make important contributions to self-confidence and maturity.	
	By end of the period (last 2 years of high school), begin to move beyond the self-consciousness and spirit of rebellion that characterize this stage.	

Sources: Hartzell, 1984; Larson & McKinley, 1987

may represent cultural and linguistic mismatches; participation in nonschool contexts; and making transitions to employment or postsecondary schooling.

Changing Roles of the Family and Continued Influence of the Primary Culture

When children reach preadolescence and the onset of puberty, dramatic changes occur in their abilities and attitudes. Although families remain important, the role of family shifts. Moving into adolescence signals the beginning of the difficult work of distancing oneself from the primary influence of family. Many youngsters want desperately to be viewed as unique individuals and to be treated as adults by their parents, yet feel a need to be as much like their peers as possible in dress, action, music preference, and speech.

When viewed from a distance, teenagers, in fact, may seem to share a culture of their own—one that cuts across ethnic and socioeconomic boundaries. When examined more closely, however, signs of cultural consistency with familial roots and the primary

culture remain. Also evident is the continued importance of many communicative opportunities within family contexts (see Personal Reflection 9.5).

Perhaps no issue is more complicated than differentiating aspects of linguistic and cultural influence in language development, particularly as related to the potential for bias in the assessment of later stage children and adolescents. Indicators of later language development are more likely to reflect a particular set of cultural and linguistic experiences and to be less predictable in time of development than are indicators of early development, which tend to be more universal.

Socialization involves "the process of growing up in a particular society," a process that involves the transmission, primarily by parents and other adults, of cultural knowledge required to operate successfully and appropriately in the everyday world (D. C. Cooper & Anderson-Inman, 1988, p. 225). The specialist's need to recognize socialization factors and to be culturally sensitive during assessment and intervention has been emphasized by Crago and Cole (1991):

The socialization of children to their culture is, indeed, an important and delicate process in which language and communication patterns have an integral and crucial role. The violation of minority cultures' cultural and socialization practices by a lack of awareness of the importance of this relationship prevents the formulation of appropriate assessment and intervention strategies for these populations. (p. 106).

Increased Interactions With Peers

Although families maintain an important role in the lives of older children and adolescents, peers occupy an increasingly important position. As D. C. Cooper and Anderson-Inman (1988) pointed out, individuals may exhibit widely different levels of communicative competence in school and other environments:

> For example, children who are judged linguistically deficient in the school environment sometimes display sophisticated and competent communication skills in the home, neighborhood, or peer group situation. Vernacular forms of speech, or ways of talking that are appropriate for the speaker's social group, may not reflect the standards of the preferred speech norms but can be judged competent because of their appropriateness for some of the situations in which they are used. It must be noted, however, that not all situationally competent communicative performances have the same influence in terms of social power, nor are they equally acceptable across a range of social contexts. (p. 232)

Language assessment and intervention for preadolescents and adolescents should involve consideration of communicative competence within multiple contexts including peer groups. Later in this chapter, several peer-to-peer discourse contexts are discussed.

Influences of Cultural and Language Mismatches at School

School continues to be a critical context for children and adolescents in the later stages of language development, but it is often a place of mixed blessings. For many individuals with language disorders, school is simultaneously a place where they find satisfying social contacts, hopes for the future, and considerable frustration. As Trapani (1990) noted, even individuals with so-called "milder impairments" experience increasing stress:

> Youths with learning disabilities encounter increasing difficulties as they progress through the school system because their poor skills do not enable them to meet the demands of an increasingly demanding curriculum. The intensity of the current high school curriculum often overwhelms the adolescent with learning disabilities who cannot read textbooks and has poor writing skills. (p. x)

The high complexity and fast pace of middle school and secondary school communicative environments can be confusing whenever language skills are wobbly, but when cultural mismatches are thrown into the mix, the risks for dropping out, low self-esteem, and reduced employment potential are magnified. As children advance in school, problems of differential diagnosis related to cultural difference increase (see Personal Reflection 9.6). It is particularly difficult to sort out the interacting influences of cultural, linguistic, educational, and economic variables that contribute to widening differences in performance on formal and informal measures of cognitive and communicative development for individuals in lower socioeconomic groups, many of whom also

---

| Personal Reflection 9.6 | "After the first few years, mismatch between the child's communication skills and the teacher's demands tend not to be attributed by the teachers to the child's cultural and linguistic background. This is especially true for English-speaking minority children. The problems children in higher grades encounter are more often attributed to low intellectual capacity and/or to a communication disorder. What teachers at this level often fail to realize is that the communicative demands of their classrooms are different from those of earlier grades, and that many of these children have not been taught, either at home or in their previous classes, the particular skills required for success in the higher grades."

Aquiles Iglesius (1985, p. 37), writing about communicative mismatches between school and home.

belong to minority groups with limited English proficiency or who speak a nonstandard dialect of English.

Whereas societal indicators and formal assessments of communicative maturity tend to be tied to a specific, standard sociolinguistic system, not all individuals are equally likely to learn that particular system. In schools, the "rich get richer" metaphor refers to the observation that children who are good at the school "game" tend to get even better as they advance through the grades. All too often, in fact, the metaphor becomes literal. Because of differential success in formal education settings, individuals from different socioeconomic groups have varied opportunities for postsecondary education and, eventually, for differential access to high-paying jobs. The problems related to this discrepancy extend far beyond problems associated with differential proficiency in the language use valued in school and business. They reach into the depths of societal problems involving poverty, racism, urban living conditions, drug culture, and other sociological complexities.

Periodically, someone observes that people whose language systems differ from those of mainstream society are not as actively involved in it. A federal judge in Ann Arbor, Michigan, for example, ruled that the district must consider the language differences of a group of African-American children whose primary language was Black English when educating them (*Martin Luther King Elementary School Children et al., v. Ann Arbor School District Board*, 1978). Furthermore, Orr (1987) hypothesized that language mismatches might explain problems in learning the science and mathematics curriculum for some African-American

students from inner-city Washington, DC, who were enrolled in her private school. Both the Ann Arbor court ruling and Orr's book have been controversial.

It is seductive, but dangerous, to link language variation too closely to indices of success in settings such as school and the workplace. It is dangerous, because it may lead to a renewed acceptance of the old, discredited **deficit theory** of language variation, in which sociolinguistic variation was equated with social disadvantage and inferiority, ignoring the more preferred **difference theory,** in which no language system or dialect is seen as inherently superior or inferior to another (see Personal Reflection 9.7).

The emphasis here is on accurate and fair, nonbiased assessment so that all the children with language disorders, and only those children, will be identified as needing language intervention. Although issues related to the effective education of minority individuals who do not have language disorders may be of interest to language specialists, they are beyond the scope of this book. What is emphasized here is the need to consider the demands of the language of school and whether mismatches between the current abilities of students with language disorders and the expectations of written and oral language processing in classrooms might be associated with their academic and social interaction difficulties. Potential language differences that might complicate the picture for these students also should be considered.

Avoid the trap of equating racial or ethnic difference with language difference. As discussed in Chapter 2, minority group membership and linguistic difference are not isomorphic. The relative indepen-

---

Personal Reflection 9.7

"As far as I can see, technical answers of the type that Orr [1987], the Ann Arbor judge [*Martin Luther King Elementary School Children et al., v. Ann Arbor School District Board, 1978*] and others give us offer no way out of the present situation in which the gap between the educational achievements of the African American poor and other poor minority groups and those of the white majority correlate so strongly with other gaps: IQ and SAT scores, dropout rates, unemployment rates, malnutrition rates, infant mortality rates, serious illness and longevity rates, violent-death rates, and so on. An understanding of the grammar of Black English will explain none of this. Perhaps the recent work that sees these differences to be the result of a caste-like structure of our society will lead to an explanation of its present disgraceful state. But still better explanations will not eliminate the Third World conditions that characterize much of urban existence in the United States."

Wayne O'Neil (1990, p. 87), linguist at Massachusetts Institute of Technology.

dence of the two conditions was highlighted by Loban (1976) in his classic longitudinal study of language development in school-age children from kindergarten through grade 12 (see Personal Reflection 9.8). Loban's results demonstrated that socioeconomic status, and not racial or ethnic diversity, correlated highly with school success. Specifically, Loban found strong correlations between both high socioeconomic status and high language ability and low socioeconomic status and low language ability. He concluded that minority group membership alone was not predictive of school success or failure.

Participating in Nonschool Contexts

Not all services to adolescents are provided in school. In many communities, adolescents receive services from private practitioners and community service agencies. Hospitals and rehabilitation centers also may provide services following traumatic brain injury or other medical crises. Other youths may be admitted to residential treatment settings or juvenile detention centers for emotional or behavioral problems.

When services are provided in acute-care centers, several factors influence assessment and intervention. If the reason for admission is crisis (e.g., vehicular accident, a suicide attempt, or delinquent behavior), the initial focus of the assessment may be on many factors other than communication. The speech–language pathologist and other learning specialists may need to focus the team on potential involvement of communicative, language, and learning impairments. Because of short admissions, more attention may be given to assessment than intervention. The transdisciplinary team then should review prior records, conduct tests including dynamic assessment of outcomes within modified communicative contexts, and generate transition plans for discharge.

When treatment is provided in long-term care centers, team members must consider individuals' needs to participate in contexts beyond the center. Many rehabilitation centers for individuals with traumatic

brain injury have "community reentry" programs with systematic strategies to help patients return to functioning in the community as much as possible. Communication specialists should play an active role, analyzing communicative demands of those contexts, the patient's current abilities in them, the potential for (and desirability of) changing contextual demands, the potential for changing the individual's abilities, and the best strategies for doing so.

In some communities, alternative school programs also are available to students who cannot make it in the regular educational system. Taff (1990) described the population from which the DeLeSalle Education Center in Kansas City, Missouri, recruits:

> To enter the school, a student must be a confirmed educational failure. We recruit from juvenile court, mental health programs, school districts that have permanently expelled students, and the inner-city streets. Our students come from neighborhoods with the highest crime rates and the lowest family incomes. Some are from families who have been unemployed for generations and on welfare for most of that time. Most have been abused. Many have a pattern of drug abuse. (p. 71)

In alternative school programs such as this, change is fostered through a combination of small class sizes; strong counseling programs with individualized goal setting; rules about attendance, drugs, and fighting; and specialized remedial programs using materials relevant to the students' interests (e.g., state driving manuals, pop music, and magazines). These programs also provide appropriate contexts to help students develop more effective communicative and language abilities and strategies.

Transitions to Higher Education, Employment, and Other Postschool Activities

Whether individuals participate in school programs or other settings, as they enter the middle stages of adolescence, the intervention team should begin deliberate planning for transitions to later adolescence

---

Personal Reflection 9.8	"Minority students who came from securely affluent home backgrounds did not show up in the low proficiency groups. The problem is poverty, not ethnic affiliation." *Walter Loban* (1976, p. 23).

and adulthood. Depending on the resources and goals of individuals and their families, transition services might focus on higher education, job training, and supported or competitive employment.

The implementation of the IDEA (PL 100–46) requires the development and evaluation of transition services as part of educational programs for special education students age 16 and older. The history of involvement of special educators in helping students make transitions beyond secondary education settings is not strong (Trapani, 1990). Even less evidence suggests that communicative specialists have played active roles to foster transitions for students with language and communicative disorders to postsecondary education and other vocational contexts. In a summary of the available literature regarding individuals with learning disabilities, Trapani reported that "it cannot be assumed that adolescents with learning disabilities will become independent upon their graduation from high school" (p. 93). Deliberate plans to consider communicative needs in consultation with academic advisers, vocational educators, vocational counselors, and job coaches during transition should increase with the new legislation. The potential for improved service delivery in this area is ripe.

TOOLS AND STRATEGIES FOR LATER STAGE ASSESSMENT

Gathering Background Information for Contextually Based Assessment

The specialist should gather a variety of background information when assessing problems of later stage language acquisition. As in early and middle stages, assessment questions related to impairment, disability, and handicap can be answered only if multiple sources of information are considered.

Information-gathering procedures for later stage assessment parallel those of middle-stage assessment. Box 9.3 presents several modifications for procedures originally introduced in Chapter 8 (Box 8.5). Primary distinctions relate to the degree to which older children and adolescents act as informants about their own problems and participate actively in formulating plans for their own future. Direct observation in classrooms may also be used less frequently in middle schools and secondary schools, partially because these students tend to have multiple teachers and to be more easily embarrassed. At these levels, interviews may be more helpful to professionals and less embarrassing to students. I have also enlisted the collaborative help of high school and junior high school teachers to audiotape record their classroom lectures by telling them that I need samples of curricular language to gauge its complexity and to identify key vocabulary.

Formal Assessment in the Later Stages

As in selecting screening instruments for later stage language disorders, a variety of problems may arise when selecting standardized instruments for later stage assessment. Problems relate to inadequate representation of later acquired language features (Nippold, 1988b); a lack of standardized instruments for measuring extended discourse production or comprehension (Constable, 1987; Launer & Lahey, 1981), and a lack of instruments that are demanding enough to be sensitive yet open-ended enough to be fair in terms of cultural and educational variation.

As pointed out by the practitioner in Personal Reflection 9.9, formal tests are mandated in schools to determine eligibility for services (Stephens & Montgomery, 1985). Third-party-pay requirements and other policies may dictate the need for formal tests in other settings as well.

In addition to meeting the need for norm-referenced tests to determine eligibility, formal testing may serve other purposes. It may identify multiple dimensions of a language disorder and related impairments, may suggest areas to address in intervention, and may identify potential strategies for doing so. Formal tests may also be used to provide ongoing assessment, particularly for documenting a continuing need for services. Norm-referenced tests, however, are generally not sensitive enough to measure changes resulting from intervention (McCauley & Swisher, 1984).

Formal tests are particularly suited to meeting certain later stage assessment needs. These include assessment of (1) written and oral language, (2) language processing and language knowledge, (3) higher order and basic language skills, and (4) the production and comprehension of connected discourse. Although similar assessment concerns are present in earlier stages of development to varying degrees, they become the hallmark of later stage assessments.

To some extent, the preceding objectives may be met with formal tests selected from Appendix A. Formal assessment works best when conducted by

Box 9.3   Procedures for gathering background information essential to the assessment of children and adolescents in the later stages of language acquisition

1. Determine the **reason for referral** by interviewing the person(s) who made the referral (or suggested that it be made). Also find out how the person being referred feels about the referral. If an older child or adolescent makes a self-referral, explore the reasons why and investigate whether others (including parents, teachers, and employers) think it was a good idea (or perhaps suggested it).

2. Gather **history information** about the nature of the problem by interviewing the adolescent as well as others who play important roles in the individual's life (e.g., parents, teachers, employers), being careful to obtain the appropriate permissions before contacting anyone beyond the person's immediate family. Information should be gathered regarding (a) family history, (b) medical history, (c) developmental history, (d) educational history, (e) social history, and (f) employment history.

3. Collaborate with others, including the client, to **identify contexts** that are particularly important in the client's life. These may be called "zones of significance" (N. W. Nelson, in press-a). Include questions about (a) places (e.g. school, social settings, or work); (b) people (teachers, employers, romantic partners, or friends); and (c) communicative events (e.g., classroom interactions, note taking, homework, or tests, social conversations, business conversations, asking assistance of strangers).

4. Use multiple strategies to **identify aspects of communicative competence in each of these important contexts.** Include both (a) observational strategies and (b) interview strategies.

5. Consider building a **profile of areas of proficiency, strength, and preference that do not involve language.** For example *The Smart Profile* (L. Miller, 1990) might be used to guide interviews with the target individual and significant others to build a profile based on strengths (rather than deficits). Miller based this profiling procedure on Gardner's (1983) theory of multiple intelligences. Using ethnographic interviewing procedures, she recommended probing for evidence of strength in each of the following eight areas (Gardner proposed seven): linguistic, musical, logical, mathematical (Gardner combined these as logical-mathematical), spatial, bodily, intrapersonal, and interpersonal.

6. Based on this initial compilation of background information, **form additional hypotheses about the child's relative areas of strength and difficulty,** which can be tested using both informal and formal assessment techniques.

multidisciplinary teams working collaboratively. Mutual planning can spread the evaluation workload but more importantly can result in mutual consideration of assessment results. Language specialists then can administer only a few formal tests but will have access to results of tests administered by others and will have others' insights about language assessment results. Particularly helpful may be the results of reading tests, processing tests (e.g., the Woodcock-Johnson Psycho-Educational Battery–Revised, Woodcock and Johnson, 1989), or academic achievement tests. If language specialists train collaborators to record verbal responses exactly, they may have a rich data source. Insights might come from qualitative reviews of test responses (not just quantitative scores) about language processing influences across multiple domains. No formal test, however, can meet all assessment needs. Informal methods also must be used.

Informal Assessment in Later Stages

Identifying zones of significance. When one attempts to understand children with language disorders within the framework of dynamic system theory, the selection of relevant contexts is central to designing assessment and intervention activities. *Disability*, by definition, is context dependent (see Chapter 1). It is defined relative to difficulty in meeting contextual demands. Therefore, reducing disability involves attempting to answer the question "What does this individual need to be able to do (communicatively) to succeed in important life contexts?"

When children reach the later stages of language development, they are expected to use language competently in a wide variety of modalities and contexts. Therefore, to be comprehensive, language sampling for most older children should include oral and written language samples (both reading and writing) and evidence of the ability to use language to think and communicate. Some prudence in selecting sampling contexts is wise, however. If all relevant contexts and modalities were sampled independently, comprehensive assessment would demand prohibitive amounts of time. Streamlining the evaluation process as much as possible therefore is important to allow assessment goals to be met without cutting into valuable intervention time. A minimalist approach involves devoting only as much time as necessary to meet goals of (1) establishing eligibility, (2) outlining critical dimensions of the problem, (3) identifying appropriate goal areas, and (4) designing appropriate intervention strategies.

The time problem may also be addressed by viewing "assessment" not as something to be completed before beginning intervention but rather as an ongoing and integral part of intervention. For most purposes, it is useful to see informal assessment and intervention as thoroughly integrated processes. When professionals adopt this attitude, they learn how to gather only as much pure assessment information as they need to make initial decisions. Then they shift to an intervention mode, implementing mediation and scaffolding strategies to assist the person to process language, and then assessing the client under the modified conditions. This "mediate and measure" approach, sometimes known as *dynamic assessment* (Feuerstein, 1979), is a key strategy of contextually based assessment. It is a critical part of keeping intervention plans updated and relevant.

Another way to narrow the sampling focus is to consider background information gathered using interview, record review, and observation. By identifying "zones of significance," professionals may gather in-depth information about areas particularly significant for the individual (N. W. Nelson, in press-a). Zones of significance are identified through participant interviews with the target person and important others (particularly parents, teachers, school administrators, and employers). Significance may stem from relevance to an individual's personal goals or to outstanding areas of ability or disability. The specialist may use the ethnographic technique of triangulation—confirmation of the same observation by interviewing several sources—to validate the selection of assessment contexts as relevant. To assist in the interview process, Table 9.2 presents some of the areas that should be probed with parents, teachers, and students. These sample questions are to be used merely as guides for areas to probe. They should not be asked verbatim, and they definitely should not be turned into a form to be filled out in writing. If a young person has a primary concern about social interactions or employment settings, the interview participants and questions should shift accordingly.

Once the professional has identified zones of significance, he or she selects specific sampling contexts to probe different aspects of those areas. During sampling, the examiner should probe an individual's language skills and strategies in certain contexts and also clarify the communicative demands and opportunities associated with those contexts. This information is used both to understand the problem and to design intervention.

If the specialist identifies impaired conversational skills and social interaction as particularly handicapping owing to social penalties from peers, he or she might gather a sample of social interaction discourse (i.e., the target student conversing with a peer, either a friend or someone recruited by the language specialist). If such an approach is objectionable to potential conversational partners or not feasible for other

TABLE 9.2
Starter questions to be asked of the key participants in the curriculum-based language assessment process

Teacher Interviews	Parent Interviews	Student Interviews
Objective information about the student's academic performance, both from achievement tests and classroom levels of performance.	Early development (Did they suspect a problem early?)	The student's description of what is hardest about school.
Descriptions of the student's classroom strengths.	Medical history (especially middle ear problems)	The student's description of what is best about school.
A prioritized review of the problems the teacher identifies as most important.	Educational history	The student's prioritized list of changes to be made.
Anecdotal descriptions of recent classroom events with which the student has experienced difficulty.	When did problems first show up at school?	Anecdotal evidence—accounts of recent classroom events that made the student feel really bad.
Descriptions of aspects of the curriculum that present the greatest difficulties to the student and the most concern to the teacher.	Did decoding problems show up early?	The student's ideas about the future.
The teacher's view of the student's potential within the current school year and in the future.	Or did the problems show up in third or fourth grade when it became more important to read longer texts for meaning?	
	Anecdotal evidence of specific problems within the past year or so.	
	A prioritized review of the problems the parents view as most critical.	
	The parents' goals for their child's future.	

© 1992 N. W. Nelson. Shared by permission of the author.

reasons, a variety of role-playing contexts may be used to set up discourse events between the examiner and the target individual (e.g., "I'm going to try to pick a fight with you, and I want you to show me what you would say in such a situation." or "How would you start a conversation with a girl you wanted to meet?"). If an adolescent is having trouble getting a job, the sampling process might involve filling out standard job applications (written language samples) or engaging in simulated job interviews. The important thing is to sample a variety of contextually based language use relevant to the concerns of the client and others who care about him or her.

Organizing an approach to later stage sampling and analysis. The nature of later stage language developments differs sufficiently from early- and middle-stage developments that specialized language sample analysis techniques are required. As in earlier stages, the advantages of naturalistic samples relate to their relevance to real-life circumstances and their opportunities for observing holistic and interactive aspects of real communication. Later

stage naturalistic language sampling and analysis, however, may be especially complex because of all of the factors in the sampling process.

Professionals need an organizational system to observe multiple variables associated with mature communication in naturalistic contexts. The system should be open enough to avoid reductionism from fitting complex behavior into a limited set of predefined categories. It should allow inference about aspects of internalized language processing as well as direct observation of oral and written language products. It should relate to appropriate contextual aspects of an individual's educational, vocational, and social world. It should address linguistic knowledge of the five basic rule systems—phonology, morphology, syntax, semantics, and pragmatics—as well as metalinguistic and other "meta-" abilities. It should be based on samples that represent multiple modalities, including listening, speaking, reading, writing, and thinking, and it should consider whether people with severe language deficits might communicate better in some other nonlinguistic modality. It should allow focus on a variety of sizes of linguistic units, from phonemes and graphemes to whole texts, and in particular, it should be appropriate for long and complex utterances. Finally, it should accomplish all of this within a variety of conversational, narrative, and expository discourse events that hold particular significance for the individual.

Table 9.3 represents an outline of most of these variables. It is an open outline, subject to revision and expansion or abbreviation, or to adaptation to allow nonbiased consideration of proficiency in more than one system. For example, Adler (1991) presented an analysis system to compare aspects of language features in multiple discourse samples. He suggested rating competence separately for the individual's native language (L1), English as a second language (L2), and nonstandard dialect (D).

The organizational system presented in Table 9.3 represents observable language production elements better than it represents internalized language processing activities, which are illustrated in Figure 9.1. Professionals may use these two organizational

frameworks together to organize the multiple factors to consider when gathering and analyzing later stage language samples.

A model of complex oral and written language processing. The primary accomplishments of later stage language acquisition are associated not so much with learning new things as with putting together known pieces in new and more complex ways for new and more varied purposes in new and more demanding contexts. When attempting to analyze later stage language processing, the specialist must do more than simply look at a limited sample of oral conversation. To understand how an adolescent's language disorder might be contributing to difficulties in the classroom or on the job, more is needed than a computation of mean length of utterance (MLU). To contribute to problem solving, language specialists need to consider the individual's internal processes as he or she attempts to process language. That is the value of a model of complex oral and written language processing.

TABLE 9.3
Organizational framework of assessment variables and contexts for later stage language sample analysis

	Metaskills[a]			
Contexts	**Rule Systems**	**Processing Modalities**	**Linguistic Units**	**Discourse Events**
School Curricula	Phonology	Listening	Sounds	Conversational
Official	Morphology	Speaking	Syllables	Informal classroom talk
Cultural	Syntax	Reading	Words	Playground or cafeteria talk
De facto	Semantics	Writing	Sentences	Peer tutoring
School culture	Pragmatics	Thinking	Simple	Peer social interactions
Hidden			Complex	Narrative
Underground				Stories from reading texts or literature
Vocational			Texts	Stories teacher reads aloud
Social				Stories students write
				Personal narratives (show and tell; oral reports)
				Expository
				Procedural directions and explanations
				Lectures
				Most textbooks
				Most worksheets and textbook assignments
				Informational papers
				Oral reports/speeches/(some show and tell)
				Note taking

[a]"Metaskills" include metalinguistic skills for talking about and manipulating linguistic symbols, metacognitive skills for monitoring and controlling thinking, and metapragmatic skills for awareness of classroom discourse rules.

Figure 9.1 presents a model of competent, mature language processing in terms of four different but interrelated, synergistic contributions.

1. **Six kinds of knowledge structures** including three linguistic (graphophonemic, semantic, and syntactic) and three additional cognitive, prag-

FIGURE 9.1
A model showing the interaction of oral and written language processing with external linguistic and nonlinguistic contextual factors to guide curriculum-based language assessment.

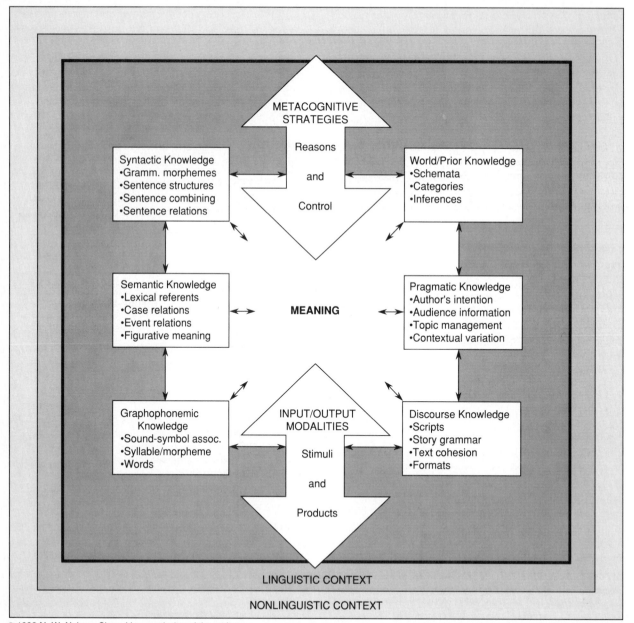

matic, and discourse rule systems. In Figure 9.1, these are represented as six modules that are loosely representational of neurolinguistic organization in the brain, in that more purely linguistic functions are shown on the left, and world knowledge, pragmatic skill, and discourse knowledge—which are not as specifically localized in the left hemisphere—are shown on the right.

2. **Peripheral processing skills** for interacting with the environment to get information in and out. In Figure 9.1, these are represented by a large bidirectional arrow at the bottom, which connects internal aspects of visual, auditory, oral–motor and graphomotor processing with the two exterior boxes that represent linguistic and nonlinguistic tasks and contexts.

3. **Central processing skills** for performing functions such as holding information in short-term memory, analyzing it, encoding it, associating it, storing it in long-term memory, and retrieving it when appropriate. In Figure 9.1, these functions are represented by small black bidirectional arrows connecting the knowledge structures with each other, enabling the formation of association pathways in the brain that might be activated in both parallel (simultaneous) or serial order, depending on the demands of the task, and relating to the central purpose of constructing meaning.

4. **Conscious metacognitive strategies** for guiding attention and for directing and organizing all of the other processes and making them work efficiently. In Figure 9.1, these are represented by a large bidirectional arrow at the top, which illustrates the interaction of internal and external forces on the executive functions of reason and control that seem to draw particularly on frontal lobe contributions in the brain.

This model is complex because human information processing systems are complex. The model represents a holistic system comprising subsystems that have boundaries but interact synergistically with each other, making the whole greater than the sum of its parts. The model is abstract because it represents many processes that can only be inferred on the basis of data from normal development, modern neuroimaging techniques, and behaviors of people with localized brain lesions. The model is practical because it pulls together many of the pieces practitioners consider when providing assessment and intervention for individuals with language disorders. It is not exhaus-

tive because the subpoints within each of the six knowledge modules are only representative of the rule systems a person must use to process complex linguistic texts. The purpose is to suggest a system for observing aspects of internalized processing that may be addressed during intervention, as discussed later in this chapter.

Contextually based language assessment. Educational, vocational, and social contexts are all relevant to the later stages of language learning. Depending on areas identified as "zones of significance" for particular individuals, some contexts may be identified as more critically in need of attention. For school-age children and adolescents with language disorders, however, school is almost always significant.

In school, where young people with language disorders spend the majority of their time, they encounter some of the most pressing language-based learning demands, and they are at great risk for failure and for damage to their self-esteem. **Curriculum-based language assessment** therefore is often the most critical form of contextually based assessment for older children and adolescents with language disorders. It is the method of focus in this section, with the expectation that readers will adapt its techniques to other contexts as appropriate when individual needs arise.

In my previous work about curriculum-based language assessment and intervention (N. W. Nelson, 1989b, 1990, in press-a, in press-b), I have been careful to differentiate it from general curriculum-based measurement (CBM). To understand the distinctions, first, consider a description of general curriculum-based assessment (CBA):

> Curriculum-based assessments are teacher-constructed tests designed to measure directly students' skill achievements at specified grades. The assessments are criterion-referenced, and their content reflects the curricula used in general education classrooms. (Idol, Nevin, et al., 1986, p. v)

Tucker (1985) commented, in addition, that CBA "includes any procedure that directly assesses student performance within the course content for the purpose of determining that student's instructional needs" (p. 200). Deno (1989) noted that "CBM is a systematic set of procedures that produces a data base for making special education decisions" (p. 1). General forms of CBM address the question "Has the student learned the curriculum?"

In contrast, curriculum-based *language* assessment refers to the more specific "use of curriculum contexts and content for measuring a student's language intervention needs and progress" (N. W. Nelson, 1989b, p. 171). It addresses the question "How does the student use language in attempting to learn the curriculum?" Although the primary distinction between the two approaches is one of specificity, some methodological distinctions also apply.

The two approaches complement each other. Questions about how well the curriculum has been learned (and which aspects are problematic) usually serve as a prelude to more specific questions about language processing. Conversely, specialists may use the in-depth probing strategies of curriculum-based language assessment to determine why a student is having difficulty learning the curriculum. It is wise, however, to keep some aspects of the two approaches separate. To understand why, consider an example: Student, parent, and teacher interviews about zones of significance for one high school student with language-learning disabilities make it fairly clear that he is competent in learning some aspects of the physical education (PE) and industrial arts curricula but that his performance is inadequate on paper and pencil or textbook tasks. He seems gifted as an athlete and when using his hands to make things. However, his language and reading deficits make it highly difficult for him to read the course textbooks, to answer questions on written assignments, and to take written tests.

Members of a diagnostic team attempting to implement general CBA for this adolescent might collaborate with the PE teacher to construct multiple-choice examination questions to assess the student's knowledge of sports rules studied and with the industrial arts teacher to construct a test with diagram labeling and true–false questions to assess knowledge of tools and methods for use in woodworking (see examples of these instruments in Idol, Nevin, et al., 1986). This team, recognizing probable negative effects of reading deficits, might design alternative forms of assessment to the paper and pencil tasks, perhaps administering the test orally, or allowing unlimited time and accepting spelling approximations. They might use the test results to draw conclusions about the extent to which the student has benefitted from the regular classroom activities, whether placement should continue in those classrooms, and whether compensatory methods should be designed for note taking, textbook reading, and test taking.

A language specialist using curriculum-based language assessment would take a slightly different approach to these same problems. This professional might work with the rest of the interdisciplinary diagnostic team to analyze the outcome of teacher-designed tests but more likely would use samples of the real curriculum rather than specially designed tests to analyze the student's curriculum-based language processing abilities.

Curriculum-based language assessment involves several kinds of data collection. The primary tools and strategies, in addition to ethnographic interviews, are **artifact analysis, onlooker observation,** and **participant observation.** *Artifacts* are products created by students in the process of regular curricular activities. For the high school student described, artifacts include classroom lecture notes and written assignments. These could be compared with class notes and homework produced by other classmates who are not having difficulty. In particular, language specialists might look for evidence of semantic organizational strategies, word knowledge, linguistic sophistication, completeness, and detail. Other artifacts that might be examined include actual responses to real classroom examinations and portfolios of representative work that classroom teachers collect for all of their students (e.g., Rief, 1990).

Onlooker observation involves sitting in the classroom with the student at a distance and observing signs of participation, including evidence of attention, listening, and communicative expression. Onlooker observation is not particularly appropriate at secondary levels because of student embarrassment, but tape recordings of classroom lectures might be used as indirect observation to gauge the level of linguistic complexity and other language demands of the classroom. Participant observation is a somewhat more intrusive form of observation. The specialist sits beside the student while the student attempts to complete a targeted curricular task (this can occur in an isolated therapy room, if appropriate). In participant observation, the adult acts not as traditional teacher, but as co-conspirator or co-learner, attempting to figure out the demands of the activity with the student.

Participant observation involves more than observation of the current status of the situation. This dynamic assessment is a deliberate exploration of the student's ability to recognize relationships, comprehend the language of an activity, and formulate appropriate responses to it, when the examiner uses facilitation strategies. Participant observation is based on Vygotsky's (1962) observation that "with assistance, every child can do more than he can by himself—though only within the limits set by the state of his development" (p. 103). Vygotsky labeled the range between what a child can do independently and what he or she can do with facilitation the "zone of proximal development."

Bruner (1978) used Vygotsky's ideas to introduce the concept of scaffolding. Scaffolding techniques, as mentioned throughout the preceding chapters, are used by parents, teachers, and supervisors at all levels of the child's development, from infancy through adulthood. Scaffolding enables individuals to reach levels of processing efficiency and success that they might not be able to reach otherwise; even more importantly, particularly in the later stages of language development, it encourages independent use of strategies after they have been modeled (Applebee & Langer, 1983; Bruner, 1978; Cazden, 1988).

An example of a scaffolding technique that might be used with the high school student described previously is modeling of "thinking aloud" or self-questioning, verbal mediation strategies. When completing assignments involving questions in the shop manual, the student is encouraged to ask a series of questions, such as "What am I supposed to do here? How many different kinds of tools am I supposed to learn this week? What are the main types and subtypes of tools? What is the function of each?" In responding to such questions, the student is taught to draw a semantic map to show major headings, subheadings, definitions, characteristics, and examples of particular types of tools. Then the student could be taught how to study with peers, using notes and diagrams to ask questions of each other and themselves.

Unique contributions by language specialists in dynamic assessment contexts come from description of students' current language knowledge, skills, and strategies when attempting to process language of the curriculum. Concurrently, language specialists informally analyze the language demands of the curriculum. The first effort might be considered an inside-out approach, and the second might be considered an outside-in approach. These assessment concerns are summarized by the two questions (outside-in and inside-out, respectively):

1. What are the external contextual demands that influence how the student processes the information?

2. What are the internal language and communicative processing abilities that the student currently brings to the task?

These two questions—oriented relatively more toward curriculum-based language assessment—are balanced by two more questions—oriented relatively more toward curriculum-based language intervention ("relatively more" because all four questions have both assessment and intervention implications). The intervention-oriented questions also have an inside-out and outside-in balance:

3. What new language knowledge, skills, and strategies might the student acquire that would improve the situation in the future?

4. What contextual modifications might be implemented to facilitate the student's processing success?

The goal of curriculum-based language assessment and intervention activities is "to facilitate the student's use of language and communicative skills and strategies for real purposes, in meaningful, functional contexts, and, as much as possible, to keep the student in the regular curriculum" (Nelson, in press-a). In planning to meet this goal, the question "What is the regular curriculum?" arises. I broadly define curriculum to include the official course of study for a school system and other less direct and less obvious aspects of school-required study. Six curricular types are summarized in Box 9.4.

Assessing linguistic and metalinguistic knowledge. In the later stages of language acquisition, the importance of assessment questions about knowledge of rule systems for phonology, morphology, syntax, semantics, and pragmatics continues. (The categories of language content, form, and use remain preferred for some purposes, particularly for communicating with teachers and parents who might be overwhelmed by linguistic labels.) Two shifts in emphasis, however, differentiate later stage language assessment from that of earlier stages. First is a greater emphasis on using linguistic knowledge to process language in multiple modalities, and second is a recognition of metalinguistic and other "meta-"abilities as primary targets of assessment.

First, consider the need to look for consistent patterns of competent or incompetent rule use across modalities. Descriptions of rule-use patterns may help an interdisciplinary team understand how a student's

Box 9.4	A summary of six curricula students must master to succeed in school	
	Official Curriculum	The outline produced by curriculum committees in many school districts. May or may not have major influence in a particular classroom. To find out, ask the teacher to show you a copy.
	Cultural Curriculum	The unspoken expectations for students to know enough about the mainstream culture to use it as background context in understanding various aspects of the official curriculum.
	De Facto Curriculum	The use of textbook selections rather than an official outline to determine the curriculum. Classrooms in the same district often vary in the degree to which "teacher manual teaching" occurs.
	School Culture Curriculum	The set of spoken and unspoken rules about communication and behavior in classroom interactions. Includes expectations for metapragmatic awareness of rules about such things as when to talk, when not to talk, and how to request a turn.
	Hidden Curriculum	The subtle expectations that teachers have for determining who the "good students" are in their classrooms. They vary with the value systems of individual teachers. Even students who are insensitive to the rules of the school culture curriculum usually know where they fall on a classroom continuum of "good" and "problem" students.
	Underground Curriculum	The rules for social interaction among peers that determine who will be accepted and who not. Includes expectations for using the latest slang and pragmatic rules of social interaction discourse as diverse as bragging and peer tutoring.

© 1992 N. W. Nelson. Shared by permission of the author.

language disorder interacts with other processing deficits. A language specialist might observe that an adolescent with a history of severe oral language delay tends to omit and transpose the same kinds of grammatical function words when reading aloud as when speaking. The team might then notice that the student ignores similar grammatical elements when listening and writing. The identification of consistency in cross-modality patterns is particularly helpful when attempting to identify basic rule system deficits that should be considered when planning intervention.

In the area of metaprocessing abilities, later stage language learners meet particular challenges. Four types of deliberate multilevel processing should be considered: metalinguistic, metapragmatic, metatextual, and metacognitive.

Metalinguistic abilities are used to reflect consciously on language, to process it on more than one level at once, and to know the labels of formal education that are used to talk about language. Metalinguistic abilities must be probed through somewhat artificial tasks, because these tasks require language

users to reflect on language and not just to use it for communication. Table 9.4 includes a set of tasks compiled by Flood and Salus (1982) to probe for metalinguistic awareness.

Another approach might be to observe evidence of metalinguistic ability (or the lack thereof) within regular curricular tasks. Opportunities to observe a student's ability to recognize anomalous language forms might arise naturally during participant editing activities. If the student fails to recognize syntactic errors independently, the language specialist might read anomalous sentences aloud to see if the student can then identify and fix difficulties.

Other metalinguistic abilities are probed more readily as responses to texts written by others. Complex and ambiguous sentences, in particular, may arise in curricular texts. For example, after a student reads a sentence such as "The teacher told us to stop talking," a participant observer might probe to determine if the student can identify "Who did the telling?" and "Who was told?" Similarly, following the reading of an ambiguous sentence such as "The fat farmer's wife cooks all day long," the observer might ask, "Who was fat?" and "Could it have been anyone else?"

The ability to paraphrase (and to recognize syntactic synonymy in paraphrases) is a metalinguistic skill that is particularly important in the middle and later school-age years. It permits students to find answers to questions at the ends of chapters when the information in the text is worded differently, and it helps them to take notes without worrying about writing a teacher's words verbatim. Therefore, observers should look especially for opportunities to probe this skill. For example, the observer might ask the student to paraphrase complex sentences such as "His mother was waiting when he arrived."

Metapragmatic abilities may be probed by asking students to describe the rules of communicative interactions. The professional might ask a student

how the rules for entering a conversation politely differ from rules for taking turns in an argument. To probe metapragmatic awareness of the school culture curriculum, students might answer direct questions about classroom routines and rules (Creaghead & Tattershall, 1985; Tattershall, 1987; Wilkinson & Milosky, 1987). A set of questions suggested by Creaghead and Tattershall is reprinted in Box 9.5. These are appropriate to ask either at the middle or later stages of language development.

Metatextual abilities may be probed by asking children to talk about the structure of stories or other discourse forms, such as expository texts. When conducting curriculum-based language assessment using samples of narrative texts, the professional might ask the student to talk about the "plot" of the story; to identify parts of the story such as the main characters, the setting, and the ending; or to tell about what

TABLE 9.4

Examples of sentences and passages that illustrate how metalinguistic abilities might be probed by asking students to reflect on language in the context of curriculum-based language assessment activities

Type	Example
Sentences anomaly	
Disjunction	Sally likes apples, but she likes bananas.
Causal	He broke his leg because he went to the hospital.
Conditional	If he puts his boots on, it will rain.
Temporal	While he stood on the shore, he waded in the water.
Nongrammaticality	
Morphological	The Martian ship unintegrated when it hit the atmosphere.
Adjective clustering	The plastic big round ball fell off the table.
Adverbial use	He wanted to play much.
Preposition	He broke the window by a hammer.
Paraphrase	
Lexical substitution	The teacher told us to stop talking.
Passive	The money for the trip was raised by the fourth grade.
Dative movement	John sent every girl a valentine.
Fronting	His mother was waiting when he arrived home.
Ambiguity	
Pronominal referent	John played with the dog while he was eating.
Lexical	The coach asked me how many times Jack beat Stuart.
Deep structure	Do you want a tiger to chase you or a lion?
Surface structure/bracketing	The fat farmer's wife cooks all day long.
Passage anomaly	
Disjunction	It had started to rain very hard. *Sally had neither a raincoat and an umbrella.* She started to run toward the building entrance and kept on running. Just as she got there, she realized it had stopped raining 2 minutes ago.

Note. From "Metalinguistic Awareness: Its Role in Language Development and Its Assessment" by J. Flood and M. W. Salus. Reprinted from *Topics in Language Disorders*, Vol. 2, No. 4, p. 62, with permission of Aspen Publishers, Inc., © 1982.

Box 9.5   Questionnaire regarding classroom routine and rules

1. What does your teacher do or say when he or she is angry with the class?
2. What really makes your teacher mad or angry?
3. What is the most important thing you should always do in class?
4. What is the most important thing you should never do in class?
5. How do you know when it is time to go inside after recess? [This question could be adapted at the secondary level to ask about the school's policy regarding tardiness.]
6. What is the first thing you should do when class begins?
7. What does your teacher do or say before he or she says something really important?
8. What is the last thing you should do before you go home at the end of the day?
9. When is it OK to talk aloud without raising your hand at school?
10. How do you know when your teacher is joking or teasing?
11. What does your teacher do when it is time for a lesson to begin?
12. When is it all right to ask a question in class?

Note. From "Observation and Assessment of Classroom Pragmatic Skills" by N.A. Creaghead and S.A. Tattershall in *Communication Skills and Classroom Success: Assessment and Therapy Methodologies for Language and Learning Disabled Students* (p. 110) edited by C.S. Simon, 1991, Eau Claire, WI: Thinking Publications. Copyright 1991 by Thinking Publications. Reprinted by permission.

---

makes a story a story. Asking for overt identification of story features differs from asking an individual to retell a story. When analyzing a student's ability to understand the language of expository text, the examiner might probe for the student's ability to recognize the organizational structure, for example, as involving temporal sequence or hierarchical categorical relationships.

Metacognitive abilities involve self-awareness and executive control of problem-solving strategies. One of the best ways to probe for metacognitive abilities is to ask students to "think aloud" as they attempt particular curricular tasks. Davey (1983) described how adults might model "think-aloud" reading comprehension techniques to make predictions, visualize meanings, develop analogies to things they already know, identify confusing points, and use repair strategies when comprehension fails. Students also may be taught to use "thinking language" during mathematics exercises. Similar metacognitive approaches involve asking students to reflect on reasons for reading certain texts and asking them questions such as "What do you have to do to get a good grade in this course?" (Burke, 1980; Westby, 1991; Wixson, Boskey, Yochum, & Alverman, 1984).

Assessing language in multiple modalities. In the later stages of language development, literacy activities gain increased importance. Language devel-

opment in the later stages involves all the modalities, listening, speaking, reading, writing, and thinking.

The importance of speech awareness related to phonological processing and word segmentation has been documented for some time as a key to normal acquisition of early reading ability (Ehri, 1975; Holden & MacGinitie, 1972; I. Y. Liberman, Shankweiler, Liberman, Fowler, & Fischer, 1977; Masaaro, 1973; Venezky, 1970). Impairment of phonological awareness has also been identified as a primary factor when children have difficulty learning to read (Kamhi & Catts, 1989; Stanovich, 1985). Recent theories, however, have emphasized the construction of meaning for social purposes as the primary link that connects different modalities of communicative processing and thinking (see Personal Reflection 9.10).

Tierney (1990) reviewed four major developments in theories of reading since 1970. First, Tierney noted that, as part of a cognitive revolution in the 1970s," a constructivist or "schema-theoretic" view of reading comprehension became dominant. This theoretical shift was based on evidence that a reader's background knowledge is a better predictor of recall than factors such as verbal intelligence, word recognition, overall reading ability, and vocabulary knowledge. Second, in the 1980s, a view of "reading as writing" began to emerge. This shift occurred largely as a result of the work of Emig (1971), Flower and Hayes

(1980), and Graves (1978; 1983), which led to emphasis on writing as process rather than product. As students began to compose, read, edit, and revise more of their own and each other's texts, it became apparent that their attitudes and approaches toward reading and thinking about texts in general changed concurrently. Reading and writing came to be viewed as activities during which students could evaluate issues, explore possibilities, adopt various perspectives, experiment with ideas, and discover new insights. Third is a recognition of "reading as engagement. . . . views of reading that connect readers to their imaginations and that reach beneath the surface to a fuller consideration of the reader's emotional, affective, and visual involvement." (Tierney, 1990, p. 39). Fourth is the recent emphasis on "reading as situation-based," moving away from the view that "comprehension processes are neatly prepackaged to the view that they are ill-structured, complex, and vary from one context to another" (p. 41).

These four views of listening, speaking, reading, writing, and thinking as interactive processes can influence diagnostic teamwork. These views move teams away from territorial beliefs that only certain professionals should assess certain modalities (e.g., speech–language pathologists should assess oral communication only). They also remove the illusion that it is possible to adequately examine different modalities in isolation. In particular, the theoretical perspective that reading is situation based is consistent with the emphasis on context throughout this book. Largely because comprehension processes are constructive and "vary from one context to another" (Tierney, 1990, p. 41), participant observers can mod-

ify contexts by what they say and do. Techniques of dynamic assessment permit identification of contextual variables that help individuals with language disorders make sense when listening, talking, reading, writing, and thinking.

Points of divergence between oral and written processing modalities also should be recognized. As Rubin (1987) noted, "Writing and speech are not merely alternative and equivalent ways of encoding language. Oral and written communication differ profoundly in both functional and structural properties" (p. 2). Rubin cited studies of written language acquisition of speakers of Black English Vernacular (BEV), which showed them to include a lower frequency of BEV features in their writing than in their speech, and to produce writing errors that were, for the most part, indistinguishable from those made by standard English (SE) speakers learning to write (see Personal Reflection 9.11).

Pragmatic distinctions also create divergence between oral and written texts. When narrative texts are written rather than spoken, differences occur in the levels of interactions and involvement of communicative partners (J. N. Britton, 1970, 1979; Westby, 1984). Literate text is structured differently from oral text partially because literate language does not involve spatial and temporal commonality, immediate ability to interact, or ability to convey meaning through prosody and gesture. In written texts, nonverbal context, prosody, and gesture are replaced by greater lexicalization of concepts (Emig, 1977) and by punctuation and other writing conventions that assist readers to parse texts and construct meanings. Intelligible spelling in written communication serves

---

Personal Reflection 9.10

"The days when reading comprehension skill was equated with reading speed or the ability to regurgitate the text have thankfully given way to a broader view of reading. Overly text-based accounts of comprehension have been displaced by multifaceted considerations of the subjectivity of meaning-making, shared understandings held by communities of readers, and reading as the flexible orchestration of problem-solving strategies in conjunction with the thoughtful consideration of ideas. Further, inference and evaluation are regarded as essential to achieving basic understanding as they are to the critical thinking that grows with interpretation and the ability to recount literal detail. In other words, a mechanical view of reading has given way to a view of reading as creative enterprise."

Robert J. Tierney (1990, p. 37), reading theorist at The Ohio State University, writing about "Redefining Reading Comprehension."

the role of intelligible speech articulation in oral communication. Writers unable to keep literate language distinctions in mind, or lacking the technical skill to execute them, may experience greater difficulty in producing written than oral language narratives.

Moran (1987) found divergence of oral and written language abilities in writing samples produced by three groups of 14- to 16-year-olds with learning disabilities, low achievement, or normal achievement. In particular, the students with learning disabilities produced more and better elaborated structures orally than in written form. Their oral language was also similar to that of their peers with low or normal achievement in terms of syntactic, morphologic, and semantic measures. Their written language samples differed from those of their low-achieving peers primarily in lower spelling performance and from samples of normal-achieving peers in lower frequency of optional words, such as adjectives. They also performed significantly lower than normal-achieving students on spelling and punctuation conventions.

Other research suggests that oral language skills of normally achieving and reading disabled children may relate differently to reading comprehension abilities at different age levels. Snyder and Downey (1991) compared word retrieval, phonological awareness, sentence completion, and narrative discourse skills of 93 reading disabled and 93 normally achieving students between the ages of 8 and 14 years. They found that variance in the younger children's reading comprehension scores was best explained by performance on sentence-completion and word-retrieval tasks. Variance in older children's reading comprehension scores was better explained by higher order inferencing skills. These results support the notion that bottom-up processing skills play a more critical role in the earlier stages of learning to read, whereas top-down processing skills play a more critical role in the later stages of written language acquisition.

The techniques for informal assessment of language in varied modalities include a combination of holistic and analytic strategies. This section presents three informal approaches for assessing reading, writing, and thinking: (1) miscue analysis for samples of oral reading, (2) procedures for analyzing written language samples, and (3) strategies for observing the ability to think aloud.

Miscue analysis was proposed originally by K. S. Goodman (1973a, 1973b) as a system for analyzing "errors" individuals produce while reading aloud. Goodman proposed that "observed responses," which differ from "expected responses," are not accidents or errors. Rather, they represent the outcome of active internal processing strategies based on the "sum total of prior experience and learning" that a reader brings to the reading process (1973a, p. 160).

Miscue analysis is based on a theory of reading that suggests that mature readers use three types of cues to predict textual meaning: semantic, syntactic, and graphophonemic. Because mature readers have considerable knowledge about language, they continually form hypotheses as they read about what they expect texts to say. First, they use semantic cues to predict words that fit textual meaning; second, they use syntactic cues to predict words that fit syntactic contexts; and third, they use graphophonemic cues to check whether the words they have predicted fit visual perceptual information sampled from the print. In this way, they confirm or disconfirm hypotheses about what the print says. If the perceptual evidence does not fit what they have predicted or if in reading on, they find that they have produced a sentence that is syntactically or semantically anomalous, mature readers retrace their steps, sample additional perceptual information, check their multiple cues against their internal knowledge systems, and correct their miscues. Miscues that maintain semantic and syntactic acceptability are usually left alone. A fourth level of cues implied by this model, although not originally discussed by K. S. Goodman (1973a) consists of textual cues. Readers must monitor not only whether elements of individual sentences maintain semantic, syntactic, and graphophonemic acceptability but also whether sentences they produce make sense within the context of the whole text they have been reading—and within the context of their knowledge of the world.

To conduct miscue analysis, the specialist selects appropriately challenging, unfamiliar, and unpracticed reading material (Y. M. Goodman, Watson, & Burke, 1987). The specialist selects material from the regular curriculum when using miscue analysis in curriculum-based language assessment. The language specialist asks students to read aloud directly from an original source "as if they were reading alone," while following along on a photocopy (or typed transcript) of the text, marking miscues as indicated in Figure 9.2. Students are also told that they should try to understand what they read because they will be expected to retell it or answer questions about it.

Miscues are then analyzed to determine their acceptability in terms of each of the four cuing systems. Miscues that violate graphophonemic, syntactic, semantic, or textual acceptability suggest that readers have weak rule systems for recognizing cues in one or more of those language areas (corresponding with four of the six knowledge modules in Figure

9.1). Alternatively, readers may have rule-based knowledge but lack proficiency for using it in complex contexts. Self-correction of miscues provides evidence that the reader is actively using at least one cuing system to construct meaning. Some problems involve integration among systems. For example, a miscue that maintains semantic sense but violates syntactic acceptability suggests that a reader is relying on the semantic rule system at the expense of the syntactic one. Other readers may demonstrate contrasting patterns.

By definition, all miscues violate graphophonemic acceptability to some degree because they are speech productions that do not match print. Therefore, analysis procedures always address the degree to which a reader's miscues are graphically or phonemically similar to the words in print. When many observed words diverge graphophonemically from expected ones, the reader probably needs help with basic decoding skills. When readers ignore minor graphophonemic miscues that do not violate semantic, syntactic, or textual meaning, they have adopted appropriate strategies to promote efficiency that are signs of strength.

FIGURE 9.2
Codes for marking miscues on oral reading transcripts.

Omissions	(circled)	He made ⓐ kite...
Substitutions		
1.	Text item substitutions.	*Her* She didn't want him to be sad.
2.	Involving reversals.	*said* "Why?" asked⟍Jane.
3.	Involving bound morphemes	*ing* ...and make kites⊘
4.	Involving nonwords	*Kansas* /kæend/ /kɑkoni/ A city is a special kind of community.
5.	Misarticulations	*$pecific* He had a specific thing in mind.
6.	Intonation shifts	*récord* He will record her voice.
7.	Split syllables	You should try cut|ting hair.
8.	Pauses	*15 sec.* Cities are╱crowded.
Insertions	(indicate with a ∧)	*her* Jane wanted to help∧Grandfather.
Repetitions and **regressions**		‖One day, Grandfather was sad.
Dialect and other language variations		*like ⓓ* ...just about everybody likes babies.
Assistance from the examiner		*Kansas* There are four special things about a ⌐city.⌐

Sources: K. S. Goodman, 1973; Y. M. Goodman et al., 1987. © 1992 N. W. Nelson. Shared by permission of the author.

The process of analyzing miscues may be more or less formal, depending on the time available. Particularly when learning to use the procedure, professionals may wish to use formal analysis procedures and recording forms such as those published by Y. M. Goodman et al. (1987). These authors suggest that examiners base their miscue analyses on either word-level or sentence-level units, with relatively more abbreviated or extensive detail. For example, the following set of questions was adapted from those suggested by Y. M. Goodman et al. to guide analysis at the sentence level:

1. *Syntactic acceptability.* Does the miscue occur in a syntactically acceptable structure in the reader's dialect? [Answer yes (Y), no (N), or partial (P), depending on the degree of acceptability.]
2. *Semantic acceptability.* Does the miscue occur in a semantically acceptable structure in the reader's dialect? [Answer yes (Y), no (N), or partial (P), depending on the degree of acceptability; Cannot be coded higher than syntactic acceptability.]
3. *Meaning change.* Does the miscue change the meaning of the text? [Answer yes (Y), no (N), or partial (P), depending on the degree of acceptability; Question is asked only if the miscues are both syntactically and semantically acceptable.]
4. *Correction.* Is the miscue corrected? [Answer yes (Y), no (N), or partial (P), depending on the degree of acceptability.]
5. *Graphic similarity.* How much does the miscue look like the text? [Answer high (H), some (S), or none (N), depending on the degree of similarity.]
6. *Sound similarity.* How much does the miscue sound like the expected response? [Answer high (H), some (S), or none (N), depending on the degree of similarity.]

Language specialists who use miscue analysis should also use evidence from other formal and informal assessment procedures to formulate and test assessment hypotheses. The outcome should be a fairly comprehensive picture of which rule systems are basically weak across modalities, which are relatively more weak in a particular modality, and which are fairly strong when used in highly controlled contexts but tend to be ignored when complex tasks demand integrated processing that draws on multiple cuing systems at one time.

Written language samples may be analyzed using a variety of strategies, including holistic qualitative scoring, analytic scoring, or quantitative scoring of countable indices (C. R. Cooper & Odell, 1977; Moran, 1987; Tindal & Parker, 1991). All three types of techniques have relative advantages and disadvantages.

Isaacson (1985) suggested a set of procedures that mixed all three. Where available, he provided normative guidelines for judging the five components (1) fluency, measured as total number of words written; (2) syntactic maturity, measured as numbers of fragments, simple, compound, and complex sentences, or as average T-unit length; (3) vocabulary, measured by counting unusual or infrequently used words that do not appear on lists of frequently used words, or by computing type-token ratios; (4) content, measured by rating global aspects of text organization, and (5) conventions, measured by counting errors in writing conventions using a checklist.

Writing is similar in many respects to speech production. It is, above all, a form of verbal expression. As noted, however, it also differs from speech in some important ways. An obvious difference is that writers must remember how to spell, which involves a complex set of cognitive linguistic processes (Frith, 1980) as diverse as sounding out words by syllable or recalling their appearance holistically.

Mature writers also must use a special kind of pragmatic knowledge to communicate with absent audiences. This involves complex decision making about how much information to encode in the text. Writers can do this well only if they have the world knowledge and metalinguistic flexibility to meet their particular purpose, the metapragmatic skills to be aware of that purpose, and the metacognitive strategies to review and revise until the purpose is met. All of this requires fairly abstract, high-level, integrated thinking.

A more informal approach for analyzing written language samples might involve questions and strategies borrowed from oral reading miscue analysis. Language specialists might observe both the writing process and products to find evidence of internalized language knowledge, skills, and information processing strategies. To guide the comparisons of observed and expected responses, examiners might use a complex model of written and oral language processing, such as that illustrated in Figure 9.1.

Language specialists may use adapted forms of miscue analysis to assess written language samples by analyzing written language evidence that the writer is actively using information from all six rule systems shown in Figure 9.1. Sample targets of observation for each of the six knowledge modules might include the following:

1. **Graphophonemic knowledge**, which shows up primarily as spelling accuracy
2. **Semantic knowledge**, which shows up as, for example, well-chosen lexical items and appropriate representation of case and event relations, use of semantic cohesion and transition devices, and use of figurative meanings
3. **Syntactic knowledge**, which shows up as, for example, syntactic acceptability, appropriate subject–verb agreement, parallel sentence structure, and appropriate use of syntactic cohesion and transition devices
4. **Discourse knowledge**, which shows up as, for example, broad text organization, formatting, and cohesion
5. **Pragmatic knowledge**, which shows up as, for example, adequate consideration of the audience's informational needs, clear management of topics, and demonstration of the ability to use different writing strategies for different communicative purposes
6. **World and prior knowledge**, which shows up as the provision of accurate and appropriately organized and elaborated information about the world

Professionals also might observe evidence of processing deficits in input–output modalities, such as fine motor coordination deficits that may influence handwriting legibility, or phonological analysis and synthesis deficits that may influence the ability to spell unfamiliar words. Examiners may select formal assessment tools to check hypotheses about language processing formed during informal assessment. The Boder Test of Reading–Spelling Patterns (Boder & Jarrico, 1982) may be used to determine the language user's ability to use both analytic (sounding out) or eidetic (visual memory) strategies to recall and to spell words. Analytic strategies work well for words spelled phonemically, but eidetic strategies are necessary for reproducing irregularly spelled words.

The written language samples gathered and analyzed will depend on the comprehensive purposes of assessment, with selections representing zones of significance identified in the interview. Samples from the student's classroom portfolios produced as regular assignments may be particularly helpful because they can be compared with those of classmates which were presumably produced under similar conditions. In other cases, the language professional may make special writing assignments to observe the writing process more directly.

Examiners and teachers must be careful when using analytical strategies to evaluate student's written language and to select intervention targets to avoid producing a fragmented picture of the student as a writer and as a communicator. As Moran (1987) commented, "The process of surveying, analyzing, and selecting priorities is abused by limiting objectives to what is readily isolated, measured, and plotted on a profile" (p. 53). To reconcile needs for quantitative and qualitative measures, C. R. Cooper (1977) proposed a set of analytic scales that could be used to make holistic judgments about complete pieces of writing.

Thinking language analysis is an informal approach for evaluating internal uses of language for thinking. Evidence of the ability to use language for thinking may be gathered simply by asking individuals to report what they are doing or thinking while performing a task. Their ability to do so without modeling may indicate the ease with which they use verbal mediation strategies. If examinees have no idea how to talk themselves through a problem-solving activity, the examiner may model the process during participant observation. It may be a direct target of language intervention (see discussion later in this chapter).

Some examples of verbal mediation language that might appear when the student is attempting to process elements of the social studies curriculum might include the following:

> "First, I have to read the directions. Then I read the first question. [Reads question aloud.] Now I have to find the part of the chapter that talks about this. Here it is. [And so forth.]"

The rationale for assessing thinking language is based on Vygotsky's (1934, 1962) views of abbreviated "inner speech." Vygotsky contrasted his own views with those of Piaget that were prevalent at the time. Whereas Piaget (1926) viewed overt self-talk as immature "egocentric speech," which needed to be replaced by social interaction discourse as the child matured, Vygotsky saw self-talk as a way of supporting mature thought, which, as the child matured, merely went underground. Vygotsky made the distinction between Piaget's position and his own explicit in the following comments:

Our experimental results indicate that the function of egocentric speech is similar to that of inner speech: It does not merely accompany a child's activity; it serves mental orientation, conscious understanding; it helps in overcoming difficulties; it is speech for oneself, intimately and usefully connected with the child's thinking. Its fate is very different from that described by Piaget. Egocentric speech develops along a rising, not a declining, curve; it goes through an evolution, not an involution. In the end, it becomes inner speech (Vygotsky, 1934/1962, p. 133).

Assessing different sizes of linguistic units. Comprehensive language sample analysis involves focus on varied sizes of linguistic units. This does not mean that separate samples are gathered but that different analysis methods are used to focus on varied sizes of units within the same samples, particularly as they are gathered in the process of curriculum-based language assessment. Table 9.3, earlier in the chapter, lists the levels sounds, syllables, words, simple sentences, complex sentences, and texts. In the later stages of development, analysis should involve looking for evidence that the individual has basic skills for using each of these units in naturalistic communication samples but also that the individual has metalinguistic awareness of them as entities.

Sound-level analysis continues to be important in the later stages of language development. The official curriculum of a school district helps to determine the degree to which language is parsed explicitly into linguistic units as small as sounds, particularly in the early grades. The current trend, as advocated by "whole-language" theorists, is to avoid fragmenting language into individual units during the initial teaching of reading (K. S. Goodman, 1986), but some theorists continue to emphasize the need for young students to be able to segment words into sounds, particularly if they seem to be having difficulty with the decoding aspects of learning to read (I. Y. Liberman & Liberman, 1990; Sawyer et al., 1985). By the time children reach the later stages of language development, they should demonstrate the ability to analyze and synthesize complex phonological sequences across modalities. When children exhibit phonological problems involving sequencing, phoneme (or grapheme) omissions, additions, or transpositions in oral or written samples, the examiner should describe these problems and should seek evidence of cross-modality commonalities.

Syllable-level analysis involves consideration of students' abilities to use syllable awareness in meeting curricular processing demands. The importance of syllabic complexity in the later grades is illustrated by readability formulas that use syllable counts to assign grade-level designations to written language samples (e.g., Fry, 1968). Some upper grade-level texts also show breakdowns of words into syllables in pronunciation guides. Indeed, when mature readers "sound out" words, they do not do it sound by sound but syllable by syllable. Without syllabication strategies, students with language-learning disabilities are more likely to panic when they see polysyllabic words in print. The analysis procedure for curriculum-based language samples should, therefore, involve identifying whether students can segment long words into syllables and whether they can recognize frequently recurring syllable patterns and the underlying meanings of syllables that encode derivational morphemes such as *pre-, dis-, -tion,* and *-ture.*

Word-level analysis is required in many later grade curricular tasks. Older students must recognize common meanings of words in complex contexts, recall words when they need them, consider alternative meanings of words when appropriate, compare and contrast word meanings, and think of alternative words for the same concept. They also must produce and understand words with abstract and figurative meanings.

Sentence-level analysis in the later stages of language development, as in the earlier stages, must determine whether students have control over a variety of simple sentence patterns, both in expression and comprehension, and with inflectional morphemes within those patterns. Especially critical in the later stages is the ability to produce and understand a rich variety of complex sentence structures with multiple embeddings and with referential and logical connections across sentence boundaries. To succeed in school, older students must be particularly good at using their sentence level skills to recognize "syntactic synonymy" (van Kleeck, 1984). Many curricular tasks require students to recognize paraphrases of what they have read, to paraphrase material themselves, to infer the relationships between two different sentences with the same or almost the same meaning, to take true–false and multiple-choice tests that require sophisticated sentence analysis strategies, and to find alternative structures for saying the same thing when revising their own written compositions. Later stage students are also expected to have the metalinguistic skill to reflect on and to formally discuss varied syntactic operations.

During the later stage development, MLU remains a valid indicator of increasing syntactic ability in both oral and written expressive language samples. In the later stages, however, the unit for dividing discourse into individual utterances should not be a sentence, because advancing maturity is not always evidenced by longer sentences. Some of the longest sentences by middle-stage language learners may be formed by the relatively immature "run-on" strategy of stringing multiple independent clauses together loosely with multiple *and then* connectors. More mature language learners generally expand utterance length by adding a variety of nonclausal structures, using embedding and phrase elaboration strategies, which allow them to say more in fewer words (Hunt, 1965, 1970, 1977).

Increasing syntactic maturity is best represented by dividing spoken or written discourse into analysis units that leave elaborated structures intact but divide immature add-on formulations into separate units. For this purpose, "communication units" were devised by Loban (1963) and "T-units" were used by Hunt (1965, 1977) in their classic studies of language development by school-age children. Loban's (1963, 1976) communication unit strategy was more semantic than syntactic. He defined a communication unit as "a group of words which cannot be further subdivided with the loss of their essential meaning" (1963, p. 6). Loban provided the following example to illustrate how three communication units would be identified within a piece of oral discourse. He marked the end of each communication unit with a slant line (/) and marked the completion of each phonological unit with a pound sign (#):

> I'm going to get a boy 'cause he hit me.#/ I'm going to beat him up an' kick him in his nose/ and I'm going to get the girl, too.#/ (p. 7)

Because semantic segmentation strategies are subjective, reliability may not be as easy to achieve as with Hunt's (1965) more syntactic "minimal terminable units" (T-units). Hunt defined a T-unit as "one main clause plus all the subordinate clauses attached to or embedded within it" (1965, p. 141). Hunt also described T-units are "the shortest grammatically complete sentences that a passage can be

cut into without creating fragments" (1977, p. 93). Hunt's research showed T-units to be a better index of syntactic maturity than sentence length, clause length, or subordination indices (see example of T-unit segmentation in Box 8.8 in Chapter 8). Average T-unit lengths for youngsters in 3rd through 12th grade (as compiled by Scott, 1988c) appear in Table 9.5.

Both Hunt (1965) and Loban (1963) recommended separate analysis of linguistic nonfluencies that intrude in the language formulations of even mature speakers and writers. Loban (1963) called linguistic nonfluencies "mazes" and described the category as including initial revisions, conjunctions, pause fillers (*um, ah, er, OK*), and part-word or whole-word repetitions not intended for emphasis. Hunt (1965) called the same kinds of behavior *garbles*. Specialists should maintain linguistic nonfluencies, although apparently extraneous to messages being conveyed, in transcripts of oral or written samples because they are evidence of internalized processing conflicts. Words in mazes or garbles, however, should not be counted when computing syntactic complexity, because they would inflate the quantitative measurements.

Box 9.6 provides a sample of discourse from a normally developing 16-year-old 10th-grader reported by Squire (1964) from his study of adolescents' responses while reading short stories. The sample primarily illustrates the marking of T-units and linguistic nonfluencies and the ability of later stage language users to talk about abstract concepts, draw inferences beyond what is stated explicitly in text, and focus consciously on how language is used to convey ideas. The number of mazes in this sample of discourse produced by a normal language user is also remarkable but not unusual. Loban (1963) found that, during the first 4 years of schooling, individuals who were rated as skillful with language did reduce both their incidence of mazes and number of words per maze but that the average number of words in mazes increased in a group of lower skilled but normally developing subjects. Similarly, Sturm (1990) found that fifth graders produced significantly more mazes in formal classroom discourse than first graders and that increases were observed in the discourse both of students and teachers. The incidence of mazes was the only discourse variable on which the teachers and students did not differ significantly from each other.

TABLE 9.5
Average T-unit length for youngsters in 3rd through 12th grades

	Research Project									
Grade	a* S†	a W	b S	b W	c S	d S	e W	f W	g W	h W
3	7.62	7.60	8.73	7.67					7.45	
4	9.00	8.02				8.52	8.60	5.21		
5	8.82	8.76	8.90	9.34					8.81	10.70
										11.40
6	9.82	9.04			9.03	8.10		7.32	8.53	
7	9.72	8.98	9.80	9.99						
8	10.71	10.37					11.50	10.34	11.68	
9	10.96	10.05								
10	10.68	11.79			10.15			10.46		
11	11.17	10.67								
12	11.70	13.27					14.40	11.45		

*(a) Loban (1976): N = 35 at each grade. Data also available for high and low language ability groups. Ages unavailable. Spoken: adult–child informal interview. Written: school compositions.

(b) O'Donnell and colleagues (1967): N = 30 at each grade. Ages available. Spoken and written: retelling/rewriting of silent fable (narrative).

(c) Klecan-Acker and Hedrick (1985). N = 24 at each grade. Retelling of a favorite film (narrative).

(d) Scott (1984b). N = 25 10-year-olds, 29 12-year-olds. Retelling of a favorite book, TV episode, film (narrative).

(e) Hunt (1965). N = 18 at each grade. School compositions.

(f) Hunt (1970). N = 50 at each grade. Sentence combining exercise.

(g) Morris and Crump (1982). N = 18 at each age (9.6, 11.25, 12.54, 14.08 years). Rewriting of silent film (narrative).

(h) Richardson and colleagues (1976). N = 257 11-year-old boys, 264 11-year-old girls, School compositions.

†S = spoken; W = written. The d, f, and g projects reported data for age only. The data were entered in the table using the following formula: Grade = Age − 6 Years.

Note. From "Spoken and Written Syntax" by C. M. Scott in *Later Language Development: Ages Nine through Nineteen* (p. 56) edited by M. A. Nippold, 1988, Austin, TX: Pro-Ed. Copyright 1988 by Pro-Ed. Reprinted by permission.

Text-level analysis in the later stages involves looking at students' abilities to use knowledge of a variety of kinds of discourse structures (conversational, narrative, and expository) and pragmatic rules to produce and understand complex texts in multiple modalities. Because this is such an important part of informal assessment in the later stages of language development, it is discussed in greater detail in the following section.

Assessing different kinds of discourse events.
Text-level language processing abilities are often critical determinants of school success (e.g., Roth & Spekman, 1989; Scott, 1989; Westby, 1989), but they are assessed minimally by formal language testing devices. Therefore, designing informal assessment tasks to analyze students' communication capabilities within a variety of kinds of discourse events is particularly important. The text used in discourse events may be categorized as one of three broad types: **con-**

versational, **narrative**, and **expository**. Some of the characteristics and examples of each are summarized in Table 9.6.

One of the major advances in language processing by older children and adolescents is their ability to manage larger units of discourse, enabling them to process both oral and written texts as coherent linguistic units (Hillocks, 1986: Pitcher & Prelinger, 1963; Scinto, 1986; Scott, 1988a, 1988c; Squire, 1987; Westby, 1982, 1984). Scinto (1986) defined text as a "functional unit of complex meaning, an extended predication that involves elaboration of ensembles of sentences by a process of composition and concatenation" (p. 108). Coherence is the distinguishing feature of organized texts. It involves three aspects: (1) microstructures, which are semantic representations of propositions, sentences, and sequences of sentences; (2) macrostructures, which are global textual structures; and (3) coherence, which results from the application of strategies for relating microstructures and macrostructures (T. Van Dijk & Kintsch, 1978). To produce written or oral extended texts, the individual must generate goal-directed intention to communicate meaning, organize meaning into appropriate information units, and integrate units into a coherent linear surface form. This discussion of connected discourse is organized under the three macrostructure headings *conversational, narrative,* and *expository.* (Although further subdivision of discourse types is possible, these three categories are conventional, and limiting the analysis to three major categories keeps the process from becoming unwieldy.)

Conversational discourse is the primary context in which young children learn language, starting when they are infants engaging in protoconversations with care givers. Because conversations are shared with partners who can help bear the communicative load, they are usually the earliest form of discourse in which children experience communicative success. In the later stages of language development, conversations continue to play an important role, but they become more demanding.

In schools, part of the underground curriculum involves learning to participate in social conversation with peers, and less frequently, with teachers. Social conversations tend to follow the usual conversational discourse rules, summarized in Table 9.6, involving balanced turn taking and negotiation of topics by the participants (these were discussed more thoroughly in Chapter 8). Somewhat different conversational rules, however, operate in the formal atmosphere of academic discussions of classrooms and in some business transactions.

Classroom conversations, in particular, with their topics and turn allocations controlled tightly by teachers, have been the object of considerable research. The well-known initiate–respond–evaluate (IRE) pattern (Mehan, 1979) has been described as "the most common pattern of classroom discourse at all grade levels" (Cazden, 1988, p. 29). The teacher takes a fairly long conversational turn to initiate a topic (I), often in the form of a question, the student takes a much shorter turn to respond (R), and the teacher follows with an evaluation (E).

The rules for this stylized form of academic conversation differ from those of more natural social conversations in three primary ways: (1) the high frequency of test-like questions (to which the teacher already knows the answers), rather than sincere questions; (2) the lack of balance in talking time by the communicative partners; and (3) the direct evaluation of what one partner says by the other, establishing a clear imbalance of power. Some business conversations between employees and employers and between service persons and customers also are influenced by a power differential. As older students with language disorders make the transition to adulthood, it is important to sample their abilities to communicate appropriately in a variety of contexts that show their sensitivity to these concerns and to sophisticated applications of the other rules of conversational interaction rules (e.g., turn-taking, interrupting, topic shading, and making polite exits from

---

Box 9.6	Sample of oral discourse produced by a 16-year-old normally developing 10th-grade girl who was describing her response to reading *Reverdy* by Jessamyn West (reported by Squire, 1964, p. 61; parentheses around mazes, including unfilled pauses (. .), and slashes (/) dividing T-units have been added)

S: I don't like her mother.
Q: Why?
S: I don't like her one bit./ I think (her mother is an . . jealous ah . .) Reverdy's mother is jealous of her because (. . perhaps she's . .)her beauty is (. .) so great and everything./ Maybe her mother didn't have boys over at her house or something,/ but (ah . . to me it just seems like her mother . .) it said here that she didn't hate her actually,/ but I think it was just plain old fashioned jealousy/ and I feel sorry for the girl for that and her mother thinking she's boy crazy/ and . . I can kinda see how she'd feel about it when she was perfectly innocent and really wasn't because I have a girl friend myself that was just about in the same predicament./ (And ah . .) I found out here that it was a little sister talking instead of a brother [laugh].

TABLE 9.6
Variations among discourse types

Conversation	Narrative	Expository
Social	Story grammars	Description
Partners take equal turns	Setting	Definition
Negotiate topics as they go	Episode structure	Division and classification
Structured with rules for:	Problem or conflict	Comparison
Initiation	Goal and intention	
Topic introduction	Plan	Illustration
Maintaining topics	Action and event	Analogy
Contingent queries	Ending	Example
Clarification requests	Other structural elements	
Contingent statements	Foreshadowing	Sequence
Changing topics	Flashback	Process
Presupposition (adapting to	Repetition	Cause and effect
listeners knowledge)	"Once upon a time"	Temporal order
termination		
	Qualities	Argument and persuasion
Instructional	Have plots made up of:	Deductive reasoning
Partners unequal	Goals	Inductive reasoning
(teachers dominate)	Actions	Persuasion
Teachers control behavior	Affective states	
and talk. Functions include:	Theme	Functional
Attract or show attention	Point	Introduction
Control amount of speech	Point of view	Transition
Check understanding		Conclusion
Summarize	Types	
Define	Fairy tale	
Edit or acknowledge but modify	Short story	
Correct	Mystery	
Specify topics	Western	
Predictable structure	Science fiction	
Initiate	Biography, diary, journal	
Respond	Drama, light or serious	
Evaluate	Parable	
Students take few and	Fable	
short turns	Advertisement	

Sources: Calfee & Carley, 1984; Cazden, 1988; Fitzgerald, 1989; Slater & Graves, 1989. *Note.* From "Performance is the prize: Language competence and performance among AAC users " by N. W. Nelson in *Augmentative and Alternative Communication* (p. 15), *8*, 3–18. Copyright 1992 by ISAAC. Reprinted by permission.

conversations). They also need to manage variations on these rules depending on the discourse's context (e.g., making a new friend, flirting, disagreeing with a teacher, apologizing to an employer).

Narrative discourse also occurs frequently in classroom oral and written language interactions and in some social settings. As noted in Chapter 8, most children know quite a bit about narrative discourse before they enter school (e.g. Applebee, 1978; McGee & Richgels, 1990; Strickland & Taylor, 1989).

In oral production, narrative and conversational forms share some of the same functions (e.g., relating personal experiences, retelling sequences of events, allowing participation by conversational partners in the recall and organizational processes). Narratives, however, also differ from conversational forms in their expression of expanded units of texts, styles of introductory and closing statements, and inclusion of sequenced events leading to a conclusion (Roth & Spekman, 1986; Westby 1984, 1985/1991).

Definitions and concepts of story grammar and narrative structure vary (see Table 9.7), but when mature language users are asked to tell what makes a story a story, certain elements—such as settings, beginnings, attempts, and outcomes—stand out. Other elements such as complex reactions and endings, are reported less often (Fitzgerald, 1989), and some cultural differences in story structure have also been found. Different strategies for opening and closing stories have been found among individuals of African-American, Chinese-American, Euro-American, and Hispanic-American descent (Heath, 1982, 1983, 1986; McClure, Mason, & Williams, 1983). Japanese folktales tend not to have goal-oriented main characters such as those appearing in Western stories (Matsuyama, 1983). When the story grammar standards associated with Anglo-Saxon culture are used to evaluate the discourse of children whose familial history is filled with influences from other native cultures (whether or not English is the first language of these children), teachers and speech–language pathologists run the risk of misidentifying multigenerational cultural differences as problems (Westby, 1991).

Most information about the normal development of narratives comes from research on the oral production of stories (Applebee, 1978; Botvin & Sutton-Smith, 1977; Peterson & McCabe, 1983; Roth & Spekman, 1986). In studying the developmental progressions of oral narratives, Applebee (1978) and

Botvin & Sutton-Smith (1977) proposed separate, but similar, schemes for rating narrative maturity. The set of criteria for making judgments of narrative maturity that appears in Figure 9.3 is based primarily on Applebee's (1978) research.

Lahey (1988) proposed a similar kind of developmental sequence for rating children's narratives on four levels: additive chains, temporal chains, causal chains, and multiple causal chains. Lahey suggested that this rating system could be used to analyze content–form interactions in self-generated narratives and to establish goals for language intervention. She emphasized that in normal development, children are concerned with more than just making sense when they tell stories, quoting Kernan (1977) (see Personal Reflection 9.12). Therefore, in addition to looking for evidence of logical–temporal structures in narratives, Lahey recommended that examiners should seek evidence that narrators can do things like entertain, adapt to listeners' needs, and express their feelings about events they are narrating.

As discussed previously, specialists should seek evidence of cross-modality influences when conducting informal analyses of children's discourse capabilities. Research on normal development demonstrated that patterns of acquisition for oral production of narrative structures for young children are analogous to text structures in material read to them (Applebee, 1978; Botvin & Sutton-Smith, 1977). By age 5 or 6 years, children can begin to produce structurally com-

TABLE 9.7
Comparison of four major story grammars to a simplified story grammar

Thomas et al. (1954)	Mandler & Johnson (1977)	Stein & Glenn (1979)	Thorndyke (1977)	Rumelhart (1975)
Setting	Setting	Setting	Setting	Setting
Problem	Beginning	Initiating event	Theme	Event
			Event	Episode, or
			+	Change of
			Goal	state, or Action,
				or Event + Event
Response	Reaction	Internal response	Plot	Reaction
	Attempt		Subgoal	Internal response
		Attempt	+	+
			Attempt	Overt response
			+	
Outcome	Outcome	Consequence	Outcome	
	Ending	Reaction	Resolution	

Note. From "Story Grammar Skills in School-Age Children" by J. L. Page and S. R. Stewart. Reprinted from *Topics in Language Disorders*, Vol. 5, No. 2, p. 18, with permission of Aspen Publishers, Inc., © 1985.

FIGURE 9.3

Criteria for rating narrative maturity based on descriptions by Applebee (1978), Westby (1982, 1984), and Botvin and Sutton-Smith (1977).

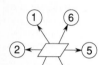

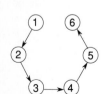

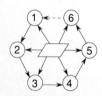

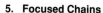

1. **Heaps**
   - Text organization comes from whatever attracts attention;
   - No story macrostructure;
   - No relationship or organization among elements or individual microstructures.

2. **Sequences**
   - Narrative has macrostructure with central character, setting, topic;
   - Activities of central character occur in particular setting;
   - Story elements are related to central macrostructure through concrete associative, or perceptual bonds;
   - Superficial sequences in time;
   - No transitions;
   - May use format A does X, A does Y, A does Z; or A does X to N, A does X to O, A does X to P;
   - No ending to narrative;
   - Trip stories may be in this category if events lack logical sequence or trip theme.

3. **Primitive Narratives**
   - Characters, objects, or events of narratives are put together because they are perceptually associated and complement each other;
   - Elements of the narrative follow logically from attributes of the center;
   - Attributes of the center are internal to the character, objects, events, and they determine the types of events that occur;
   - May use inference in narrative;
   - Narrative goes beyond perceptual and explicit information, but stays concrete, with links forged by shared situation rather than abstract relationship;
   - May talk about feelings;
   - Interactive narrative elements;
   - Organized trip stories fall in this category if they include multiple comments on events, including interpretive feelings.

4. **Unfocused Chains**
   - Events are linked logically (cause-effect relationship);
   - Elements are related to one another;
   - No central theme or character, no plot or story theme;
   - Lack of evidence of complete understanding of reciprocal nature of characters and events;
   - True sequence of events.

5. **Focused Chains**
   - Organized with both a center and a sequence;
   - Actual chaining of events that connect the elements;
   - Does not have a strong plot;
   - Events do not build on attributes of characters;
   - Characters and events of narratives seldom reach toward a goal;
   - Weak ending, no ending, or end does not follow logically from the beginning;
   - May be problems or motivating events that cause actions;
   - Transitions are used;
   - More because–then chains are used;
   - May be a trip story if the events follow logically from each other more than just occurring next on the same trip.

6. **True Narratives**
   - Integrated chaining events with complementary centering of the primitive narrative;
   - A developed plot;
   - Consequent events build out of prior events and also develop the central core;
   - Ending reflects or is related to the issues or events presented in the beginning of the narrative;
   - Intentions or goals of characters are dependent on attributes and feelings.

Note. From N. W. Nelson & Friedman, 1988. © 1988 by N. W. Nelson. Shared by permission of the author.

Personal Reflection 9.12	"Narratives, however, are concerned with more than making sense. They are also concerned with being appreciated, being amusing, being considered well done, and so on."
	Keith T. Kernan (1977, p. 100), writing about "Semantic and Expressive Elaboration in Children's Narratives."

plete fantasy narratives in oral story telling, but they reach a peak in the ability to tell narratives that use episode structures embedded within stories by 11 to 12 years of age (Botvin & Sutton-Smith, 1977).

In my own research (N. W. Nelson, 1988), and in my work with Friedman (N. W. Nelson & Friedman, 1988), we rated written personal narratives produced by 4th-, 7th-, 10th-graders, and college freshmen, with a scoring system from 1 to 6, using categories based on Applebee's (1978) stages with criteria shown in Figure 9.3. We found that writers in regular classes still produced personal narratives with average story scores of 3.77 and 3.74 in 4th and 7th grade, respectively (63% of the 7th-graders still produced primitive narratives that scored 3); the mean story score (5.11) for the 10th-graders was significantly higher (46% of the 10th-graders produced focused chains, and 39% produced *true narratives*; by the time they were college freshmen, the majority of the writers spontaneously produced true narrative texts (25%, focused chains, and 75%, true narratives).

Expository discourse competence is critical to success in school because expository text structure is used in most content textbooks and teacher lectures to give directions or to present information about theories, predictions, persons, facts, dates, specifications, generalizations, limitations, and conclusions. Students who cannot understand the complex language of expository discourse are at great risk for school failure.

During a comprehensive curriculum-based language assessment, students may read a selection aloud, sound out complex words syllable by syllable, summarize the text, paraphrase selected passages, answer factual and inferential questions about it, and formulate questions that could be asked about the discourse on a test. The examiner's level of focus may shift fluidly from sound, to word, to sentence, to passage, to text, and back again. Examiners might ask some students specific questions designed to elicit evidence about processing ability on one or

more levels, or examiners might draw inferences about unit processing from holistic behavior.

Examiners also might observe multiple contexts. Students might be observed as they listen to lectures and take notes in class or as they listen to a tape-recorded lecture that simulates the classroom experience. Some examples of expository contexts and discourse events to be used for varied purposes (depending on the student's own zones of significance) include the following:

1. Oral classroom discourse related to procedure and material presented in lectures (e.g., following directions, taking notes, making transitions between activities)
2. Expository discourse from textbooks, worksheets, and handouts (e.g., science textbook, social studies textbook, written homework assignments)
3. Mathematics discourse activities (e.g., self-talk while solving computational problems, sketching referents while solving story problems)

To probe for internalized models of text organizational structure and for comprehension of the complex semantic and syntactic relationships represented in expository text, the examiner might ask students to use visual–spatial strategies to outline or sketch organizational relationships they detect in examples of expository text. Most students are unlikely to be able to do this unless the process is modeled for them first (dynamic assessment). The examiner might select text excerpts from the student's curriculum that provide clear examples of two or three different organizational structures of expository text. A variety of expository text structures are diagrammed in Figure 9.4 (Calfee & Chambliss, 1988; Meyer, 1975; Pehrsson & Denner, 1988; Richgels, McGee, Lomax, & Sheard, 1987; Westby, 1991). Elements of hierarchical structure (with each organizational scheme having at least two or three levels) and sequencing may become evident to students only when these elements are diagrammed spatially. "The reader who is

FIGURE 9.4
Expository text macrostructures used.

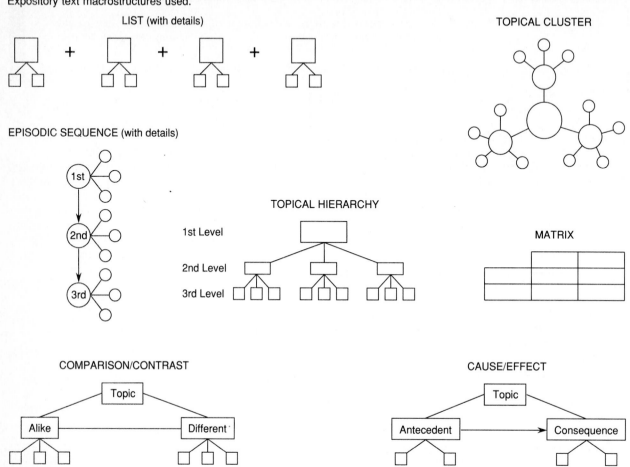

Sources: Calfee & Chambliss, 1988; Meyer, 1975; Pehrsson & Denner, 1988; Richgels et al., 1987; Westby, 1991.

able to uncover the author's top-level structure can organize ideas in ways that more or less match the pattern used by the author" (Pehrsson & Denner, 1988, p. 27).

The primary objective when assessing knowledge of expository text structure is to observe whether the student can grasp intuitively the concept of mapping elements of factual information from texts into spatial organizations. For example, if the examiner sets up the structure, can the student continue to fit additional pieces of text information into the arrangement? If so, the examiner may infer that the student has some internalized recognition of common text organizational strategies and needs only to acquire more metatextual ability to use those strategies con-

sciously for comprehending, studying, and remembering text-based information. If not, the student may need some basic instruction about how language is organized in different texts, using examples from the student's own curriculum.

The language of mathematics represents a special case of expository discourse. Across grade levels, some of the language in mathematics textbooks and much of the language in oral explanations by teachers is organized as direction-giving language. These directions sometimes are given primarily in words but often also include mathematical symbols that students have to learn to "read." The ability to use short-term memory span and reauditorization of the teacher's directions (facilitated by visual memory) to maintain instructional steps in proper sequence is particularly critical when attempting to understand directional expository discourse. The ability to use verbal mediation strategies to "read" mathematical symbols to oneself may also be an important key to performing steps in the correct sequence when attempting to solve similar problems later without assistance. Verbal mediation comes into play particularly when a set of problems does not require application of the same operation but requires varied operations (e.g., multiplication, subtraction, division). In these cases, the student cannot work on "automatic pilot," without thinking about what a particular problem demands. Requesting the student to use thinking language may help the examiner observe whether the student misreads symbols (either linguistic or mathematical) or fails to use verbal mediation strategies in problem solving.

Other investigational strategies may be appropriate when examining how a student's language impairment might interfere with the ability to solve story problems. Asking the student to sketch the elements of the problem may allow the examiner to see whether the student comprehends the language of the problem sufficiently to imagine its referents. Accurate understanding of the elements of story problems and their relationships is a key to setting up strategies to solve the problems. During this part of curriculum-based language assessment, the examiner asks the student to read the problem aloud (and observes for reading miscues and self-correction strategies) and then asks the student to show what he or she thinks the problem means by drawing a very rough sketch of the important pieces in it (the examiner may need to model this for the student to demonstrate that the quality of the drawings is not

important). Often, story problems require the student to represent referents in two stages: first, before the mathematical operation is applied, and again afterward, to show how the situation has changed. If the student either misreads or misrepresents the meaning of language of the problem, the examiner should probe further whether the student did not understand the meaning of individual words (e.g., *each, neither, most*) or whether the student misunderstood the relationship represented by the word combination. See Box 9.7 for example.

Language specialists who conduct curriculum-based language assessment should remember that their role is not to assess the child's understanding of mathematical principles and operations (that role belongs to the academic diagnostician) but to assess whether the student has the language capabilities and strategies to understand the language of the text and to direct his or her own thinking. It will be easier to design relevant intervention plans if the dimensions of the problem are better understood.

SUMMARY

This section presented the measurement of later stage needs and abilities and covered a wide range of territory. To focus on later stage needs, the discussion addressed various contexts for later stage assessment and intervention. Family and cultural concerns are still important in the later stages, but interactions with peers are increasingly important as well, as is increased participation outside school and home. The culmination of the later stages of child development are marked by transition to higher education, employment, and other postschool activities.

Box 9.7	Curriculum-based language assessment for a fifth-grade girl having difficulty understanding the language of math story problems

She read aloud the language of the problem without error:

"There are seven bike racks. If each bike rack has eight bikes, how many bikes in all?"

Then said, "eight."
When asked to sketch the problem, she first drew representations of the seven bike racks correctly: ___ ___ ___ ___ ___ ___ ___

But then, she drew only one cross mark (representing one bike) on each of the racks:
_|_ _|_ _|_ _|_ _|_ _|_ _|_

How might language processing difficulty have interfered with her understanding of what the language of the problem meant?

A wide variety of tools and strategies particularly suited to later stage assessment were discussed. Most initial diagnostic evaluations and 3-year comprehensive reevaluations involve a combination of formal and informal assessment procedures. If the assessment process is to be relevant to individualized needs, the first step must be to gather contextually based background information. This procedure leads to the selection of appropriate formal assessment devices and to the design of informal assessment activities tailored to the individual's needs.

Informal assessment in the later stages is based on the philosophy of dynamic assessment, which suggests that abilities are not found in static, identifiable quantities that can be labeled and numbered but are fluid, variable, interactive, and contextually sensitive. Abilities may be facilitated (scaffolded) to reach higher levels by certain contextual conditions but impeded by others. A major goal of the dynamic assessment process is to identify the conditions that result in these varied outcomes. The goals and activities of assessment and intervention are at times indistinguishable.

Because informal assessment of later stage language developments can become quite complex, I suggested several organizational strategies. Examiners need to keep in mind at least three factors: (1)

their plan to set up and administer participant assessment tasks, (2) a complex model of oral and written language processing that allows examiners to infer intactness and operation of internalized language processing abilities by guiding observations of external evidence, and (3) a system for organizing observations so that examiners can cover all of the bases without spending forever gathering evidence piece by piece.

Suggested procedures of contextually based language assessment included asking multifaceted questions about contextual demands and examinees' current functioning in those contexts and about the potential for modifying language learning contexts and individuals' basic abilities and strategies through intervention. Ethnographic interviewing, artifact analysis, and onlooker and participant observation techniques may be used to gather data. These data include information about linguistic and metalinguistic processing, the use of language in multiple modalities (through miscue analysis, written language sample analysis, and thinking language analysis); the ability to process different sizes of linguistic units (sounds, syllables, words, sentences, and texts); and specialized processing strategies for differing texts (conversational, narrative, and expository) within differing discourse events.

METHODS AND TARGETS OF LATER STAGE INTERVENTION

The methods and targets of intervention for the later stages of language acquisition are designed to encourage the integrated and complex use of language knowledge and skills, most of which have been acquired to some degree in earlier stages. The later stages are a time for consolidating and fine-tuning foundation skills, for acquiring conscious strategies for using language for academic and vocational purposes, and for developing the automaticity and experience to communicate with confidence in a variety of modalities and circumstances.

Language processing and language strategies, as well as more basic aspects of language knowledge, are all appropriate targets of later stage intervention. The model of complex oral and written language processing presented in Figure 9.1 represents these varied factors. Competent performance, according to this model, depends on synergistic contributions from

the following four different but interrelated elements: (1) background knowledge to recognize and manipulate six kinds of linguistic and nonlinguistic units, rules, events, and relationships; (2) peripheral processing skills to interact with the environment and to get information in and out; (3) central processing skills to encode, store, remember, and retrieve information; and (4) conscious strategies to guide the processes efficiently. Mature communicative competency depends on partnership among these elements, and intervention strategies should be designed accordingly.

Discussions of intervention in this chapter are consistent with the view that language processing differs somewhat when using different units in different modalities. This discussion is also consistent, however, with the view that during real-life communicative events, boundaries are easily blurred, and it is not always clear what kinds of symbols (e.g., auditory word images, graphemes, or phonemes) a person might be manipulating internally. Intervention directed toward improving processing in one modality may facilitate processing in another (D. J. Johnson, 1985; N. W. Nelson, 1981). For example, helping a student acquire strategies for sounding out words syllable-by-syllable from print and for spelling from memory may help the student hear sequences of syllables and remember new multisyllabic words during a lecture. This may help the student to take notes during class and to recall important words when responding on a test.

MODIFYING LANGUAGE LEARNING CONTEXTS

When most children reach the later stages of language development, parents play a relatively minor role in fostering their development compared to teachers and peers. Even when children and adolescents in the later stages of child development have language disorders, most have acquired sufficient language for communicating basic meanings and performing most communicative functions, but their developmental pathways are considerably rockier than for individuals developing normally.

Summaries of longitudinal studies of individuals with developmental language impairments (D. S. Weiner, 1985) points to continued limitations in understanding and producing the complex language of regular classrooms; frequent problems with social–emotional development and behavioral adjustment; and many cases of special classroom placement with concurrent diagnoses of mental retardation and learning disabilities. The evidence for adolescents with significant hearing losses also documents their continued academic struggles (Geers & Moog, 1989). By extension, individuals with a history of impaired language development from any cause may have exaggerated risks for failing to meet the communicative demands of adult work settings and independent living (Records, Tomblin, & Freese, 1992; Tomblin, Freese, & Records, 1990).

Professionals may use a variety of strategies to assist individuals with language weaknesses to develop competencies for meeting important daily communicative demands. The traditional focus has been on "fixing" communicative processes. Newer approaches recognize the critical importance of designing language learning contexts to help students improve their competence as communicators. Educational and intervention approaches designed to foster development by providing facilitative learning contexts are often called *mediated learning approaches*. Teachers and speech–language pathologists using these techniques act more as facilitators than instructors, leading students to make their own decisions and draw their own conclusions as they learn. The unique contribution of language specialists to this approach is their ability to be highly cognizant of the interactions of the activity's language demands with the student's language abilities and to design scaffolding questions and cues accordingly. Language demands of tasks, however, must be considered within even larger sociocultural contexts.

Starting With Respect for Sociocultural Backgrounds of Learners

Mediational techniques start when one or more key adults in a young person's life communicates respect for the individual as a learner and as a person who brings strengths to the learning process. This respect should extend to the participant's sociocultural background.

In the United States, more than one in five schoolchildren come from families living in poverty, and despite commitment of federal and local resources, many of these children continue to experience disproportionate failure of school (Knapp, Turnbull, & Shields, 1990). Although some poor children have language disorders, many do not. Knapp and colleagues (1990) noted that traditional explanations for discouraging educational outcomes for poor children tend to locate the problem in the learner and his or her background. The child's language system may be implicated as the primary problem, which is inappropriate when the problem is language difference, not language disorder. Knapp et al. proposed an alternative view that locates parts of both the problem and the solution in the attitudes and practices of adults in school. Students whose families are socioeconomically disadvantaged are better able to meet the academic challenges of school when

❏ Teachers respect the students' cultural/linguistic backgrounds and communicate this appreciation to them in a personal way;
❏ The academic program encourages students to draw and build on the experiences they have, at the same time that it exposes them to unfamiliar experiences and ways of thinking;

❏ The assumptions, expectations, and ways of doing things in school—in short, its culture—are made explicit to these students by teachers who explain and model these dimensions of academic learning. (Knapp et al, 1990, p. 5)

Whether or not they come from poor, linguistically different, and/or culturally different families, students with language disorders will likely also benefit from these educational principles. A part of the intervention process for all students with language disorders involves helping them, in collaboration with classroom teachers, to consciously recognize aspects of classroom communication expectations that many more "typical" students acquire without explicit assistance.

Being sensitive to cultural differences also means that professionals should design learning contexts that take advantage of children's and adolescents' strengths from their home cultures. For example, Kawakami and Au (1986) noted that Hawaiian children, and particularly those from lower income families, were more likely to have participated in group interaction communication at home than in dyadic interactive experiences with adults. A talk-story format strongly facilitated reading and language development in these children.

Using Mediational Discourse in Curriculum-Based Language Intervention

One technique for assisting students to make more sense of varied classroom language is to teach them verbal mediation discourse for self-talk. This can be done with individuals, small groups, or classrooms by mediational teachers and clinicians who model thinking language for students to organize approaches to curricular tasks and to understand the language of those tasks.

Mediational discourse is a special form of scaffolding to facilitate "inner speech," as Vygotsky (1962) discussed it, to support mature thought. To some extent, the ability to use self-questioning strategies may depend on maturation. In a 3-year longitudinal study of students in first, second, and third grades, Bivens and Berk (1990) found that, in accordance with Vygotsky's theory, private speech moved from externalized to more internalized task-relevant forms as they worked on their math seatwork. These results suggest that children above third grade should be reasonably adept at using self-talk, encouraged in inter-

vention. Language intervention using verbal mediation is a top-down processing approach. Students are taught to process language better by using their world knowledge and sense-making expectations to direct their other attentional and perceptual processes and to begin doing this overtly, gradually learning to do it covertly with practice.

Psychologist Reuven Feuerstein (1979) defined mediated learning as an interactional process between a developing individual and "an experienced intentioned adult"; the adult mediates the world to the child by "framing, selecting, focusing, and feeding back environmental experiences" to produce in the child "appropriate learning sets and habits" (p. 179). The mediational strategies developed by Feuerstein, Rand, and Rynders (1988) for work with mentally retarded individuals, which they called instrumental enrichment (IE), have been adapted for persons with other problems.

For example, Haywood, Towery-Woolsey, Arbitman-Smith, and Aldridge (1988) reported a study using Feuerstein's IE methods with 53 deaf adolescents in residential schools. The results showed that the children who had received the experimental approach made significant gains (and greater gains than control subjects) on most measures (Haywood et al., 1988).

Haywood and his colleagues (1988) emphasized that the teacher's role during IE shifts from being a giver of information to being the mediator of experiences for children:

Mediational teachers elicit understanding from the children by asking guiding questions, supplying needed information, directing activity, challenging answers, requiring logical evidence for conclusions, and, most important, emphasizing the processes of thinking, learning, and problem solving rather than the products (answers). (p. 27)

When applying these techniques, mediational teachers often respond, even to correct answers, with more questions. They might ask the children how they knew which one to select, why that choice was better than another one, and what they had to do to solve the problem—also whether there might be another way, to approach the problem. In addition to process-oriented questions, mediational teachers elicit "bridges" from the children. Teachers ask children to think of analogous contexts in which the same thinking operations and strategies might be used. Finally, mediational teachers seek to engage children in understanding that the universe has an order, structure, and predictability that they can grasp by applying generalized principles of thinking.

Because question-asking is central both to traditional classroom discourse and to mediated learning interactions, a closer look at the use and misuse of questions in mediation is appropriate. Marion Blank and her colleagues have contributed much to the understanding of how questions can be used to facilitate language and cognitive development, both in the preschool years and beyond (Blank, 1975; Blank, Rose, & Berlin, 1978; Blank & White, 1986). Blank and White (1986), however, also pointed out several ways that questions might be misused in instructional discourse, leading to confusion and bad feelings. They commented that a "situation that is unfortunate for any child is almost unbearable for learning-disabled children, given the insecurities and failures that they face elsewhere" (p. 11).

Blank and White (1986) noted the failure of teachers to provide scaffolding questions appropriate to the individual's level of development. Teachers may have learned, as a general principle, that higher order, open-ended processing questions are best to elicit elaborate answers (e.g., *how* and *why* questions), but this strategy may go astray in a couple of ways. First, it may suggest to students that a wide range of responses is acceptable when a teacher has a very specific topic or response in mind. Only students who are tuned into the "hidden curriculum" of the teacher's own pet topics and peeves then can infer what the teacher really wants. For example, one teacher asked older students simply to talk about current events, suggesting that the topic was wide open, but then ignored a student's mention of Pablo Casals, the famous cellist, while accepting another student's topic of war in the Middle East. Blank and White commented that it would have been better for the teacher to state directly that she wanted to talk about the war in the Middle East in the first place. (Indirect communication of teachers' personal preferences make up a large part of the "hidden curriculum" described earlier in Box 9.4.)

A related problem may result when higher order questions require abstract reasoning at levels beyond the student's capabilities. Then, higher order questions are likely to result in unacceptable responses, putting teachers in a dilemma about whether to correct errors. Again, teachers may have learned well the

lesson not to criticize directly anything students say. As a result, teachers may consequate inappropriate or incorrect responses from students with vague and ambiguous evaluative comments. For example, they may ask the same question of another child, or they may ask the same child again, perhaps repeating the child's erroneous response in an incredulous tone. This is what happened in the following example, reported by Blank and White (1986) from an exchange between a teacher using a poster of a jungle consumed by fire:

Teacher: How could grass in a jungle get on fire?
Child: Cause they (*referring to animals*) have to stay in the jungle.
Teacher: (*in an incredulous tone*) You mean the grass gets on fire because the animals stay in the jungle?
Child: Yeah. (p .4)

A common teaching strategy is to identify areas a student does not understand and ask about them. In the preceding situation, this student was known to have difficulty with causal reasoning. The strategy of focusing on the area of deficit, in this case, only led to frustration for both the student and the teacher. After a few more attempts to get the student to identify causal relationships, the teacher abandoned the effort. A better strategy might have been to provide more concrete product-oriented questions, such as "What is happening in the picture?" or "What are the animals doing in this picture?" (Blank & White, 1986). Then the student could have experienced some success in answering and would have been assisted in focusing on the topic. The teacher then could have asked the entire group to brainstorm possible causes of fire in jungles. By using such strategies, skilled teachers can work with heterogeneous groups of students so that all can participate in constructing meaning at levels appropriate to their own ability.

Mediational strategies are appropriate across communicative modalities. For example, Hoskins (1990) described common guidelines for acting as "facilitator" for oral language conversation groups and written language mediation:

These same principles are relevant in facilitating print literacy: (a) intervention is based on the participant's communication; (b) language is learned in interaction; and (c) the facilitator acts as a metalinguistic guide. (p. 55)

Facilitative strategies to guide written language production were studied formally by Bernice Wong and her colleagues (Wong, Wong, Darlington, & Jones, 1991). They reported two studies of *interactive teaching* (another term for *mediated learning*) aimed at helping adolescents with learning disabilities learn to revise their written compositions. Written language problems of adolescents with learning disabilities have been documented to include "lower-order cognitive problems in spelling, punctuation, and grammar, and higher-order cognitive and metacognitive problems in planning, writing fluency, revising, and awareness of audience" (Wong et al., 1991, p. 117). Interactional teaching uses oral disclosure with adolescent writers to help them to identify ambiguities in their essays and to make their themes salient. An example of this strategy appears in Box 9.8.

Mediated Reading and Miscue Analysis

Mediated reading is a special case of mediational language intervention. The educator frames and focuses students' attention, first, on whether or not what they say when they read aloud makes sense, and second, on whether it matches the printed data. This approach uses the basic principles of miscue analysis presented earlier in this chapter, coupled with mediational efforts designed to teach self-questioning strategies.

The general technique involves repeating a piece of text the child has just read when the child has produced an observed response that does not match an expected response. The purpose is to focus the child on one or more key features of the mismatch. Questions about bigger units of text, for example, might include the following:

❏ Does this make sense?
❏ Does this fit with what we have been reading?
❏ Does it fit with what we see on the page?
❏ When you say _____, I expect to see _____. Is that what you see?

Depending on the individual students' needs, some mediational efforts may be designed to develop bottom-up abilities for decoding smaller units of text, perhaps by drawing students' attention to mismatches involving graphophonemic miscues at the word level. For example, when a student reads *was* for *saw*, the language interventionist might attempt to get the student to focus on the graphophonemic nature of the miscue by saying, "When you read this word as *was*, I expect to see a /w/ at the beginning of this word; Is that what you see?" If attempting to help the student focus on syntactic cues, the adult mediator might say, "Listen to what you read, 'The boy *was* a huge truck'; Does that make sense? Can

---

Box 9.8	An examples of interactive teaching strategies to help an adolescent with language-learning disabilities to develop an awareness of audience informational needs

This student was writing about the most scary event of his life, which concerned his daredevil antics on his mountain bike. He wrote, "I hit the ramp so hard my XKJ475 fell off." Upon reading this sentence, the experimenter-teacher stopped and hummed and sighed loudly. With a puzzled expression on her face, she turned to the student and said: "What on earth do you mean here? You're writing nicely and all of the sudden, you got this chunk of capital letters and numbers!" The student quickly inspected the offending sentence and with surprise exclaimed: "That's the license of my mountain bike!" "Oh, I see," said the experimenter, now totally demystified. "You mean to say your mountain bike hit the ramp so hard, it got its license plate knocked off. You see, it's all clear in your own head what you intend to say to the reader. You know what it's about, you understand what you have written. But I didn't! I don't know a thing about mountain bikes or their license numbers, so I wouldn't know what you were writing about! You see now, when you write, you've got to make yourself clear so people know what you mean, O.K.? So how can we fix this part so readers would understand what you want to say?" The student returned to the screen and added "my mountain bike license XKJ475 fell off."

_____

(Wong, Wong, Darlington, & Jones, 1991, p. 120)

we say that?" When students with speech–language impairments have significant and ongoing difficulty making sound–symbol associations, they may need highly systematic multi-modality practice in articulating, tracing, writing, reading, and sequencing more isolated bits of print and related speech sounds and syllables before they can use graphophonemic cues reliably in contextual reading.

Decisions about which miscues to point out, which to let go, and how often to interrupt are not easy. If the student reads along fairly smoothly and appears to comprehend the text, it may be most appropriate to ignore the minor graphophonemic miscues. Letting the student read past a rough spot without correction may also leave the student more in charge of the process of creating meaning and more likely to self-correct. Cazden's (1988) review of the literature on correction showed that teachers tend to interrupt poorer readers more immediately and frequently than better readers. When language interventionists see themselves as guides and facilitators of the language acquisition process, rather than as individuals who must monitor for errors and let none get by, they can relax about jumping in too frequently and can begin to enjoy reading with the student for the central purpose of constructing meaning.

Using Other Strategies to Modify the Language Learning Contexts of Classrooms

Some methods for modifying learning contexts focus on one-on-one interactions between adult facilitators and students with special language-learning needs. Others focus on modifying broader aspects of classroom contexts or coordinating them with therapy room contexts.

Hughes (1989) provided suggestions for helping students with language-learning disabilities generalize newly acquired linguistic abilities from therapy room to classroom. She emphasized the need for speech–language pathologists and classroom teachers to collaborate to accomplish mutually set goals in slightly different ways. For example, when a student's problem has been identified through the collaborative process as failing to comprehend or follow the teacher's multistep directions, the following therapy room objectives and activities might be used:

> Objectives: to increase comprehension of multistep directions that include terms used in classroom instructions; to increase readiness to listen; to teach

compensatory strategies, such as writing down page numbers, problem numbers, due dates.
> Activities: in small groups, students take turns role playing teacher, giving common classroom directives that require multiple steps; verbal rehearsal of listening strategies for particular teachers, subject periods, or assignment. (p. 226)

The corresponding strategy for modifying classroom contextual demands might include the following:

> Teacher asks student chosen at random to orally repeat directions; writes specific details on the board; reinforces direction following specifically; cues student to write down details. (p. 226)

Similarly, Maxon and Brackett (1987) pointed out how contextually based solutions might be designed for students with hearing impairments by analyzing specific problems (called "zones of significance" in this chapter) and their probable causes. Areas they identified as frequently problematic for students with hearing impairments included exchanges in the hallway, changes in teachers, spelling, language-based subjects such as social studies and science, class discussion, test taking, reading groups, classroom lectures on specific content material, independent desk work, group projects, peer-to-peer social interactions, homework, and announcements over the loudspeaker. Possible problems occurring in the hallway might include taking off amplification after every class and giving no response to greetings. Possible causes might include embarrassment about wearing amplification and inability to hear in noisy, reverberant hallways. Possible solutions might include provision of less obvious amplification along with consultation with peers and teachers to teach them about the function and purposes of amplification and the importance of being in close proximity when conversing in hallways.

The common elements of all of these contextually based intervention strategies are (1) identify "zones of significance" (contextually based needs); (2) analyze the communicative demands of the event or situation; (3) observe the individual's current attempts to meet those demands; (4) provide intervention to assist the individual to acquire new knowledge, skills, and strategies; (5) mediate the contextual demands to make them more accessible; and (6) keep in mind the desired outcome of independent functioning in the real world to avoid "the forest and the trees problem" (raised in Chapter 1).

FOSTERING "METASKILLS" AND OTHER EXECUTIVE STRATEGIES

The acquisition of mature strategies for directing one's own behavior is an important contributor to adult independence. The adoption of systematic "strategies" can enable learners to order input, make sense of it, remember it, and recall it. Such individuals have learned how to learn a particular kind of information. Language plays an important role in this process.

The Prevalence of Learning Strategies Models

The current emphasis on learning strategies in intervention programs for students with language-learning disabilities in secondary school programs is relatively recent (Larson & McKinley, 1987; Schumaker, Deshler, Alley, Warner, & Denton, 1982). A review of earlier programming approaches in a large school district (Deshler, Lowrey, & Alley, 1979) showed a preponderance of other instructional models: basic skills remediation (45%), tutorial approaches (24%), functional curriculum approaches (17%), and work–study approaches (5%). Learning strategies approaches accounted for only 4% of the programs.

Intervention programs that target the development of deliberate processing strategies are probably more common now than in 1979, when Deshler and his colleagues conducted their original study (Deshler et al., 1979). However, obtaining data about current programming is difficult, even for high-incidence disorders such as learning disabilities. McKenzie (1991) surveyed all 50 states; Washington, DC; the Bureau of Indian Affairs; the Virgin Islands; and Puerto Rico to ask questions about the degree to which the service-delivery system in a particular state or territory was based on a model of "basic skill" instruction or "content area" instruction. McKenzie defined *the basic skill model* as *instruction to students with learning disabilities* "to improve their basic reading, writing, computational, and social skills for the purpose of improving their performance in mainstream content area classes" (p. 116). McKenzie described *the content area model* as instruction

in core content areas such as English, math, social studies, science, etc., to those students who are assumed unable to benefit from inclusion in one or more mainstream content area classes. (p. 116)

McKenzie, in addition, differentiated both of these models from a third, *learning strategies model*. However, he indicated that

although instruction in "learning strategies" may occur within either model, a program focused exclusively on learning strategies should not be considered representative of either a "skill" or a "content" model. (p. 116)

McKenzie (1991) found wide variability by geographic region, as well as evidence that many state directors of special education were not sure about instructional methods used in their states. He did find that, of 49 respondents, 41 reported that content area instruction occurred within their state or territory. Unfortunately, he did not ask about strategy instruction. McKenzie concluded that "although the question of 'which approach is better' may never be adequately answered, there is a pressing need to identify the efficacy of each." (p. 121)

The Rationale for Learning Strategies Models

Most aspects of purposeful "executive control" are acquired normally in the later stages of childhood (Forrest-Pressley & Waller, 1984; Nippold, 1988a; Pressley & Harris, 1990). They enable young people to become increasingly organized and self-directed as they move toward adulthood.

Executive control strategies often rely on the use of "meta-" skills. A variety of metaprocessing skills were described previously in this chapter, with suggestions for assessing individuals' conscious awareness of language (metalinguistic knowledge), pragmatics (metapragmatic knowledge), texts (metatextual knowledge) and their own cognitive processes (metacognitive knowledge). A primary reason for assessing these areas relates to the role they play in determining whether individuals can succeed in school and other formal communication contexts (Chabon & Prelock, 1989; Ehren & Lenz, 1989; Silliman, 1987; Wallach, 1989).

Although executive control involves systematic, strategic approaches to problem solving, not all strategy learning is highly conscious or deliberate; some is relatively automatic and unconsidered (Chabon & Prelock, 1989). The seemingly automatic acquisition of strategy learning by most normally developing children may make the process appear to occur without assistance. However, the need to teach strategic approaches to information processing and problem solving deliberately is currently recognized in the literature of general education as well as special education. Pressley and Harris (1990) noted that "We realize now that many students do not learn strategies automatically" (p. 31). Pressley and Harris pointed to research findings that even some adults do not use self-questioning strategies automatically when they need to learn a set of facts.

Children and adolescents with certain conditions associated with language disorders, such as attention deficit hyperactivity disorder or traumatic brain injury (Ylvisaker & Szekeres, 1986), may have exaggerated risks for failure to acquire and apply strategies on their own. Others, such as youths with hearing impairments or deafness, may not have strong enough language skills to support strategies although they attempt to apply them (Andrews & Mason, 1991). Similarly, many individuals with language-learning disabilities are at risk for learning to use self-mediational language to direct their own behavior and thinking because of their lack of strong underlying language competencies (Hagen, Barclay, & Schwethelm, 1982; Torgesen, 1982).

Silliman (1987) ascribed some of the individual differences in classroom performance by language-impaired students to their strategic planning limitations. Silliman contrasted two kinds of knowledge—declarative knowledge for knowing about things, and procedural knowledge for knowing how to do things. She noted that "communicative strategies might be considered part of the procedural component" (p. 359). When children have difficulty in school, intervention will be most effective if efforts are first made to sort out the degree to which problems may be attributed to each of several factors, including inefficient processing, inadequate management of available processing resources, or insufficient content knowledge (Silliman, 1987). Wallach (1989) also proposed that "individual strategy preferences of language learning disabled students must be understood over a variety of contexts and discourse types" (p. 213).

Children who take passive approaches to learning have been described as "inactive learners" (Silliman, 1987; Torgesen & Licht, 1983). These children may have relatively intact intellectual abilities but fail to take advantage of them, particularly in school. Wallach (1989) also noted that many learners with language learning disabilities are passive but argued that they could become "constructive

comprehenders" if they were taught how to draw on existing background knowledge and to use learning strategies.

Using Metapragmatic Strategies to Develop School Survival Skills

Success in school largely depends on knowing how to follow unspoken rules for classroom interactions. When students understand the school culture curriculum and have efficient strategies for getting organized, they have greater attentional and information processing resources to devote to understanding the official academic curriculum. When they do not, they risk being inefficient, disorganized, inappropriate, and "lost" during a major portion of the school day. The problem is that much of what I call the "school culture curriculum" and "hidden curriculum" is never explained to students. R. J. Sternberg and his colleagues called this *the tacit knowledge of school* (R. J. Sternberg, Okagaki, & Jackson, 1990; see Personal Reflection 9.13).

Tattershall (1987) noted that "Just as most students learn their syntax and phonology without explicit teaching, many students extract the critical rules of classroom participation without direct instruction. However, there are some students who have to be taught these classroom interactional/instructional rules" (p. 182). Tattershall emphasized the importance of the critical 1st month of school, when students begin to learn the routines of new classrooms. She commented that parents may be valuable partners in monitoring whether their children are learning school rules. They may do this by observing whether their children seem vague when asked about classroom routines. If so, parents may urge their children to be more assertive in determining teachers' expectations about homework, asking clarification questions, and talking in class (see Box 9.5). By discussing classroom expectations with their youngsters, parents may stimulate them to recognize classroom rules they might otherwise overlook. Conveying the expectation that children are in charge may avoid the pitfalls of becoming too dependent on (and resentful of) the parents' rescuing efforts. Parental intervention, which may have been appropriate at earlier grade levels, is not as appropriate later. When children appear uncertain of classroom expectations, parents may alert others who may be in a better position to make them explicit. This in turn may contribute to

Personal Reflection 9.13

"Teachers have a wide array of expectations for students, many of which are never explicitly verbalized. Students who cannot meet these implicit expectations may suffer through year after year of poor school performance without knowing quite what is wrong. Their teachers expect them to know how to allocate their time in doing homework, how to prepare course papers, how to study for tests, how to talk (and not to talk) to a teacher—if they never learn these things, they will suffer for it."

Robert J. Sternberg, Lynn Okagaki, and *Alice S. Jackson* (1990, p. 35), writing about the need for what they called "practical intelligence" to succeed in school. Sternberg, who is IBM Professor of Psychology and Education at Yale, proposed the triarchic theory of human intelligence, with componential, contextual, and experiential operations (R. J. Sternberg, 1985, 1988).

consultation between speech–language pathologists and teachers as they seek to recognize how language-learning difficulties influence inappropriate behavior. By identifying misunderstanding as the source for inappropriate behavior, it may be possible to "change a student's premature 'bad' reputation" (Tattershall, 1987, p. 183), and to avert a destructive spiral of negative feedback from teachers and increasingly sullen attitudes from students.

Without intervention, students with learning disabilities are at risk for increased problems with school culture rules as they advance in grade level. In research by Schumaker, Sheldon-Wildgen, and Sherman (1980), classroom rule violations by students with learning disabilities exceeded those for students without learning disabilities by 9% in seventh grade, 17% in eighth grade, and 26% in ninth grade. When teachers left the classroom, the students with learning disabilities engaged in rule-violating episodes during 92% of the intervals; whereas students without learning disabilities did not participate in a single rule-violating episode.

One possible reason for the increase at the secondary level is that the processing demands of the school culture curriculum become particularly intense during those years. Students must deal with changing classrooms and multiple teachers. Ehren and Lenz (1989) discussed the executive demands of secondary school settings in conjunction with the executive characteristics of many adolescents with learning disabilities.

1. Students are expected to work independently with little feedback.

2. Students are expected to apply knowledge across the content areas.
3. Students are expected to solve problems on their own.
4. Students are expected to organize information and a variety of resources independently to solve problems. (p. 197)

A comparison of this list of expected characteristics with the corresponding set of observed characteristics that Ehren and Lenz (1989) noted among students with learning disabilities highlights the mismatch that gives so many of these students difficulty:

1. LD [learning disabled] adolescents often do not invent appropriate strategies or approaches that lead to successful task completion.
2. They have difficulty learning how to solve problems.
3. They often do not generalize what they have learned.
4. They often fail to take advantage of prior knowledge when facing new problems. (p. 198)

Lists of expected school survival skills provided by Ehren and Lenz (1989) are supported by other research. Schaeffer, Zigmond, Kerr, and Farra (1990) surveyed principals, school administrators, special education teachers, mainstream teachers, and over 4,000 high school students to identify skills important to school success. Of a list of 69 items, they identified six skills as most critical to school survival:

1. Going to class every day.
2. Arriving at school on time.
3. Bringing pencils, paper, and books to class.
4. Turning in work on time.
5. Talking to teachers without using "back talk."
6. Reading and following directions. (p. 198)

Skills like these were targeted in an alternative adolescent language classroom described by G. M. Anderson and Nelson (1988). Students learned about teachers' "unspoken contract" with their students, such as "I will live up to my part of the bargain and will continue to support and encourage you if you will also live up to yours and *attempt* to do the work" (p. 349). The students placed in the alternate adolescent language classroom had a variety of disabilities ranging from hearing loss to emotional disturbance. All learned to say that the most unacceptable form of student behavior was failure to turn in required work. To avoid that problem and to help them organize themselves, these students learned strategies involving notebooks and assignment sheets to keep track of their responsibilities. They also participated in metapragmatic exercises observing the "student-like behaviors" exhibited by the successful students in their regular education classes and emulating them. They observed, labeled, and practiced paying attention, acting interested, asking questions, and taking notes. While they were in the alternative language classroom daily (for which they received grades and credit), the students constantly repeated to themselves and to each other their main goal of acquiring the skills they needed so that they would no longer need the alternative class. Of the initial seven students enrolled in the classroom, only one was unable to meet this goal after 1 year in the program (two moved out of the district and four were successfully mainstreamed in regular education programs). That student needed an additional year in the more structured classroom. Anderson and Nelson reported:

> Teachers began to indicate both verbally and on report cards that the students were "doing better, making an effort, interested, working harder," and "catching on." In many cases, the teachers felt that the students had been immature and had suddenly matured. Teachers also perceived that the students' attitudes toward school had actually changed. (1988, p. 351)

Using Metacognitive Strategies to Improve Memory and Higher Order Thinking

Not all students learn equally well in the same ways. At least since D. J. Johnson and Myklebust (1967) published their classic text on learning disabilities, speech–language pathologists and other special educators have been aware of the need for becoming attuned to the varied learning strengths of individual students. However, professionals have now surpassed the simplistic models of "visual learners" and "auditory learners" and the faddish models of "left-hemisphere learners" and "right-hemisphere learners" and recognized that many factors together determine how an individual learns specific content in a particular context.

Students in the later stages of child development may benefit from direct instruction in understanding their own intelligence and that of their fellow students. A school curriculum on "practical intelligence," with this purpose, was developed through collaboration between Howard Gardner, at Harvard, and Robert Sternberg, at Yale University (R. J. Sternberg et al., 1990) (see Table 9.8). Gardner and Sternberg developed separate but relatively compatible theories of intelligence (Gardner, 1983; R. J. Sternberg, 1985, 1988). Gardner's theory addresses the multiple relatively autonomous forms of intelligence, and his seven modular intelligence forms include linguistic, logical-mathematical (L. Miller, 1990, separated logical and mathematical), musical, spatial, bodily-kinesthetic, interpersonal, and intrapersonal. (See L. Miller's 1990, "Smart Profile" system for helping students recognize the different ways they are smart.) Sternberg's (1985, 1988) triarchic theory of intelligence includes *componential operations* (mental processes), *contextual operations* (practical applications), and *experiential operations* (transfer to new situations).

Langer (1982) suggested that teachers assist students to gain knowledge from written texts by using a prereading plan (PREP) to clarify students' prior knowledge on a topic so teachers can judge how much additional information must be taught. For example, by asking students to "Tell me everything you think of when you hear . . ." teachers prompt students to free associate and access their prior knowledge. By asking, "What made you think of . . . ?," teachers prompt students to reflect on their thought processes and organization of knowledge. By asking, "Do you want to add to or change your first response?" teachers prompt students to reformulate and refine their responses. Based on Langer's work, Westby (1991) summarized response characteristics that teachers or language specialists might use to judge children's prior knowledge as little knowledge, some knowledge, or much knowledge. For example, little knowledge is judged when students respond to teachers' questions with associative tangential comments, with tangential first-hand experiences, or with no apparent knowledge at all. Some knowledge is

TABLE 9.8
A "practical intelligence" curriculum for success in school

I. Managing Yourself	II. Managing Tasks	III. Cooperating With Others
A. Overview of Managing Yourself 1. Introductory Lesson 2. Kinds of Intelligence: Definitions and Principles 3. Kinds of Intelligence: Multiple Intelligences 4. Kinds of Intelligence: Academic or Practical Intelligence 5. Understanding Test Scores 6. Exploring What You May Do 7. Accepting Responsibility 8. Collecting Your Thoughts and Setting Goals **B.** Learning Styles 9. What's Your Learning Style? 10. Taking in New Information 11. Showing What You Learned 12. Knowing How You Work Best 13. Recognizing the Whole and the Parts **C.** Improving Your Own Learning 14. Memory 15. Using What You Already Know 16. Making Pictures in Your Mind 17. Using Your Eyes—A Good Way to Learn 18. Recognizing the Point of View 19. Looking for the Best Way to Learn 20. Listening for Meaning 21. Learning by Doing	**A.** Overview of Solving Problems 22. Is There a Problem? 23. What Strategies Are You Using? 24. A Process to Help You Solve Problems 25. Planning a Way to Prevent Problems 26. Breaking Habits 27. Help with Our Problems **B.** Specific School Problems 28. Taking Notes 29. Getting Organized 30. Understanding Questions 31. Following Directions 32. Underlining—Finding the Main Idea 33. Noticing the Way Things Are Written 34. Choosing Between Mapping and Outlining 35. Taking Tests 36. Seeing Likenesses and Differences in Subjects 37. Getting It Done on Time	**A.** Communication 38. Class Discussions 39. What to Say 40. Tuning Your Conversation 41. Putting Yourself in Another's Place 42. Solving Problems in Communication **B.** Fitting into School 43. Making Choices— Adapting, Shaping, Selecting 44. Understanding Social Networks 45. Seeing the Network: Different Roles 46. Seeing the Network: Figuring Out the Rules 47. Seeing the Relationship Between Now and Later 48. What Does School Mean to You?

Note. From "Practical Intelligence for Success in School" by R. J. Sternberg, L. Okagaki, and A. S. Jackson, 1990, *Educational Leadership, 48*(1), p. 37. Reprinted with permission of the Association for Supervision and Curriculum Development. Copyright 1990 by ASCD. All rights reserved.

judged when students respond with specific examples from the appropriate classification, with attributes subordinate to the larger concept, or by citing defining characteristics of the concept. Much knowledge is judged when students place the concept within a superordinate (higher class) category, provide precise definitions of it, explain it by analogy, or appropriately link one concept with another on the same level. In a related approach, Marzano, Hagerty, Valencia, and DiStefano (1987) suggested that stu-

dents categorize their own prior knowledge (and learned knowledge) using a chart format with the headings "What We Think We Know," "What We Want to Know," and "What We Found Out."

Many approaches that relate language and thinking in the later stages of language learning use B. S. Bloom's (1956) taxonomy of educational objectives. Bloom's taxonomy has influenced efforts to teach thinking strategies in both regular classrooms (e.g., Lundsteen, 1979; Tonjes & Zintz, 1987) and language intervention programs (Boyce & Larson, 1983; N. W. Nelson, 1988b; L. Schwartz & McKinley, 1984; Simon, 1985; Westby, 1991). Westby (1991) gave examples of questions that might be used in a social studies lesson to probe each of the six levels of Bloom's taxonomy:

Knowledge: Where did the Alaskan oil spill occur? What company owned the boat that caused the spill?

Comprehension: Describe how the Alaskan oil spill occurred.

Application: What are some other ways that the wildlife could have been rescued?

Analysis: What types of problems were created by the spill?

Synthesis: What kinds of problems would occur if there were a chemical spill in our town?

Evaluation: Discuss who should be responsible for the cleanup and why they should be responsible. (p. 19)

N. W. Nelson and Gillespie (1991) devised three sets of "Analogies for Thinking and Talking" that can be used as a framework to encourage similar kinds of cognitive–linguistic interactions in a social learning context. We designed one set of figurative analogies to tap visual-spatial analysis and synthesis abilities; a second to tap the ability to recognize and talk about analogical word meanings; the third set was represented entirely by pictures. We conducted field tests with adults with acquired brain injuries and with students who had language-learning disabilities, mild mental retardation, emotional problems, and varying degrees of hearing impairment. With mediational teaching and practice, almost everyone improved in the ability to complete the analogies correctly and to tell why other choices were not as good. One of the nicest outcomes was the development of confidence and skill in talking about and evaluating ideas in cooperative learning groups. The ability to engage in verbal analogical reasoning is one of the hallmarks of later language development (Nippold, 1986; 1988e) and one that deserves further attention.

Does research evidence show that intervention approaches designed to teach meta-awareness of language and learning strategies work? An overview of research on "talking about talking" (metalinguistics) and "thinking about thinking" by Chipman, Segal, and Glaser (1984) suggested that it is possible to change problem solving, memory, and abstract thinking by focusing consciously on the steps and strategies used to accomplish them. Research evidence

gathered in the process of implementing the practical intelligence curriculum with 100 seventh-grade students (R. J. Sternberg et al., 1990) (contrasted with a control group) also supported the conclusion that it is possible to teach tacit knowledge and learning strategies.

Making aspects of the school culture curriculum and the hidden curriculum part of the official curriculum, as Sternberg and his colleagues did (R. J. Sternberg, et al., 1990) (see Table 9.8) sometimes may be the best pathway to building increased metacognitive proficiency. For other students, acquiring purposeful strategies of "executive control" through the use of mediational strategies may be preferred (described previously in one-to-one interactions with an "experienced, intentioned adult"; Feuerstein, 1979, p. 179). The adult mediators influence the acquisition of metacognitive strategies by modeling the language of mediated learning and then systematically assisting children to acquire self-mediating functions. Instructional techniques such as these have even been shown to influence the thinking of retarded learners (Feuerstein et al., 1988; Hagen et al., 1982) and of individuals with hearing impairments (Haywood et al., 1988).

It is impossible to talk about thinking without drawing on concepts of **memory.** In the complex processing model illustrated in Figure 9.1, two types of memory, short-term and long-term memory, are represented as different entities. Long-term memory is noted in Figure 9.1 as the mechanism for storing knowledge about events, things, abstract ideas, symbols, and rule systems within six rather different schemata (represented as boxes). Short-term memory is represented by the small black bidirectional arrows connecting all of the other components of the model. Rohwer and Dempster (1977) described the different kinds of storage functions this way:

Short-term memory represents information on a temporary basis and long-term memory represents information on a permanent basis. Moreover, since the contents of short-term memory are transitory, information can be continuously added and deleted in order to meet changing task demands. For example, in attempting to solve a problem it is often necessary to store and discard one partial result after another, while simultaneously coordinating these changes with the resources of long-term memory. Given these functions, it is clear why short-term memory is commonly referred to as the system's "working memory." By contrast, long-term memory plays a passive role in information processing; its primary importance arises from the fact that it represents the products of the individual's experience. These products range from the particular, such as individual letter codes, to the general, including strategies for processing and transforming new information. (p. 410)

The trick, in using metacognitive resources for intervention, is to get learners to draw more actively and deliberately on experiential resources stored in long-term memory. Because short-term memory is marked by a limited storage capacity, the learner must use storage and retrieval strategies while working on more complex and extensive sets of information. *Storage* is a person's mental representation of information in long-term memory. *Retrieval* is the process of returning to that information. The load on short-term memory capacity can be reduced by collapsing the number of units the person must remember. This can be done by applying conscious efforts to chunk or group together isolated bits of information into patterns that are easier to remember. Encoded information (sometimes using language) or information associated with other information already held in long-term storage may be easier to remember. Teachers and other professionals can encourage this process by arranging and organizing information to encourage the discovery and use of organizational processes, by instructing students directly in how to use such strategies and by providing opportunities for practice (Rohwer & Dempster, 1977). B. Britton, Glynn, and Smith (1985) suggested that teachers could reduce the processing load associated with reading and remembering expository texts by (1) using titles, outlines, abstracts, and explicit descriptions to increase predictability; (2) priming students to pay attention to certain structure and content; (3) signaling transitions from phrase to phrase; and (4) controlling the number of concepts presented at one time.

Wiig (1984) compared the development of memory and memory strategies for academically achieving students and students with language-learning disabilities (see Table 9.9). She drew on descriptions of concept formation proposed by Bruner, Oliver, and Greenfield (1966), including (1) discrimination of the salient properties of objects, actions, and events; (2) categorization on the basis of those properties; (3) forming a superordinate concept for the category; and (4) generalizing this superordinate concept to other cases or contexts. Wiig noted that students with language-learning disabilities might differ from other students in several ways. Bruner et al. (1966) described four approaches to forming new concepts:

(1) simultaneous scanning, (2) successive scanning, (3) conservative focusing, or (4) focused gambling. Wiig suggested that students with language-learning disabilities might have limited use of the first three strategies because of inadequate memory capacity and that they might rely excessively on the fourth, focused gambling, as a more impulsive approach, even though it often leads to blind alleys.

Instruction aimed specifically at teaching students to tie new information to old as a way to facilitate retrieval is called **mnemonic instruction.** Scruggs and Mastropieri (1990) described mnemonic techniques, including key-word strategies (using acoustically and semantically similar words, such as viper, to remember vituperation); peg-word strategies (using rhyming words to facilitate recall of numbered or ordered information); acronym strategies (using acronyms such as HOMES to remember the names of the Great Lakes, Huron, Ontario, Michigan, Erie, and Superior); reconstructive elaborations (using familiar and concrete associations to build elaborations of concepts); phonemic mnemonics (using sound patterns to build associations); and spelling mnemonics (using spelling patterns to build associations). Although mnemonic strategies have been employed for thousands of years (dating back to ancient Greek scholars), Scruggs and Mastropieri reported that they have only been employed recently with students with learning disabilities. Preliminary results of research are highly encouraging. L. Schwartz and McKinley (1984) agreed that it may be helpful for students with language-learning disabilities to practice using mnemonic strategies. They cautioned, however, against teaching such strategies as isolated skills, and against making assumptions about background linguistic and nonlinguistic knowledge that may not be available to these learners. Mnemonic strategies often make use of culturally based knowledge as well, which is not equally available to all participants (I remember when my husband tried to teach our daughter to associate *Bismarck* as the capital of North Dakota with jelly doughnuts, but first he had to teach her to call jelly doughnuts *Bismarcks*).

Using Metacognitive, Metalinguistic, and Metatextual Strategies to Focus on Process Rather Than Product

In arguing that adolescents with language-learning disabilities should be taught strategies rather than specific course content, McKinley and Lord-Larson

TABLE 9.9
Overview of memory and memory strategy developmental patterns, with notation about delays among children and adolescents with learning disabilities

Age Level	Population	Selective Attention/Rehearsal	Organization/Serial Recall	Metamemory
7–9 yr	Academic achievers	Can be taught to label and rehearse verbal labels/items at 6-7 yr.	Phonologically similar (goat–boat) are more often misrecognized than categorically related words (goat-sheep) at age 7.	Recognize that something should be done to facilitate memory but do not employ strategies spontaneously at age 7.
	Language-learning disabled	Show developmental delays in selective attention and in the acquisition of rehearsal strategies.	Can benefit from external organization by semantic category of pictured stimuli.	Show approximately a two-year delay in the use of past experiences and/or present context (complementary relations) and in the shift to using generic (semantic) category for grouping.
10–13 yr	Academic achievers	Demonstrative efficient cumulative rehearsal at age 10, and verbal labeling, rehearsal, and chunking strategies at age 11.	Categorically related words (goat–sheep) are misrecognized more often than phonologically related words (goat–boat) at age 12. Central recall increases while incidental recall decreases significantly between ages 12 and 14.	Recognize and spontaneously employ rehearsal and categorization strategies.
	Language-learning disabled	Rehearsal strategies can be induced by reinforcement and verbal direction. Spontaneous rehearsal occurs with greater frequency for monosyllables than for multisyllabic words. Selective attention abilities better among reflective children and high modelers than among impulsive and low modeler counterparts.	External grouping and categorization of pictured stimuli can facilitate recall. Show random shifts in recalling foods but use grouping strategies for recalling animals.	The shift from using complementary relations to using generic category for grouping (thematic to taxonomic) was not completed at age 11.

Note. From "Language Disabilities in Adolescents: A Question of Cognitive Strategies" by E. H. Wiig. Reprinted from *Topics in Language Disorders*, Vol. 4, No. 2, p. 46, with permission of Aspen Publishers, Inc. ©1984.

(1985) emphasized the importance of learning how to learn rather than what to learn. They commented that programs built on strategy acquisition would be more likely to help such students "generalize basic skills across situations, settings, and curricula" (p. 4). This philosophy is consistent with current general educational approaches that emphasize the value of process over products in the development of mature reading and writing.

Processes of mature reading and writing are guided metacognitively (as represented by the large upper arrow in the model in Figure 9.1). Purves (1981) noted that literacy involves more than simply reading words off a page—"one doesn't just read; one has a purpose for one's reading, and one reads for many purposes" (p. 77). Similarly, Odell (1981) noted that effective writers have something to communicate and that the process of writing involves discovering what they wish to say and how to say it. Nystrand (1982) emphasized purpose and control as important pragmatic factors associated with both reading and writing as communicative acts.

Theorists have varied, however, in the degree to which they believe that cognitive awareness should be called into play for controlling literacy processes. LaBerge and Samuels (1987), for example, emphasized that automaticity is important because it allows mature readers to focus their attention on deriving meaning rather than decoding words. Many other researchers, however, emphasized that metacognitive monitoring of process may be essential for constructing meaning (e.g., Baker & Brown, 1984). Perhaps different processes are important at different developmental stages and for different purposes.

Automaticity might be associated differentially with different stages of learning and different types of learning. Tharp and Gallimore (1988) diagrammed four stages that involve differing degrees of automaticity. First, beginning capacity is fostered by mediating teachers and parents who help the child reach upward within the zone of proximal development, described by Vygotsky (1962). Second, the child learns to assist his or her own processing by using overt or covert verbal monitoring (also within the zone of proximal development). Third, automatization occurs through internalization of the strategy (extending learning beyond the zone of proximal development). Fourth, the child has the ability to deautomatize the task, analyzing the strategy and using it to learn new concepts. The final three stages may occur in recursive loops in which the child can use current understanding to become an active participant in further learning.

Recursive development patterns appear to be typical of much later learning and language processing. When researchers have used "thinking aloud protocols" (Emig, 1971; J. R. Hayes & Flower, 1980), for example, to get normally developing secondary students to talk while composing written language, they have found that writing does not occur as a solid, evenly paced, uninterrupted activity from planning to proofreading. Rather, writing has a recursive rhythm that involves bursts of fluency, interspersed with pauses and revisions (Emig, 1971). This research has led to the development of "process-oriented" (rather than "product-oriented") instructional models.

Writing process intervention models. According to process-oriented instructional models, writers generate the best products when they have "authentic" purposes for writing. Based on this philosophy, programs have been designed for both general educational and special education students using the multiple processing stages: planning, drafting, revising, editing, sharing, and publication—not as isolated exercises but for real communicative purposes (Bos, 1988; J. R. Hayes & Flower, 1987; N. W. Nelson, 1988a, 1988b, 1988c).

Simply providing the opportunity to complete each of these steps with classmates who read and edit each others' work may encourage written language development among most students. Other students who have special education needs may require more direct modeling and explanation, using language they can understand and clear steps for planning. In addition, acceptance and encouragement from the teacher may be critical to encourage students who have experienced failure to risk expressing themselves in writing and to overcome learned helplessness (Winograd & Niquette, 1988). Individuals who have experienced failure in learning to read also need to experience literacy as a process with its own rewards rather than as a product evaluated for acquisition (see Personal Reflection 9.14).

A staff member of a high school special services team (Carignan-Belleville, 1989) demonstrated the potential power of interactive literacy approaches with a seventh-grade student named Jason. Jason

---

Personal Reflection 9.14	"Poor readers who suffer from learned helplessness need to spend more time interacting with books that interest them. These children, in particular, need to understand that success in reading is defined as the fulfillment of one's own purposes, not as one's placement relative to others."
	Peter Winograd and *Garland Niquette* (1988, p. 52).

was described as having "writing paranoia" and a hearing impairment when Carignan-Belleville was brought in as a teacher consultant to work with him for 1 hour/week. Jason had previously announced to his teachers and the hearing specialist that he did not plan to write any more journals, essays, or book reports. The reason he gave was that he simply could not do it. Carignan-Belleville started the intervention by discussing with Jason a game of baseball his team had recently won. She asked him to give her three reasons why his team had deserved to win. After he had done so orally, she said, "Let's put that in writing," and provided him with the following format for organizing his short essay:

Question: Who won Saturday's baseball game?

Five-sentence paragraph
1. Topic sentence: (Answer to the question)
2. Reason #1
3. Reason #2
4. Reason #3
5. Conclusion: (Restate topic sentence in different words.) (1989, pp. 57–58)

The clear organizational strategy and oral language rehearsal of this approach gave Jason sufficient support to write an acceptable essay. Over time, Jason's writing continued to improve. Carignan-Belleville (1989) gave him story starters (e.g., "If I had more money . . ."), and these made him willing to attempt the journal writing he had once hated. He also was encouraged to dictate his stories first into a tape recorder and then transcribe them. As Jason began to experience more success, he also began to want to read books. A particularly interesting aspect of Jason's case study for language specialists is the way that improved competency in one modality encouraged increased effort in others.

Improving reading comprehension with metacognition. Metacognitive techniques have also been recommended to improve reading comprehension (A. L. Brown & Palincsar, 1982; Palincsar & Brown, 1987; Palincsar & Ransom, 1988). The association of metacognition with mature reading is supported by research on normal development. For example, when Forrest-Pressley and Waller (1984) studied third- and sixth-graders who were poor, average, and good readers, they found that only older and better readers employed metacognitive strategies effectively.

Metacognitive intervention techniques to improving written language comprehension may take a vari-

ety of forms, some previously discussed in this chapter. Students might be taught strategies for using advance organizers, self-questioning, and self-monitoring of their own comprehension.

Providing students with objectives before they read is an example of an advance organizer. Evidence shows that when objectives are provided in advance, students are more likely to learn targeted material (Tierney & Cunningham, 1984). Other advance organizers include pretests, prequestions, and the PREP described previously (Langer, 1982). These may also alert students to the nature of particular tasks and help them acquire strategies to evaluate, categorize, and generalize information as they read.

A related metacognitive technique involves guiding students to become conscious of the purpose of a particular reading activity. For example, Tierney and Cunningham (1984) summarized four steps found to increase reading comprehension:

Step 1: Establish purposes(s) for comprehending.
Step 2: Have students read or listen for the established purposes(s).
Step 3: Have students perform some task which directly reflects and measures accomplishment of each established purpose for comprehending.
Step 4: Provide direct informative feedback concerning students' comprehension based on their performance of that (those) task(s). (p. 625)

The metacognitive strategy of self-questioning relies on mediational techniques described previously in this section. When using self-questioning approaches, remember that asking good questions may not come automatically, particularly for students with language disorders. These students may need intensive modeling before they can use self-questions effectively on their own. For example, Wong and Jones (1982) taught a group of 120 learning disabled eighth- and ninth-graders and normally achieving sixth-graders to use self-questioning strategies to monitor their understanding of important textual units. They did this in five steps:

(a) What are you studying this passage for? (So you can answer some questions you will be given later); (b) Find the main idea/ideas in the paragraph and underline it/them; (c) Think of a question about the main idea you have underlined. Remember what a good question should be like. (Look at the prompt); (d) Learn the answer to your question; (e) Always look back at the questions and answers to see how each successive question and answer provides you with more information. (p. 231)

The results (Wong & Jones, 1982) showed an increased awareness of important textual units by the students with learning disabilities. Those students also learned to monitor their own understanding of text units and to formulate good questions about them, and their comprehension performance improved. The procedure did not increase the metacomprehension or comprehension performance of the normally achieving sixth-graders to a similar degree. Wong and Jones interpreted this as evidence that the normally achieving students were already processing the texts actively compared to the inactive approaches taken by the learning disabled adolescents.

A related strategy-based approach to enhance written language comprehension of expository texts is called *multipass* (Schumaker et al., 1982), which is based on an adaptation of a widely known procedure originally published in 1946 to train soldiers rapidly for specialized jobs during World War II (Robinson, 1970). The acronym SQ3R represents the five strategic steps of this approach. As summarized by Just and Carpenter (1987), readers should (a) **survey,** by skimming the table of contents, major headings, illustrations, summary paragraphs, and the like, to become familiar with the text's general outline, main topics, and organization; (b) generate **questions** based on headings and topics discovered during the survey step, to learn to be attentive and to think about what is already known about the topic; (c) **read** one section of the chapter at a time, while trying to answer the question posed for that section; (d) **recite** possible answers to the questions, citing examples from notes or memory; and (e) **review,** by going over main points with the help of brief notes, citing major subpoints, and trying to memorize both the main points and subpoints.

Other specialized forms of self-questioning training include a program that taught students to identify task demands to guide comprehension (Raphael & Pearson, 1982). Students learned to examine textbook questions and to label them differentially depending on whether they required the students (a) to locate an answer in the text ("right there"); (b) to derive an answer from the student's own background knowledge ("on my own"); or (c) to derive an answer that involved inferring relationships among text segments ("think and search").

The ability to monitor one's own comprehension is a strategy that can be acquired. Research has shown that, apparently as a result of disparate task demands,

comprehension monitoring may appear as early as age 2 or as late as age 12 in normal development (Dollaghan, 1987b). As Dollaghan cautioned, "trying to understand a message requires effort on the part of the listener, and even normal listeners do not try to construct meaning representations for all the messages they receive" (p. 47). The failure to construct an adequate representation of message meaning cannot be detected unless a receiver has made an attempt to understand the message. (The comprehension monitoring program designed by Dollaghan & Kaston, 1986, was described in Chapter 8.)

Summary of Metaskills and How to Teach Them

This review has provided examples of intervention programs designed to teach students to use learning strategies, including metapragmatic strategies to manage expectations of classroom communication events, metacognitive strategies to learn, think, and remember, and multiple metastrategies to focus on processes within writing and reading tasks.

Professional across disciplines may be involved in implementing such programs. The contribution of speech–language pathologists or other language specialists is their awareness of the unique relationships between individuals' language abilities and their related ability to acquire and use learning strategies. Particularly when task expectations include highly language-related components such as discourse knowledge and verbal mediation techniques, individuals with intrinsic language disorders may need more deliberate efforts to learn how to analyze the task and to remember the steps in their problem-solving strategies. Westby (1991) reported that many of the young adults in her program who have acquired strategies and can use them, nevertheless do not use them in real life. When she asked the students why not, they gave reasons that suggested that they thought the strategies might take too much time or that they liked doing it their old way better.

To overcome some of these barriers, Seidenberg (1988) suggested that strategy instruction should be systematic. The seven steps Seidenberg suggested for teaching cognitive strategies for complex academic tasks follow: (1) Introduce the strategy and review the student's current performance. (2) Explain the relevance of the strategy by using real-life examples. (3) Describe the strategy and provide a "help sheet" that lists its steps. (4) Model the strategy and rehearse it with students as a group. (5) Provide opportunity to practice the strategy using controlled materials, with prompts and corrective feedback as necessary. (6) With the student, evaluate the data gathered during practice with controlled materials. (7) Provide further practice using textbook materials drawn from the regular curriculum. In my experience, children can use their own textbook materials for learning strategies. Starting at step 4 in this sequence and using the regular curriculum as the source of all practice materials may be advantageous to their motivation and to their ultimate carryover of new strategies.

DEVELOPING COMPETENCE IN VARIED DISCOURSE GENRES AND EVENTS

Three kinds of discourse genres, conversational, narrative, and expository, were discussed previously in this chapter as contexts to probe during informal assessment. Decisions to target language knowledge and skills within one or more of these discourse contexts are made when participants identify zones of significance that require their competent use. If getting along with and being accepted by peers is identified as an area of particular concern, the specialist may target social conversational discourse with peers. If a student has difficulty comprehending written language stories, the specialist may probe the student's intrinsic and explicit knowledge of narrative structure. If concerns expressed by students, teachers, and parents center around academic difficulties in science and social studies, targeting new skills to understand expository texts about them may be most appropriate.

Development of intervention plans might also involve choices of communicative events using one or more discourse type. Contextually based language intervention involves analyzing the demands and opportunities of currently available communicative events and deciding whether new communicative opportunities should be provided. Communicative events involving one or more of the three discourse types may be found throughout the regular curriculum and as students make transitions into employment settings.

Interacting for Business or Pleasure: The Conversational Genre

Conversation may be defined broadly as uses of language for social interaction. Conversation is the primary context for all natural language learning and a key context for language intervention. Hoskins (1990; see Personal Reflection 9.15) pointed out that reading and writing are also social interactive phenomena. She noted that written language interactions between authors and readers may be targeted for intervention as conversational events, just as oral interactions between speakers and listeners are. Students may be encouraged to act as conversational partners, imagining the absent audience for a piece they are writing or imagining the author of the work they are reading. Some of the techniques described in the previous section on metaskills may help to encourage such perspective taking.

Later stage children may benefit from strategies for targeting conversation in assessment and intervention with middle-stage language-impaired children similar to the strategies in Chapter 8 (e.g. Brinton & Fujiki, 1989). This section presents a consideration of the specialized needs of later stage language learners for interacting in classrooms, with peers, and in family conversations.

Conversing in classrooms. Participating in classroom conversations, as considered earlier in this chapter, requires a special set of linguistic and social skills but not a uniform set of skills. Part of the complexity of knowing how to participate in classroom conversations stems from the fact the rules for conversational access vary across classrooms and across

---

| Personal Reflection 9.15 | "We not only are continuously learning language, but, in our interactions in language, we are constantly developing the narratives that comprise who we are, how we think of ourselves, and how we present ourselves to others."

Barbara Hoskins (1990, p. 60), Language/Learning Disabilities Consultant in Pasadena, California. |

discourse events (Bloome & Knott, 1985). Even within a single event, individual children may experience communicative demands and opportunities differently (Cazden, 1988; F. Erickson & Schultz, 1981; N. W. Nelson, 1986; Silliman & Lamanna, 1986).

Some aspects of classroom discourse superficially might seem to be less demanding than other forms of social interaction discourse. If only syntactic demands are considered for explaining the demands of answering teachers' questions, the lack of complexity might seem remarkable at first. In her analysis of formal classroom discourse, Sturm (1990) found that MLU counts for students did not vary significantly among first- (mean = 3.7), third- (mean = 4.6), and fifth-grade (mean = 4.8) classrooms. None of these expressive language means surpassed a level of complexity expected for preschoolers, but looks may be deceiving.

To be appropriate in classroom conversations, students need to keep their responses short and to the point. As Leonard and Fey (1991) pointed out, ellipsis is one of the bulwarks of conversation. It allows speakers to converse without repeating information already contained in prior utterances. Considerable syntactic sophistication, however, is required for a speaker to analyze specific grammatical elements that should be retained and replaced during ellipsis processes. For example, when an adult asks, "Who eats worms?," and a child responds, "I don't," the child must have analyzed the verb phrase as the focus of the question and have selected the appropriate auxiliary verb to replace it. Children with language impairments may need special practice in making their responses accurate, relevant, and brief. Language specialists should take particular note of these classroom conversation demands because of their more natural tendency to require students to give complete and elaborated responses to questions.

Not only expressive but receptive demands of classroom conversations must be understood. With advancing grade level, children are faced with advancing syntactic complexity in their teachers' language (N. W. Nelson, 1984). Both Sturm (1990) and Cuda (1976) found significant increments in syntactic complexity of teacher talk beyond third grade, and neither found significant differences between first and third grades (Sturm's data resulted in mean T-unit MLUs of 7.5, 7.9 and 9.7 for first-, third-, and fifth-grade teachers, respectively). Although teachers have been found to use considerable figurative language even in the early grades (Lazar, Warr-Leeper, Nicholson, & Johnson, 1989; N. W. Nelson, 1984), the demands on cognitive processing of teacher talk probably also increase with grade level. Students must learn to listen, take notes, organize their own thoughts, follow classroom rules for talking and not talking, think about what they are hearing and relate it to what they already know, and imagine absent contexts and textbook authors as they try to understand classroom language.

When children in classroom conversations have opportunities to do more than answer teachers' questions, the demands on their pragmatic and syntactic systems increase accordingly. Ervin-Tripp and Gordon (1986) studied children's skill in making requests. They found that before the age of 8 years, children had sufficient control of advanced syntactic structures and politeness markers to modulate features such as urgency, force, friendliness, and demand. Children above third grade demonstrated clear advantages in classroom strategies for making effective requests, such as requesting marker pens and other supplies from busy adults. The younger children used fairly direct strategies that tended to assume that the adults had the materials and would comply:

> I need a blue marker.
> Where's the marker?
> Can I have the letter to my parents? (Ervin-Tripp & Gordon, 1986, p. 87)

The older children seemed to acknowledge the possibility that the addressee might not comply with the request and to recognize that they might be intruding on the listener. Their strategies were relatively more indirect:

> Are there any more markers?
> Do you have a green marker I could use?
> She told me to get a letter for my parents. (Ervin-Tripp & Gordon, 1986, p. 87)

Wilkinson, Milosky, and Genishi (1986) observed slightly different strategies for making classroom requests, depending on the backgrounds of individual children, some aspects of which are cultural. Those authors expressed concern that therapeutic activities aimed at teaching students mainstream strategies for looking at an intended listener, addressing the listener by name, and waiting to begin speaking until attention clearly has been secured may conflict with some students' cultural customs. Nevertheless, Wilkinson and her colleagues found more similarities than differences among small-group academic conversations between monolingual English-speaking and bilingual Hispanic students. They suggested that effective speakers could be defined by their ability to elicit a response from their partners. Box 9.9 summarizes general behaviors that might be targeted in the intervention process, as long as cultural differences are respected.

Silliman and Lamanna (1986) studied the strategies that elementary school children use to get and keep the floor in classroom discussion, including turn overlaps and interruptions. They noted that teachers may

conrol these turn disruptions to some extent but that children need systematic opportunities to practice turn taking in the classroom.

Teachers can increase the opportunity for private dialogue with individual students by interacting with them in writing using dialogue journals. Lindfors (1987) noted that dialogue journals give students a chance to express their personal wonderings, opinions, grievances, anger, and anticipation. C. W. Hayes and Bahruth (1985) described a fifth-grade classroom where teachers interacted in a dialogue with a reluc-

---

Box 9.9   **Request characteristics of effective speakers**

A successful request is likely to be:

1. *Direct:* Use of linguistic forms that directly signal the speaker's needs. For requests for action, the imperative or *I want/I need* statements; for requests for information, the *Wh-, yes–no* or tag question.

   Direct requests: *How do you do this one?, I need a pencil;*
   Indirect requests: *I don't get this, Anybody have a pencil?*

2. *Designated to a listener:* Unambiguously indicates the intended listener through verbal or nonverbal means:

   C: Sally, where do you put the dollar sign? *or*
   C: (*looking at P*) Did you get that one?

3. *Sincere:* According to Labov and Fanshel (1978), a request is sincere if (a) the action, purpose, and need for the request are clear; for example, in a request for information, the listener believes that the speaker really wants the information and does not already know the information; (b) there is both an ability and an obligation of the listener to respond to the request; and (c) the speaker has a right to make the request.

   Sincere: "John, I can't find the price for hamburger."
   Insincere: "Well, slow-poke, what one are you finally up to now?"

4. *Revised if unsuccessful:* A restatement of a request previously made by the same speaker to the same listener who had not responded appropriately:

   A. "Bob, I need a pencil:"
   B. "Uh:"
   A. "Bob, can I borrow a pencil?"

5. *On task:* Related to the academic content or procedures and materials of the assignment.

   On task: "Is this one add or subtract?"
   Off task: "Whaddya gonna do at recess?"

6. *Responded to appropriately:* The requested action or information was given or else a reason was given why the action and/or information could not be given.

   Appropriate response: C: "Alice, what's five?"
                               A: "I got 22 for that one."
   Inappropriate response: C: "Alice, what's five?"
                               A: "What did you get for it?"

Note. From "Second Language Learners' Use of Requests and Responses in Elementary Classrooms" by L.C. Wilkinson, L.M. Milosky, and C. Genishi. Reprinted from *Topics in Language Disorders*, Vol. 6, No. 2, p. 59, with permission of Aspen Publishers, Inc., ©1986.

tant writer. On the 1st day, when the children turned in their journals, Larry's first page was blank. The ensuing written conversation:

> T: How can we answer you if you don't write?
> L: I don't like writing.
> T: Does anything bother you about writing?
> L: I don't like to write because I can't not spell right. that's bother me about writing.
> T: Don't worry about it right now. The more you read and write the better your spelling will get. Just worry about getting your ideas written down. (p. 99)

Speech–language pathologists might use similar dialogue journals to interact with their students; using journals written during regular classroom experiences may be more advantageous (Swoger, 1989). The speech–language pathologist who is granted access to writing produced during the regular or special classroom might have a rich source of data about the child's continuing language development. The naturalistic quality of conversing with a known partner in writing might also provide a powerful context for learning more elaborate language forms and vocabulary when previous language learning experiences have not been positive.

Conversing with peers. Wiig and Semel (1976) viewed social perception as a component language skill. Donahue and Bryan (1984) commented:

> *Perhaps in no other developmental phase is the relationship between communicative skills and peer group membership as apparent as in adolescence.* (p. 11)

Donahue and Bryan (1984) particularly mentioned the importance of slang in identifying group membership and also noted its importance to language and learning disabled youth who are often cast as "outsiders" (learning from peers was identified as the "underground curriculum" earlier in this chapter). Based on informal observation (owing to a lack of research data on the topic), Donahue and Bryan reported that the use of slang by students with learning disabilities related to the amount of interaction of these students with students who had no disabilities and appeared to lag by about 6 months to 1 year.

Donahue and Bryan (1984) commented that this problem might be partially remedied by structuring social and academic experiences of students with learning disabilities to increase their opportunities to learn adolescent social skills through satisfying peer interactions. Those authors commented that peers make the best coaches and that "No adult could keep up with the rapid changes in slang nor fully appreciated the fine nuances of its meaning" (p. 19).

In summarizing approaches to intervention for peer interaction problems, T. Bryan (1986) recognized three types: direct instruction, structured situations, and group-training programs. The structured situations that involved peer modeling seemed to be the most effective (although it is difficult to generalize across studies). The problem with the direct instruction approaches was that practicing a verbal behavior in one kind of discourse event (direct instruction) was insufficient to encourage its generalization to others. Bryan concluded that, "Not only particular verbal skills must be taught but also the parameters of the situations in which the child is expected to display these skills" (p. 251). Structured situations in which peers served as models of the targeted behaviors (e.g., asking open-ended questions in the talk show format), however, were found to be highly effective. The fact that students with learning disabilities could abstract conversational rules by listening to a model present very few examples suggested that the students already had elements of the conversational skills in their repertoires and only needed to be taught the parameters of social situations in which they were appropriate. Bryan interpreted the results from large-group teaching programs as mixed.

Several programs aimed at helping adolescents with communicative disorders to acquire social communication skills have now been published (Hazel, Schumaker, Sherman, & Sheldon-Wildgen, 1981; Hoskins, 1987; LaGreca & Mesibov, 1981; Minskoff, 1982; Wanat, 1983; Wiig, 1982). However, clear evidence regarding their effectiveness is not yet available. To evaluate these programs, Donahue and Bryan (1984) suggested asking the following questions:

❏ Will the acquisition of these skills allow students to meet peer as well as adult norms for appropriate communicative style? It is important to recognize that target behaviors are likely to be selected because they appeal to adult expectations. For example, should educators be teaching rules for polite requests or how to engage in friendly exchanges of insults?

❏ Will this training program enable students to discern how and when to use their newly acquired skills in naturalistic settings?

❏ Will use of these communicative skills enhance the adolescent's social acceptance with peers and adults? (p. 19)

One modeling program successful in encouraging adolescent students to exhibit greater competence in conversations is the model, analyze, practice (MAP) approach described by Hess and Fairchild (1988). A group of adolescents with learning disabilities participated in six weekly, 1-hour sessions. The adolescents viewed videotaped models of desirable and undesirable interactions, analyzed the models, and practiced the targeted skills of topic initiation, topic maintenance, and using open-ended questions and follow-up questions and comments to sustain the dialogue. In one segment, the students observed a videotaped sample in which each exchange consisted of one utterance per participant and one turn exchange:

Speaker 1: What are your hobbies?
Speaker 2: I like to build models and play basketball.
Speaker 1: Do you go to movies?
Speaker 2: Yes.
Speaker 1: How is your marching band doing?
Speaker 2: Okay.

After analyzing this sample, the students were shown a version where more effective conversational strategies were used:

Speaker 1: What are your hobbies?
Speaker 2: I like to build models and play basketball.
Speaker 1: Do you play basketball for your school team?
Speaker 2: No. I play for fun with my friends. I'm not tall enough for the school team.
Speaker 1: I didn't think so. I play basketball on one of the YMCA teams.
Speaker 2: Oh yeah. How did you get on that team?

The students then were assisted to analyze and compare the two samples, writing down their observations. They were encouraged to return to the first videotaped sample when necessary to check details. The third step in the procedure was to practice the better conversational techniques and to analyze their effectiveness. They videotaped themselves conversing about self-chosen topics so that they could practice the desirable features they had identified and critique their own performance when finished. If they identified problems, they retaped their conversations, again attempting to incorporate the group's suggestions, and again, analyzing the improvement. This approach is consistent with many of the principles of mediated learning and of strategy acquisition discussed previously.

Problems with peer acceptance have been consistently noted in the literature on learning disabilities (e.g., Bruininks, 1978; J. H. Bryan & Sherman, 1980; C. L. Fox, 1989; Vaughn, McIntosh, & Spencer-Rowe, 1991), and occasionally for individuals with other disabilities, such as hearing impairment (Gagné, Stelmacovich, & Yovetich, 1991) (see Personal Reflection 9.16). Peer acceptance is a central problem of the syndrome of autism (e.g., Schopler & Mesibov, 1986). Gallagher (1991) noted that negative social consequences were among the first problems identified in the early literature on speech–language pathology. Gallagher also noted that despite this fact, and despite the centrality of language as the primary means of interpersonal contact and socialization of children, "the profession has been slow to develop assessment and intervention programs that deal with language disorders in social interaction terms" (p. 11).

Numerous factors influence the degree of peer acceptance that might be subject to modification through language intervention. To identify specific skills to target for an individual student the specialist must thoroughly understand expected social interaction patterns within that child's culture and potential influences of the child's disability, and should investigate peer reactions to current interaction behaviors.

| Personal Reflection 9.16 | "Peer interaction is an essential component of the individual child's development. Experience with peers is not a superficial luxury to be enjoyed by some children and not others, but is a necessity in childhood socialization. And among the most sensitive indicators of difficulties in development are failure by the child to engage in the activities of the peer culture and failure to occupy a relatively comfortable place within it."

William Hartup (1983, p. 220), child development specialist, writing in a chapter entitled "Peer Interaction and the Behavioral Development of the Individual Child." |

For example, Gagné et al. (1991) staged scenes in which a group of "hearing impaired" actors interacted with normal-hearing college students. Gagné et al. asked another group of students to rate the acceptability of the clarification requests dramatized by "hearing impaired" students. The researchers found that reactions were more favorable when the "hearing impaired" actors used specific rather than nonspecific requests.

Similar studies might be conducted on a smaller scale for individual students within their own communities. For both assessment and intervention, aspects of the MAP sequence (Hess & Fairchild, 1988, described previously) could be implemented. However, instead of providing the group experience only for children with disabilities, professionals could include normally developing peer volunteers as partners to obtain insights about how the child with a disability might develop more acceptable communicative strategies.

Peers may be enlisted in conversational skills intervention programs in a variety of roles. Gallagher (1991) noted that "they can become directly involved in the intervention program by serving as peer partners or be involved more indirectly through their participation in cooperative group experiences" (p. 32). Some training of peer partners is probably necessary to teach them to use verbal and nonverbal communication strategies to facilitate partner participation.

A conversational skills intervention program might be used in the regular curriculum in early adolescent life skills classes that tend to be taught at the junior high school level. Even youngsters presumably developing normally may benefit from direct instruction in social interaction skills. D. W. Johnson and Johnson (1990) found, for example, that before children could succeed in working toward mutual goals in cooperative learning groups, they needed to

(1) get to know and trust one another, (2) communicate accurately and unambiguously, (3) accept and support one another, and (4) resolve conflicts constructively. (p. 30)

To teach such skills, teachers need to help students see the need to work cooperatively and to believe that they will be better off if they know how to do so. Teachers can assist the process by making the use of strategies for encouraging participation explicit. For example, D. W. Johnson and Johnson (1990) suggested using a chart, with the heading "encouraging

participation" across the top and two vertical columns labeled "looks like" and "sounds like." The cue for the nonverbal *smiles* may be paired with the verbal suggestion, "What is your idea?"; *eye contact* may be paired with "Awesome!"; *thumbs up* with "Good idea!"; and *pat on back* with "That's interesting" (p. 30).

As Donahue and Bryan (1984) pointed out, not all peer interactions are equally appealing to adults. Normal social interactions among peers may include ritualized insults and dispute behavior as well as other kinds of exchanges. Although adults may not wish to encourage children's disputes because they seem to be mostly negative, learning to argue fairly and effectively can have positive outcomes and is part of achieving adult communicative competence.

Brenneis and Lein (1977) studied arguments among children in third- and fourth-grade classrooms who were all white, primarily middle class, and normally developing. The researchers categorized the content of 70 role plays of verbal arguments and found that a limited set of categories accounted for virtually all assertions or responses made by the children in disputes (see Box 9.10).

Although the examples in Box 9.10 are probably familiar to anyone who remembers childhood, such categories appear rarely if ever in assessment protocols, formal or informal. They serve here as reminders to consider the range of contexts in which children need to participate and the varied skills they need to become competent communicators. Other behaviors of interest that Brenneis and Lein (1977) identified were the overt labeling of some speech acts, such as threats and insults, by participants (e.g., "Don't you threaten me"). This metapragmatic awareness might also be encouraged through direct modeling and role play. Children with disabilities could be taught to identify and to participate as more competitive partners in dispute discourse if they learn how to recognize it and label it, as well as how to use appropriate language and speech acts to participate.

Another form of peer interaction discourse that is not often sanctioned by adults, but which may be a rich context for learning to communicate through writing, is surreptitious passing of social notes (Lindfors, 1987; N. W. Nelson, 1988c). In Personal Reflection 9.17, Lindfors considers the rationale for discouraging the passing of social notes and recommends encouraging them (unless removing the forbidden aspect of the process lessens its desirability for children and adolescents, in which case it should just be ignored).

Box 9.10   Content categories observed in the verbal arguments of third- and fourth-graders (summarized from Brenneis & Lein, 1977, pp. 51–53):

1. Threats: "I'll kill you." "I'm going to tell the teacher on you."
1'. Bribes: "I'll give you a dollar if you can." "I'll give it right back to you."
2. Insults: "You dummy." "Your shirt is filthy."
2'. Praise: "You are smart." "You sure look pretty today."
3. Command: "Give it back." "Don't say that."
3'. Moral persuasion: "I had it first." "It's my brother's."
4. Negating or contradictory assertion: JULIE: "I'm the strongest."
                                        JOHN: "*I'm* the strongest."
4'. Simple assertion: "That's my shirt you're wearing." "I'm so strong I can lift you up."
5. Denial response: "No, you can't." "Unh-unh."
5'. Affirmative (often delivered ironically): "Yes." "Yes, I want it."
6. Supportive assertion: (It's mine) "Because I bought it." (I'm stronger) "Because I'm bigger than you."
6'. Demand for evidence: "Prove it." "How do you know?" "I bet you can't."
7. Nonword vocal signals: "Nyeeh-nyeeh." "Aaaargh."

Lindfors described the kind of rich communicative interactions in notes that she had been privileged to read, including a series of lengthy personal Eskimo-style ritual insults that the teacher had taught them. Do children with disabilities have the same kinds of opportunities for learning through written conversational exchanges where no red pencil is expected? If not, can we facilitate similar opportunities without spoiling their essence? It is worth a try.

Conversing in families. The quality of conversational contexts within and across families of children with disabilities is no more uniform than it is for any of us. Family's conversations are influenced by the age and gender relationships of participants, power and autonomy concerns, topics being discussed, the family's cultural history, and a thousand other variables.

Regardless of variability (and perhaps because of it), family conversations may provide a fruitful context for fostering later language learning. Intervention strategies for using family conversations might be two-pronged. Family conversations could help children acquire some of the middle-stage foundation skills they might have missed during therapeutic practice sessions (see discussion in Chapter 8 of conversational interaction strategies). They also could help parents acquire more deliberate scaffolding skills to ensure that their child participates actively in the conversation.

Personal Reflection 9.17   "To me, one of the most intriguing types of personal writing that children seem to engage in so naturally is note passing. I find it interesting that we try so hard to stamp out this activity that is written personal communication at its very best! That it is so resistant to our stamping out efforts should tell us how meaningful this activity is to our children. Note passing is alive and well—thriving—in most of the classrooms I visit. And it should be! It involves everything we would ask of a communication experience; it is purposeful and relevant communication for the child; it is language used for a valid function (personal); it receives relevant and immediate feedback in the response of the receiver. Why, then, do we pounce with such zeal on the note being passed from hand to hand under the desks and across the aisles?"

From Judith Wells Lindfors, *Children's Language and Learning,* Second Edition. Copyright © 1987. Reprinted with permission of Allyn and Bacon.

An example of suggestions for modifying family conversational contexts comes from research by Bodner-Johnson (1991). She studied 10 families, each of which included one deaf child between the ages of 10 and 12.75 years. All of the children had prelingual unaided hearing losses exceeding 70 dB in the range of 250 to 2,000 Hz in the better ear and no other disability. The hearing parents and siblings of these youngsters used either a simultaneous method of signed and oral communication (four families) or oral–aural communication only (six families). Bodner-Johnson videotaped the families at home during their evening meals and found that deaf children were responsive participants in their families' dinner-table conversations. However, the deaf children participated significantly more often when the family member focused the topic with a two-question scaffold, such as "Did you like it? Did you like the street?" (p. 507). When the family asked *wh-* questions, children's responses tended to be more complex and elaborated, for example, "What was the favorite thing you did on the trip? Did you ride the roller coaster?" (p. 507). Although these deaf children tended to respond following sequences of two questions in family conversations, they were less responsive following a barrage of questions. Compared with their

family, they were also more responsive and less likely to initiate topics of their own or to contribute to the development of ideas or topics suggested by other family members. Bodner-Johnson interpreted the results as having practical implications for teachers and families of deaf children. (see Box 9.11).

Understanding and Telling Stories: The Narrative Genre

Previously (here and in Chapters 7 and 8), narrative discourse was emphasized as an important language learning context, relevant across the age span from infancy through adolescence. Milosky (1987) summarized the processing demands of narrative discourse:

> When narrating, the child must recall and organize content, take into account the listener by determining shared background, formulate new utterances, relate them to what has already been said, and introduce referents and distinguish unambiguously among them in subsequent utterances. The need to balance all these demands makes narration cognitively demanding and requires extensive mental resources. (p. 331)

As they enter the later stages of language development, normally developing children exhibit qualitative advances in their stories. In particular, "the sense of a plotted story becomes increasingly clear after the age

---

Box 9.11   **Suggestions for encouraging participation of children who are deaf in the conversations of their families**

❑ Conversation is a functional mechanism for facilitating the deaf child's access to an important aspect of family life. Families have their child's attention during dinnertime conversation. Children are at the ready for participation. Parents should make the most of that initiative by being responsive receptors, by paying attention to the flow of conversation, and by expressing interest and having fun.

❑ Mine the possibilities of questions but don't let go of a good idea. Questions seem to invite the greatest participation for the child—perhaps because their structure makes meaning clearer and, therefore, easier to respond to. Families should be encouraged to be their own researchers and observe how their children respond to comments/ideas they make versus questions they ask. Perhaps family members should rephrase or simplify the language of these comments to be sure the deaf child is understanding the content. The goal is to engage the child into more conversation on the same topic.

❑ "Mix it up" so that questions and ideas are integrated more evenly in conversation. The best strategy for encouraging participation in family conversation is to avoid a high rate of questioning relative to other conversation moves. Questions strung together seem to have a cumulative effect that diminishes the child's participation. (p. 508)

Note. From "Family Conversation Style: Its Effect on the Deaf Child's Participation" by B. Bodner-Johnson, *Exceptional Children, 57,* 1991, p. 508. Copyright 1991 by The Council for Exceptional Children. Reprinted with permission.

of 8 years" (Sutton-Smith, 1986, p. 9), and mature narratives with multiple embedded episodes emerge in normal development at around 11 to 12 years of age (Botvin & Sutton-Smith, 1977). Older story tellers

> have all the verbal devices of turn-taking, argumentation, teasing, rebuttal, introduction, asides, giving back-ground, summaries, morals, scandalous content, evaluations, dramatizations, and prosody to keep their audiences under control and in an appreciative state. When older children tell stories, they have conrol of both management and matter. (p. 9)

Children with language-learning disabilities and other language disorders, however, may not fare as well. Children with learning disabilities, in particular, have been shown in many studies to have difficulty with various aspects of narrative comprehension and production. Garnett (1986) reviewed a series of studies showing that the original stories told by students with learning disabilities had more restricted vocabulary, less complex linguistic patterns, and more immature text construction. Data gathered by Roth and Spekman (1986) for children between the ages of 8 and 14 years confirmed that they were more like younger control subjects in that they tended to tell original stories that had fewer propositions and fewer complete episodes than did older and normally achieving students.

As Garnett's (1986) review showed, students with learning disabilities also tend to leave out key information about things such as settings (time, place, and characters) and endings when they retell stories. They often fail to use syntactic connectors to mark temporal and causal relations explicitly; they tend to produce sequencing errors; they are more likely to use a descriptive format tied to pictures; and they often have difficulty rephrasing when listeners fail to understand. When asked comprehension questions about stories, children with learning disabilities tend to have particular difficulty making use of cohesive ties that organize discourse and direct its flow. They are more likely to have difficultly identifying pronoun antecedents embedded in simple short paragraphs than their peers (Garnett, 1986).

Children with hearing impairments perhaps have even greater difficulty with the narrative genre. Yoshinaga-Itano and Downey (1986) attributed a major portion of the difficulty to the limiting effects of severe hearing loss on incidental hearing, experiences that enable children to gain a wide variety of language-based schema knowledge about the world.

Components of stories that are not heard are missed, and then, a "child either fills in the gaps by making appropriate or inappropriate inferences, or simply stores incomplete information" (p. 47). As a result, hearing impaired children often have underdeveloped concepts and verbal labels for those concepts. They also seem to have difficulty grasping the idea that scripts can be embedded within scripts and concepts within concepts. When they write stories, they tend to write primarily descriptive, immature sequence stories.

On the other hand, the basic concept of narrative structure seems to be relatively resistant to disruption across disorder types. Even in the studies reviewed by Garnett (1986) for children with learning disabilities, the findings regarding narrative structure tended to be subtle. Garnett concluded that there seemed to be "no pervasive lack in these children's understanding of simple narratives" (p. 52). The narrative genre, because of its basis in universal human experience, may be a particularly appropriate context for language intervention with children with varied needs. As Heath (1986) pointed out, different cultures emphasize different subtypes and structures of narrative genre, but "the fundamental genres in every socio-cultural group are narratives that capture verbally remembered or projected experiences" (p. 87).

Preliminary data suggest that the narrative genre may be a particularly useful intervention context for older children and adolescents with traumatic brain injury because of its relative resistance to the negative effects of brain damage. F. M. Jordan, Murdoch, and Buttsworth (1991) studied two groups of children in Australia who had been injured in accidents and were matched at age (8 to 16 years), sex (11 boys and 9 girls each), and socioeconomic status. One group of children had experienced closed head injuries in their accidents and the other had not. Jordan et al. examined both story grammar and inter-sentential cohesion by giving the children and adolescents a GI Joe figure and asking them to "tell me a story about this man—the sort of story you might write if you had to write a story for school; it can be a short story or as long as you like" (p. 575). Even though the head-injured children had previously performed differently from their matched controls on standard measures of language, their story grammar and text cohesion skills did not differ significantly on the narrative measures.

Many of the first intervention programs designed for children and adolescents with traumatic brain injuries were aimed at remediation of isolated perceptual and memory deficits. Focusing treatment instead on an area of integrated language and cognitive processing may be the most appropriate intervention for facilitating movement beyond the initial stages of confusion and fragmentation following brain injury (Ylvisaker, 1985).

For intervention directed at using narrative discourse strengths or at improving narrative comprehension and construction, where appropriate, adult facilitators must thoroughly and explicitly understand narrative structure and cohesion and the contexts in which narratives are normally found (R. C. Anderson, 1985; Botvin & Sutton-Smith, 1977; Bransford & Johnson, 1972; Halliday & Hasan, 1976; Mandler & Johnson, 1977; Rumelhart, 1975; Stein & Glenn, 1979; van Dijk & Kintsch, 1978). In the model of complex language processing that appears in Figure 9.1, the major subcomponents that contribute to the discourse knowledge module are (1) scripts, including nonlinguistic event knowledge whose predictability contributes to discourse knowledge as a form of shared experience; (2) story grammars (Stein & Glenn, 1979) and other ways of representing narrative text organizational maturity (Applebee, 1978); (3) text cohesive devices, including knowledge of both grammatical and semantic strategies (Halliday & Hasan, 1976) for building transitions and representing relationships among elements of texts (e.g., redundant, contrastive, or illustrative relationships); and (4) formats, including such variations as dramatic narratives in the form of plays and other subcategories, such as narrative jokes, science fiction stories, or murder mysteries. The question that remains is whether students also need explicit metatextual knowledge of scripts, story grammar, text cohesion, and formats to become competent adult language processors.

The essence of the argument that students need explicit knowledge is that individuals who can activate predictions to replay certain familiar scripts may be able to use those predictions to help them comprehend and produce texts structured similarly. Some of the advantages of encouraging individuals to use metacognitive awareness of text organization strategies were considered in the previous discussion of metaskills and executive control strategies. Familiarity with narrative structure through exposure to many stories with clear narrative elements may help prepare individuals to adopt such strategies (Page & Stewart, 1985). Quality literature for children and ado

lescents, rather than "controlled language" books and stories, may be particularly effective to help children "respond cognitively and aesthetically to the stories they hear and read" (Van Dongen & Westby, 1986, p. 80). Children may also be able to learn more about narrative structure by writing and acting in plays (Milosky, 1987), where plot and character motivations are central.

Once individuals are familiar with narrative structure through repeated exposure in different contexts, they can practice making predictions and drawing inferences about characters, motivations, and events, based on a combination of world knowledge, discourse knowledge, and information gleaned from reading or hearing the initial parts of stories. Page and Stewart (1985) suggested a variety of techniques for helping students develop prediction abilities. One frequently used technique involves having students sequence parts of a scrambled story. Depending on reading level, students may use cut-apart paragraphs or pictures to complete this task. Milosky (1987) cautioned, however, that commercially available picture sequencing sets might be confusing to children because the sequences they depict are somewhat arbitrary and do not necessarily depict real cause–effect relationships driven by problem-solving efforts of characters with clear motivations (e.g., what does it matter whether a child washes his face or brushes his teeth first). If children do need extra assistance to recognize narrative structure, other techniques involve "story frames" (Stewart, 1985) that provide fill-in tasks about story topics, main characters, motivating problems, first attempts, subsequent attempts, and problem resolutions. A story frame might include items such as "This story is about _____," and "The problem is solved when _____" (p. 351). Such structures and other "macrocloze" (fill-in-the-blank) techniques help children with language disorders focus on aspects of narratives they may not recognize on their own.

Many researchers have investigated instructional strategies that involve explicit instruction regarding story grammar structure. Stewart (1985), for example, recommended teaching children to use simplified outlines of story grammar elements (including, setting, problem, response, and outcome) to help them organize their internalized schemas for reading and writing stories. B. L. Miller (1988) taught a group of severely to profoundly hearing impaired adolescents the five parts of a "complete story." She taught the component labels *setting, problem, action, outcome,* and *ending.* She also taught that "*feelings* make a story interesting." Miller illustrated these components by displaying model personal narratives she had written with an overhead projector so groups of six or seven students could read and discuss them. The students used color-coded marking pens to identify parts of stories, using Miller's model stories (sometimes with key components deliberately omitted), stories they wrote themselves, and stories written by their peers. A matched control group spent the same amounts of time with Miller, learning about indefinite pronouns and noun modifiers and practicing written language only at the sentence level. The experimental group made greater improvement from pre- to post-test in the maturity of their written narratives than did the control group. The experimental group also was able to use "metatextual" strategies to tell a friend how to write a story, whereas the control group tended to respond to the directions more directly, simply by writing about a friend.

Montague, Graves, and Leavell (1991) designed a similar program to teach junior high students with learning disabilities to write more mature narratives by providing them with a "story grammar cue card." When Montague et al. gave students with learning disabilities cue cards to structure their writing, along with sufficient planning time, the students wrote stories that did not differ along quantitative or qualitative measures when compared with stories of normally achieving students. When extra time and structure were not provided, the learning disabled students' stories were not as sophisticated.

Not only structure but other elements of narrative discourse may be drawn to the conscious attention of later stage language learners. B. L. Miller (1988) taught her students to pay attention to feelings expressed in the stories they read and wrote. Westby (1985/1991) emphasized that discussions of narrative texts provide opportunities not only to build comprehension of factual elements but also to consider the feelings and motivations of characters. Lahey (1988) also reminded professionals of the need to help students appreciate uses of narratives to entertain.

An intervention program that uses narrative discourse as one context for targeting language change should encourage alive, shared, and communicative narratives. Children mostly need multiple opportunities to read, write, act out, and talk about stories. They need to work with interesting and entertaining

stories, not sterile stories constructed to illustrate some grammatical feature, graphophonemic pattern, controlled set of vocabulary, or in response to a particular "story starter." As Hoskins (1990) commented (in Personal Reflection 9.15), "in our interactions in language, we are constantly developing the narratives that comprise who we are, how we think of ourselves, and how we present ourselves to others." (1990, p. 60). This is not the same as completing exercises to please a teacher or a clinician.

Getting and Giving Information: The Expository Genre

A summary of research on comprehension of expository texts by Slater and Graves (1989) showed that students (1) increasingly develop their ability to use expository text structure to facilitate comprehension and recall from fourth grade through college; (2) remember more of what they read when they can identify and use text structures; (3) generally retain main ideas better than lower level ideas from expository texts; (4) can be taught to identify expository text structure and main ideas; (5) can benefit from training in the use of text structures and main ideas to improve reading comprehension; and (6) are particularly disadvantaged when they fail to use expository text structure to comprehend if the topic is unfamiliar.

When children and adolescents have difficulty handling the processing demands of expository texts, the problem may appear in several different classroom events. From at least third grade on, children are expected to spend considerable time reading, understanding, and recalling key facts from expository texts. They are also expected to discuss, describe, define, and use other expository discourse strategies to talk about ideas in the whole class, small group, and individual learning, studying, and testing environments. As they listen to lectures, complete daily assignments, and prepare for tests, students might take notes from spoken lectures and from written work on the chalkboard. They might also review, outline, highlight, and answer factual and discussion questions from their textbooks. They may be expected to write expository texts of their own, doing research from multiple sources, and organizing information in an expository text format appropriate for the topic and purpose. Many of these activities require complex language and information processing strategies simultaneously on multiple levels, guided by an executive system to decide which questions to ask and strategies to use to understand the text, remember important parts, and recall them.

Identifying expository text structures to assist comprehension.   Several authors recommend starting intervention for expository text problems by ensuring that individuals with problems can recognize different discourse structures, beginning with narrative structure (N. W. Nelson, 1988b; Scott, 1988a; Wallach, 1990; Westby 1985/1991, 1988). Then students may be taught to contrast narrative and expository structures. Those who have difficulty grasping the distinctions might be shown examples of their favorite narrative stories rewritten as expository texts (see Piccolo, 1987, for examples). When content is held relatively constant, some students may more easily recognize variations in form and talk about how different structures might be used for different purposes. Eventually, students might learn to recognize and diagram different expository discourse structures (e.g., those shown earlier in this chapter, Figure 9.4) and talk about why an author might have chosen to write in a particular style (Wallach & Miller, 1988).

Many researchers have demonstrated that reading comprehension improves when students learn to recognize text organizational structures (B. M. Taylor & Beach, 1984). Bos and Anders (1990) taught students with learning disabilities to build graphic representational "maps" of expository text structures and then to enter specific ideas from the text onto the text structure maps. P. L. Smith and Friend (1986) showed that training learning disabled adolescents to use a text structure-recognition strategy improved the students' ability both to recognize the structures and to recall instructional content, an effect that remained stable over at least 1 week.

Wallach (1990) pointed out that sensitivity to text structure is a skill that develops in interaction with other abilities and with demands of a particular text from the late elementary years through high school. Older students have advantages over younger ones because of their greater familiarity with how textbooks are usually structured and because of their accumulated world knowledge and greater experience learning certain subject matter. Being able to "read better" involves more than just having better decoding and word-recognition skills.

If the textbooks in the students' curriculum are not written with explicit structure, and if the student has difficulty inferring the structure without assistance,

the adult's job is not to rewrite the textbooks (although, sitting on curriculum committees and influencing textbook selection decisions is not a bad long-term idea). Rather, the facilitator's job is to help frame the existing cues so that the student can recognize them as independently as possible, to arrange opportunities to practice the strategies with scaffolding support, then systematically to withdraw that support until the student can use the strategies independently in the regular classroom.

Identifying key words and other text cohesion devices.   Westby (1991) pointed out that the framing and focusing process should help students recognize key words that may cue them to recognize different kinds of expository text. Key words in the form of conjunctions and logical connectors serve as one type of syntactic–semantic text cohesion device, which along with others such as pronoun reference, are particularly difficult for children with developmental language disorders (Liles, 1985; Norris & Bruning, 1988). Westby's summary of particular text functions, key words, and formats for testing for six types of expository text appears in Table 9.10.

Part of the curriculum-based language assessment and intervention process for students having difficulty with expository texts may be to focus students on key words and to make sure students comprehend their meaning. The specialist can do this by giving students experience in noticing such words and highlighting them when they appear in texts. Another is to teach students to use similar words and structures to write their own expository texts for similar purposes.

Writing expository texts.   Expository text writing assignments should come fairly early in the educational or intervention process. Calkins (1983) provided an example of expository text written by a 5-year-old about how to make a robot in a kindergarten classroom that encouraged such writing. Several of the boy's steps, shown with his own invented spellings, follow:

1. get a hed
2. atuch one liot
3. atach the athr liot
4. get the boty
13. put a sekrt hand in the boty (p.11)

Children with language-learning disabilities should be given similar opportunities to write expository texts early in their educational experiences, and they

TABLE 9.10
Guide for monitoring expository texts

Text Pattern	Text Function	Key Words	Test Formats
Description	The text tells what something is	is called, can be defined as, is, can be interpreted as, is explained as, refers to, is a procedure for, is someone who, means	Define . . . Describe . . . List the features of . . . What is . . . Who is . . .
Collection/ enumeration	The text gives a list of things that are related to the topic	an example is, for instance, another, next, finally, such as, to illustrate	Give examples of . . . What is . . . and give some examples
Sequence/ procedure	The text tells what happened or how to do something or make something	first, next, then, second, third, following this step, finally, subsequently, from here . . . to, eventually, before, after	Give the steps in doing . . . When did . . . occur?
Comparison/ contrast	The text shows how two things are the same or different	different, same, alike, similar, although, however, on the other hand, contrasted with, compared to, rather than, but, yet, still, instead of	Compare and contrast . . . and . . . How are . . . and . . . alike and different
Cause/effect explanation	The text gives reasons for why something happened	because, since, reasons, then, therefore, for this reason, results, effects, consequently, so, in order to, thus, depends on, influences, is a function of, produces, leads to, affects, hence	Explain . . . Explain the cause(s) of . . . Explain the effect(s) of . . . Predict what will happen . . . Why did . . . happen? How did . . . happen? What are the causes (reasons for, effects, results, etc) of . . .?
Problem/solution	The text states a problem and offers solutions to the problem	a problem is, a solution is	Describe the development of the problem and the solutions. What are the solutions to the problem . . .?

Note. From *Steps to Developing and Achieving Language-Based Curriculum in the Classroom* (p. 12) by C. E. Westby, 1991, Rockville, MD, American Speech-Language-Hearing Association. Copyright 1991 by C. E. Westby. Reprinted by permission.

should be given similar latitude in meeting writing conventions. As students mature into the later stages of development, they may benefit from explicit instruction in organizing their own writing that parallels their instruction in analyzing the macrostructures of texts that they read. In turn, the explicit instruction and practice in writing expository texts may make it easier for students to recognize similar structuring strategies used by other authors.

Englert and Raphael (1988) noted that successful writers seem to engage in both task-specific strategies and executive control functions simultaneously. Task-specific strategies include planning, monitoring, and revising, while carefully considering the needs

and questions of the audience, using awareness of text structure to serve as a map to decide what information to include and what signals to use to indicate the relationships among various elements of the texts (e.g., cohesive devices, such as *in contrast to, but, like, different*). Executive functions used during expository discourse writing include implementing, monitoring, and sustaining various subprocesses, including the ability to self-instruct or to ask oneself questions, considering and choosing among various strategies and subprocesses, monitoring performance, and making modifications or corrections as necessary. To teach students to develop skills at both levels, Englert and Raphael advocated a dialogic approach (referred to here as *mediational teaching*, or *scaffolding*) that included teacher modeling and the use of a series of "think sheets" to organize ideas. For example, students might use a series of four different think sheets for four different stages of the writing process:

STAGE ONE. *Plan think sheet* with categories and questions such as

> Focus on audience—Who am I writing this for?
>
> Purpose—Why am I writing this?
>
> Background knowledge—What do I know about my topic?
>
> Organization—How can I organize my brainstormed or collected ideas?

STAGE TWO. *Organize think sheet* with categories and questions that change according to the type of text structure composed. For example, if a sequential–procedural text structure is being taught, the think sheet might ask

> What is being explained?
>
> What are the materials you need?
>
> What are the steps?
>
> What do you do first, second, next, then, etc.?

STAGE THREE. *Self-edit think sheet* with guides to focus students on both the content and structure of their work:

> First, star the parts I like best and put a question mark by something my readers might not understand.
>
> Then, check whether I answered the text structure questions (rate this *yes, no,* or *maybe*); for example, Did I tell . . . what is being explained? . . . what materials are needed? . . . the steps? . . . what you do first, next, etc.?

STAGE FOUR. *Editor think sheet* to be completed by a peer editor with the same categories on it as on the *self-edit think sheet*. Following its completion, the peer editor and author compare and discuss their observations, and revisions are made as needed.

Note taking, summarizing, and studying. Interactions among the language modalities—listening, speaking, reading, writing, and thinking—have been emphasized throughout this book. Nowhere is that relationship more apparent than in activities involving expository texts in classrooms. Learning to read and write expository texts involves opportunities to talk about expository texts, to ask and answer questions about them, and to take notes from written and oral presentations.

Williams (1988) pointed out that learning to abstract important points from larger units of text is a developmental skill that rests heavily on the ability to categorize. Development data gathered by A. L. Brown and Day (1983) showed that text-summarizing rules are acquired over the years from fifth grade to college in the sequence (1) delete unimportant information, (2) delete redundant information, (3) substitute category names for lists, (4) select a topic sentence from the text, and (5) invent a topic sentence. Fifth graders could use only the delete strategy, and college students were differentiated from expert writers in their abilities to use the invention rule.

Teaching students to take notes from material they read and hear involves helping them to make categorical decisions quickly and to build hierarchical and sequencing maps of important information for review, study, and recall on tests. This intervention relies heavily on information processing theories of language acquisition. Suritsky and Hughes (1991) pointed out that most studies of note taking ability have been conducted with nondisabled college students as subjects and that most were designed to test one of two theories. The level of processing theory (F.I. Craik & Lockhart, 1972) is based on the idea that information retention is a function of the depth of cognitive processing applied to the input stimulus. The information processing memory model (Ladas, 1980) suggests that the preparation of information for long-term memory storage involves a series of processing steps: (1) giving attention in response to orienting stimuli; (2) using search and associate behaviors, such as differentiating relevant from irrelevant information and associating incoming lecture information with previous knowledge (this process may fail if the student possesses insufficient prerequisite knowledge); (3) coding the information, for example, by using shorthand notes, mnemonic devices, and varied levels of headings to represent superordinate and subordinate information; and (4) deliberately deciding which information to place in long-term storage in preparation for a test.

Intervention for note-taking problems may target changes in behavior of both lecturers and listeners.

Through consultation, the language specialist may encourage lecturers to use strong orienting cues that a new topic is being introduced, to use strategically placed pauses to help students group together related pieces of information and to give them additional processing time at regular intervals, to write key words and to list outline headers and major subpoints on the chalkboard, and to review and summarize periodically. The professional might teach listeners to write down main points using abbreviations and other coding strategies, rather than to attempt verbatim encoding of the lecture, and, if possible, to paraphrase key points to ensure deeper cognitive processing of information. Because of their significantly slower "tool rates" (i.e., number of letters written per minute), most students with learning disabilities also need to learn to use shorthand abbreviations and symbols as primary strategies (Suritsky & Hughes, 1991).

Larson and McKinley (1987) noted that many adolescents with language disorders and learning disabilities, because of their slowness and other deficits, may also need compensatory support to compete in regular classroom settings. For example, lecturers might provide main points of lectures on preprinted "listening guides," to take some of the pressure off note taking. Students might use a "buddy system" to gain access to notes taken by a classmate who is a particularly proficient note taker, by using machine, carbon, or hand copying. My experience with the note-sharing approach at the university level suggests that the student with the disability still should be required to take some notes "on-line." Otherwise, the student may too easily assume a passive listening posture in the classroom, knowing that he or she will get the notes later. This observation is consistent with the research review by Suritsky and Hughes (1991) that showed that "students who record notes during lectures benefit more from the lectures than students who simply listen" (p.14).

Tape recording of classroom lectures has often been suggested for helping students with learning disabilities compensate for listening and note-taking deficits. Tape-recorded lectures are not automatically helpful, however, primarily because listening to taped lectures takes time, and time is often already a problem for students with learning disabilities. Some teachers also may object to having to having their lectures recorded, although the right to listen to tape-recorded lectures may be interpreted as a reasonable accommodation that must be made for a student with learning disabilities under Section 504 (Larson &

McKinley, 1987) (see Chapter 5 for a discussion of Section 504).

Note taking and review sheets may be constructed from analysis and review of tape-recorded lectures and written texts. Special arrangements may need to be made to allow students with learning disabilities to highlight key points in school textbooks as they read (not allowed for many regular education students in public schools). Again, however, students may need direct instruction to learn how to select pieces of text to highlight or underline as they read. Otherwise, they are likely to highlight everything! Larson and McKinley (1987) suggested that students might highlight main ideas in yellow, relevant details in blue, and new vocabulary words in green. They also recommended that teachers and clinicians should collaborate to decide on one color-coding system so as not to confuse students and that early highlighting might be done by teachers in the students' books so that students will have their own teachers' models for identifying what is important. Williams (1988) reviewed several studies in which students were given explicit instruction and practice to identify important points, using a variety of strategies, including rules for summarizing, and strategies for circling main topics and underlining details. All of the studies yielded some success in helping students to recognize main ideas and become more attentive to details (see Figure 9.5 for a set of objectives from N.W. Nelson, 1988b, for guiding intervention in this area).

In the first chapter of this book and previously in this chapter, I identified questions as having a key function in orienting attention and higher order thinking skills. Knapczyk (1991) designed an intervention strategy to teach three ninth-grade students with learning disabilities better strategies for asking and answering questions in their regular education world geography class. The instructional program started with a series of sessions in the controlled environment of the resource room before moving into the regular classroom. From the beginning, however, the regular curriculum (in the form of videotape-recorded class sessions) provided the content for the intervention sessions. Knapczyk organized sessions for learning to ask questions as follows:

SESSION ONE. The student and resource teacher viewed the videotape together. The student was asked to identify places where he did not understand what the teacher said, was unclear about what was being asked, or was unfamiliar with the

FIGURE 9.5
A sequence of objectives for targeting note-taking ability.

WRITTEN LANGUAGE: LATER STAGES

Date: _____

PART C. EXPOSITORY TEXTS

CHILD: _____

OBJ WL2

SHORT-TERM OBJECTIVES:

THE CHILD WILL:

	INTERVENTION SETTING							COMMENTS/ TECHNIQUES/ EVALUATION
	INDIVIDUAL THERAPY		MINICLASSROOM		CLASSROOM			
	Date In.	Date Accom.	Date In.	Date Accom.	Date In.	Date Accom.		
1. listen and take notes from expository lectures, showing the ability to detect organization and major points by using a variety of strategies adapted to lecture style, time available, familiarity with topic, and related variables, and the ability to use the notes for studying in order to answer test questions based on the lecture (notes should match major content of notes taken on the same lecture by a highly competent learner [such as the speech–language pathologist or a successful fellow classmate] and a passing percentage of questions based on the lecture must be answered correctly for 3 lectures in each target setting):								
a. by using listening skills, to abstract major points and organizational relationships in notes taken during the lecture;								
b. by developing and practicing a set of abbreviations and symbols for particular classes that the student can recognize and expand later;								
c. by recopying notes in a neater form, cleaning up their organization and detail in the process, asking clarification questions of fellow students or teacher as needed and appropriate, to make the notes complete;								
d. by referring to related written texts to fill in missing information, and to check spellings of key words;								
e. by referring to an audiotape of the lecture (if available) to check notes for completeness and accuracy;								
f. by using a highlighter pen or other color-coding strategy to box off information the teacher might emphasize on a test;								
g. by using the notes to ask a peer (or someone role-playing a peer) possible test questions, and to answer them, in a group study atmosphere;								
h. by taking an actual or contrived written test on material covered in the lecture.								

Note. From *Planning Individualized Speech and Language Intervention Programs* (2nd ed., p. 368) by N .W. Nelson, 1988, Tucson AZ: Communication Skill Builders. Copyright 1988 by Communication Skill Builders, Inc. Reprinted by permission.

information being discussed. At that point, the tape was stopped and the student was directed to ask a question that met these criteria:

1. Timed at a natural break where it is appropriate to ask questions, or
2. Timed following a teacher prompt that it is appropriate to ask questions
3. Formulated to solicit the desired information
4. Formulated to be relevant to the lesson content

The resource teacher stopped the tape at several points and asked whether the student had any questions. Appropriately timed and formulated questions were reinforced. If problems arose, parts of the tape were replayed to demonstrate examples of appropriate performance.

SESSION TWO. The same tape was viewed again. The student was directed to stop the tape when appropriate and ask the clarification question, which the resource teacher answered.

SESSIONS THREE, FOUR, FIVE. Additional practice was provided using different taped lectures, with feedback about performance and additional demonstration as necessary.

LAST 2 DAYS OF TRAINING. These sessions consisted of regular classroom interactions. Before going into the classroom, students met with the resource teacher, who reviewed with them the major elements of asking questions. (In the research study, the teacher was not aware that the students had been working on question asking and answering.)

Knapczyk (1991) organized sessions for learning to answer questions using a similar format but asked students to

(a) identify points in class activities where the teacher asked questions of the students, (b) repeat or paraphrase the question that was asked, (c) formulate an answer to the questions, (d) attend to examples of how other students recited answers, and (e) evaluate his and the other students' performance. (p. 78)

Knapczyk (1991) reported positive results both in terms of numbers of questions asked and answered appropriately and in increased accuracy on assigned seat-work activities.

Combining strategies for complex multimodality processing. The final approach reviewed in this section combines many of the techniques discussed previously. It involves using aspects of the procedure called "reciprocal teaching," in which students take turns acting as teachers to guide their own learning and that of their peers. In original descriptions, during reciprocal teaching (Palincsar & Brown, 1984) students lead discussions about short sections of texts using the four strategies *predicting, questioning, clarifying,* and *summarizing.*

As developed further by Englert and Mariage (1991), the approach is combined with text structure mapping and note-taking strategies. Englert and Mariage used the mnemonic acronym, POSSE, to represent the text processing steps predict, organize, search, summarize, and evaluate. The researchers worked with fourth-, fifth-, and sixth-grade students with learning disabilities and their teachers. As part of the intervention, the teachers modeled the strategies and then selected a student leader to guide aspects of the POSSE sequence. Student leaders were provided cue cards to help them know what to ask, for example:

PREDICT. Students learned to activate background knowledge by attending to cues in titles, headings, pictures, and initial paragraphs, prompting each other:

"I predict that. . . ." "I'm remembering. . . ."

ORGANIZE. Students learned to brainstorm their ideas into a semantic map, prompting each other:

"I think one category might be. . . ."

SEARCH–SUMMARIZE. Students read short segments of text and looked for text structure and predicted information, prompting each other:

"I think the main idea is. . . ." "My question about the main idea is. . . ."

EVALUATE. Students learned to compare, clarify, and predict what the next section of the text will be about, prompting each other:

"I think we did [did not] predict this main idea [compare]." "Are there any clarifications? [Clarify]" "I predict the next part will be about . . . [predict]."

In the study conducted by Englert and Mariage (1991), teachers continued to participate in the sense-making process even after students began to take turns using the cue cards to guide discussion. Teachers facilitated and scaffolded the discussions and decided which of and how the students' comments would be written in the group summary (see Figure 9.6), but gradually they turned over as much control to the students as possible.

Summary

This section presented a variety of strategies for using language to participate in different kinds of discourse—conversational, narrative, and expository. You have probably noticed that the discussions of this section have overlapped considerably with those of earlier sections in their joint focus on modifying the learning context, using mediational teaching approaches, and developing learning strategies and metaskills for processing different aspects of communicative events. That is no accident. These are com-

mon themes among many varieties of intervention systems used with later language learners.

ENCOURAGING LATER STAGE SYNTACTIC–SEMANTIC DEVELOPMENTS

Most later stage learners with language disorders need fairly direct instruction to acquire strategies to manage information and direct their own thinking and learning processes. Some later stage language learners also may be struggling excessively with both oral and written syntactic construction and comprehension. These students may need intervention that focuses specifically on complex syntactic structures and on syntactic–semantic strategies for comprehending and producing elements of text cohesion.

FIGURE 9.6
Partially completed POSSE strategy sheet.

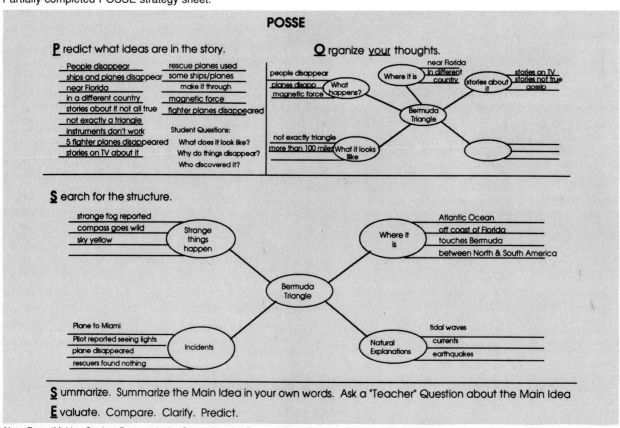

Note. From "Making Student Partners in the Comprehension Process: Organizing the Reading 'POSSE' by C. S. Englert and T. V. Mariage, 1991, *Learning Disability Quarterly, 14,* p.129. Copyright 1991 by The Council for Learning Disabilities. Reprinted by permission.

Problems of Later Stage Syntactic Development

Klecan-Aker (1985) reviewed the research on the syntactic abilities of school-age children with language disorders. A summary of those findings includes evidence that (1) the syntactic abilities of adolescents with language-learning disabilities may plateau at levels expected for 5- or 6-year-olds; (2) children with language disorders are less proficient in paraphrasing sentences than their normally developing peers, often repeating stimulus sentences rather than paraphrasing them; (3) children with language disorders are less proficient in using rules of linguistic cohesion; and (4) the linguistic cohesion problems they exhibit are characterized by a lower frequency of subordinating conjunctions (rarely using conjunctions such as *which, after, where,* and *since*) and a higher frequency of ambiguous reference.

Judging Level of Syntactic Development

Several cautions should be observed when making developmental level decisions about later stage needs. Scott (1988c) observed that, although predictable schedules of morphological and syntactic development are established for the preschool years:

> it is much more difficult to construct comparable syntactic schedules for the 9-through-19 age range because the concern now is not with the presence or absence of high-frequency structures, but with the gradual acquisition of low-frequency structures and the ability to form unique combinations of structures. To uncover later syntactic developments, finer grained methods of analysis are needed. (pp. 50–51)

Later stage syntactic developments are measured as changes in written and oral language samples. Individual differences exceed those of children in earlier stages, and the influences of both the immediate context and prior educational experiences must be considered in any quantification efforts. As Rubin (1984) noted, "research aimed at providing developmental descriptions of children's writing abilities must tread cautiously in formulating age-norm generalization that fail to provide for the effects of communicative context" (p. 227).

Appropriate, nontrivial indices of advancing maturity are difficult to identify, in part because some syntactic characteristics of written language samples appear to represent developmental improvements but are not necessarily valid signs of greater language

maturity. For example, Rubin (1984) noted that although composition length often predicts judged quality, under certain circumstances, mature writers employ strategies that reduce verbosity rather than increase it (Rubin, 1982). Similarly, although syntactic complexity has often been used to measure composition quality (C. R. Cooper, 1976), complex syntax may not be appropriate in certain contexts (Crowhurst, 1980), and overly complex syntax may indicate that the writer has not judged the reader's needs. Normal growth in child writers is often accompanied by errors involving both syntactic and semantic rules. As Weaver (1982) noted, when developing writers "start adding to or elaborating their ideas, they may produce fragments consisting of compound or explanatory phrases. And when they begin using a variety of subordinate clauses, they may punctuate some of these as if they were complete sentences" (p. 443). Based on a review of the literature on written language development, Brannon (1985) also concluded that "when writers push toward intellectual complexity in their work, their texts may not demonstrate the formal and technical competence of their previous, less complex texts" (p. 20).

Predicting the difficulty of syntactic structures for individuals in receptive language also is not easy. Bransford and Nitsch (1985) reviewed studies exploring contextual or situational constraints on ease of comprehension and concluded that "the same sentence may differ in ease of comprehension depending on the contextual situations to which it refers" (p. 91). They also commented that "syntactic structure has semantic implications and that syntactic appropriateness is determined relative to the situation in which the sentence is uttered" (p. 91).

Potential Targets and Methods for Later Stage Syntactic Intervention Programs

Syntactic knowledge is closely tied to linguistic strategies for representing meaning. Four subcomponents are represented in the syntactic module of the complex processing model shown in Figure 9.1. Any of these might be targeted in language intervention. They include knowledge of (a) grammatical morphemes (including bound morphemes and function words); (b) sentence structures (e.g., declaratives, questions, passives, imperatives, and negative sentences); (c) sentence combining (including phrasal and clausal embedding and other types of complex and compound sentences); and (d) relations among sentences (including syntactic elements that can be used to build text cohesion). (See Scott's, 1988b, summary of types of complex sentences in Figure 9.7.)

Targeting grammatical morpheme learning in written language. Blank and Bruskin (1982) pointed out that most reading programs have neglected the level of the sentence, focusing on content word identification instead. To overcome the limitations of these approaches, Blank and Bruskin provided suggestions for a sentence-based program of instruction in which equal, but separate, segments of time were devoted to teaching content and noncontent function words,

such as grammatical morphemes and connector words, such as those used to build text cohesion (see Table 9.10 for sets of these suggested by Westby, 1991). Blank and Bruskin taught the structures within the context of a special series of books that allowed them to introduce grammatical elements in a set of controlled, "sensible" sentences.

The problem with "language-controlled" materials (in which language is chosen for its form, rather than for its ability to convey an intended meaning) is that the controlled forms often end up being awkward, uninteresting, or marginally appropriate to a particular

FIGURE 9.7
Structural relationships for categories of English sentence complexity. (Note: Numbers refer to examples of complex sentences on p. 471)

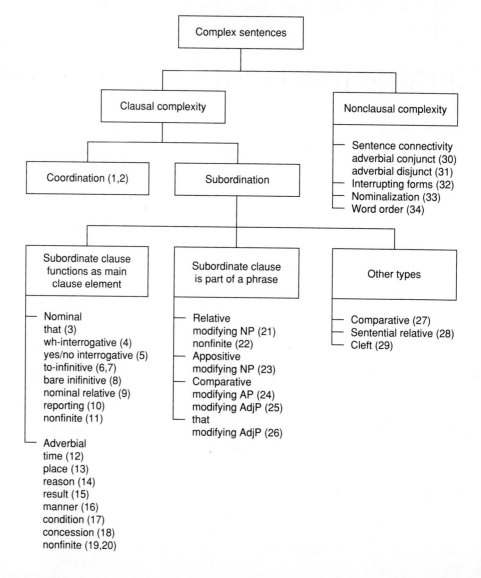

Personal Reflection 9.18

"We need to remember that syntax mirrors the mind at work, wrestling with thought; and we need to expect that students, particularly those with weak backgrounds in reading or little practice in writing, will write many disastrous sentences before writing good ones."

William Strong (1986, pp. 18–19), Utah State University, author of *Creative Approaches to Sentence Combining.*

FIGURE 9.7
continued

1. and then the giant weed grows up *and* knocks out all the windows. (3, p. 29)*
2. she loves soccer *but* hates softball.
3. and he found out that this man was paying the other man for *insurance or something.* (4, p. 22)
4. he didn't know *where the breaks were.* (3, p. 185)
5. and he asked his father *if he could do part pony exchange for a pony with one of the cars.* (3, p. 67)
6. he wanted *to tell his father about it.*
7. so he didn't want *her to come home till another two weeks.* (3, p. 227)
8. and she wouldn't let *anybody buy the house.* (4, p. 110)
9. and the hospital was *where the Zulus were waiting.* (3, p. 38)
10. then this boy goes *there's the brakes.* (3, p. 185)
11. the horse could hear *the boy shouting.* (4, p. 307)
12. *so when he got out* then they gave him the present of the pony. (3, p. 64)
13. they found nothing *wherever they went.*
14. and they couldn't get at him *because there was gates going round.* (3, p. 197)
15. he didn't pay any attention *so she left.*
16. she acts like *my mother did.*
17. *if you can't take me* I'll have to take the bus.
18. she tells good stories *even if sometimes they're too long.*
19. then in the end it was like they just sat there you know *getting everything out of the boat.* (4, p. 158)
20. *having tried the pizza before* they ordered spaghetti this time.
21. and there was this friend *that always brought cookies.*
22. it's this reporter *following the Hulk.* (3, p. 170)
23. and he took this vase thing *it was like an ornament* as proof and these papers from the safe. (4, p. 238)
24. she talks better *than she used to.*
25. you must have been sicker *than I was.*
26. she was sure *it was her lunchbox.*
27. they have more cookies in their house *than we ever did.*
28. the horse just disappeared *which made all the others very sad.*
29. it was in school *that they told him.*
30. I've never had nightmares/not as far as I know *anyway.* (4, p. 89)
31. *personally* I think I'm getting pretty good.
32. Harold *whose army had just marched across England after fighting an invading group of Norwegians back* was tired and sore.
33. the *development* of this beach makes me sick.
34. *there stood* a little tiger cub.

*All sentences referenced with a page number have been taken from the Fawcett and Perkins corpus (1980) of spoken language of children 6 to 12 years.

Note. From "Producing Complex Sentences" by C. M. Scott. Reprinted from *Topics in Language Disorders,* Vol. 8, No. 2, pp. 47, 62, with permission of Aspen Publishers, Inc., © 1988.

context. They may also lead students to develop erroneous ideas about the nature of reading and purposes for reading. "Formula writing" of paragraphs with a certain number of sentences with a specified number of words has similar drawbacks. Further, as suggested throughout this book, using language intervention materials relevant to an individual's needs in other areas (e.g., materials from the classroom curriculum based on zones of significance identified in consultation with teachers and students) usually is preferred.

Targeting syntactic comprehension and production. Some regular educators also have recommended teaching grammar through written materials drawn from children's regular textbook series and writings (Vavra, 1987). For example, the educator might teach prepositions by deleting them from a textbook passage and then asking students to replace them in a cloze procedure exercise. Alternatively, the instructor might ask students to place parentheses around structures such as prepositional phrases in their course texts or to highlight them. Students' own writing might also provide practice material for the acquisition and application of syntactic knowledge. Students might practice adding complexity to their writing by adding prepositional phrases where appropriate, if those forms are consistent with their general purpose.

Individuals with written language syntax problems may also have a history of oral language learning impairment. The comprehensive intervention program then should address problems of both oral and written syntactic knowledge. An advantage of using written language in intervention efforts stems from its relative permanence. Because written sentences are not transient, as oral sentences are, they may be reviewed and revised, which may help students overcome short-term memory deficits that make it difficult for them to monitor their oral syntactic productions. When using regular curricular materials to help students learn to use syntactic knowledge to receive or convey meanings, the instructor may give them practice in paraphrasing to develop fluency and flexibility in syntactic processing. Paraphrasing skill is often necessary to understand the questions at the ends of textbook chapters and to relate them to sections of the text where information for answering questions is found (N. W. Nelson, 1989b).

Moran (1988) suggested an intervention approach for helping students be more productive in their writ-

ing. Moran's approach focused on synthesis rather than analysis of sentences. She encouraged students to acquire new syntactic knowledge by starting with the smallest meaningful unit (the independent clause or proposition) and gradually adding length by expanding T-units (Hunt, 1970), "culminating in alternative arrangements of T-units to form paragraphs according to patterns dictated by expressive, descriptive, narrative, expository, or persuasive purpose" (Moran, 1988, p. 554). Moran's approach thus encouraged the activation of interactions among the various aspects of mature written language processing, with a focus on using syntactic knowledge to serve the construction of meaning.

Moran's (1988) approach starts with small-group discussions, during which writers brainstorm topics, mentioning some person, object, place, or idea that they know. Teachers print the student-generated topics on the left side of a chalkboard or overhead transparency and then guide the students to provide a comment about each. One student gave the comment, "lives next door," to go with the topic, "my friend Gloria." Another produced the comment, "is the best car," to go with the topic, "a Porsche."

In the next step, Moran (1988) helps students to expand the topics and to produce clauses, which aides write on strips of paper without capital letters or end punctuation to mark their boundaries. This allows the students to reorder their sentence elements differently. When they learn to produce a variety of clauses, the students are taught to combine clauses into complex T-units using the set of subordinating terms *because, when,* and *after,* and the relative pronouns, *who, which,* and *that.* Finally, the students learn to generate additional T-units and to arrange them in paragraphs in more than one way, again to help them appreciate the flexibility of being able to say basically the same thing in different ways. Ultimately, the students learn to produce paragraphs with expressive, descriptive, narrative, expository, and persuasive purposes.

Targeting sentence combining and paraphrasing. Sentence-combining strategies, such as those incorporated by Moran (1988) in her approach, are not new. Strong (1986), who is credited with developing many of the modern approaches to sentence-combining exercises, pointed out that the 14th century rhetorician Erasmus "showed how a single sentence could be expressed 150 ways by altering syntax or diction" (p. 3).

Strong (1986) noted that sentence-combining exercises come in a variety of formats, both oral and written, and both "cued" (with a limited set of right answers) and "open" (with more divergent possibilities being accepted). Strong provided the following example of a cued exercise:

Sentence combining is an approach.
The approach is for *teaching*.
Some teachers find it useful. (THAT)
Others regard as it dangerous. (BUT)

This sentence, when combined, would yield "Sentence combining is a teaching approach that some teachers find useful but (that) others regard as dangerous" (p. 5). As an example of an open strategy, Strong provided this:

SC [sentence combining] is a means to an end.
The end is clear syntax.
The end is controlled syntax.
SC is not an end in itself. (p. 5)

This exercise is "open" because several possible solutions might be acceptable for combining these propositions, including, "SC is a means to an end, not an end in itself; that end is clear, controlled syntax," and "Rather than being an end in itself, SC is a means to an end: syntactic control and clarity."

Both special educators and regular educators may use sentence-combining exercises for a variety of purposes and to teach a variety of syntactic structures inductively. The primary identifying characteristic is that they start with a set of given language propositions, followed by play with the language to vary its form. Sentence-combining exercises have been criticized as being artificial formula writing. Strong (1986) agreed:

SC works best when done two or three times a week for short periods, when students use exercises as springboards for journals or controlled writing, when teachers and students monitor problem sentences, and when transfer is made to real writing—either through decombined student drafts or marginal notations. (p. 22)

Targeting text cohesion. To produce intelligible connected written discourse, writers must develop complex strategies to process ideas in text to form a cohesive whole (Halliday & Hasan, 1976). As Halliday and Hasan defined it, *cohesion* is a semantic system of ties across sentence boundaries that bind a text together.

Cohesion strategies represent a true marriage between syntax and semantics. Halliday and Hasan (1976) described three cohesion processes: Lexical cohesion involves semantic linkage among vocabulary items; grammatical cohesion involves the three syntactic-semantic operations of reference, substitution, and ellipsis; and conjunction strategies relate ideas with a cohesion process that is largely grammatical but also lexical (see Box 9.12) for a summary.

The common feature among these strategies is that cohesion is established in words, so that linguistic items "point" to each other. Cohesive devices may be used to point backward to previously introduced lexical items (anaphora) or ahead to new information (cataphora), and they can provide immediate cohesion between two linguistic items; they can be chained in a sequence of immediate ties; or they can

---

Box 9.12	Cohesive devices	
	Type	**Example**
	Reference	<u>Jack</u> went to the park. <u>He</u> played ball.
	Substitution	Jack <u>went</u>. Everyone <u>did.</u>
	Ellipsis	The <u>roses</u> were red. There were twelve.
	Conjunction	I left <u>after</u> he did.
		I left <u>because</u> he did.
	Lexical reiteration	The <u>cat</u> was black. It was a good <u>cat</u>.
	Lexical collocation	I had 50 <u>cents</u>. That made a <u>dollar</u>.

Note. From "Linguistic Cohesion and the Developing Writer" by J. W. Irwin. Reprinted from *Topics in Language Disorders,* Vol. 8, No. 3, p.15, with permission of Aspen Publishers, Inc., © 1988.

be remote, in that they are separated by one or more sentences.

Text cohesion is built both within and between sentences. Paragraphs may also be made more or less cohesive by arranging and rearranging clauses. Subordinating terms (e.g., *because, when, after*) and relative pronouns (e.g., *who, which, that*) are examples of cohesive devices that Moran (1988) targeted as she helped students learn to write cohesive texts.

Irwin (1988) pointed out that most cohesion instruction probably occurs incidentally, as teachers help students resolve their problems during normal reading and writing tasks. For example, teachers may help students to identify the correct referents for confusing pronouns as they read, or they may help students replace redundant nouns with appropriate pronouns when they write. Irwin noted that "there is general agreement that students need not learn the names for any of these devices; instead, instruction can be planned in which skills are explained to the students and modeled by the clinician, followed by guided practice" (p. 20). An example of the three steps explaining, modeling, and practice is included in Box 9.13.

DEVELOPING ABSTRACT AND NONLITERAL MEANINGS

As mentioned at the beginning of this chapter, by traditional accounts, most language development was considered complete by the time children entered school. That notion has been countered throughout much of this chapter. Even in those earlier accounts, development of the semantic system was recognized to continue into adulthood. In the later stages of development, acquisition of a mature literate lexicon and acquisition of figurative language are two major accomplishments (Nippold, 1988a, 1988b, 1988d).

Acquiring a Literate Lexicon

To describe the special characteristics of lexical acquisition in the later stages of language learning, Nippold

(1988d) used the term *literate lexicon*, which acknowledges the symbiotic relationship between lexical growth and literate activities. Nippold explained that "whereas literacy requires knowledge and use of a wide variety of words, the process of lexical growth itself is facilitated by literate activities" (pp. 29–30).

This is part of the "rich-get-richer" phenomenon. Children who read have the means to acquire new words. Children who have large vocabularies like to read. Full capacity seems never to be reached. The more words one knows, the easier it seems to acquire additional ones. That is the good news. Unfortunately, the bad news is that many individuals with language impairments are unable to hook into this positive spiral and instead, slip further and further behind their normally developing peers as they advance through school.

Older children and adolescents with language disorders may fall short in acquiring a literate lexicon on two levels: (1) They may have difficulty acquiring increasingly abstract words and concepts for use in basic comprehension and production. (2) They may have difficulty using metalinguistic strategies to talk about meanings and definitions. Both levels are part of competent, mature language functioning, and either may be targeted appropriately for some individuals in language intervention (N. W. Nelson, 1988b).

Wiig's (1984) review of the limited literature in this area suggested that differences in semantic acquisition by children with specific language disabilities are primarily quantitative. Children with language-learning disabilities tend to know fewer words and have less elaborated meanings for those words. Qualitative problems have also been found, however, particularly in the problems of concept formation (reflected in restricted word definitions), categorization, semantic associations and contrasts, interpreting lexical ambiguities, and processing multiple meaning words. As in other areas, children with language disorders tend to perform more like younger children than their same-age peers. For example, Table 9.11 includes Wiig's (1984) summary of the similarities between

---

Personal Reflection 9.19	"The status of the sentence as the sole unit of analysis when studying complexity in child language has changed with the advent of discourse analysis." *Cheryl Scott* (1988b, p. 45), Oklahoma State University, in an article entitled "Producing Complex Sentences."

Box 9.13   Direct teaching of implicit connective inference

Explaining the Skill

Clinician: It is very important when you read to know how the sentences fit together. Sometimes there are things for you to infer that the author doesn't state directly. This is especially true when one sentence tells why the event in the next sentence happened. You will need to infer many of these in the story we are about to read.

Modeling the Skill

Clinician: Let me show you how I do this. Read the first paragraph silently while I read it aloud (*read paragraph*). Now, let's see. The first sentence tells me that Janice loved the store. The second sentence tells me that it had a lot of pretty things. Now, I ask myself, how do these sentences fit together? Well, I know that most people love pretty things. So, she probably loved the store because . . .
Student: It had pretty things!!

Guided Practice

Clinician: Good! Now, let's read the next two sentences. How do these fit together?
Student: They sold the candy so they could get money.
Clinician: Good! One thing was the reason for another. Now, let's read on until we find another place where we can find reasons like this.

Note. From "Linguistic Cohesion and the Developing Writer" by J. W. Irwin. Reprinted from *Topics in Language Disorders*, Vol. 8, No. 3, p. 20, with permission of Aspen Publishers, Inc., © 1988.

---

word definitions produced by adolescents with language-learning disabilities and younger children, based on their levels of cognitive development.

New words are generally acquired in normal development through direct teaching or contextual abstraction (Werner & Kaplan, 1950). The rate at which new words are acquired in normal development is incredible. G. A. Miller and Gildea (1987) estimated that the average high school graduate has learned the meanings of at least 80,000 different words. This rate of learning would be impossible if words were acquired only through direct teaching (18-year-olds would have had to acquire an average of 12 words per day, including during infancy, to reach this total). Therefore, the majority of words must be acquired by the majority of learners by abstracting their meanings from contextual uses rather than through direct instruction (G. A. Miller & Gildea, 1987).

Several factors complicate the lexical learning picture for all individuals, regardless of language disorder. Evidence from normal development suggests complex interactions between internalized organizational capabilities and externalized lexical learning opportunities. For example, the well-known syntagmatic–paradigmatic shift (Entwisle, Forsyth, & Muus, 1964), which occurs between the ages of 5 and 9 years in the children's verbal responses to free-association tasks, suggests that children's semantic systems undergo some type of semantic reorganization during these years. (Younger children's responses to stimulus words, e.g., *go*, are often "syntagmatic" words, e.g., *home*, which might follow the stimulus word in a sentence; beyond age 7, older children's responses to stimulus words, e.g., *go*, are more often paradigmatic, categorically related words, including antonyms, e.g., *come*.)

During this period, methods for teaching words within the official curriculum also shift. At around second grade, definitional learning begins to be emphasized as dictionary skills are introduced. By fourth grade, written language becomes a major source of new word learning (Nippold, 1988d). Official vocabulary lists often accompany reading assignments of formal textbook series (part of the *de facto* curriculum).

The second level of lexical learning then becomes obvious. Students talk about the meanings of words, look them up in dictionaries, write down varied definitions, and take tests on them. Learning new words and definitions places considerable demands on students' metalinguistic systems. When Crais (1987)

TABLE 9.11
Overview of cognitive stages and the acquisition of word meanings

Stage/Age	Child's Word Meanings	Examples of Age-Expected Definitions	Definitions by Adolescents With Language-Learning Disabilities
Preoperational intuitive thinking (2–7 yr)	Meanings are tied to concrete actions. Child begins to compile a dictionary of word meanings.	Bird: "Something that flies in the sky." Bottle: "Where you pour something out." Mother: "She feeds me and gives me a bath."	Apple: "Something you eat." History: "Something you learn in school."
Concrete operational (7–11 yr)	Perceives more complex relationships and has broader meanings, has difficulties in conversing about events that are not visible. Word definitions are tied to sentence contexts.	Bird: "It's like an airplane only it's little and chirps." Bottle: "It's like a can only you can see through it.' Mother: "She has babies and takes care of them."	Apple: "It's something you eat that grows on trees." History: "It's something you learn in school that tells about a long time ago."
Formal operational (11+ yr)	Word definitions are essentially at adult levels. Talks about complex processes from an abstract point of view.	Bird: "It's a warmblooded animal that uses its wings to fly." Bottle: "A hollow glass container that holds liquid." Mother: "A lady who is a parent."	

Note. From "Language Disabilities in Adolescents: A Question of Cognitive Strategies" by E. H. Wiig. Reprinted from *Topics in Language Disorders*, Vol. 4, No. 2, p. 45, with permission of Aspen Publishers, Inc., © 1984.

studied children's and adults' comprehension of novel and familiar words in stories, she found that third- and fifth-graders were the most likely to provide definitions when they were asked to tell what they remembered about common words. Four of 20 third-graders and eight of 20 fifth-graders did this, whereas none of the 20 first-graders or adults did the same. Crais hypothesized that the difference was related to the educational emphasis on definition tasks in these middle grades.

Learning a common dictionary meaning does not mean that an individual has full adult understanding of a word with all of its multiple, abstract, and figurative connotations (see Chapter 2 for a discussion of these features). That takes time and exposure. Language learners must encounter new words in multiple contexts, must recognize new words each time they are encountered, and must be able to relate new shades of meaning to old, thus enhancing and modifying existing schemata as appropriate.

Targeting lexical learning. Wiig and Semel (1976, 1980) outlined several categories of words and lexical

relationships to be probed and encouraged for older students with language-learning disabilities. N. W. Nelson (1988b) provided intervention objectives based on these same categories including (1) varied parts of speech (verbs, adjectives, pronouns), with particular focus on subtle differences between exemplars (e.g., *strike, slug*); (2) abstract word relationships (e.g., antonyms, synonyms, homonyms); (3) semantic classification (e.g., functional word definitions, multifaceted word definitions); (4) verbal analogies; (5) words signaling logicogrammatical relationships of time (e.g., *when, while, after*), and space or order (e.g., *"John was in front of Bill."*); (6) figurative language (e.g., idioms, metaphors, similes); and (7) semantic relationships (e.g., inconsistencies and absurdities).

Wiig and Semel (1980) provided a set of 12 principles to assist children and adolescents with language-learning disabilities to acquire new lexical concepts: (1) Use information from normal development to decide when to introduce words, concepts, and relational terms. (2) Introduce new words with their prototypical referents. (3) Introduce words with more general meanings before those with more specific meanings. (4) Introduce words that are less complex before those that are more complex semantically. (5) Introduce the positive member of antonymous pairs before the negative one. (6) Introduce new words in sentences with controlled syntax. (7) Use pictorial or concrete referents to illustrate the concept whenever possible. (8) Emphasize the critical components of meaning when illustrating a new concept with a picture or other means. (9) Use multiple (at least 10 typical but different), clear referential contexts to introduce and elaborate the new concept. (10) Extend the concept to at least 10 more specific and abstract semantic contexts. (11) Extend the range of application and control of newly established words, concepts, and relationships. (12) Extend the range of application and control of new concepts to curricular areas.

Crais (1990) summarized several methods for targeting lexical knowledge in language intervention programs. She noted that, although much lexical learning occurs in normal development through naturalistic contextual experiences used by children to relate world and word knowledge, children with language learning difficulties may not be able to benefit as readily from such experiences. They may need more explicit instruction, for which Crais reviewed the following options: (1) Conduct mediational discussions to build on existing vocabulary by finding out what a student currently knows about a word, helping the student to elaborate that knowledge and to correct any misconceptions. (2) Expand the characteristics students associate with a word, perhaps by filling in a grid that lists words on one axis and common attributes on another with plus (+) or minus (−) symbols for characteristics that are either present or absent on a semantic feature chart. (3) Introduce alternative meanings of words, particularly facilitating students' recognition that words can have different meanings in different contexts. (4) Teach students to use morphological strategies to recognize word roots and to modify them by adding derivational morphemes like un- and -less. (5) Introduce semantically related information.

N. W. Nelson (1989b) suggested that regular curricular contexts provide the most relevant source of new words to be targeted. Targeting words in the regular curriculum provides a lexicon within a linguistic context shared with classmates, where alternative meanings and shades of meaning can be discussed

and within a value system reinforced by the regular classroom teacher. A sequence of IEP objectives for a high school student might be written as follows (N. W. Nelson, 1988b):

❏ The student will recall target words and use them appropriately in structured intervention activities of the following types (at least 2 different tasks correct for 18 of 20 target words; 3 sets of target words):
  a. Fill-in tasks
  b. Synonym and antonym tasks
  c. Definition tasks
  d. Rephrasing tasks
  e. Alternate meaning tasks.
❏ The student will use context to figure out meanings of words that are newly introduced in paragraph contexts and will define them or use them correctly in a related context (8 of 10 new words for 3 sets of new words). (pp. 248–249)

These are rather traditional-looking objectives. The content for meeting them, however, can be obtained from collaborative meetings with classroom teachers or on-line participant observations with the student and his textbooks. When new content words, descriptive words, derivational morphemes (e.g., hypo-; hyper-), connectives, or directional words (e.g., discuss; compare) are encountered within the context of curricular language, they can become the word sets mentioned in the objectives. The reason for teaching new words in sets is that they tend to be learned better in association and contrast to each other. A notebook with divided sections might be used to organize aspects of the student's new word-learning and related information, such as semantic maps and study outlines. New words, concepts, and definitional characteristics may be added as they are encountered, and previously taught words may be reviewed periodically to make sure that they are still active. Other curricular activities may also provide rich opportunity for new vocabulary acquisition. When students engage in process writing activities with peers, the activities may motivate them to need new words in a way that sterile exercises cannot (see Personal Reflection 9.20).

Semantic organizers (Pehrsson & Denner, 1988) or semantic mapping (Heimlich & Pittelman, 1986) techniques provide a graphic demonstration that may help students begin to conceptualize and remember categorical relationships among words and their definitive characteristics. Semantic organizers allow students to visualize superordinate and subordinate relationships,

Personal Reflection 9.20	"One day, later in the year, he came to my desk and asked if there were two meanings of the word 'hospital.' He wrote: 'The friend's sister had a lot of people over to celebrate Mardi Gras. I met a lot of them and they were very hospitable.' Scott seemed to be noticing words. He needed words; he was a writer.
	He also needed details. 'Scott notices everything,' his mother told me. His writing began to show this attention to detail. He wrote: 'It was the first time I ate crawfish. You suck the inside of the head and eat the tail. It was very spicy.' These details were certain to entertain his classmates."
	Peggy A. Swoger (1989, pp. 62–63), Regular Education English Teacher, Mountain Brook Junior High School, Mountain Brook, Alabama, writing about Scott's gift, which appeared when he participated in a regular writing class.

to identify defining traits, component parts, and to provide examples. They may be used as study sheets and to engage in question asking and answering exchanges with fellow classmates. Semantic maps may be used to organize semantic elements from a variety of discourse genre. Figure 9.8 is a semantic map that organizes information about a narrative story, "Rattlesnakes," along with expository information that was embedded in the text.

Another option to help students extend their vocabularies, which is currently in its infancy, is computer-assisted instruction. As video-disk technology and software become more widely available, some truly effective programs may be provided. Meanwhile, some initial attempts have been made. For example, to help develop definitional word learning, Torgesen and Torgesen (1985) developed a computer program called *WORDS*. Each word in a practice set of 10 words is presented first individually along with a picture that represents its meaning. As each word is presented, the child pronounces the name of the picture orally and then types the word into a computer. In a second activity, children select the correct word from two choices and type it into the computer to match each picture. Levels of difficulty are controlled based on the nature of the distractor words. In a third activity, three choices are provided, again with distractors of increasing difficulty. A follow-up study by Cohen, Torgesen, and Torgesen (1988), using a "no-typing" version of the program, found that, like the first version, this one was effective in improving speed and accuracy of reading words but that students liked the second version more and obtained mastery levels sooner on new word sets.

Figurative Language

Nippold (1985) commented that "learning the correct interpretation and appropriate use of figurative language is important to youths aged 10–18 in both the academic and personal-social realms" (p.1). In other words, older children and adolescents need to learn teenage slang (see discussion of social interaction conversation with peers earlier in this chapter) as well as the figurative language of idioms, similes, and metaphors. Other authors (e.g., D. K. Bernstein, 1986; Lund & Duchan, 1988; N. W. Nelson, 1988b) have included humor among the categories of figurative language acquired in the later stages of language learning.

Figurative language requires the language user to recognize nonliteral meanings of words and phrases (and often to make metalinguistic judgments about multiple levels of meaning). Because such meanings do not relate to referents in the usual ways, they generally require experience in a social context before their meaning can be discovered. Idioms, particularly, have a fixed or conventional meaning in the language (Ackerman, 1982) and, to be understood, must be encountered in meaningful contexts. Hyperbole is a related figurative language strategy that is sometimes so stereotypic it becomes idiomatic.

Metaphor and simile are closely related figurative language forms because they both compare two unlike entities on some shared quality. A metaphor typically has three parts that may be labeled, *topic, vehicle,* and *ground*. For example, in the sentence, "After the new permanent, her hair was a rat's nest," *hair* is the topic, *rat's nest* is the vehicle, and *messiness* is the ground. Metaphors may be structured

FIGURE 9.8
Semantic map generated around the topic *rattlesnakes,* in preparation for reading a story.

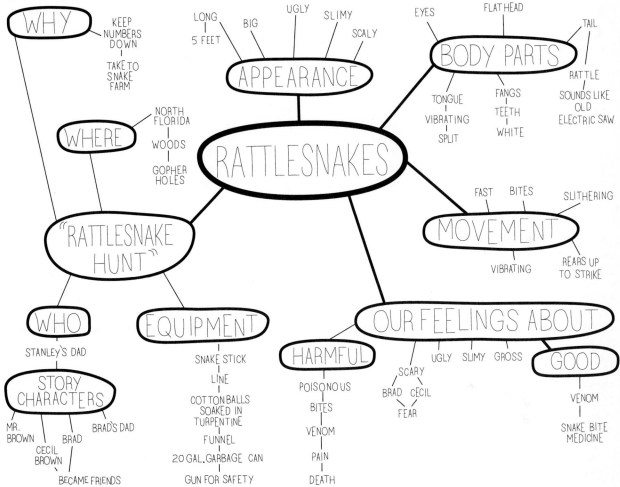

Note. From *Semantic Mapping: Classroom Applications* (p. 28) by J. E. Heimlich and S. D. Pittelman, 1986, Newark, DE, International Reading Assoc. Reprinted with permission of Joan E. Heimlich and the International Reading Association.

either as predicative metaphors (similarity) or as proportional metaphors. Predicative metaphors have one topic and one vehicle, with both stated, "Her eyes were deep blue pools." Proportional metaphors have two topics, but the second is only inferred, based on an analogical relationship in the ground (e.g., "The party was a balloon that never got off the ground"). Some aspects of metaphors may be perceptual, and some may be psychological.

Similes have much in common with metaphors, but differ in that the comparison between the literal and nonliteral meanings is made explicit. Most studies have shown similes to be easier for younger children and children with language disorders than metaphors are, probably because of this explicitness (Nippold, 1985, 1988a).

Many variables influence the relative ease or difficulty of understanding figurative language (Nippold, 1985; 1988a). Variables to be controlled in assessment and intervention task design include frequency of occurrence, syntactic complexity, semantic analyzability, and inclusion of linguistic and nonlinguistic context (Nippold & Martin, 1989). Nippold's (1985) review showed that, if appropriate testing methods are used, preschoolers can understand some metaphoric meanings; first-graders can give interpretations for some idioms; and figurative language skills continue to develop throughout the school-age years and into adulthood (Nippold & Martin, 1989).

Several studies have shown, however, that children with language-learning disabilities in the later grades of elementary school and later do not fare as well as their normal-language-learning peers (Nippold & Fey, 1983; Seidenberg & Bernstein, 1986). Rather, they tend to process figurative language more like younger children do, needing additional contextual support and more explicit linguistic markers to understand the relationships conveyed. Nippold (1985) reported that research findings tend to show high correlations between figurative language proficiency, reading ability, and vocabulary development; however, experience seems to play a major role as well. Ezell and Goldstein (1991) found that a group of 9-year-old children with mild mental retardation performed worse than age-matched peers on an idiom-comprehension task, as expected, but rather surprisingly, they performed better than a group of younger children matched for receptive vocabulary age. The children with mental retardation did particularly well matching pictures to frequently occurring idioms such as "got cold feet" and "got carried away."

These results highlight perhaps the most important intervention strategy for encouraging the development of figurative language—*exposure.* Language specialists must ensure that older children and adolescents have the opportunity to hear examples of idiomatic and metaphoric language in meaningful and natural contexts. They also may need opportunities to practice telling jokes even before they fully understand them (Lund & Duchan, 1989). Studies of regular classroom environments show that such opportunities do occur as early as kindergarten in teachers' language (Lazar et al., 1989). However, teachers may not always provide the scaffolding necessary for all children to benefit. Children in special education classrooms are even less likely to have the opportunity to hear figurative language in natural contexts, and their isolation from teenage slang has already been discussed. Newton (1985) compared the teacher talk of three groups of teachers, a group of teachers of the deaf who used oral communication strategies, a group who used total communication

strategies, and a group of teachers of normal hearing students. She found no differences between the uses of idiomatic language in the teachers of oral-communicating deaf and normal-hearing children, but she found reduced idiomatic expression in both the oral and signed portions of communication in the total communication classrooms.

Language acquisition is not achieved by simple exposure. Otherwise, children having difficulty in this area would be rare, because figurative language is so prevalent. Many individuals with language disorders need to be shown how to abstract meaning from context through repeated exposure with mediation to make sure figurative meanings are grasped, they need repeated practice in similar and new contexts, and they need application in new settings (Nippold, 1991). Learning how to learn has been a major topic of much of this chapter. One might imagine a whole class of children becoming "idiom detectives" and creating a classroom master list of all of the idioms they hear or read, identifying the source, and noticing opportunities to reuse the idioms in their own exchanges. A language-rich environment is one of the enticements for including more children with language disorders in regular classrooms with students of mixed ability levels.

HELPING INDIVIDUALS WITH SEVERE DISABILITIES MOVE INTO ADULTHOOD

Providing Equal Opportunity

In the past, students with severe disabilities that interfered significantly with their ability to communicate and to benefit from education commonly were segregated from their normal-learning peers into separate classrooms and separate buildings. As discussed in Chapter 5, educators and parents now recognize that separate is generally not equal, and educators are providing more opportunities for people with severe disabilities to interact in significant ways within educational and social situations (Lipsky & Gartner, 1989; Murray-Seegert, 1989). However, as Asch (1989) points out in Personal Reflection 9.21, the United States has a long history of providing services to individuals with disabilities that are insufficient to allow them to gain the experience they need to become independent adults.

Now most professionals agree that change is needed. Strong advocacy and a few success stories

Personal Reflection 9.21

"With very rare exceptions, today's adults with disabilities who recall segregated facilities, separate classes, or home instruction cannot say enough about how inadequate was their academic training. They compare their education with that of siblings or neighbors who were not disabled and speak only of gaps. For example, they mention subjects, such as science, that they never studied, maps they never saw, field trips they never took, books that were never available, assignments that were often too easy, expectations of their capacity (by nearly all teachers) that were too low."

Adrienne Asch (1989, p. 183) writing about what some adults with disabilities (primarily physical or sensory ones) say about their experiences in special education in the United States. Asch is herself a blind adult who went to school with sighted children.

currently outweigh solid models backed by extensive research. Professionals therefore are mostly left to glean what they can from anecdotal reports, attempting to use philosophy to guide practice, and experimenting in their own work settings. This section presents suggestions to facilitate movement into adulthood by individuals with severe disabilities in the later stages of child development.

The complex nature of severe and multiple disabilities demands collaboration among persons with disabilities, their parents, their regular and special educators, and possibly others. The contributions of speech–language pathologists and other communication specialists to the collaborative process are based on expertise in analyzing the communicative aspects of diverse events, as well as the speech, language, and communicative abilities of people who participate in them. Some of the intervention efforts of these professionals may aim directly at changing behaviors, thereby reducing impairment. Others may aim to help individuals meet important communicative demands through acquisition of new abilities or compensatory techniques, thereby reducing disability. Still others may aim to expand environmental opportunities for persons with disabilities to participate in educational and community activities, thereby reducing handicap.

Perhaps one of the greatest challenges facing professionals as they attempt to implement multifaceted intervention programs is to balance the need to modify contexts, so that individuals can experience some communicative successes, without creating new contexts that are so different that they practically ensure continued isolation of people with handicaps. The

challenges apply across academic, social, and vocational settings.

In academic settings, what may look like harmless accommodations may actually "deprive students of achieving their full potential" (Asch, 1989, p.186). In secondary schools, for example, note taking is a critical skill. As much as possible, students with severe disabilities involving peripheral sensory and motor systems should take their own notes rather than relying on the note-taking skills of others. Students with visual impairments may be provided with lap-top computers. Students with physical impairments may be provided with microcomputers with special accessing, abbreviation characteristics, and printers. Students with hearing impairments or deafness may be provided interpreters. As Asch (1989) commented:

If students are to develop the ability to sift out the essential from the illustrative in a lecture, they must themselves have the full text of that lecture communicated to them. If they are to join in class discussions, they must know what other students have said. For the student who must get information from lip-reading or sign, the only efficient and equivalent substitute for hearing is the interpreted class lecture and discussion. (p. 186)

In social settings, opportunities also may be limited, particularly when severe central processing deficits are involved, such as mental retardation or autism. Lack of opportunity may be exacerbated by the inappropriate and sometimes frightening communicative behaviors that appear when young people with these severe disabilities are placed in settings with their normally developing peers. Schuler and

Goetz (1981) pointed out that a lack of appropriate social and communicative skills may cause individuals with severe disabilities to communicate by using behaviors that others find unpleasant or frightening (e.g., tantrums or inappropriate hugging to communicate "I'm tired of doing this," or "Pay attention to me").

The social interaction problems of individuals with severe disabilities have been summarized as failure to initiate, maintain, and terminate social interactions in ways that others perceive as socially acceptable (Murray-Seegert, 1989). Recognizing this, a first step in intervention might be to teach socially acceptable behaviors. However, because such behaviors tend to be learned best in the context of natural social interactions, and because their absence may limit those interactions, by the adolescent years, a vicious cycle may be well established, which is hard to break.

Murray-Seegert (1989) wrote about one attempt to break this cycle. By acting as a classroom aide in a San Francisco Bay area high school, Murray-Seegert used participant observation techniques to conduct an ethnographic study of social interactions in a program designed to integrate students with severe disabilities with regular education students. Adolescents with disabilities participated actively with regular education students, many of whom could themselves be considered at risk for school failure. The "regulars" volunteered to work with the students with disabilities, receiving course credit for their enrollment in the Internal Work Experience (IWE).

One part of the program involved peer tutoring. Murray-Seegert (1989) reported that it "proved to be an important variable influencing the development of social relations between disabled and nondisabled students" (p. 114). A variation on peer tutoring involved what Murray-Seegert called "mediated interactions," which were identified when nondisabled "helpers" promoted positive proximal or reciprocal contact between another nondisabled student and a student with a severe disability. One day Anita (a member of the group the students dubbed the "Popular People") asked to bring her "Thug" boyfriend, Denard (who had dropped out of school), to class. After a card game with several special education students, including Phuc Sanh and Dwayne, Murray-Seegert, described what happened when Denard wanted to try out the computer:

> Anita says, "Phuc Sanh knows how to do it," and so the two boys go to work. Phuc Sanh uses a single word utterance to help Denard: "Load . . . run . . . 5." Anita comes to sit with them. Dwayne comes over to watch and puts his hand on Anita's shoulder. Denard says, "Hey! Don't you touch my woman!" Dwayne removes his hand. Denard says, "I was just kiddin'." (p. 90)

The program was not always successful in meeting its primary objective of developing intergroup social relations. Ten of the 42 IWE students dropped out after a few weeks, but many students in both groups benefitted from the interaction. Personal Reflection 9.23 describes how one of the IWE stu-

---

Personal Reflection 9.22

"Wouldn't you hate it if people were always helping you? Wouldn't it be awful if everybody pretended to accept everything you did, even when you were boring or obnoxious, just because you were "special"? How would you like it if other people always initiated and terminated the interactions that involved you? Worst of all, how would it feel to experience that omnipresent strained politeness, lingering like a damp fog that obscured your individuality from every new person you met?"

Carola Murray-Seegert (1989, p. 91), encouraging perspective taking in her book *Nasty Girls, Thugs, and Humans Like Us*, in which she reports an ethnographic study of an inner-city high school integration project that benefitted students with obvious disabilities and the regular education students who volunteered to work with them.

Note. From *Nasty Girls, Thugs, and Humans Like Us: Social Relations Between Severely Disabled and Nondisabled Students in High School* (p. 91) by C. Murray-Seegert, 1989, Baltimore, MD: Paul H. Brookes. Copyright 1989 by Paul H. Brookes. Reprinted by permission.

Personal Reflection 9.23

"Dear Darryl,

How you been I been fine. I'm just out here in frisco going to school and waiting to graduate out of High School.

I go to my first period to sixth and I'm out at 2:00 pm. But in my third period class I have a Special Ed class. It's students with a disability. Like one student Juan he's a student that's a little slow in the mind and can't all the way speak yet. He's about 59 inches and black hair he's Spanish and he dress average. Sometimes he likes to play games or go out side for a walk, but sometimes he just likes to Kick back. When he wants something he yells and gives you sign language. He can go to the restroom by his self he know his way around the school and sometimes he goes to lunch with a peer tutor or to the wash house or to the store. He's kind of slow learning but he catches on sooner or later. He needs a little help with yelling out loud or whistling, and he needs help with his way of approaching people. Sometimes I will go to the church and he likes to come along with me. He likes too go just about everywhere with any of the peer tutors. I like to take him places with me because even though he's disabled we still are good friends and I wouldn't mind taking him anywhere with me. I like to play games and baseball or running after each other. I can tell he's happy because everyday he comes in smiling about anything. And he always wants to go somewhere with me or play a game of battleship with me.

P.S. Write back soon. Sincerely yours, Preston."

Preston was a "Peer Tutor" writing to a hypothetical friend about his disabled classmate in an assignment which he and fellow peer tutors were given. (Quoted by Murray-Seegert, 1989, pp. 112–113.) Murray-Seegert noted the matter-of-fact way the regular students accepted behaviors that are often cited as evidence of lack of readiness for inclusion in integrated settings. The letters written by peer tutors also showed that "dressing okay" was at least as important to teenage peers as "acquisition of social skills" was to adult supervisors.

Note. From *Nasty Girls, Thugs, and Humans Like Us: Social Relations Between Severely Disabled and Nondisabled Students in High School* (pp. 112–113) by C. Murray-Seegert, 1989, Baltimore, MD: Paul H. Brookes. Copyright 1989 by Paul H. Brookes. Reprinted by permission.

dents in the program described his disabled peer. As Murray-Seegert noted, "remarks like 'sometimes they get on my nerves' or 'sometimes I get bored' by the Regulars showed that they were relating to disabled students as fallible, multidimensional 'humans like us' rather than as idealized, infantilized Poster Children" (p. 105).

In some inclusion programs, techniques for promoting positive peer tutoring may be relatively more structured than those used in Murray-Seegert's (1989) study. Some studies have used refinements of behavioral technology to structure interactions between adolescents with and without disabilities. In one two-study series, a group of researchers taught peer tutors to work with three young men with autism,

first, in their integrated high school, and then, in their off-campus jobs. In the first study (Gaylord-Ross, Haring, Breen, & Pitts-Conway, 1984), the peer tutors taught the young men to initiate, maintain, and terminate social interactions that were object centered in that they revolved around things like offering chewing gum or listening to a personal stereo. After training, the students with autism had generalized the social skills across persons and were more often being approached themselves for social interaction. In the second study (Breen, Haring, Pitts-Conway, & Gaylord-Ross, 1985), nondisabled schoolmates taught the disabled individuals to participate in social interactions with co-workers during coffee breaks at their job sites. In this intervention program, the peer tutors learned to teach a social skill chain that involved greeting a familiar co-worker, offering a cup of coffee, and elaborating the social exchange when the co-worker showed a willingness to continue the interaction. The results again supported improvement in the students' abilities to make effective social bids. Few avoidance reactions occurred, and the bids "did lead to meaningful social responses of different types by the co-workers" (p. 14).

Facilitating Transitions

One of the primary rites of passage in Western societies from childhood to adulthood involves making the transition from school to work. The data on employment of students with disabilities after leaving school are generally discouraging. For many, the transition process from school to work is far from complete.

> Few handicapped students move from school to independent living in communities. Secondary special education programs appear to have little impact on students' adjustment to community life. More than 30% of the students enrolled in secondary special education programs drop out. (Edgar, 1987, p. 40)

Comprehensive vocational transition programs for persons with severe handicaps have several characteristics. As summarized by Moon, Diambra, and Hill (1990), these include (1) a written, formal plan with goals and objectives, time lines, and responsible agencies and persons; (2) a functional school curriculum that uses community-based vocational instruction; and (3) concrete outcomes that include job placements. The development of Individualized Transition Plans (ITPs) requires a collaborative effort by a team of professionals. Sometimes missing from those plans is the consideration of the communicative demands of job settings and the students' related abilities. Contextually based assessments may increase the likelihood that students will succeed in their job placements.

Some students with severe disabilities may make transitions to higher education settings rather than jobs. Some make transitions to both (see Personal Reflection 9.24). When students with severe disabilities attend postsecondary educational programs, they often need additional support from student-service programs in their vocational training programs, community colleges, or universities. Language specialists may provide some of those services.

Fostering Independence

Strategies for encouraging adult independence among people with severe disabilities, including mental retardation, are often based on principles articulated by Lou Brown and his colleagues (L. Brown, Nietupski, & Hamre-Nietupski, 1976). As summarized by Falvey, Bishop, Grenot-Scheyer, and Coots (1988), these include (1) preparation to function as independently as possible across as many integrated, heterogeneous environments as possible; (2) planning for generalization by teaching activities in environments that require them, using natural cues, corrections, and reinforcers specific to each environment; and (3) designing instructional strategies to be sufficiently

---

Personal Reflection 9.24

"When J-P began college, he needed to find work to help support himself. He had never worked outside our home before, and again, we wondered if he ever could or would. I convinced a woman in the Microfiche Dept. of the college library to give J-P a chance. When he began to work, it took a lot of her time and patience to train him. He memorized the Microfiche system in several days, but he had to be painstakingly taught to do visual/motor tasks like using keys to unlock doors. J-P managed to create a niche for himself in the library over his four years there. He was always prompt and dependable. He worked hard and was willing to take on extra work when demand was high. He talked to and became friends with his co-workers."

Julia Donnelly (1991, p. 14), parent of Jean-Paul, a young man with autism, in an excerpt from a biographical series Donnelly wrote for *The Advocate*, the newsletter of the Autism Society of America.

flexible and individualized to meet the diverse needs of students with mental retardation.

Chapter 8 presented a set of functional goals (Mire & Chisholm, 1990) in seven different functional-outcome areas. Each was related to a specific functional context, and each was analyzed into a series of component sub-behaviors. Those behaviors are appropriate for continued development throughout adolescence and adulthood. For example, one of the goal areas was communicating needs independently while traveling. After analysis of a particular contextual demand, intervention in this area might target (1) requesting amount of bus fare and where to deposit it, (2) phoning for a taxi, (3) responding to questions about destination, and (4) requesting directions.

The strategies of contextually based assessment and intervention discussed throughout this book mainly involve assessment of the abilities of persons with disabilities within specific ecological contexts. L. Brown et al. (1979) called similar analyses, "Ecological and Student Repertoire Inventories." These inventories are charts that include three columns of information: (1) a contextually based ecological inventory of the demands of a key task, (2) an inventory of the student's current repertoire within that environment, and (3) recommendations for fostering a better match between the two. One student's vocational plan included the need to interact with customers in the grocery store where he worked. Brown et al. analyzed the task demands to include three skills: (1) Look in the direction of a customer requesting assistance. (2) Answer the customer's question if possible, and if not possible, (3) direct the customer to the manager's desk at the front of the store. The student's current repertoire for dealing with each of these situations was often hampered by problems that included looking at the floor when someone approached, insufficient verbal skills, and failure to direct customers when they needed it. Intervention for this student involved provision of extensive experiences for interacting with others, the development of augmentative communicative aids, techniques, and strategies, and teaching him to use them in actual communicative interactions.

What about literacy expectations? Historically, educators assumed that individuals with severe disabilities were not "ready" to learn to read and write during their preschool and early elementary school years. Often, they have never been considered "ready." Parents have urged professionals to move beyond a strictly developmental model to write literacy goals in their children's IEPs even when they still could not tie their shoes or zip their pants. (Recall the personal reflections of parent reported in Chapter 1—"We'll buy him velcro!," Personal Reflection 1.5—and Chapter 5—"You listen to me politely, but you never write it down!"—Personal Reflection 5.10.)

Current trends are to include children with severe disabilities in activities where they will have opportunities to become literate and, if necessary, to provide them with microcomputer word processing systems with special switch access to help them learn to write. It is difficult, at this point, to establish a prognosis for learning to read and write because so many individuals with developmental disabilities did not have access to writing systems (Light, Kelford-Smith, & McNaughton, 1990), or the same experiences to encourage emergent literacy as their peers (Koppenhaver, Coleman, Kalman, & Yoder, 1991).

Following tradition, older individuals with severe cognitive and linguistic impairments should be taught to recognize written symbols and the international symbols needed for personal safety and daily living. Deliberate and early attempts should also be made to surround children who have severe disabilities with literate language and print, as discussed in Chapters 7 and 8. As programs are developed to incorporate literacy goals and related activities for older students with severe disabilities, new discoveries may be made about their capacity to learn.

Still in the early stages of exploration, facilitated communication is used with individuals who have autism and other severe developmental disabilities. Biklen (1988, 1990) has been the primary proponent of the approach. He adapted the method from a program developed by Rosemary Crossley in Melbourne, Australia. Crossley used the program with a young girl with cerebral palsy who had been institutionalized all her life but left the institution successfully when Crossley worked with her as she learned to read and write using facilitated communication (Crossley & MacDonald, 1984).

Using facilitated communication, as developed further by Biklen (1988, 1990, 1992), the adult facilitator provides a keyboard writing system with print output (the Cannon communicator, an augmentative communication device, was used in the early studies). The adult supports the child's forearm, wrist, and index finger (if necessary). The adult then uses systematic steps to introduce the child to sound–letter corre-

Personal Reflection 9.25   "He does have talent, interest, and desire to pursue being a history professor. All his life I have taught, guided, and supported him. I have smoothed his path in what I thought were the best directions. Now he is 21 and I can no longer make his decisions. We have talked very honestly about his future. Jean-Paul is aware of his disabilities and the limited job market. He still chooses to work in the field that he loves and has ability in. What more can I say to him? His life has been a series of challenges, none of them easy, but he has always been willing to try. He has surprised us all with what he has achieved. All I can tell him now is, 'Yes, Jean-Paul, Go for it.'"

Julia Donnelly (1991, p. 15), parent of Jean-Paul, a young man with autism, in the closing comments of her biographical series about her son.

spondences, to teach simple words, to request simple words in response to fill-in tasks, and ultimately, to converse with the child in writing. In a significant proportion of cases, children have typed written messages that far exceeded expectations based on the child's ability to communicate orally. It is an intriguing phenomenon and one that deserves much further investigation.

When a person with a severe disability acquires sufficient communicative ability to live independently, it is a challenge to the parents and professionals who have guided the person's development along the way to let go. Eventually, and to varying degrees, letting go, however, may be the best form of intervention (see Personal Reflection 9.25).

SUMMARY

This chapter presented consideration of the communicative contexts, abilities, and needs of children at later stages of language development. During this period, children consolidate their earlier language learning and gain confidence in using oral and written language for new and varied purposes. They expand their contacts with their peer group, and they work toward independence from their families.

For later stage children and adolescents, both formal and informal assessment contexts remain important. Techniques of curriculum-based language assessment and intervention were emphasized for working with language learning needs within the context of real academic experiences, both written and oral. A complex model of written and oral language processing was presented to guide assessment and intervention decisions to help individuals with childhood language disorders move toward adult competence and independence.

Examples of later stage intervention targets and strategies include the following: modify language learning contexts with mediational and scaffolding techniques; foster "metaskills" and other executive strategies for school survival, higher order thinking, and focus on process rather than product; develop competence in varied discourse genres and events (conversational, narrative, and expository); encourage syntactic sophistication; develop abstract and nonliteral meanings; and help individuals with severe disabilities move into adulthood.

As in previous chapters, no one intervention approach was advocated as best for all abilities and all children and adolescents. At the secondary level, however, strategy-based intervention approaches are particularly appropriate. The role of adults in the process is as mediator or facilitator to help students gain access to more communicative events. The underlying message in this final chapter is consistent with the message conveyed throughout the book. *Problems are not just within children—and neither are solutions.*

Appendix A

ANNOTATED BIBLIOGRAPHY OF SELECTED SCREENING AND ASSESSMENT TOOLS APPROPRIATE FOR MEASURING THREE STAGES OF LANGUAGE DEVELOPMENT

EARLY STAGE ASSESMENT DEVICES

Note: Sources include Sparks and Clark (1990); Hill and Singer (1990); Roberts and Crais (1989).

Assessing Prelinguistic and Early Linguistic Behaviors in Developmentally Young Children. Olswang, L. B., Stoel-Gammon, C., Coggins, T. E., & Carpenter, R. L. (1987). Includes five scales of cognitive antecedents to word meaning, play, communication intention, language comprehension, and language production. A training videotape is also available. Based on 3-year longitudinal study of prelinguistic and early linguistic behaviors of 37 normally developing children.

Assessment in Infancy. Uzgiris, I. C., & Hunt, J. C. (1975). Chicago: University of Illinois Press. Six scales are used to assess sensorimotor behaviors expected in the range from birth to 2 years.

Assessment of Children's Language Comprehension. (ACLC). Foster, R., Giddan, J., & Stark, J. (1983). Palo Alto, CA: Consulting Psychologists Press. Establishes recognition of single-word vocabulary, then uses this vocabulary to test comprehension of 2-, 3-, and 4-word phrase (e.g., "Happy little girl jumping), using picture-pointing task.

Assessment of Premature Infant Behavior (APIB). Als, H. (1984). Boston: The Children's Hospital. Behavioral evaluation scale (adapted and expanded from Brazelton's 1984 *Neonatal Behavioral Assessment Scale*) for rating behaviors in visual, auditory, tactile, organization, and reflexes categories. Used with medically stable neonates until they react to environment similar to full-term infants.

Autism Screening Instrument for Education Planning (ASIEP). Krug, D. A., Arick, J. R., & Almond, P. J. (1980). Portland, OR: ASIEP Education Company. Assessment and educational planning system for persons with autism, severe handicaps, and developmental disabilities who are between 18 months and adulthood but have low language abilities. Includes five components: autism behavior checklist; sample of vocal behavior; interaction assessment (including self-stimulation, crying, laughing, gesturing, manipulation of toys, conversation, and tantrums); educational assessment; and prognosis of learning rate.

Battelle Developmental Inventory (BDI). Newborg, J., Stock, J. R., Wnek, L., Guidubaldi, J., & Svinicki, J. (1984). Allen, TX: DLM. Comprehensive, standardized assessment (requiring 1 to 2 hours) for children from birth to 8 years in the domains of personal-social, adaptability, motor, communication, and cognition. Spanish version is available.

Battelle Developmental Inventory Screening Test. Newborg, J., Stock, J. R., & Wnek, L. (1984). Allen, TX: DLM. Screens personal-social, adaptive, motor, communication, and cognitive areas from birth to age 8 years.

Bayley Scales of Infant Development. Bayley, N. (1969). San Antonio, TX: Psychological Corporation. This diagnostic norm-referenced assessment instrument assesses mental, motor, and behavioral development in children ages 2 through 30 months and can be used for making placement decisions. It uses two scales, mental and motor, and yields standard scores for 14 age groups. Requires 45 minutes to administer.

Birth to Three Developmental Scales. Bangs, T., & Dodson, S. (1979). Allen, TX: DLM. Observation, direction following, motor and verbal imitation, object and picture naming, and pointing are used to build a development profile for the age range 0:0 to 3:0 years.

Communication and Symbolic Behavior Scales (CSBS). [Research ed.]. Wetherby, A. M., & Prizant, B. M. (1990). *Communication and Symbolic Behavior Scales* [Norm-referenced ed.] Wetherby, A. M., & Prizant, B. M. (1991). Chicago, IL: The Riverside Publishing Company. (Reviewed extensively in Chapter 7.) The CSBS is designed to be used with children whose functional communication ages are 9 months to 2 years. Uses a care-giver questionnaire, direct sampling of verbal and nonverbal communicative behaviors, and observation of relatively unstructured play activities. Scoring of the CSBS is accomplished by assigning a rating of 1 to 5 for each of 20 separate scales. Includes 16 communication scales (subdivided into four areas) and 4 scales for rating symbolic behavior (subdivided into two areas).

Denver Developmental Screening Test (DDST). Frankenburg, W. K., Dodds, J. B., & Fandal, A. W. (1969). (Manual revised, 1970). Denver, CO: University of Colorado Medical Center. Designed to screen children from the general population to identify children from birth to age 6 years in four areas, including language, who need further evaluation. Standardized on 1,036 Denver children. Items are marked as to when 25%, 50%, 75%, and 90% of the normative sample passed them.

Developmental Communication Curriculum (DCC). Hanna, R. P., Lippert, E. A., & Harris, A. B. (1982). San Antonio, TX: Psychological Corporation. This curriculum is designed for children of developmental ages birth to 5 years. It includes an assessment component, the Developmental Communication Inventory, for assessing four levels: prelinguistic, symbolic, symbolic relationships, complex symbolic relationships. Uses play contexts to observe form, content, and function. Encourages teacher and parent input.

Early Language Milestone Scale (ELM Scale). Coplan, J. (1987). Austin, TX: Pro-Ed. A norm-referenced validated screening instrument for children from birth to 36 months. Includes 42 items (most to be completed per parental report). Percentile values may be reported for each item, arranged in three divisions: auditory expressive (prelinguistic—cooing, reciprocal vocalization, babbling; linguistic—single words, two-word phrases, complex utterances; intelligibility—percentage of child's speech understood by strangers); auditory receptive (prelinguistic—alerting and orienting to sounds; linguistic—execution of verbal commands); and visual (prelinguistic—eye contact, visual tracking, visual recognition of faces; linguistic—informal and formal gestures, e.g., pointing).

ECOScales. MacDonald, J. D., & Gillette, Y. (1989). Chicago: The Riverside Publishing Company. Five separate scales are used to assess the five competencies of social play, turn taking, preverbal communication, language, and conversation. Results may be displayed on the competencies profiles or the interaction profile to address developmental goals or adult–child interaction patterns. Takes 10 to 30 minutes.

Environmental Language Intervention Program (ELIP). MacDonald, J. D. (1978). San Antonio, TX: Psychological Corporation. This assessment/diagnostic/ remediation program includes the Oliver (Parent-Assisted Communication Inventory) of prelanguage and early language skills. The Environmental Prelanguage Battery (EPB) is an assessment tool for children who have no oral language skills, designed to assess readiness behaviors (e.g., play) for learning language. The Environmental Language Inventory (ELI) assesses early language development (two or more word phrases) in conversation, imitation, and free play.

Evaluating Acquired Skills in Communication (EASIC). Riley, A. M. (1984). Tucson, AZ: Communication Skill Builders. This assessment can be used with severely impaired clients with skills in the 3-months to 8-years range. It can be used to rate behaviors at the levels: prelanguage, receptive I (noun labels, action verbs, and basic concepts); expressive I (emerging modes of communication); receptive II (more complex language forms); and expressive II (using more complex communication). Criterion referenced.

Hawaii Early Leaning Profile (HELP). Furuno, S., O'Reilly, K., Inatsuka, T., Hosaka, C., Allman, T., & Zeisloft-Falbey. (1979) Palo Alto, CA: VORT Corporation. Charts are provided for 650 skills developed from birth to 3 years in the six areas of cognitive, language, gross motor, fine motor, social, and self-help. A sequenced checklist can be used to select objectives.

The MacArthur Communicative Development Inventory: Infants. (1989). San Diego, CA: San Diego State University, Center for Research in Language, The Developmental Psychology Lab. Uses a parental checklist format to assess first signs of understanding, comprehension of early phrases, and starting to talk. Vocabulary checklist (for both understanding and saying) includes sound effect and animal sounds, animal names, vehicles, toys, food and drink, clothing, body parts, furniture and rooms, small household items, outside things and places to go, people, games and routines, action words, words about time, descriptive words, pronouns, question words, prepositions and locations, quantifiers. Early gestures, play, pretending, and imitating behaviors are also probed.

The MacArthur Communicative Development Inventory: Toddlers. (1989). San Diego, CA: San Diego State University, Center for Research in Language, The Developmental Psychology Lab. Uses a parental checklist format to assess vocabulary (similar to the infant inventory, but with additions): sentences and grammar, including morphological endings, and varied ways of expressing two-word meanings.

Neonatal Behavioral Assessment Scale. Brazelton, T. B. (1984). Philadelphia, PA: J. B. Lippincott. Behavioral evaluation scale for use with neonates. Requires 30 to 60 minutes to assess visual, auditory, tactile, organization, motor maturity, and reflexes.

Observation of Communicative Interactions (OCI). (Klein, M. D., & Briggs, M. H., 1987). Los Angeles: Mother–Infant Communication Project, California State University, Los Angeles. Designed specifically to measure care-giver responsivity to infant's communicative cues. Includes a continuum of 10 categories of responsiveness ranging to basic care-giving responses to more sophisticated efforts to facilitate language and conceptual development. It can also be used to guide intervention efforts.

Oral-Motor/Feeding Rating Scale. Jelm, J. M. (1990). Tucson, AZ: Communication Skill Builders. This observational scale can be used for combined assessment and intervention purposes with persons of all ages to summarize oral-motor and feeding functioning in eight areas: breast feeding, bottle feeding, spoon feeding, cup drinking, biting (soft cookie), biting (hard cookie), chewing, and straw drinking.

Parent–Infant Interaction Scale. Clark, G. N., & Seifer, R. (1985). Assessment of parents' interaction with their developmentally delayed infants. *Infant Mental Health Journal, 6*(4), 214–225. The areas addressed by this scale include care-giver interaction behaviors, care-giver and child social referencing, reciprocity, and care-giver affect.

Preverbal Assessment Intervention Profile (PAIP). Connard, P. (1984). Austin, TX: Pro-Ed. This is a standardized Piagetian assessment of sensorimotor (stages I to III) prelinguistic behavior. It can be used with severely, profoundly, and multiply handicapped individuals of all ages.

Program for the Acquisition of Language With the Severely Impaired (PALS). Owens, R. E., Jr. (1982). San Antonio, TX: Psychological Corporation. A three-step assessment program precedes individualized training. Care-giver interview and environmental observation are used to identify communication partners, communication content, communication behaviors. The Diagnostic Interview Survey is used with nonspeaking or minimally verbal clients. The Developmental Assessment Tool is a more formal evaluation instrument that may be administered in whole or in part in one or more sittings.

The Receptive–Expressive Emergent Language Scale (REEL-scale). Bzoch, K., & League, R. (1971). Austin, TX: Pro-Ed. Also Bzoch, K., & League, R. (1978). *Assessing language skills in infancy: A handbook for use with the Receptive-Expressive Emergent Language Scale (2nd ed.)* (REEL-2) (1991). Austin, TX: Pro-Ed. Designed to help public health nurses, pediatricians, and educators identify children up to 3 years of age who have specific language problems based on interview of "significant others" (usually a parent). Results are presented as expressive, receptive, and combined language ages.

Reynell Developmental Language Scales. Reynell, J. K. (1985). Los Angeles: Webster Psychological Services. Uses observation, picture identification, object identification, and object manipulation to measure general language receptive and expressive skills among 1:0- to 5:0-year-olds.

The Rossetti Infant–Toddler Language Scale. Rossetti, L. (1990). East Moline, IL: LinguiSystems. Designed for infants and toddlers, birth to 3 years, this is a criterion-referenced assessment scale covering multiple developmental areas: interaction and attachment, gestures, pragmatics, play, language comprehension, and language expression. Includes three to seven items for each domain at each 3-month interval.

Sequenced Inventory of Communication Development (2nd ed.). (SICD). Hedrick, D. L., Prather, E. M., & Tobin, A. R. (1984). Seattle: University of Washington Press. Designed for children functioning between 4 months and 4 years of age. Includes receptive and expressive scales. Cuban-Spanish Edition (by L. R. Rosenberg) is available.

Transdisciplinary Play-Based Assessment (TPBA). Linder, T. W. (1990). Baltimore, MD: Paul H. Brookes. This set of criterion-referenced informal assessment scales (reviewed extensively in Chapter 7) is designed for children functioning developmentally between the ages of 6 months and 6 years. It uses a play interaction context to observe four domains: social–emotional, cognitive, language and communication, and sensorimotor. A 1-hour to 1½ -hour session of videotaped play interaction with facilitator, parent, and peer is observed and scored by multiple professionals. No standardized scores are computed with the TPBA. The outcome is an analysis of developmental level, learning style, interaction patterns, and other relevant behaviors that can become an integral part of intervention planning.

MIDDLE STAGE ASSESSMENT DEVICES

Note: Sources include Deal and Rodriguez (1987) and McCauley and Swisher (1984), who reviewed tests summarized in Table 8.4.

Analysis of the Language of Learning (ALL). Blodgett, E. G., & Cooper, E. G. (1987). East Moline, IL: LinguiSystems. Provides standardized scores for 5- to 9-year-olds based on their ability to display metalinguistic knowledge of what a word is, a syllable, and a sentence, and understanding of directions. It is appropriate for nonreaders.

The ALPHA (Assessment Link Between Phonology and Articulation) Test of Phonology. Lowe, R. J. (1986). East Moline, IL: LinguiSystems. Designed to relate articulation assessment results to phonological analysis. It takes 10 to 15 minutes to administer and 15 minutes to score. It provides norms based on 1,300 subjects.

Assessment of Children's Language Comprehension (ACLC). Foster, R. Giddan, J., & Stark, J. (1973). Palo Alto: Consulting Psychologists Press. Measures comprehension of single words, two–, three–, and four-element utterances, with a picture pointing task.

Assessment of Phonological Processes—Revised (APP-R). Hodson, B. (1986). Austin, TX: Pro-Ed. Can be administered in 15 to 20 minutes and scored in 30 minutes. Results in categorization of phonological processes that is useful for intervention planning.

ASSET (Assessing Semantic Skills through Everyday Themes). Barrett, M., Zachman, L., & Huisingh, R. (1988). East Moline, IL: LinguiSystems. Uses a thematic approach to assess receptive and expressive vocabulary for 3- to 9-year-olds in 10 tasks: understanding labels, identifying categories, identifying attributes, identifying functions, understanding definitions, expressing labels, expressing categories, expressing attributes, expressing functions, expressing definitions. Yields standard scores, percentile ranks, and age equivalencies.

Bankson-Bernthal Test of Phonology (BBTOP). Bankson, N. W., & Bernthal, J. E. (1990). Chicago, IL: The Riverside Publishing Company. Assesses articulation and phonological processes among children ages 3 to 9 years.

Bankson Language Text (2nd ed.) (BLT-2). Bankson, N. W. (1990). Austin, TX: Pro-Ed. In the revised version, test results may be reported for children from ages 3 through 7 years as standard scores or percentile ranks. Organized into three general categories: semantic knowledge (body parts, nouns, verbs, categories, functions, propositions, opposites); morphological/syntactic rules (pronouns, verb tense, auxiliaries, modals, copulas, plurals, comparatives/superlatives, negation, questions); and pragmatics (ritualizing, informing, controlling, imagining). Standardized on 1,200 children in 19 states.

Bilingual Syntax Measure I and II. Medida de Sintaxis Bilingue (BSM). Burt, M. K., Dulay, H. C., & Chavez, E. H. (1978). San Antonio, TX: Psychological Corporation. Assesses mastery of basic oral syntactic structures in both English and Spanish. Provides a criterion-referenced measure of proficiency.

Boder Test of Reading-Spelling Patterns. Boder, E., & Jarrico, S. (1982). San Antonio, TX: Psychological Corporation. This criterion-referenced test uses word reading and spelling tasks to identify students in elementary and secondary grades as having one of four types of reading disability: nonspecific, dysphonetic, eidetic, and mixed dysphonetic-eidetic.

Boehm Test of Basic Concepts (BTBC). Boehm, A. (1971). San Antonio, TX: Psychological Corporation.

Boehm Test of Basic Concepts—Revised (BTBC-R), and *Boehm Test of Basic Concepts—Preschool Version* Boehm, A. (1986). San Antonio, TX: Psychological Corporation. The preschool version is for children ages 3 to 5 years. It is individually administered to test comprehension of basic relational concepts. The BTBC-R is for children ages kindergarten to grade 2. It is group administered and tests concepts generally considered important for following teacher instructions. Yields percentile rankings.

Bracken Basic Concept Scale (BBCS). Bracken, B. A. (1984). San Antonio, TX: Psychological Corporation. Designed to be used with preschool- and primary-age children and children with receptive language difficulties. Items require either short verbal responses or pointing. Eleven subtests of colors, letter identification, numbers/counting, comparisons, shapes, direction/position, social/emotional, size, texture/material, quantity, and time/sequence. Yields percentile ranks, z-scores, and standard scores with a mean of 10 and standard deviation of 3 based on national norms.

Carolina Picture Vocabulary Test (CPVT). Layton, T. L., & Holmes, D. W. (1985). Austin, TX: Pro-Ed. Norm-referenced test of receptive sign vocabulary for deaf and hearing impaired children between 4 and 11:6 years.

Carrow Auditory–Visual Abilities Test (CAVAT). Carrow-Woolfolk, E. (1991). Allen, TX: DLM. Norm-referenced test with 14 subtests to measure auditory and visual perceptual, motor, and memory skills for children ages 4 to 10 years. Entire test takes 1½ hours. Yields percentile ranks and T-scores.

Carrow Elicited Language Inventory (CELI). Carrow E. (1974). Allen, TX: DLM. Designed for children ages 3:0 to 7:11. This norm-referenced test uses elicitation tasks to assess productive use of imitated grammatical structures. Yields percentile ranks and standard scores.

Clinical Evaluation of Language Fundamentals—Revised (CELF-R). Semel, E., Wiig, E., & Secord, W. (1987). San Antonio, TX: Psychological Corporation. This test is now standardized for children ages 5 to 16+. For children ages 5 to 7, a receptive language score is based on the subtests linguistic concepts, sentence structure, and oral directions. An expressive language score is based on the subtests word structure, formulated sentences, and recalling sentences. Supplemental subtests include listening to paragraphs, word associations, word classes, semantic relationships, and sentence assembly. The significance of receptive/expressive subtest differences can be tested statistically. (A screening test is available.)

Communication Abilities Diagnostic Test (CADeT). Johnston, E. B., & Johnston, A. V. (1989). Chicago, IL: The Riverside Publishing Company. Uses informal assessment tasks involving stories, a board game, and conversational contexts with children ages 3 to 9 to assess language development in the areas of syntax, semantics, and pragmatics. Used to observe abilities to identify feelings, make choices, give directions, predict outcomes, and verbalize problems. Yields norm-referenced language comprehension and expression scores.

Conner's Teacher Rating Scales (CTRS) and *Conner's Parent Rating Scales* (CPRS). Conners, C. K. (1989). Austin, TX: Pro-Ed. These scales provide both short and long versions to help identify hyperactive children. They can be used with children ages 3 to 17.

Denver Articulation Screening Examination (DASE). Drumright, A. (1971). Denver, CO: Ladoca Project and Publishing Foundation.

Detroit Tests of Learning Aptitude—Primary (DTLA-P). Hammill, D. D., & Bryant, B. R. (1986). Austin, TX: Pro-Ed. Designed for ages 3 through 9. Includes 11 subtests: articulation, conceptual matching, design reproduction, digit sequences, draw-a-person, letter sequences, motor directions, object sequences, oral directions, picture fragments, picture identification, sentence imitation, and symbolic relations. Yields standard scores, percentile ranks, composite scores, and a total score.

Developmental Assessment of Spanish Grammar (DASG). Toronto, A. S. (1976). *Journal of Speech and Hearing Disorders, 41,* 150-171. Adaptation of Lee's (1974) Developmental Sentence Scoring technique for Spanish speaking children.

Developmental Indicators for the Assessment of Learning—Revised (DIAL-R). Mardell-Czudnowski, C., & Goldenberg, D. S. (1990). Circle Pines, MN: AGS. A preschool and prekindergarten screening instrument that screens children ages 2 to 6 in three developmental skill areas (motor, concepts, and language) in 20 to 30 minutes. Includes statistical data from the three norming groups, 1990 census, caucasian, and minority. Results can be compared with cut-off scores at ±1, ±1.5, or ±2 *SD*.

Early Screening Profiles (ESP). Harrison, P., Kaufman, A., Kaufman, N., Bruininks, R., Rynders, J., Ilmer, S., Sparrow, S., & Cicchetti, D. (1990). Circle Pines, MN: AGS. Comprehensive screening instrument for children aged 2:0 to 6:11 years. Yields screening indexes or standard scores in cognitive/language, motor, or self-help social areas to identify at-risk or gifted children.

Expressive One Word Picture Vocabulary Test (EOWPVT). Gardner, M. (1979). Austin, TX: Pro-Ed. Assesses expressive vocabulary in children ages 2:0 to 11:11. (Can be administered with ROWPVT.)

Fisher-Logemann Test of Articulation Competence. Fisher, H.B., & Logemann, J. A. (1971). Chicago: The Riverside Publishing Company. Provides a picture test and sentence test for examining all English phonemes according to syllabic function—prevocalic intervocalic, and postvocalic—with frequent reliability checks. Preschool to adult.

Full Range Picture Vocabulary Test (FRPVT). Ammons, R., & Ammons, C. (1948). Missoula, MT: Psychological Test Specialists.

Goldman-Fristoe Test of Articulation (G-FTA). Goldman, R., & Fristoe, M. (1972, 1986). Circle Pines, MN: AGS. Measures articulation of sounds-in-words, sounds-in-sentences, and stimulability. Yields percentile ranks for the sounds-in-words and stimulability subtests for children ages 2 to 16+.

Goldman-Fristoe-Woodcock Auditory Skills Test Battery (GFW-Battery). Goldman, R., Fristoe, M., & Woodcock, C. W. (1976). Circle Pines, MN: AGS. For persons 3 years to adult, this is a battery of four 15-minute tests: auditory selective attention, diagnostic auditory discrimination, auditory memory, and sound–symbol association. Yields age-based standard scores, percentile ranks, stanines, and age equivalents.

Goldman-Fristoe-Woodcock Test of Auditory Discrimination (GFW). Goldman, R., Fristoe, M., & Woodcock, C. W. (1970). Circle Pines, MN: AGS. To be used with persons 3 years old and up, this is a test of closed-set word identification in quiet and in noise. Yields standard scores and percentile ranks.

Illinois Children's Language Assessment Test (ICLAT). Arit, P. (1977). Danville, IL: Interstate Printers and Publishers.

Illinois Test of Psycholinguistic Abilities (ITPA) (rev. ed.). Kirk, S., & Kirk, W. (1968). Urbana, IL: University of Illinois Press. This classic norm-referenced test includes 10 subtests (and two supplementary subtests) to evaluate auditory reception, visual reception, auditory association, visual association, verbal expression, manual expression, grammatic closure, visual closure, auditory sequential memory, visual sequential memory, auditory closure, and sound blending for children ages 2 to 10 years.

Kahn-Lewis Phonological Analysis (KLPA). Khan, L., & Lewis, N. (1986). Circle Pines, MN: AGS. To be used with the Goldman-Fristoe Test of Articulation (G-FTA) to analyze articulatory responses for the presence of 15 phonological processes. Percentile ranks, speech simplification ratings, and age equivalents can be computed for composite scores for children ages 2 through 5:11 years.

The Language Processing Test (LPT). Richard, G., & Hanner, M. A. (1985). East Moline, IL: LinguiSystems. This test is designed for 5- to 11-year-olds, yielding standard scores, percentile ranks, and age equivalencies for language processing tasks: associations, categorization, similarities, differences, multiple meanings, and attributes. Analysis yields information about processing deficits such as word retrieval difficulties, inappropriate word substitutions, nonspecific word usage, inability to correct errors, response avoidance, rehearsing responses, and unusual pauses.

Laradon Articulation Scale (LAS). Edmonston, W. (1963). Beverly Hills, CA: Western Psychological Services.

Let's Talk Inventory for Children (LTI-C). Bray, C. M., & Wiig, E. H. (1987). San Antonio, TX: Psychological Corporation. Helps identify preschool- and early ele-

mentary-age children who have inadequate or delayed social-verbal communication skills. Children are asked to formulate speech acts to go with pictured situational contexts. Items require formulation or association. Means and standard deviations are reported by age groups.

McCarthy Scales of Children's Abilities. McCarthy, D. (1972). San Antonio. TX: Psychological Corporation. Used with children ages 2:6 through 8:6, subscales may be used for differential diagnosis in six areas: verbal scale, quantitative scale, perceptual performance scale, general cognitive index, memory, and motor development.

Merrill Language Screening Test (MLST). Mumm, M. Secord, W., & Dykstra, K. (1980). San Antonio, TX: Psychological Corporation. Used with kindergarten and first-graders as a 5-minute screening test of language and articulation. Children retell a 3-minute story using six corresponding picture cards. Screens receptive and expressive language performance in five areas: production of complete sentences, utterance length, verb–tense agreements, elaboration, and communication competence.

Miller Assessment for Preschoolers (MAP). Miller, L. J. (1982). San Antonio, TX: Psychological Corporation. This comprehensive preschool screening instrument can be individually administered to children between 2:9 and 5:8 years in approximately 20 to 30 minutes per child. It yields percentiles for six age groups based on a standardization of 1,200 preschoolers across the United States.

Miller-Yoder Language Comprehension Test (MY). Miller, J. F., & Yoder, D. (1984). (Manual by G. Gill, M. Rosin, N. O. Owings, & K. A. Carlson). Austin, TX: Pro Ed. Includes three sets of pictures that can be used to assess comprehension of short simple sentences with a variety of grammatical structures. Can be administered to normally developing, developmentally delayed, or mentally retarded children. Results allow comparison to performance of same-age peers between 4 and 8 years.

Multilevel Informal Language Inventory (MILI). Goldsworth, C. L. (1982). San Antonio, TX: Psychological Corporation. Provides an informal assessment of level of language function for children from kindergarten through grade 6 in the production of critical semantic relations and syntactic constructions. Uses three types of tasks: survey scenes (elicit short but spontaneous language sample), survey stories (elicit storytelling and paraphrasing), and probes (of key syntactic structures).

Muma Assessment Program (MAP) (rev. 2nd ed.). Muma, J. R. (1981). Austin, TX: Pro-Ed. This criterion-referenced test may be used as a follow-up or alternative to standardized tests. It uses a "testing for teaching" approach with assessment of cognitive-linguistic-communication systems, which was developed for preschool through early elementary ages but can be used across age ranges. Taps multiple areas: different learning styles, sensorimotor skills, rule- and nonrule-governed learning, concepts of conservation, quantity, and likeness.

Northwestern Syntax Screening Test (NSST). Lee, L. (1971). Evanston, IL: Northwestern University Press. Uses a picture pointing task to measure receptive language and a delayed imitation task to measure expressive language for children from 3:0 to 8 years.

Peabody Picture Vocabulary Test (PPVT). Dunn, L. (1965). Circle Pines, MN: American Guidance Service.

Peabody Picture Vocabulary Test—Revised (PPVT-R). Dunn, L. M., & Dunn, L. M. (1981). Circle Pines, MN: AGS. Measures receptive vocabulary of standard American English. Yields standard scores ($M = 100$: $SD = 15$), percentile ranks, stanines, and age equivalents.

Photo Articulation Test (PAT). Pendergast, K., Dickey, S., Selmar, J., & Soder, A. (1984). Austin, TX: Pro-Ed. Color photographs are used to test articulation of all consonants, vowels, and diphthongs. Six Articulation Age Overlays (AAOs) are included to allow comparison of test results with norms.

Preschool Language Assessment Instrument (PLAI). Blank, M., Rose, S., & Berlin, L. (1978). San Antonio, TX: Psychological Corporation. This is not a standardized test but can be used to assess a variety of language skills: label objects and actions, role play, respond to conversational interactions, describe object functions, solve problems, define, and perform other language skills related to academic success. Can be used with Spanish-speaking children.

Preschool Language Scale (PLS). Zimmerman, I. L., Steiner, V. G., & Pond, R. E. (1979). San Antonio, TX: Psychological Corporation. This is not a standardized test, but raw scores can be converted to language age scores. It includes tasks for measuring auditory comprehension and verbal ability.

Preschool Language Scale—3 (PLS-3). Zimmerman, I. L., Steiner, V. G., and Pond, R. E. (1992). San Antonio, TX: Psychological Corporation. Revised and standardized for use with children from birth to age 6:11. Takes 20 to 30 minutes and yields total language, auditory comprehension, and expressive communication standard scores, percentile ranks, and language-age equivalents. A Spanish-language version, with norms based on Spanish-speaking children throughout the United States, is also available.

Preschool Language Screening Test (PLST). Hannah, E., & Gardner, J. (1974). Northridge, CA: Joyce Publications.

Prueba del Desarrollo Inicial del Lenguaje (PDIL). Hresko, W. P., Reid, D. K., & Hammill, D. D. (1982). Austin, TX: Pro-Ed. This is a standardized test of the Spanish spoken language for children ages 3 to 7 years. It includes 38 items used to assess receptive and expressive language through a variety of semantic and syntactic tasks.

The Quick Test (QT). Ammons, R., & Ammons, C. (1962). Provisional manual. *Psychological Reports Monograph Supplement* (Suppl. 1–7).

Receptive One Word Picture Vocabulary Test (ROWPVT). Gardner, M. (1985). Austin, TX: Pro-Ed. Assesses receptive vocabulary in children ages 2:0 through 11:11 years. (Can be administered with EOWPVT.)

Receptive Expressive Emergent Language Scale (REEL—scale). Bzoch, K., & League, R. (1971). Austin, TX: Pro-Ed. (See "Early Stage" for description).

Rhode Island Test of Language Structure (RITLS). Engen, E., & Engen, T. (1983). Austin, TX: Pro-Ed. This test of English language development emphasizes understanding of language structure. It was primarily designed for use with children with hearing impairments (ages 3 to 20 years) but can also be used with other children (ages 3 to 6 years), including those who have mental retardation or learning disabilities or who are bilingual.

Screening Kit of Language Development (SKOLD). Bliss, L. S., & Allen, D. V. (1983). East Aurora, NY: Slosson Educational Publications. Screening test that can be administered to 2- to 5-year-old children in 15 minutes by paraprofessionals. Assesses preschool language development in six areas: vocabulary, comprehension, story completion, individual and paired sentence repetition without pictures, and comprehension of commands. It is norm-referenced for both Black English- and Standard English-speaking children.

Screening Test for Auditory Processing Disorders (SCAN). Keith, R. W. (1986). San Antonio, TX: Psychological Corporation. This test of auditory processing is designed for children ages 3 to 11 years. It consists of three subtests, which may be presented using a regular portable stereo cassette player: filtered words (two lists of 20 monosyllabic low-pass filtered words); auditory figure-ground (two lists of 20 monosyllabic words presented to the same ear as multitalker speech babble); and competing words (two lists of 25 monosyllabic words presented simultaneously to right and left ears.

Screening Test for Developmental Apraxia of Speech (STDAS). Blakely, R. W. (1980). Austin, TX: Pro-Ed. Designed to assist in the differential diagnosis of speech apraxia in children ages 4 through 12. Uses eight subtests: expressive language discrepancy, vowels and diphthongs, oral-motor movement, verbal sequencing, motorically complex words, articulation, transposition, and prosody.

Slingerland Screening Tests for Identifying Children With Specific Language Disability. Slingerland, B. H. (1970). Cambridge, MA: Educators Publishing Service. Group-administered screening test for identifying specific language disability in reading, writing, and spelling in children in grades 1 through 6. (Spanish version by L. R. Strong, 1989.)

Stephens Oral Language Screening Test (SOLST). Stephens, M. I. (1977). Peninsula, OH: Interim Publishers.

Structured Photographic Expressive Language Test–Preschool (SPELT-P). Werner, E. O., & Kreshech, J. D. (1983). Sandwich, IL: Janelle Publication. Uses snapshots to elicit early developing morphological and syntactic forms, including prepositions, plurals, possessive nouns and pronouns, present progressive, regular/irregular past tense, contractible, uncontractible copula, negation. It can be administered in 10 to 15 minutes to children from ages 3:0 to 5:11. Guidelines are provided for analyzing productions from speakers of Black English.

Spanish Structured Photographic Expressive Language Test—Preschool (Spanish SPELT-P). Werner, E. O., & Kresheck, J. D. (1989). Sandwich, IL: Janelle Publications. This version uses snapshots to elicit early developing Spanish morphological and syntactic forms. It can be administered in 10 to 15 minutes to children from ages 3:0 to 5:11. The manual addresses issues in assessing children with limited English proficiency and provides developmental guidelines for Spanish morphology and syntax.

Structured Photographic Expressive Language Test—II (SPELT-II). Werner, E. O., & Kresheck, J. D. (1983). Sandwich, IL: Janelle Publications. This version of the test is for children ages 4:0 to 9:5. It elicits prepositions, plurals, possessive nouns and pronouns, reflexive pronouns, present progressive, regular/irregular past tense, future, contractible/uncontractible copula, contractible/uncontractible auxiliary, and secondary verbs. It also elicits syntactic structures: affirmatives, negatives, conjoined sentences, imperatives, *Wh*-questions and interrogative reversals. Guidelines are provided for analyzing productions from speakers of Black English.

Spanish Structured Photographic Expressive Language Test—II (Spanish SPELT-II). Werner, I. O., & Kreshech,

J. D. (1989). Sandwich, IL: Janelle Publications. This Spanish version of SPELT-II elicits articles; prepositions; plural and possessive nouns; possessive and reflexive pronouns; future, present, present progressive, and preterit (past) tenses of regular and irregular verbs; singular and plural present and past forms of copulas; secondary verbs; *Wh*- and Y/N interrogatives; and negatives. It can be administered in 10 to 15 minutes to children from ages 4:0 to 9:5. The manual addresses issues in assessing children with limited English proficiency and provides developmental guidelines for Spanish morphology and syntax.

Templin-Darley Tests of Articulation (T-D) (2nd ed.). Templin, M. & Darley, F. (1969). Iowa City, IA: University of Iowa.

Test of Auditory Comprehension of Language (TACL). Carrow, E. (1973). Austin, TX: Teaching Resources.

Test of Auditory Comprehension of Language—Revised (TACL-R). Carrow, E. (1985). Allen, TX: DLM. The revised test provides age and grade norms for ages 3:0 through 9:11. Assesses auditory comprehension of word classes and relations, grammatical morphemes, elaborated sentence constructions. Yields standard scores, percentile ranks, age equivalents. (A computerized scoring system is also available.)

Test of Auditory-Perceptual Skills (TAPS). Gardner, M. F. (1985) Burlingame, CA: Psychological and Educational Publications. This test can be administered in 10 to 15 minutes to children between 4 and 12 years. It assesses auditory discrimination, sequential memory, word memory, sentence memory, interpretation of directions, and processing (based on learning and thinking) and provides a measure of hyperactivity. Scores may be converted to stanines, percentiles, auditory age equivalents, and auditory standard scores for each subtest.

Test of Awareness of Language Segments (TALS). Sawyer, D. J. (1987). Austin, TX: Pro-Ed. A screening test that can be administered to children from 4:6 through 7 years. Includes 46 items distributed across three subtests: sentences-to-words, words-to-syllables, and words-to-sounds. Cut off scores permit inferences about readiness to meet instructional demands of beginning reading programs, and which types of introductory reading approach might be easier for an individual child to master.

Test of Early Language Development (TELD). Hresko, W. P., Reid, D. K., & Hammill, D. D. (1981). Austin, TX: Pro-Ed. Measures spoken language abilities of children ages 3:0 through 7:11 in the areas of semantics and syntax in about 15 minutes using 38 items. Yields standard scores, percentile ranks, and age equivalent scores.

Test of Early Reading Ability—2 (TERA-2). Reid, D. K., Hresko, W. P., & Hammill, D. D. (1989). Austin, TX: Pro-Ed. Measures reading abilities of children between the ages 3:0 and 9:11. Items measure knowledge of contextual meaning, alphabet, and conventions. Standard scores with $M = 100$ and $SD = 15$ result.

Test of Early Written Language (TEWL). Hresko, W. P. (1988). Austin, TX: Pro-Ed. Measures emerging written language abilities of children ages 3:0 through 7:11. Standard scores and percentiles may be particularly helpful for identifying mildly handicapped students.

Test for Examining Expressive Morphology (TEEM). Shipley, K. G., Stone, T. A., & Sue, M. B. (1983). Tucson, AZ: Communication Skill builders. Evaluates use of expressive morphemes by 3- to 8-year-olds (in 7 minutes). Assesses present progressives, plurals, possessives, past tenses, third-person singulars, derived adjectives. Norms based on more than 500 children.

Test of Language Competence—Expanded Edition (TLC-Expanded). Wiig, E. H., & Secord, W. (1988). Identifies language and communication deficits in children ages 5 through 19 years. Includes two levels. Level 1 is designed for ages 5 through 9 years. It includes subtests: ambiguous sentences, listening comprehension (making inferences), oral expression (recreating speech acts), figurative language. Yields subtest and composite standard scores, and age-equivalent scores.

Test of Language Development (TOLD). Newcomer, P., & Hammill, D. (1977). Austin, TX: Pro-Ed. (Earlier version of TOLD-2).

Test of Language Development—2 Primary (TOLD-2 Prim.). Newcomer, P. L., & Hammill, D. D. (1988). Austin, TX: Pro-Ed. To be used with children ages 4:0 to 8:11, this test requires approximately 40 minutes. It yields standard and percentile scores. Seven subtests measure different components of spoken language: picture vocabulary (understanding words); oral vocabulary (defining words); grammatic understanding (understanding sentence structures); sentence imitation (generating proper sentences); grammatic completion (using acceptable morphological forms); word discrimination (noticing sound differences); and word articulation (saying words correctly).

Test of Nonverbal Intelligence—2 (TONI-2). Brown, L., Sherbenou, R. J., & Johnsen, S. K. (1990). Austin, TX: Pro-Ed. The administration of this test requires no reading, writing, speaking, or listening by the test subject. It measures intelligence, aptitude, and reasoning and may be used with individuals from age 5:0 through 85:11, including individuals with severe speech impairments, brain injury, and deafness or hearing loss.

Test of Pragmatic Skills—Revised. Shulman, B. B. (1986). *Computerized Test of Pragmatic Skills.* Shulman, B. B., & Fitch, J. L. (1987). Tucson, AZ: Communication Skill Builders. Assesses communicative intentions in 10 categories, including naming/labelling, reasoning, denying. Provides mean and percentile data.

Test of Problem Solving (TOPS). Zachman, L., Barrett, M., Huisingh, R., & Jorgensen, C. (1984). East Moline, IL: LinguiSystems. This standardized test for 6- to 11-year-olds assesses expressive reasoning in the areas explaining inferences ("How does the family know the electricity just went off?"); determining causes of events ("How did the boy's bike get a flat tire?"); answering "why" questions ("Why shouldn't he ride his bike with a flat tire?"); determining solutions ("The losing team has lost three games in a row. What could they do to improve the way they play?"), and avoiding problems ("The boy dripped all over his shirt. What could he have done to keep from getting his shirt dirty?").

Test of Relational Concepts (TRC). Edmonston, N. K., & Thane, N. L. (1988). Austin, TX: Pro-Ed. Tests understanding of 56 relational concepts among children between the ages 3:0 to 7:11, including dimensional adjectives, spatial, temporal, and quantitative words. Takes approximately 15 minutes to administer and yields standard scores and percentile ranks for 10 six-month age groups.

Test of Word Finding (TWF). German, D. J. (1986; manual revised, 1989). Allen, TX: DLM. This is a standardized test of word finding skills for 6:6- to 12:11-year-olds with naming tasks organized into five sections: picture naming (nouns); sentence completion; description naming; picture naming (verbs); and picture naming (categories). A sixth section is used to assess comprehension or concept deficits. Analysis includes both accuracy and response time, yielding standard scores, percentile ranks, and grade standards.

Test of Word Finding in Discourse (TWFD). German, D. J. (1991). Allen, TX: DLM. Includes standardized procedures for assessing word finding in discourse for individuals from 6:6 to 12:11 years and nonstandardized procedures for individuals outside the normed age range.

Token Test for Children (TTC). DiSimoni, F. (1978). Allen, TX: DLM. Used for children ages 3 to 12 years. Yields age and grade scores.

Test de Vocabulario en Imágenes Peabody (TVIP). Dunn, L. M., Lugo, D. E., Padilla, E. R., & Dunn, L. M. (1986). Circle Pines, MN: AGS. A test of receptive Spanish vocabulary (modified from the vocabulary of the PPVT-R to be culturally appropriate) for 2:6- to 18-year-olds. Separate and combined norms are available for children with either Mexican or Puerto Rican backgrounds.

Utah Test of Language Development (UTLD). Mecham, M., Joy, J. & Jones, J. (1967). Salt Lake City: Communication Research Associates.

Utah Test of Language Development—3 (UTLD-3). Mecham, M. J. (1989). Austin, TX: Pro-Ed. This revision can be administered to children from ages 3:0 to 10:11 years. It yields subtest standard scores with $M = 10$ and $SD = 3$ in the areas of language comprehension and language expression. It also yields a language quotient score with $M = 100$ and $SD = 15$.

Vane Evaluation of Language Scale (VANE-L). Vane, J. (1975). Brandon, VT: Clinical Psychology Publishing.

Verbal Language Development Scale (VLDS). Mecham, M. (1958). Circle Pines, MN: AGS.

Visual-Aural Digit Span Test. Koppitz, E. M. (1977). San Antonio, TX: Psychological Corporation.

Vocabulary Comprehension Scale. Bangs, T. E. (1975). Allen TX: DLM. Criterion-referenced checklist of 95 vocabulary words and phrases in a developmentally sequenced order based on performance by 542 preschool and kindergarten children. Includes pronouns, quantity, quality, position, direction, size, time, possessives, category words, negation, identification of objects by function. Takes 20 minutes to 1 hour to administer.

Wechsler Intelligence Scale for Children—Revised (WISC-R). Wechsler, D. (1974). San Antonio, TX: Psychological Corporation. This intelligence test is a used for testing the verbal scale and performance scale intelligence of children ages 6 to 16 years.

Wechsler Preschool and Primary Scale of Intelligence (WPPSI). Wechsler, D. (1967). San Antonio, TX: Psychological Corporation. This intelligence test is a downward extension of the WISC-R, used for testing children ages 4:0 to 6:6 years.

Wide Range Achievement Test—Revised (WRAT-R). Jastak, S., & Wilkinson, G. S. (1984). San Antonio, TX: Psychological Corporation. Level 1 assesses reading (at the single word level), spelling, and arithmetic abilities for children ages 5 through 11 years. Level 2 is for persons ages 12 through 75. Yields standard scores, percentiles, and grade equivalents.

Wiig Criterion-Referenced Inventory of Language (Wiig CRIL). Wiig, E. H. (1990). San Antonio, TX: Psychological Corporation. This criterion-referenced assessment can be used as follow-up to norm-referenced testing to obtain baseline information and plan intervention in the areas of semantics, morphology, syntax, and pragmatics. For children ages 4 through 15 years.

Woodcock-Johnson Psycho-Educational Battery—Revised (WJ-R). Woodcock, R. W., & Johnson, W. B. (1989). Allen, TX: DLM. Includes two batteries: *Tests of Cognitive Ability* and *Tests of Achievement*. Based on extensive standardization information for persons in the age range 2 to 90+ years. It is a lengthy test, but it is divided into standard and supplemental batteries. The standard battery of the cognitive test can be used to yield a full-scale cognitive score in 40 minutes. The standard cognitive subtests are memory for names, memory for sentences, visual matching, incomplete words, visual closure, picture vocabulary, and analysis-synthesis. The supplemental cognitive subtests are visual-auditory learning, memory for words, cross out, sound blending, picture recognition, oral vocabulary, concept formation, delayed recall for names, delayed recall for visual-auditory learning, sound patterns, spatial relations, listening comprehension, and verbal analogies. The standard achievement subtests are letter–word identification, passage comprehension, calculation, applied problems, dictation, writing samples, science, social studies, humanities. The supplemental achievement subtests are word attack, reading vocabulary, quantitative concepts, proofing, writing fluency, punctuation, spelling, usage, and handwriting.

The Word Test—R. Huisingh, R., Barrett, M., Zachman, L., Blagden, C., & Orman, J. (1990). East Moline, IL: LinguiSystems. This test is designed for 7- to 11-year-old children. It uses six subtests to assess associations, antonyms, synonyms, definitions, semantic absurdities, and multiple definitions. Standard scores, percentile ranks, and age equivalencies are provided for individual subtests and the total test.

LATER STAGE ASSESSMENT DEVICES

Note: Sources include Deal and Rodriguez (1987) and McCauley and Swisher (1984).

Adapted Sequenced Inventory of Communication Development for Adolescents and Adults with Severe Handicaps (A-SICD). McClennen, S. E. (1989). Seattle: University of Washington Press. Retains theoretical basis for SICD-R but uses tasks, materials, and interactions appropriate for adolescents and adults, including those with severe hearing loss, legal blindness, epilepsy, spastic-quadriplegia, and nonambulation.

Adolescent Language Screening Test (ALST). Morgan, D. L., & Guilford, A. M. (1984). Austin, TX: Pro-Ed. Requires less than 15 minutes to screen speech and language for 11- to 17-year-old students. Includes seven subtests: pragmatics, receptive vocabulary, concepts, expressive vocabulary, sentence formulation, morphology, and phonology.

Assessing Asian Language Performance: Guidelines for Evaluating Limited-English-Proficient Students (2nd ed.). Cheng, L.-R. L. (1991). Oceanside, CA: Academic Communication Associates. Provides information about nonbiased assessment, cultural values, and communicative behaviors for individuals who are Vietnamese, Korean, Chinese, Japanese, Filipino, and members of other Asian populations.

Boder Test of Reading–Spelling Patterns. Boder, E., Jarrico, S. (1982). San Antonio, TX: Psychological Corporation. This criterion-reference test uses word reading and spelling tasks to identify students in elementary and secondary grades as having one of four types of reading disability: nonspecific, dysphonetic, eidetic, and mixed dysphonetic-eidetic.

Classroom Communication Screening Procedure for Early Adolescents (CCSPEA) (rev. ed.). Simon, C. S. (1987). Tempe, AZ: Communi-Cog. Designed for screening large groups of upper elementary students before their entering junior high school. It is recommended for students who score below the 40th percentile on standardized reading assessments and other students whose underachievement might stem from oral language deficits. Assesses abilities to scan an assignment for answers, follow oral and multipart written directions, use metalinguistic and metacognitive skills, and match vocabulary items with definitions/synonyms.

Clinical Evaluation of Language Fundamentals—Revised (CELF-R). Semel, E., Wiig, E., & Secord, W. (1987). San Antonio, TX: Psychological Corporation. This test is now standardized for children ages 5 to 16+. For children ages 8 to 16, a receptive language score is based on the following subtests: oral directions, word classes, and semantic relationships. An expressive language score is based on the following subtests: formulated sentences, recalling sentences, and sentence assembly. Supplemental subtests include listening to paragraphs, word associations, linguistic concepts, sentence structure, and word structure. The significance of receptive/expressive subtest dif-

ferences can be tested statistically. (A screening test is available.)

Conner's Teacher Rating Scales (CTRS) and *Conner's Parent Rating Scales* (CPRS). Conners, C. K. (1989). Austin, TX: Pro-Ed. These scales provide both short and long versions to help identify hyperactive children. They can be used with children ages 3 to 17.

Detroit Tests of Learning Aptitude—2 (DTLA-2). Hammill, D. D. (1985). Austin, TX: Pro-Ed. Designed for 6- through 17-year-olds. Includes 11 subtests: word opposites, sentence imitation, oral directions, word sequences, story construction, design reproduction, object sequences, symbolic relations, conceptual matching, word fragments, and letter sequences. Yields nine composite scores of specific abilities in linguistic, cognitive, attention, and motor domains.

Evaluating Communicative Competence: A Functional Pragmatic Procedure (rev. ed.). Simon, C. S. (1986). Tucson, AZ: Communication Skill Builders. Uses 21 informal evaluation tasks to assess the skills of 9- to 17-year-olds as communicators. Includes tasks to measure language processing, metalinguistic skills, and functional uses of language for varied communicative purposes. A videotape is also available.

Expressive One Word Picture Vocabulary Test: Upper Extension (EOWPVT-UE). Gardner, M., & Brownell, R. (1983). Austin, TX: Pro-Ed. Assesses expressive vocabulary in children ages 12 to 15 years. (Can be administered with ROWPVT-UE.)

Goldman-Fristoe-Woodcock Auditory Skills Test Battery (GFW-Battery). Goldman R., Fistoe, M., & Woodcock, C. W. (1976). Circle Pines, MN: AGS. For persons 3 years to adult, this is a battery of four 15-minute tests: auditory selective attention, diagnostic auditory discrimination, auditory memory, and sound–symbol associations. It yields age-based standard scores, percentile ranks, stanines, and age equivalents.

Goldman-Fristoe-Woodcock Test of Auditory Discrimination (GFW). Goldman, R., Fristoe, M., & Woodcock, C. W. (1970). Circle Pines, MN: AGS. To be used with persons 3 years old and up, this is a test of closed-set word identification in quiet and in noise. It yields standard scores and percentile ranks.

Gray Oral Reading Tests—Diagnostic (GORT-D). Bryant, B. R., & Wiederholt, J. L. (1990). Austin, TX: Pro-Ed. This test is designed for children in kindergarten through grade 6 who have trouble reading print. The first subtest requires the student to orally read passages and respond to comprehension questions. If the student performs poorly on this subtest, the remaining subtests are administered: decoding (consonant/cluster recognition, phonogram recognition, blending); word identification (word recognition and vocabulary); word attack, morphemic analysis; contextual analysis; and word ordering. Scores are reported as grade equivalents, standard scores ($M = 100$; $SD = 15$), and percentiles.

Gray Oral Reading Tests (3rd ed.) (GORT-3). Wiederholt, J. L., & Bryant, B. R. (1989). Austin, TX: Pro-Ed. This revisions yields a passage score and standard scores and percentile rankings for oral reading comprehension for students' ages 7:0 through 18:11. The manual provides a system for performing a miscue analysis. Analysis provides information in the following four areas: meaning similarity, function similarity, graphic/phonemic similarity, and self-correction.

Let's Talk Inventory for Adolescents (LTI-A). Bray, C. M., & Wiig, E. H. (1982). San Antonio, TX: Psychological Corporation. Helps identify inadequate or delayed social-verbal communication skills among 9-year-olds to young adults. Probes ability to formulate speech acts appropriate for pictured situational contexts for the functions: ritualizing, informing, controlling, feeling. Pictures represent interaction both with adolescent peers and with an authority figure. Means and standard deviations are reported for 2-year intervals.

Lindamood Auditory Conceptualization Test (LAC). Lindamood, C., & Lindamood, P. (1979). Allen, TX: DLM. Criterion-referenced test for ages preschool to adult. Measures auditory discrimination and perception of number and order of speech sounds in sequences. Takes 10 minutes. Spanish cue sheets are available.

Matrix Analogies Test—Short Form and *—Expanded Form.* Naglieri, J. A. (1985). San Antonio, TX: Psychological Corporation. This test can be used with students ages 5 through 17 years. It uses a task in which a missing element must be selected from six options to fit into an analogical matrix. Yields percentile ranks, stanines, and age equivalents by half-year intervals.

Picture Story Language Test (PSLT). Myklebust, H. R. (1965). San Antonio, TX: Psychological Corporation. Used with children ages 7 to 17, this test is used for differential diagnosis of learning disabilities, mental retardation, emotional disturbance, reading disability, and dyslexia. Individuals are asked to write the best story possible about a picture. Five scores are obtained: total words, total sentences, words per sentence, syntax, abstract-concrete meaning.

Prueba de Lectura & Lenguaje Escrito (PLLE). Hammill, D. D., Larsen, S. C., Wiederholt, J. L., & Fountain-Chambers, J. (1982). Austin, TX: Pro-Ed. This is a standardized battery of reading and writing in Spanish for children in grades 3 through 10. Its 6 subtests measure reading vocabulary, paragraph reading, thematic maturity, writing vocabulary, writing style, and spelling.

Pupil Rating Scale–Revised. Myklebust, H. R. (1981). San Antonio, TX: Psychological Corporation. Can be used to screen for learning disabilities with students ages 5 to 14. Teachers complete the scales, using a 5-point scale, in 5 to 10 minutes in five areas: auditory comprehension and memory, spoken language, orientation, motor coordination, and personal-social behavior.

Raven Progressive Matrices. Raven, J. C. (1986). San Antonio, TX: Psychological Corporation. Designed for age range 8 to 65 years. Assesses mental ability by requiring the examinee to solve problems in abstract figures and designs that assess nonverbal analogical reasoning ability. Percentiles are available for British children and adults.

Receptive One Word Picture Vocabulary Test: Upper Extension (ROWPVT-UE). Gardner, M., & Brownell, R. (1987). Austin, TX: Pro-Ed. Assesses expressive vocabulary in children ages 12 to 15 years. (Can be administered with EOWPVT-UE.)

Ross Information Processing Assessment (RIPA). Ross, D. G. (1986). Austin, TX: Pro-Ed. This test is designed to assess cognitive linguistic deficits following traumatic brain injuries to adolescents and adults. It allows quantification of cognitive deficits, establishment of severity ratings, development of rehabilitation goals and objectives, and profiles in 10 areas: immediate memory, recent memory, temporal orientation (recent memory), temporal orientation (remote memory), spatial orientation, orientation to environment, recall of general information, problem solving and abstract reasoning, organization, and auditory processing and retention.

Speech and Language Evaluation Scale (SLES). Fressola, D. R., & Hoerchler, S. C. (1989). Columbia, MO: Hawthorne Educational Services. Includes a teacher rating scale and speech and language scale, which can be completed in approximately 20 minutes and used for screening, referral, and follow-up in areas of articulation, voice, fluency, form, content, and pragmatics.

Stanford Diagnostic Reading Test, Third Edition (SDRT). Karlsen, B., & Gardner, E. F. (1984). San Antonio, TX: Psychological Corporation. Provides diagnostic reading tasks at four levels (red, green, brown, blue) to measure specific strengths and needs in reading. Yields standard scores, percentile ranks, stanines, and grade equivalents.

Test of Adolescent Language—2 (TOAL-2). Hammill, D. D., Brown, V. L., Larsen, S. C., & Wiederholt, J. L. (1987). Austin, TX: Pro-Ed. A revision of the TOAL (originally published in 1981), in which easier items have been added to each subtest. Yields an adolescent language quotient (ALQ) and composite scores in 10 areas: listening, speaking, reading, writing, spoken language, written language, vocabulary, grammar, receptive language, and expressive language. Normative information for students ages 12:0 through 18:5.

Test of Language Competence—Expanded Edition (TLC-Expanded). Wiig, E. H., & Secord, W. (1989). San Antonio, TX. Psychological Corporation. Identifies language and communication deficits in children ages 5 through 19 years. Includes two levels. Level 2 is designed for ages 9 through 18 years. It includes the following subtests: ambiguous sentences, listening comprehension (making inferences), oral expression (recreating speech acts), figurative language, remembering word pairs (supplemental subtest). Yields subtest and composite standard scores, and age-equivalent scores.

Test of Language Development—2 Intermediate (TOLD-2 Int.). Newcomer, P. L., & Hammill, D. D. (1988). Austin, TX: Pro-Ed. To be used with children ages 8:6 to 12:11, this test requires approximately 40 minutes to give. It yields standard and percentile scores. Has six subtests that measure different components of spoken language: sentence combining (constructing sentences); vocabulary (understanding word relationships); word ordering (constructing sentences); generals (knowing abstract relationships); grammatic comprehension (recognizing grammatical sentences); and malapropisms (correcting ridiculous sentences).

Test of Nonverbal Intelligence—2 (TONI-2). Brown, L., Sherbenou, R. J., & Johnsen, S. K. (1990). Austin, TX: Pro-Ed. The administration of this test requires no reading, writing, speaking, or listening by the test subject. It measures intelligence, aptitude, and reasoning, and may be used with individuals from ages 5:0 through 85:11, including individuals with severe speech impairments, brain injury, and deafness or hearing loss.

Test of Reading Comprehension (TORC). Brown, V. L. Hammill, D. D., & Wiederholt, L. J. (1986). Austin, TX: Pro-Ed. This is a multidimensional test of silent reading comprehension for students ages 7 through 17 years. The four major subtests measure general vocabulary, syntactic similarities, paragraph reading, and sentence sequencing. Five supplemental subtests measure abilities to read the vocabulary of math, science, and social studies, and the language of written directions.

Test of Adolescent/Adult Word Finding (TAWF). German, D. J. (1990). Allen, TX: DLM. This is a standardized test of word-finding skills for adolescents from 12 to 19:11 years, and adults from 20 to 80 years. It also includes a 10-minute brief test. Naming tasks are organized into five sections: picture naming (nouns), picture naming (verbs), sentence completion naming, description naming, and naming categories of words. Analysis includes both accuracy and response time, yielding standard scores, percentile ranks, and grade standards.

Test of Written Language—2 (TOWL-2). Hammill, D. D., & Larsen, S. C. (1988). The revision provides two forms and new stimulus pictures for the spontaneous writing task that are analyzed for thematic maturity, contextual vocabulary, syntactic maturity, contextual spelling, and contextual style. Contrived writing tasks are also used to assess vocabulary, style and spelling, logical sentences, and sentence combining. Normative data are available for students ages 7:0 through 17:11 years.

Wide Range Achievement Test—Revised (WRAT-R). Jastak, S., & Wilkinson, G. S. (1984). San Antonio, TX: Psychological Corporation. Level 1 assesses reading (at the single-word level), spelling, and arithmetic abilities for children ages 5 through 11 years. Level 2 is for persons ages 12 through 75. Yields standard scores, percentiles, and grade equivalents.

Woodcock-Johnson Psycho-Educational Battery-Revised (WJ-R). Woodcock, R. W., & Johnson, W. B. (1989). Allen, TX: DLM. Includes two batteries: *Tests of Cognitive Ability* and *Tests of Achievement*. This battery is based on extensive standardization information for persons in the age range 2 to 90+ years. It is a lengthy test, but it is divided into standard and supplemental batteries. The standard battery of the cognitive test can be used to yield a full-scale cognitive score in 40 minutes. The standard cognitive subtests are memory for names, memory for sentences, visual matching, incomplete words, visual closure, picture vocabulary, and analysis-synthesis. The supplemental cognitive subtests are visual-auditory learning, memory for words, cross out, sound blending, picture recognition, oral vocabulary, concept formation, delayed recall for names, delayed recall for visual–auditory learning, sound patterns, spatial relations, listening comprehension, and verbal analogies. The standard achievement subtests are letter-word identification, passage comprehension, calculation, applied problems, dictation, writing samples, science, social studies, and humanities. The supplemental achievement subtests are word attack, reading vocabulary, quantitative concepts, proofing, writing fluency, punctuation, spelling, usage, handwriting.

Woodcock Language Proficiency Battery, English Form and *Spanish Form.* Woodcock, R. W. (1980). Allen, TX: DLM. This battery measures oral language, reading, and written language for persons ages 3 to 80+. It uses eight subtests in areas of oral language (picture vocabulary, antonyms and synonyms, analogies); reading (letter–word identification, word attack, passage comprehension); and written language (dictation, proofing, punctuation and capitalization, spelling, usage). The English form can be used with students for whom English is a second language if the Spanish form is also administered.

Woodcock Reading Mastery Tests—Revised (WRMT-R). Woodcock, R. W. (1987). Circle Pines, MN: AGS. This test may be used with persons ages 5 to 75+. Form G includes the following subtests: visual-auditory learning, letter identification, word identification, word attack, word comprehension (antonyms, synonyms, analogies), and passage comprehension. Form H includes word identification, word attack, word comprehension (antonyms, synonyms, analogies), and passage comprehension. Test scores are combined to form five clusters, with age and grade based on standard scores, percentile ranks, and equivalency scores.

The Word Test—Adolescent. Zachman, L., Huisingh, R., Barrett, M., Orman, J., & Blagden, C. (1989). East Moline, IL: LinguiSystems. This is a norm-referenced test for 12- to 17-year-olds that uses four tasks to assess semantic knowledge tapped by academic expectations and everyday life: brand names (explaining why a semantically descriptive name of a product is appropriate); synonyms; signs of the times (telling what a sign or message means and why it is important); and definitions. Yields standard scores, percentile ranks, and age equivalencies for both subtests and total test.

Appendix B

**SUMMARY AND REFERENCE CHARTS TO USE IN MAKING
SERVICE-DELIVERY AND AUGMENTATIVE AND ALTERNATIVE
COMMUNICATION DECISIONS ABOUT CHILDREN WITH SEVERE
COMMUNICATION IMPAIRMENTS**

Name: _____   BD: _____   Speech–Language Clinician: _____

Date: _____   Classroom Teacher: _____

SUMMARY CHART

COGNITIVE BASES	RECEPTIVE LANGUAGE	EXPRESSIVE LANGUAGE	SOCIAL INTERACTION & PLAY
Preintentional (Birth to 8 months) *Sensorimotor I, II, III* ___ Infant moves from being purely re-flexive to showing the initial beginnings of goal-oriented behavior ___ Developing object permanence	___ Startles to sound ___ Turns to sound ___ Reacts to human voice ___ Responds to tone of voice	___ Cry ___ Reflexive Vocalizations	___ Engages in interaction ___ Maintains interaction ___ Initiates interaction ___ Indicates preference for familiar people and objects
Early intentional (8 to 12 months) *Sensorimotor IV* ___ Uses familiar means to achieve novel ends	___ No word comprehension yet ___ Imitates on-going action ___ Looks where parent looks	___ Differentiated cries ___ Syllabic babbling	___ Plays nursery games ___ Plays with toys
Late intentional (12 to 18 months) *Sensorimotor V* ___ Invention of new means to achieve familiar ends	___ Responds appropriately to single words in context	___ Hi/bye routines ___ First words ___ Words used as 'performatives' (to manipulate environment)	___ Solitary or onlooker play ___ Hugs doll, pulls toy
Representational (18 to 24 months) *Thought* *Sensorimotor VI* ___ Begins symbolic thinking	___ Understands words without context (points to pictures) ___ Follows 2-word commands	___ Novel one-word utterances ___ Asks "What's that?" ___ Onset of 2-word utterances	___ Parallel play
Early Preoperations (2 to 3½ yrs.) ___ Thought is preconceptual ___ Inference is sometimes but not always correct	___ Begins to understand Wh-questions ___ Answers yes/no questions	___ Two-word utterances ___ Basic sentences develop ___ Morphological markers develop	___ Symbolic play
Late Preoperations (3½ to 7 yrs.) ___ Beginning of intuitive thought ___ Problem solves by trial & error (not always correct)	___ Points to pictures representing sentences ___ Uses word order to understand agent–object relationships	___ Uses compound and complex sentences ___ Uses language to relate experiences ___ Talks about remote experiences ___ Adequate voice, articulation, fluency	___ Plays in small groups
Concrete Operations (7 to 12 yrs.) ___ Classifies on 2 characteristics	___ Understands conditional causal sentences	___ More clauses per sentence ___ Uses language to converse, persuade, tease	___ Genuine cooperative play

Recommendations:

Instructions:
1. Place a check mark beside characteristics demonstrated (reference chart or other evaluation tools may be used as necessary)
2. Shade in areas which describe functioning (areas may be partially shaded)
3. Refer to program decision chart

REFERENCE CHART

COGNITIVE BASES	RECEPTIVE LANGUAGE	EXPRESSIVE LANGUAGE	SOCIAL INTERACTION & PLAY
Preintentional (Birth to 8 months) *Sensorimotor Stages I, II, III* ___ Little evidence of goal oriented actions at beginning of period ___ Assimilates new objects into reflex exercises ___ Explores objects by mouthing or banging ___ By end of period infant moves from being purely reflexive to showing the initial beginnings of goal oriented behavior ___ Gradually develops object permanence ___ Early: eyes focus on empty space where object was when it is dropped; fails to look under scarf for object ___ Later: eyes follow object as it is moved; looks under scarf for hidden object	*Precursors* (Birth to 8 months) ___ Startles to noise ___ Orients to sound source ___ Looks at person who calls name	*Precursors* (Birth to 8 months) ___ Undifferentiated cry ___ Reflexive vocalizations and comfort sounds	(Birth to 8 months) ___ Stares at large masses ___ Grasps object placed in hand ___ Makes eye contact briefly ___ Quiets when picked up ___ Actively seeks sound source ___ Looks intently and shakes toy in hand ___ Smiles at mirror image, familiar faces ___ Sobers at sight of strangers ___ Increases activity at sight of toy, familiar caretaker ___ Works for toy out of reach ___ Returns to activity after interruption
Early Intentional (8 to 12 months) *Sensorimotor IV* ___ Uses familar means to achieve novel ends (tries to repeat or prolong an effect he/she has discovered) ___ Imitates ongoing actions already in repertoire (e.g., pattycake, kiss mommy, peekaboo) ___ Object permanence now established (looks for object previously seen) ___ Looks at pictures in a book with adult ___ Stares to gain information ___ Reacts in anticipation prior to familiar event	*Precursors* (strategies used prior to actual linguistic comprehension) (8 to 12 months) ___ Looks at objects that mother looks at ___ Acts on objects noticed ___ Imitates ongoing action or sound if it is already within repertoire ___ Laughs at familiar interaction sequences ___ Inhibits action in response to "no" ___ Responds to "bye-bye" ___ Follows caretaker's gaze to common objects when labelled	*Precursors* (8 to 12 months) ___ Differentiated cries ___ Syllabic babbling ___ Communication games ___ Intentional action	(8 to 12 months) ___ Responds to facial expressions ___ Frequently cries when parent leaves room ___ Drinks from cup, feeds self crackers ___ Imitates arm movements for games like peekaboo, pattycake ___ Squeezes toy to make it squeak ___ Drops toys and watches them fall ___ Puts small objects in and out of container ___ Stacks rings on peg ___ Holds crayon, imitates scribbling ___ Cooperates in dressing ___ Kisses, waves, holds out hands

Note: Columns and boxes of Reference Chart correspond to those of the Summary Chart

REFERENCE CHART, continued

COGNITIVE BASES	RECEPTIVE LANGUAGE	EXPRESSIVE LANGUAGE	SOCIAL INTERACTION & PLAY
Late Intentional (12 to 18 months) *Sensorimotor V* ___ Uses novel means to achieve familiar ends (e.g. communicative gestures and stereotyped vocalization used to achieve adult attention, particular object, object's removal) ___ Figures out ways to overcome some obstacles (opens door, reaches high objects)	*Lexical comprehension* (12 to 18 months) ___ Understands one word in some sentences when referents are present ___ Points to objects in response to "Show me _____" (e.g. body parts) *Nonverbal comprehension strategies used to respond to commands:* ___ Attend to object mentioned ___ Give evidence of notice ___ Do what is usually done in a situation	*First words* (12 to 18 months) ___ Performatives (gesture accompanies vocalization or word) ___ Hi/bye routines ___ Comment ___ Request object or attention ___ Reject ___ Communicates immediate needs by pulling or pointing	(12 to 18 months) ___ Reacts to emotions of others ___ Solitary or onlooker play, self play ___ Scribbles spontaneously with crayon ___ Points to objects he/she wants and claims certain objects as own ___ Imitates sweeping, hair combing, etc. ___ Hugs doll, pulls toy

Representational Thought (18 to 24 months) *Sensorimotor VI*
 ___ Begins to replace sensorimotor activity of previous stages with internalized problem solving using images, memories, and symbols to represent actions and objects
	Lexical comprehension (18 to 24 months)
	 ___ Understanding of words when referent is not present
	 ___ Understanding of action verbs out of routine context; carries out two-word commands, but often fails to understand three lexical elements
	 ___ Understanding of routine forms of questions for agent, object, locative, and action
	 Nonverbal comprehension strategies used to respond to commands:
	 ___ Locate the objects mentioned
	 ___ Give evidence of notice
	 ___ Do what you usually do: objects into containers, conventional use
	 ___ Act on the objects in the way mentioned
	 ___ Child as agent
		Transition to two word combination (18 to 24 months)
		 ___ New semantic roles
		     Early: action–object relations; agent, action, object, recurrence, disappearance
		     Later: object–object relations, location, possession, nonexistence
		 ___ Asks a "What's that" question
		 ___ Answers some routine questions
		 ___ Rapid acquisition of vocabulary
		 ___ Successive one-word utterances
		 ___ Increased frequency of talking
		 ___ Onset of two-word utterances (MLU 1.5)
			(18 to 24 months)
			 ___ Parallel play (near others but not with them)
			 ___ Talks to self while playing
			 ___ Little social give and take—hugs, pushes, pulls, snatches, grabs, but pays little attention to what others say or do
			 ___ Relates action to object or another person—washes, feeds doll in addition to self
			 ___ Listens to short story
			 ___ Demonstrates pleasure in make believe games (e.g., 2 sticks to represent "airplane")

REFERENCE CHART, continued

COGNITIVE BASES	RECEPTIVE LANGUAGE	EXPRESSIVE LANGUAGE	SOCIAL INTERACTION & PLAY

COGNITIVE BASES

Early Preoperations (2 to 3½ yrs)
- ___ Arranges objects in patterns but not in categories
- ___ Initiates drawing of vertical line (by 30 mos)
- ___ Imitates drawing of horizontal line and circle (by 36 mos.)
- ___ Matches identical objects
- ___ Draws 2 or more lines imitating a cross (by 3½ yrs)
- ___ Copies short line of beads by matching individual items but fails to put them in correct order, getting only adjacent pairs correct
- ___ Matches similar objects
- ___ Ability to represent one thing by another increases speed and range of thinking, particularly as language develops, but thinking remains tied closely to actions
- ___ Thought is preconceptual; inferences sometimes but not always correct

RECEPTIVE LANGUAGE

Lexical comprehension (2 to 3½ yrs)
- ___ Accepts or rejects, confirms or denies in response to yes/no questions

2½ yrs
- ___ What for object
- ___ What-do for action
- ___ Where for location (place)

3 yrs.
- ___ Whose for possessor
- ___ Who for person
- ___ Why for cause or reason
- ___ How many for number
- ___ Understanding of gender contrasts in third person pronouns

2-3 yrs. - *Comprehension strategies*
- ___ Does what is usually done
- ___ Probable location strategy for in, on, under, beside
- ___ Probable event strategy for simple active reversible sentences
- ___ Supplies missing information (2 years)
- ___ Supply explanation (3 years)
- ___ Infers most probable speech act in context
- ___ Sequence for understanding Wh-questions

EXPRESSIVE LANGUAGE

Typ Age	Brown's Stage	New Development	MLU (morph)
		(2 to 3½ yrs)	
2	I	Basic semantic relations	1.75
		___ Agent–action	
		___ Action–object	
		___ Agent–object	
		___ Possessive	
		___ Entity–locative	
		___ Action–locative	
		___ Existence	
		___ Recurrence	
		___ Nonexistence	
		___ Rejection	
		___ Denial	
		___ Attributive	
	II	Grammatical inflections	2.25
		___ Some articles, plurals, possessives	
		___ -ing on verbs	
		___ What doing? questions	
2½	III	Differentiation of sentence	2.75
		___ Modalities	
		___ Possession	
		___ Number (noun plural)	
		___ Locative containment and support (in, on)	
		___ Temporary duration (ing)	
3	IV	Sentence embedding	3.50
		___ Immediate future (gonna)	
		___ Regular past -ed	
		___ Inflects verb *be* (am, was, are)	

SOCIAL INTERACTION & PLAY

(2 to 3½ yrs)
- ___ Parallel play predominates (24 mos)
- ___ Dramatization, imagination and symbolic play (make believe and pretend)
- ___ Takes turns
- ___ Watches cartoons on TV
- ___ Associative group play begins (3½ yrs)
- ___ Organizes doll furniture accurately and plays imaginatively
- ___ Builds bridge from model

REFERENCE CHART, continued

COGNITIVE BASES	RECEPTIVE LANGUAGE	EXPRESSIVE LANGUAGE	SOCIAL INTERACTION & PLAY
Late preoperations (3½ to 7 yrs)	*Lexical comprehension* (3½ to 7 yrs)	*Typ* *Brown's* (3½ to 7 yrs) *MLU* *Age* *Stage* *New Development* *(morph)* — 3½ — V — 3.75	(3½ to 7 yrs)
___ Applies systematic trial and error problem solving strategies to classification and seriation tasks	___ Understands contrasts for topological locatives (in, on, under, beside)	___ Sentence Conjoining	___ Increased dramatization in play
___ Sorts set of blocks varying in size, shape, and color into 2 piles on basis of single attribute (50% can do by age 3½)	___ Answers how questions with manner or instrument responses ("What do we eat with")	___ Regular past -ed	___ Suggests turns, but often bossy
___ Places seven blocks varying in height in order and places 3 missing blocks in sequences (50% can do by age 4½)	___ Comprehension of word order as cues to understand agent-object in active sentences (word order strategy)	___ Third pers. singular	___ Plays in group of 2 to 3 children
___ Begins differentiating open and closed shapes in drawings, and squares may have corners (by age 4½)	___ Responds to two-stage action commands	*Event relations* (sequence of emergence from 3½ to 7 years)	___ Shows off
___ Develop concepts of time and space		___ And (coordinate and temporal)	___ Friendships stronger
___ Identifies one of the three pictures not in the same category		___ Because, so (causal)	___ Plays in groups of 2 to 5
___ Matches pictures that "go together"		___ But (contrastive)	___ Able to play games by rules (by age 6)
___ Draws person with 2 parts		___ When (conditional)	___ Spends hours at one activity
___ Copies square (by age 4½)		___ While (simultaneity)	___ Demands more realism in play (age 7)
___ Cuts and pastes—may finish project next day		___ After	
___ Copies triangle (by age 5)		___ Before	
___ Draws person with body, arms, legs, feet, nose, and eyes		___ Past time (-ed)	
		___ Possibility (might)	
		Syntactic rule emergence from 4 to 6 years	
		___ N + cont + cop + PN/PA/loc (He's sick)	
		___ There's expleture (There is a table)	
		___ Poss + N + V (Jim's dog bites)	
		___ Adj + N + V (the big truck rolled)	
		___ N + N + V (Joe and Jim race cars)	
		___ Reflexive (He sees himself)	
		___ S because S (He went because he wanted to)	
		___ S + V + indirect + N (He gave her a book)	
		___ When S + S (When I go to town, I will buy an ice cream cone)	
		___ Obligatory & emphatic do (He does not feel good. He does feel good)	
		___ Noninversion of aux/modal (Where daddy is?)	
		___ Aux/modal + aux modal (How can he can look? Is that's a rocket?)	
		___ Continued use of double negation.	
		___ Some problems in the truth value of negatives.	
		___ Continued regularization of irregular forms.	
		Syntactic rule emergence from 6 to 7 years	
		___ Passive transform (The boy was hit by the girl)	
		___ If transformation (If it rains, we won't go)	
		___ N + V + particle (He jumped up)	
		___ S/V concord (He likes candy)	
		___ Pronominalization (John knew he would win the race. He knew John would win the race)	
		___ Inversion of aux/modal + main V (When's going to be the party?)	
		___ Noninversion of aux/modal (Where she's going?)	

REFERENCE CHART, continued

COGNITIVE BASES	RECEPTIVE LANGUAGE	EXPRESSIVE LANGUAGE	SOCIAL INTERACTION & PLAY
Concrete Operations (7 to 12 yrs) — Formation of series and classes takes place mentally; physical actions are internalized as mental actions or 'operations' — Classifies in two ways at once (e.g., can sort by both color and shape in matrix) — Still solves problems primarily through trial and error rather than establishing general rules and testing hypotheses — Able to correct misconceptions through discussion	(7 to 12 yrs) — Understanding of conditional conjunctions *if* and *when* (usual rather than logical sense) — Probable relation of events strategy for causal conjuctions — Understanding of causal conjunctions *because* and *so* (8 years) — Understanding of contrastive conjunctions *but* and *although* as though they mean *and* (8 years) — Contrastive conjunctions *but* and *although* (10 years)	(7 to 12 years) *Marks of maturity in language* — Longer sentences — More clauses per sentence—8th graders use 150% more than 4th graders — Use of adverbial clauses (He was sleeping when I walked in the door) — Use of adjective clauses (The man with the broken foot limped along the highway) — Nominals (Flying airplanes is fun) — Sentence complements (They elected Jim president) — Infinitive complements (He told Jim to feed the dog) — Reduction of mazes and tangles (characteristic of younger children who begin a sentence which does not fulfill a communication unit and eventually drop it as if it is beyond them.) — Uses language to converse, persuade, tease	(7 to 12 years) — Genuine cooperation with others replaces isolated play or play in the company of others — Reduction in imaginary play but development of theatrical entertainment — Makes accurate replicas and working models — Enjoys categorizing collections of various sorts

Note. From *The Michigan Decision-Making Strategy for Determining Appropriate Communicative Services for Physically and/or Mentally Handicapped Children* by N. W. Nelson, J. C. Silbar, and E. L. Lockwood, 1981, November, presented at the annual conference of the American-Speech-Language-Hearing Association, Los Angeles. Copyright 1981 by N. W. Nelson, J. C. Silbar, and E. L. Lockwood. Reprinted by permission.

Appendix C

**DEVELOPMENTAL SENTENCE SCORING AND
BLACK ENGLISH SENTENCE SCORING**

Developmental Sentence Scoring (DSS) criteria.

	INDEFINITE PRONOUNS OR NOUN MODIFERS	PERSONAL PRONOUNS	MATH VERBS	SECONDARY VERBS	
1	it, this, that	1st and 2nd person: I, me, my, mine, you, your(s)	A. Uninflected verb: I <u>see</u> you. B. copula, is, or 's: <u>It's</u> red. C. is + verb + ing: He <u>is coming</u>.		
2		3rd person: he, him, his, she, her, hers	A. -s and -ed: <u>plays</u>, <u>played</u> B. Irregular past: <u>ate</u>, <u>saw</u> C. Copula: <u>am</u>, <u>are</u>, <u>was</u>, <u>were</u> D. Auxiliary <u>am</u>, <u>are</u>, <u>was</u> <u>were</u>	Five early-developing infinitives I wan<u>na</u> <u>see</u> (want <u>to</u> <u>see</u>) I'm gon<u>na</u> <u>see</u> (going <u>to</u> <u>see</u>) I got<u>ta</u> <u>see</u> (got <u>to</u> <u>see</u>) Lem<u>me</u> [to] see (let me [<u>to</u>] <u>see</u>) Let's [to] play (let [us <u>to</u>] <u>play</u>)	
3	A. no, some, more, all, lot(s), one(s), two (etc.), other(s), another B. something, somebody, someone	A. Plurals: we, us, our(s), they, them, their B. these, those		Non-complementing infinitives: I stopped <u>to</u> <u>play</u>. I'm afraid <u>to</u> <u>look</u>. It's hard <u>to</u> <u>do</u> that.	
4	nothing, nobody, none, no one		A. can, will, may + verb: <u>may</u> <u>go</u> B. Obligatory do + verb: <u>don't</u> <u>go</u> C. Emphatic do + verb: I <u>do</u> <u>see</u>.	Participle, present or past: I see a boy <u>running</u>. I found the toy <u>broken</u>.	
5		Reflexives: myself, yourself, himself, herself, itself, themselves		A. Early infinitival complements with differing subjects in kernels: I want you <u>to</u> <u>come</u>. Let him [<u>to</u>] <u>see</u>. B. Later infinitival complements: I had <u>to</u> <u>go</u>. I told him <u>to</u> <u>go</u>. I tried <u>to</u> <u>go</u>. He ought <u>to</u> <u>go</u>. C. Obligatory deletions: Make it [<u>to</u>] <u>go</u>. I'd better [<u>to</u>] <u>go</u>. D. Infinitive with wh- word: I know what <u>to</u> <u>get</u>. I know how <u>to</u> <u>do</u> it.	
6		A. Wh- pronouns: who, which, whose, whom, what, that, how many, how much I know <u>who</u> came. That's <u>what</u> I said. B. Wh- word + infinitive: I know <u>what</u> to do. I know <u>who(m)</u> to take.	A. could, would, should, might + verg: <u>might</u> <u>come</u>, <u>could</u> <u>be</u> B. Obligatory does, did + verb C. Emphatic does, did + verb		

NEGATIVES	CONJUNCTIONS	INTERROGATIVE REVERSALS	WH- QUESTIONS
it, this, that + copula, or auxiliary is, 's, + not: It's <u>not</u> mine. This is <u>not</u> a dog. That is <u>not</u> moving.		Reversal of copula: <u>Isn't</u> <u>it</u> red? <u>Were</u> <u>they</u> there?	
			A. who, what, what + noun: <u>Who</u> am I? <u>What</u> is he eating? <u>What</u> <u>book</u> are you reading? B. where, how many, how much, what . . . do, what . . . for <u>Where</u> did it go? <u>How</u> <u>much</u> do you want? <u>What</u> is he <u>doing</u>? <u>What</u> is a hammer <u>for</u>?
	and		
can't, don't		Reversal of auxiliary be: <u>Is</u> <u>he</u> coming? <u>Isn't</u> <u>he</u> coming? <u>Was</u> <u>he</u> going? <u>Wasn't</u> <u>he</u> going?	
isn't, won't	A. but B. so, and so, so that C. or, if		when, how, how + adjective <u>When</u> shall I come? <u>How</u> do you do it? <u>How</u> <u>big</u> is it?
	because	A. Obligatory do, does, did: <u>Do</u> <u>they</u> run? <u>Does</u> <u>it</u> bite? <u>Didn't</u> <u>it</u> hurt? B. Reversal of modal: <u>Can</u> <u>you</u> play? <u>Won't</u> <u>it</u> hurt? <u>Shall</u> <u>I</u> sit down? C. Tag question: It's fun, <u>isn't</u> <u>it</u>? It isn't fun, <u>is</u> <u>it</u>?	

Developmental Sentence Scoring (DSS) criteria, continued.

7	A. any, anything, anybody, anyone
	B. every, everything, everybody, everyone
	C. both, few, many, each, several, most, least, much, next, first, last, second (etc.)
		(his) own, one, oneself, whichever, whoever, whatever
		    Take <u>whatever</u> you like.
			A. Passive with <u>get</u>, any tense
			    Passive with <u>be</u>, any tense
			B. must, shall + verb: must come
			C. have + verb + en: <u>I've</u> <u>eaten</u>
			D. have got: <u>I've</u> <u>got</u> it.
				Passive infinitival complement:
				With <u>get</u>: I have <u>to get dressed</u>.
				        I don't want <u>to get hurt</u>.
				With <u>be</u>: I want <u>to be pulled</u>.
				        It's going <u>to be locked</u>.	

8			A. have been + verb + ing
			    had been + verb + ing
			B. modal + have + verb + en
			    <u>may</u> <u>have</u> <u>eaten</u>
			C. modal + be + verb + ing
			    <u>could</u> <u>be</u> <u>playing</u>
			D. Other auxiliary combinations:
			    <u>should</u> <u>have</u> <u>been</u> <u>sleeping</u>
				Gerund
				    <u>Swinging</u> is fun.
				    I like <u>fishing</u>.
				    He started <u>laughing</u>.	

Note. From *Developmental Sentence Analysis* (p. 67) by L. L. Lee, 1974, Evanston, IL: Northwestern University Press. Copyright 1974 by Northwestern University Press. Reprinted by permission.

All other negatives:
A. Uncontracted negatives:
    I can <u>not</u> go.
    He has <u>not</u> gone.
B. Pronoun-auxiliary or pronoun-
   copula contraction:
    I'm <u>not</u> coming.
    He's <u>not</u> here.
C. Auxiliary-negative or copula-
   negative contraction:
    He was<u>n't</u> going.
    He has<u>n't</u> been seen.
    It could<u>n't</u> be mine.
    They are<u>n't</u> big
			why, what if, how come
			how about + gerund
			   <u>Why</u> are you crying?
			   <u>What if</u> I won't do it?
			   <u>How come</u> he is crying?
			   <u>How about</u> coming with me?

	A. where, when, how while,
	   whether (or not), till, until,
	   unless, since, before, after, for,
	   as + adjective + as, as if, like,
	   that, than
	     I know <u>where</u> you are.
	     Don't come <u>till</u> I call.
	B. Obligatory deletions:
	     I run faster <u>than</u> you [run].
	     I'm <u>as</u> big <u>as</u> a man [is big].
	     It looks <u>like</u> a dog [looks].
	C. Elliptical deletions (score 0)
	     That's <u>why</u> [I took it].
	     I know <u>how</u> [I can do it].
	D. Wh- words + infinitive:
	     I know <u>how</u> to do it.
	     I know <u>where</u> to go.
		A. Reversal of auxiliary have:
		   <u>Has</u> <u>he</u> seen you?
		B. Reversal with two or three
		   auxiliaries:
		    <u>Has</u> <u>he</u> <u>been</u> eating?
		    <u>Couldn't</u> <u>he</u> <u>have</u> waited?
		    <u>Could</u> <u>he</u> <u>have</u> <u>been</u> cry-
		    ing?
		    <u>Wouldn't</u> <u>he</u> <u>have</u> <u>been</u>
		    going?
			whose, which, which + noun
			   <u>Whose</u> car is that?
			   <u>Which</u> <u>book</u> do you want?

Black English Sentence Scoring (BESS) criteria.

	INDEFINITE PRONOUNS OR NOUN MODIFIERS	PERSONAL PRONOUNS	MAIN VERBS	SECONDARY VERBS	
1	— these/this: <u>these</u> many.	— mine's/my, you/your: That <u>you</u> book? — y'all (plural <u>you</u>) — me/I (in compound subj.): Me and my brother went in it.	— Ø copula <u>is</u>, <u>am</u>, <u>are</u>: That boy my friend. Or hypercorrect: I'm is six. — Ø aux <u>be</u> + Ving: The girl singin'. — locational <u>go</u> or existential <u>it's</u>: Here <u>go</u> some lights. <u>It's</u> two dimes stuck on the table. — <u>got</u> as uninflected <u>have</u>: You gotta take it home.		
2		— he, she (in apposition): My brother, <u>he</u> bigger than you. — they/he: They my uncle. — he, he's/his: He's name is Terry. — she, she's/her	— third person singular and regular past tense markers deleted. — have/has: It have money on it. — Regularization of -s and -ed: Trudy and my sister hides. (hypercorrect) — Aux was/were: We <u>was</u> <u>gon'</u> rob some money. — Irreg. past tense — Uninflected: He <u>find</u> the money; Past form as participle: We <u>have</u> <u>went</u>; Participle as past form: He <u>done</u> it first.	— I'm, I'mon, I'ma pronunciation of I'm gonna + V: I'm play. I'ma be tired. — <u>go</u> pronunciation of gonna: His nose <u>go</u> bleed. — fixin' to (used like gonna): I'm fixin' to take him to jail. (sometimes pronounced as /fʌtə/)	
3	— <u>no</u> (when 2nd or 3rd neg. marker): He don't like me <u>no</u> more.	— we, they (in apposition): The boys, <u>they</u> get in trouble. — they/their: <u>They</u> name is Tanya and Bryan. — them/they or their: I know what <u>them</u> is. One of 'em name is Caesar. — them/those: <u>them</u> kids.			
4	— nothing, nobody, none, no one (when 2nd or 3rd neg. marker): Ain't nobody got none.		— Ø modal <u>will</u> or <u>'ll</u>: I be five when my birthday come. — don't + verb (3rd pers. sing.): My mama, she don't like it. — <u>do</u> uninflected: <u>Do</u> he still have it? (Score inc. in My sister <u>do</u>.) — Ø <u>do</u> in Qs: You still have it? — ain't (as copula or aux): Ain't no dirt in it. Nobody ain't got no more. — can't, don't, won't as preposed neg. aux.: Can't nobody do it. — could/can: He could climb that tree.	— Participle with deleted -en: She has a state name Tennessee. (phonological cluster reduction rule) — I found the toy broke. (morphological difference)	
5		— personal datives me, him, her: I'm gonna buy <u>me</u> some candy. He make <u>him</u> a lot of 'em. — reflexives: hisself, theirselves, themself, theyselves.		— Deleted <u>to</u> in infinitval complements: My grandma tell me stay away from him. I like go shopping. My mommy used do it.	

NEGATIVES	CONJUNCTIONS	INTERROGATIVE REVERSAL	WH- QUESTIONS
— it, this, that + Ø copula/aux + not/ain't: That <u>not</u> mine. It <u>ain't</u> on?		— rising intonation with deleted or unreversed copula: You my friend? Where the gas at? What that is? — is/are: Derrick, is you?	
			— who, what, what + noun (with deleted aux or copula) — where, how many, how much, what . . . do, what . . . for (with deleted aux or copula): Where the man? — Wh- Qs formed without interrogative reversal: What that is?
	— and plus — Ø and (when intonation makes sentence combination clear): He pointed his finger at him, (with rising intonation) he pointed his finger at him (with falling intonation).		
— don't (with 3rd pers. sing. as 2nd or 3rd neg. marker): He <u>don't</u> want none. No, nobody <u>don't</u> live with me. — can't, don't (as preposed aux): Can't nobody make me. — Ø copula/aux + not + V: My mama <u>not</u> gonna pick me up today. He <u>not</u> a baby. — ain't (as negative copula or aux. <u>be</u>): He <u>ain't</u> my friend.		— Ø auxiliary be: My voice gonna come out of here? You gonna tell my mama? — was/were: Was you throwin' rocks?	
— won't (as preposed aux): <u>Won't</u> nobody help him.	— for/so: The dog make too much noise for they won't catch many fish. — conditional <u>and</u>: You do that <u>and</u> I'm gonna smack you. — <u>if</u> with phrase deletions: He lookin' if he see the money. — aux. inversion in indiret Qs (instead of <u>if</u>): She ask me do he want some more.		— when, how (with deleted aux, copula or do): How you do this?

Black English Sentence Scoring (BESS) criteria, continued.

6		— what (in apposition): My voice gonna come out of here <u>what</u> I said on that book? — what/that or who: He's the one <u>what</u> I told you about. — Deleted relative pronoun: I saw a little girl was on the street.	— did + nt + verb (when 2nd or 3rd neg. marker: Nobody didn't do it. — could, would, should + nt + verb (preposed neg. aux): Couldn't nobody do it. — Ø contracted could or would (phonol. deletions): You('d) burn your head off. — might/will: Who might be the baby?		
7	— many a: <u>Many</u> a people likes to give him a nickel.		— passive verb + en with <u>getting</u> (aux. deleted): Leroy <u>getting</u> dressed. — passive verb ± be ± en: One is name Brick. They named Chief and JoJo. — done + verb + en (completive aspect): I <u>done tried</u>. — ± (neg.) aux. + supposed: He don't supposed to do it. What toy you supposed to play with? — ± have ± verb ± en: We seen him already. He have made him mad.	— Passive with phonological deletions: I'm be dressed up real cute. I'ma be tired. She gonna be surprise, ain't she? I want it cut on.	
8			— invariant <u>be</u>: My daddy know I skip school 'cause I be home with him. He be mad when somebody leave him home. — double modals: We might could come. — other expanded aux. forms: He be done jumped out the tub. He been going. (<u>have</u> has undergone phonological deletion) You shouldn't did that. — remote past aspect: She been whuptin' the baby. I been wanted this.	— gerund with <u>go to</u>, <u>got to</u>, <u>start to</u>: When I cry, she goes to whipping me. He started to crying. He got to thinking.	

Note. From *Black English Sentence Scoring: Development and Use as a Tool for Nonbiased Assessment* by N. W. Nelson and Y. D. Hyter, 1990, unpublished manuscript, Western Michigan University, Kalamazoo. Copyright 1990 by N. W. Nelson. Reprinted by permission.

	— or either, or neither (as disjunctives): He will go <u>or either</u> he will stay. He told her that he wouldn't be bad <u>or neither</u> get in trouble. — preposed why phrase (with because): Why he's in here, cause baby scared the dog.	— Ø do: You know that one with the tractor? Where you work? You got blue eyes? — do (with 3rd pers. sing.) Do he still have it? — Ø or unreversed modal: Now, what else I be doin? Why you can't talk on that? — Tag question with ain't: It gonna be fun, ain't it?	
— ain't (for have + not) ± uninflected V: I <u>ain't</u> taste any. — ain't (for did + not) ± uninflected V: Yesterday, he <u>ain't</u> go to school. I ain't found Marge in the school. — couldn't, wouldn't, shouldn't (as preposed aux) — wasn't/weren't: The brakes wasn't workin' right. — weren't/wasn't: There weren't no money. — uncontracted, uninflected neg. aux.: Lester <u>do</u> <u>not</u> like it.			— why, what if, how come (with deleted or unreversed aux, copula or do, or with got): Why she turn that way? Hey, why you got a dress on mama?
	— less'n (for unless) — to/till: I didn't get to sleep <u>to</u> I had to come in the morning. — ± as + adjective + as: He sock Leroy in the arm hard as he could.	— deleted have: He seen it? How you been? What you been doing? — have with 3rd pers. sing.: Have he seen you?	— whose, which, which + noun (with deleted aux, copula or do) — who/whose: Who this bed? Who baby is that?

TABLE 1

Example scoring form and partial sample for Black English Sentence Scoring (BESS) using Developmental Sentence Scoring (DSS; Lee, 1974) as a base.

Name Eric
Age 4;0
Date May 31, 1993 DSS 3.73 BESS 6.55

	Indef. Pron.	Pers. Pron.	Prim. Verb	Sec. Verb	Neg.	Conj.	Inter. Rev.	WH Ques.	Sent. Point	Total
1. That the food that grandma ate.	1	6	1 / -, 2						1[c] / 0	11[b] / 9[a]
2. I goin' to nursery school.		1	1 / -						1 / 0	3 / 1
3. I putting my sister on a motorcycle.		1,1	1 / -						1 / 0	4 / 2
4. I listening.		1	1 / -						1 / 0	3 / 1
5. I watched him yesterday.		1,2	2						1	6
6. I like these.		1,3	1						1	6
7. I push all these buttons, ok?	3	1,3	4 / -						1 / 0	12 / 7
8. They try catch me.		3,1	2 / -	5 / -					1 / 0	12 / 4
9. I had a spoon.		1	2						1	4
10. Who this on the phone?	1		1 / -				1 / -	2 / -	1 / 0	6 / 1
11. Where the gun?			1 / -				1 / -	2 / -	1 / 0	5 / 0

Total DSS for this partial sample:
  41 divided by 11 = 3.73
Total BESS for this partial sample:
  72 divided by 11 = 6.55

[a] Sentence total for DSS.
[b] Sentence total for BESS.
[c] Point earned for BESS but not DSS. (Numbers above DSS attempt markers (—) represent credit awarded for BESS but not DSS.)

Note. From *Black English Sentence Scoring: Development and Use as a Tool for Nonbiased Assessment* by N. W. Nelson and Y. D. Hyter, 1990, unpublished manuscript, Western Michigan University, Kalamazoo. Copyright 1990 by N. W. Nelson. Reprinted by permission.

TABLE 2
Means and standard deviations for Developmental Sentence Analysis (DSS) and Black English Sentence Scoring (BESS) scores at 6-month intervals from normative studies

Age Range	N	Mean DSS	SD	Mean BESS	SD
3:0 – 3:6	8	5.63	0.91	7.44	1.15
3:6 – 4:0	8	5.73	1.04	7.71	0.98
4:0 – 4:6	8	7.47	1.58	9.33	1.26
4:6 – 5:0	8	7.51	1.68	8.85	1.48
5:0 – 5:6	8	8.86	1.93	10.79	1.92
5:6 – 6:0	8	8.31	2.04	10.02	2.16
6:0 – 6:6	8	9.12	2.43	11.08	1.61
6:6 – 7:0	8	9.47	1.72	11.17	2.17

Note. From *Black English Sentence Scoring: Development and Use as a Tool for Nonbiased Assessment* by N. W. Nelson and Y. D. Hyter, 1990, unpublished manuscript, Western Michigan University, Kalamazoo. Copyright 1990 by N. W. Nelson. Reprinted by permission.

References

Abikoff, H., & Gittelman, R. (1985). The normalizing effects of methylphenidate on the classroom behavior of ADDH children. *Journal of Abnormal Child Psychology, 13,* 33–44.

Ackerman, B. P. (1982). On comprehending idioms: Do children get the picture? *Journal of Experimental Child Psychology, 33,* 439–454.

Adler, S. (1991). Assessment of language proficiency of limited English proficient speakers: Implications for the speech–language specialist. *Language, Speech, and Hearing Services in Schools, 22,* 12–18.

Aitchison, J. (1976). *The articulate mammal: An introduction to psycholinguistics.* New York: Universe Books.

Algozzine, B., Morsink, C. V., & Algozzine, K. M. (1989). What's happening in self-contained special education classrooms? *Exceptional Children, 55,* 259–265.

Allen, J. P. B., & Van Buren, P. (1971). *Chomsky: Selected readings.* London: Oxford University Press.

Allen, R. E., & Oliver, J. M. (1982). The effects of child maltreatment on language development. *Child Abuse and Neglect, 6,* 299–305.

Allen, R. E., & Wasserman, G. A. (1985). Origins of language delay in abused infants. *Child Abuse and Neglect, 9,* 335–340.

Alley, G., & Deshler, D. (1979). *Teaching the learning disabled adolescent: Strategies and methods.* Denver: Love Publishing.

Als, H., Lester, B. M., Tronick, E., & Brazelton, T. B. (1982). Toward a research instrument for the assessment of preterm infants' behavior (APIB). In H. E. Fitzgerald, B. M. Lester, & M. W. Yogman (Eds.), *Theory and research in behavioral pediatrics, Vol. 1* (pp. 35–132). New York: Plenum Press.

American Psychiatric Association. (1980). *Diagnostic and statistical manual of mental disorders, third edition (DSM III).* Washington, DC: Author.

American Psychiatric Association. (1987). *Diagnostic and statistical manual of mental disorders, third edition—revised (DSM III–R).* Washington, DC: Author.

American Psychological Association. (1985). *Standards for educational and psychological testing.* Washington, DC: Author.

American Speech-Language-Hearing Association Committee on Amplification for the Hearing Impaired. (1991). Amplification as a remediation technique for children with normal peripheral hearing. *Asha, 33* (Suppl. 1), 22–24.

American Speech-Language-Hearing Association Committee on Language. (1983, June). A definition of language. *Asha, 25*(6), 44.

American Speech-Language-Hearing Association Committee on Language Learning Disabilities. (1989, March). Issues in determining eligibility for language intervention. *Asha, 31,* 113–118.

American Speech-Language-Hearing Association Committee on Language, Speech, and Hearing Services in Schools. (1982). Definitions: Communicative disorders and variations. *Asha, 24,* 949–950.

American Speech-Language-Hearing Association Committee on Language, Speech, and Hearing Services in Schools. (1984). Guidelines for caseload size for speech-language services in the schools. *Asha, 26*(4), 53–58.

American Speech-Language-Hearing Joint Committee on Infant Hearing. (1991). 1990 Position statement. *Asha, 33* (Suppl. 5), 3–6.

Amochaev, A. (1987). The infant hearing foundation—A unique approach to hearing screening of newborns. *Seminars in Hearing, 8* (2), 165–168.

Anderson, G. M., & Nelson, N. W. (1988). Integrating language intervention and education in an Alternate Adolescent Language Classroom. *Seminars in Speech and Language, 9* (4), 341–353.

Anderson, R. C. (1985). Role of the reader's schema in comprehension, learning, and memory. In H. Singer & R. B. Ruddell (Eds.), *Theoretical models and processes of reading* (3rd ed., pp. 372–384). Newark, DE: International Reading Association.

Andreasen, N. C. (1984). *The broken brain: The biological revolution in psychiatry.* New York: Harper & Row.

Andrews, J. F., & Mason, J. M. (1991). Strategy usage among deaf and hearing readers, *Exceptional Children, 57,* 536–545.

Applebee, A. N. (1978). *The child's concept of story.* Chicago: University of Chicago Press.

Applebee, A. N., & Langer, J. A. (1983). Instructional scaffolding: Reading and writing as natural language activities. *Language Arts, 60,* 168–175.

Aram, D. M. (1988). Language sequelae of unilateral brain lesions in children. In F. Plum (Ed.), *Language, communication, and the brain* (pp. 171–197). New York: Raven Press.

Aram, D. M. (1990, June). *Definition of child language disorders.* Paper presented at the 11th symposium for research on child language disorders, The University of Wisconsin.

Aram, D. M., & Ekelman, B. L. (1987). Unilateral brain lesions in children: Performance on the Revised Token Test. *Brain and Language, 32,* 137–158.

Aram, D. M., & Ekelman, B. L. (1988). Scholastic aptitude and achievement among children with unilateral brain lesions. *Neuropsychologia, 26,* 903–916.

Aram, D. M., Ekelman, B. L., & Gillespie, L. L. (1989). Reading and lateralized brain lesions in children. In K. von Euler, I. Lundberg, & G. Lennerstrand (Eds.), *Brain and reading* (pp. 61–75). Hampshire, England: Macmillan Press Ltd.

Aram, D. M., Ekelman, B. L., & Nation, J. E. (1984). Preschoolers with language disorders: 10 years later. *Journal of Speech and Hearing Research, 27,* 232–244.

Aram, D. M., Ekelman, B. L., & Whitaker, H. A. (1986). Spoken syntax in children with acquired unilateral hemisphere lesions. *Brain and Language, 27,* 75–100.

Aram, D. M., Ekelman, B. L., & Whitaker, H. A. (1987). Lexical retrieval in left and right brain lesioned children. *Brain and Language, 31,* 61–87.

Aram, D. M., Morris, R., & Hall, N. E. *Validity of discrepancy criteria for identifying children with developmental language disorders.* Manuscript submitted for publication.

Aram, D. M., & Nation, J. E. (1975). Patterns of language behavior in children with developmental language disorders. *Journal of Speech and Hearing Research, 18,* 229–241.

Aram, D. M., & Nation, J. E. (1980). Preschool language disorders and subsequent language and academic difficulties. *Journal of Communication Disorders, 13,* 159–170.

Armbruster, B. B. (1984). The problem of "inconsiderate" text. In G. G. Duffy, L. R. Roehler, & J. M. Mason (Eds.), *Comprehension instruction: Perspectives and suggestions* (pp. 202–217). New York: Longman.

Aronson, E., Blaney, N., Stephan, C., Sikes, J., & Snapp, M. (1978). *The jigsaw classroom.* Beverly Hills, CA: Sage Publications.

Arwood, E. (1983). *Pragmaticism: Theory and application.* Rockville, MD: Aspen.

Asch, A. (1989). Has the law made a difference? What some disabled students have to say. In D. K. Lipsky & A. Gartner (Eds.), *Beyond separate education: Quality education for all* (pp. 181–205). Baltimore, MD: Paul H. Brookes.

Augoustinos, M. (1987). Developmental effects of child abuse: Recent findings. *Child Abuse and Neglect, 11,* 15–27.

Augustine, D. K., Gruber, K. D., & Hanson, L. R. (1990). Cooperation works! *Educational Leadership, 47* (4):4–7.

Austin, J. (1962). *How to do things with words.* London: Oxford University Press.

Autism Society of America Board of Directors. (1988). Autism Society of America Resolution on abusive treatment and neglect. *Advocate (newsletter of the ASA),* 20(3), 17.

Aylward, E. H. (1987). Psychological evaluation. In F. R. Brown III & E. H. Aylward (Eds.), *Diagnosis and management of learning disabilities* (pp. 33–57). Boston: College-Hill.

Aylward, E. H., & Brown, F. R. III. (1987). Interdisciplinary diagnosis. In F. R. Brown III & E. H. Aylward (Eds.), *Diagnosis and management of learning disabilities* (pp. 109–125). Boston: College-Hill.

Bailey, D. B., Jr., & Brochin, H. A. (1989). Tests and test development. In D. B. Bailey & M. Wolery (Eds.), *Assessing infants and preschoolers with handicaps* (pp. 22–46). Columbus, OH: Merrill/Macmillan.

Bailey, D. B., Jr., & Simeonsson, R. J. (1988). Home-based early intervention. In S. L. Odom & M. B. Karnes (Eds.), *Early intervention for infants and children with handicaps* (pp. 199–215). Baltimore, MD: Paul H. Brookes.

Bailey, D. B., Jr., Simeonsson, R. J., Yoder, D. E., & Huntington, G. S. (1990). Preparing professionals to serve infants and toddlers with handicaps and their families: An integrative analysis across eight disciplines. *Exceptional Children, 57,* 26–35.

Bailey, D. B., Jr., & Wolery, M. (1989). *Assessing infants and preschoolers with handicaps.* Columbus, OH: Merrill/Macmillan.

Baker, L., & Brown, A. L. (1984). Metacognitive skills and reading. In P. D. Pearson (Ed.), *Handbook of reading research* (pp. 353–394). New York: Longman.

Baker, L., & Cantwell, D. P. (1982). Psychiatric disorder in children with different types of communication disorders. *Journal of Communication Disorders, 15,* 113–126.

Baker, L., & Cantwell, D. P. (1987a). Comparison of well, emotionally disordered and behaviorally disordered children with linguistic problems. *Journal of the American Academy of Child and Adolescent Psychiatry, 26,* 193–196.

Baker, L., & Cantwell, D. P. (1987b). A prospective psychiatric follow-up of children with speech/language disorders. *Journal of the American Academy of Child and Adolescent Psychiatry, 26,* 546–553.

Baldwin, D. A., & Markman, E. M. (1989). Establishing word-object relations: A first step. *Child Development, 60,* 381–398.

Baltaxe, C. A. M., & Simmons, J. Q., III. (1985). Prosodic development in normal and autistic children. In E. Schopler & G. B. Mesibov (Eds.), *Communication problems in autism* (pp. 95–125). New York: Plenum Publishing.

Baltaxe, C. A. M., & Simmons, J. Q. (1988). Communication deficits in preschool children with psychiatric disorders. *Seminars in Speech and Language, 8,* 81–90.

Baratz, J. C. (1969). Language and cognitive assessment of Negro children: Assumptions and research needs. *Asha, 10,* 87–91.

Barber, P. A., Turnbull, A. P., Behr, S. K., & Kerns, G. M. (1988). A family systems perspective on early childhood special education. In S. L. Odom & M. B. Karnes (Eds.), *Early intervention for infants and children with handicaps* (pp. 179–198). Baltimore, MD: Paul. H. Brookes.

Barbero, G. (1982). Failure-to-thrive. In M. H. Klaus, T. Leger, & M. A. Trause (Eds.), *Maternal attachment and mothering disorders: Pediatric Round Table: 1* (pp. 3–6). Skillman, NJ: Johnson & Johnson Baby Products Company.

Barkley, R. A. (1988). Poor self-control in preschool hyperactive children. *Medical Aspects of Human Sexuality, 21*(6), 176–180.

Baroff, G. S. (1986). *Mental retardation: Nature, cause, and management* (2nd ed.). New York: Hemisphere Publishing.

Barrie-Blackley, S., Musselwhite, C. R., & Rogister, S. H. (1978). *Clinical oral language sampling.* Danville, IL: Interstate Printers and Publishers.

Bashir, A. S. (1989). Language intervention and the curriculum. *Seminars in Speech and Language, 10*(3), 181–191.

Bashir, A. S., Wiig, E. H., & Abrams, J. C. (1987). Language disorders in childhood and adolescence: Implications for learning and socialization. *Pediatric Annals, 16,* 145–156.

Bass, P. M. (1988, November). *Attention deficit disorder/Management in preschool, adolescent, and adult populations.* Miniseminar presented at the annual conference of the American Speech-Language-Hearing Association, Boston.

Bates, E. (1976). *Language and context: Studies in the acquisition of pragmatics.* New York: Academic Press.

Bates, E. (1979). *The emergence of symbols: Cognition and communication in infancy.* New York: Academic Press.

Bates, E., Benigni, L., Bretherton, I., Camaioni, L., & Volterra, V. (1979). *The emergence of symbols: Cognition and communication in infancy.* New York: Academic Press.

Bates, E., Bretherton, I., & Snyder, L. (1988). *From first words to grammar: Individual differences and dissociable mechanisms.* New York: Cambridge University Press.

Bates, E., Camaioni, L., & Volterra, V. (1975). The acquisition of performatives prior to speech. *Merrill-Palmer Quarterly, 21,* 205–226.

Bates, E., & MacWhinney, B. (1979). A functionalist approach to the acquisition of grammar. In E. Ochs & B. Schieffelin (Eds.), *Developmental pragmatics* (pp. 167–211). New York: Academic Press.

Bates, E., & MacWhinney, B. (1982). Functionalist approaches to grammar. In E. Wanner & L. Gleitman (Eds.), *Language acquisition: The state of the art* (pp. 173–218). New York: Cambridge University Press.

Bates, E., & MacWhinney, B. (1987). Competition, variation, and language learning. In B. MacWhinney (Ed.), *Mechanisms of language acquisition* (pp. 157–194). Hillsdale, NJ: Lawrence Erlbaum.

Bates, E., & Snyder, L. (1985). The cognitive hypothesis in language development. In I. Uzigiris & J. M. Hunt (Eds.), *Research with scales of psychological development in infancy.* Champaign-Urbana: University of Illinois Press.

Bateson, M. (1971). The interpersonal context of infant vocalizations. *Quarterly Progress Report, Research Laboratory of Electronics, MIT, 100,* 170–176.

Bateson, M. (1975). Mother–infant exchanges: The epigenesis of conversational interaction. In D. Aronson & R. Rieber (Eds.), *Developmental psycholinguistics and communication disorders* (pp. 101–113). New York: New York Academy of Sciences.

Bayley, N. (1969). *Bayley Scales of Infant Development.* San Antonio, TX: Psychological Corporation.

Bean, C., Folkins, J. W., & Cooper, W. E. (1989). The effects of emphasis on passage comprehension. *Journal of Speech and Hearing Research, 32,* 707–712.

Beitchman, J. H., Nair, R., Clegg, M., & Patel, P. G. (1986). Prevalence of speech and language disorders in 5-year-old kindergarten children in the Ottawa-Carlton Region. *Journal of Speech and Hearing Disorders, 51,* 98–110.

Bellack, A. A., Kliebard, H. M., Hyman, R. T., & Smith, F. L., Jr. (1966). *The language of the classroom.* New York: Columbia University Teachers College Press.

Bellugi, U., & Klima, E. (1982). The acquisition of three morphological systems in American Sign Language. *Papers and Reports on Child Language Development, 21,* 135.

Benedict, H. (1979). Early lexical development: Comprehension and production. *Journal of Child Language, 6,* 183–200.

Bennett, C. W. (1989). *Referential semantic analysis* [Computer program]. Woodstock, VA: Teaching Texts.

Bennett, C. W., & Alter, K. S. (1985). *Word class inventory for schoolage children* [Computer program]. San Diego, CA: College-Hill Press.

Bennett, C. W., & James, C. (1990, November). *TTR revisited: Selecting remedial targets.* Paper presented at the meeting of the American Speech-Language-Hearing Association, Seattle, WA.

Benson, D. F. (1967). Fluency in aphasia: Correlation with radioactive scan localization. *Cortex, 3,* 373–394.

Benson, D. F., & Geschwind, N. (1976). Aphasia and related disturbances. In A. B. Baker (Ed.), *Clinical Neurology* (Vol. 1, pp. 1–28). NY: Harper & Row.

Berko, J. (1958). The child's learning of English morphology. *Word, 14,* 150–177.

Bernstein, B. B. (1972). A critique of the concept of compensatory education. In C. B. Cazden, V. P. John, & D. Hymes (Eds.), *Functions of language in the classroom* (pp. 135–154). New York: Columbia University Teachers

College Press.

Bernstein, D. K. (1986). The development of humor: Implications for assessment and intervention. *Topics in Language Disorders, 6* (4), 65–72.

Bertalanffy, L. von. (1968). *General system theory: Foundations, development, applications.* New York: George Braziller.

Bess, F. H. (1982). Children with unilateral hearing loss. *Journal of Academy of Rehabilitation Audiology, 15,* 131–144.

Bess, F. H., Freeman, B., & Sinclair, J. S. (Eds.). (1981). *Amplification in education.* Washington, DC: A. G. Bell.

Bess, F. H., & McConnell, F. (1981). *Audiology, education, and the hearing impaired child.* St. Louis: C. V. Mosby.

Bettelheim, B. (1967). *The empty fortress.* New York: Free Press.

Beukelman, D. R. (1987). When you have a hammer, everything looks like a nail. *Augmentative and Alternative Communication, 3,* 94–96.

Beukelman, D. R., & Mirenda, P. (1992). *Augmentative and alternative communication: Management of severe communication disorders in children and adults.* Baltimore, MD: Paul H. Brookes.

Beukelman, D. R., & Mirenda, P. (1988). Communication options for persons who cannot speak: Assessment and evaluation. In C. A. Coston (Ed.), *Proceedings of the national planners conference on assistive device service delivery: Planning and implementing augmentative communication service delivery* (pp. 151–165). Washington, DC: Association for the Advancement of Rehabilitation Technology.

Beukelman, D. R., & Tice, R. (Programmer). (1990). *The vocabulary toolbox* [computer program]. Field test version under development at the University of Nebraska-Lincoln, Lincoln, NE.

Beukelman, D. R., Tice, R., Garrett, K., & Lange, U. (1988). *Cue-write: Word processing with spelling assistance and practice* [Computer software]. Tucson, AZ: Communication Skill Builders.

Beukelman, D. R., & Yorkston, K. M. (1991). Traumatic brain injury changes the way we live. In D. R. Beukelman & K. M. Yorkston (Eds.), *Communication disorders following traumatic brain injury: Management of cognitive, language, and motor impairments* (pp. 1–13). Austin, TX: Pro-Ed.

Bickerton, D. (1983, July). Creole languages. *Scientific American, 249,* pp. 116–122.

Biklen, D. (Producer). (1988). *Regular lives* [Videotape]. Washington, DC: State of the Art.

Biklen, D. (1990). Communication unbound: Autism and praxis. *Harvard Educational Review, 60,* 291–314.

Biklen, D. (1992). Typing to talk: Facilitated communication. *American Journal of Speech-Language Pathology, 1*(2), 15–17.

Bishop, D. V. M., & Edmundson, A. (1987). Language-impaired 4-year-olds: Distinguishing transient from persistent impairment. *Journal of Speech and Hearing Disorders, 52,* 156–173.

Bivens, J. A., & Berk, L. E. (1990). A longitudinal study of the development of elementary school children's private speech. *Merrill-Palmer Quarterly, 36,* 443–463.

Bjorkland, D., & Bjorkland, B. (1988, January). Cultural literacy. *Parents,* p. 144.

Blackstone, S. (1989) Life is not a dress rehearsal. *Augmentative Communication News, 2*(5), 1–2.

Blager, F. B. (1979). The effect of intervention on the speech and language of abused children. *Child Abuse and Neglect, 5,* 991–996.

Blager, F. B., & Martin, H. P. (1976). Speech and language of abused children. In H. P. Martin (Ed.), *The abused child: A multidisciplinary approach to developmental issues and treatment* (pp. 83–92). Cambridge, MA: Ballinger Publishing.

Blank, M. (1973). *Teaching learning in the preschool: A dialogue approach.* Columbus, OH: Merrill/Macmillan.

Blank, M. (1975) Verbalization from young children in experimental tasks. *Child Development, 46,* 254–257.

Blank, M. (1982). Language and school failure: Some speculations on the relationship between oral and written language. In L. Feagans & D. Farran (Eds.), *The language of children reared in poverty* (pp. 75–93). New York: Academic Press.

Blank, M., & Bruskin, C. (1982). Sentences and non-content words: Missing ingredients in reading instruction. *Annals of Dyslexia, 32,* 103–121.

Blank, M., Rose, S. A., & Berlin, L. (1978). *The language of learning: The preschool years.* New York: Grune & Stratton.

Blank, M., & White, S. J. (1986). Questions: A powerful but misused form of classroom exchange. *Topics in Language Disorders, 6* (2), 1–12.

Bliss, L. S. (1987). "I can't talk anymore; My mouth doesn't want to." The development and clinical applications of modal auxiliaries. *Language, Speech, and Hearing Services in Schools, 18,* 72–79.

Bloom, B. S. (Ed.). (1956). *Taxonomy of educational objectives. Handbook I. Cognitive domain.* New York: David McKay.

Bloom, L. (1967). A comment on Lee's "Developmental sentence types: A method for comparing normal and deviant syntactic development." *Journal of Speech and Hearing Disorders, 32,* 294–296.

Bloom, L. (1970). *Language development: Form and function in emerging grammars.* Cambridge, MA: MIT Press.

Bloom, L. (1973). *One word at a time: The use of single word utterances before syntax.* The Hague, Netherlands: Mouton.

Bloom, L. (1975). Communication skills of abused children (Doctoral dissertation, University of Pittsburgh, 1975) *Dissertation Abstracts International, 36,* 7728A.

Bloom, L. (1988). What is language? In M. Lahey, (Ed.), *Language disorders and language development* (pp. 1–19). New York: Macmillan.

Bloom, L., Hood, L., & Lightbown, P. (1974). Imitation in language development: If, when, and why. *Cognitive Psychology, 6,* 380–420.

Bloom, L., & Lahey, M. (1978). *Language development and language disorders.* New York: John Wiley & Sons.

Bloom, L., Lahey, M., Hood, L., Lifter, K., & Fiess, K. (1980). Complex sentences: Acquisition of syntactic connectives and the semantic relations they encode. *Journal of Child Language, 7,* 235–261.

Bloome, D., & Knott, G. (1985). Teacher–student discourse. In D. N. Ripich & F. M. Spinelli (Eds.), *School discourse problems* (pp. 53–76). San Diego, CA: College-Hill.

Boder, E., & Jarrico, S. (1982). *Boder Test of Reading–Spelling Patterns.* San Antonio, TX: The Psychological Corporation.

Bodner-Johnson, B. (1991). Family conversation style: Its effect on the deaf child's participation. *Exceptional Children, 57,* 502–509.

Boehm, A. E. (1971). *Boehm Test of Basic Concepts.* San Antonio, TX: Psychological Corporation.

Boehm, A. E. (1986). *Boehm Test of Basic Concepts—Revised.* San Antonio, TX: Psychological Corporation.

Bohannon, J. N., III, & Warren-Leubecker, A. (1989). Theoretical approaches to language acquisition. In J. B. Gleason (Ed.), *The development of language* (2nd ed., pp. 167–223). Columbus, OH: Merrill/Macmillan.

Bond, D. J., & Chandley, A. C. (1983). The origin and causes of aneuploidy in man. In *Aneuploidy: Oxford monographs on medical genetics* (pp. 55–76.) Oxford, England: Oxford University Press.

Boothroyd, A. (1982). *Hearing impairments in young children.* Englewood Cliffs, NJ: Prentice-Hall.

Bos, C. S. (1988). Process-oriented writing: Instructional implications for mildly handicapped students. *Exceptional Children, 54,* 521–527.

Bos, C. S., & Anders, P. L. (1990). Interactive practices for teaching content and strategic knowledge. In T. E. Scruggs & B. Y. L. Wong (Eds.), *Intervention research in learning disabilities* (pp. 116—185). New York: Springer-Verlag.

Botvin, G. J., & Sutton-Smith, B. (1977). The development of structural complexity in children's fantasy narratives. *Developmental Psychology, 13,* 377–388.

Bouvier, L. F., & Gardner, R. W. (1986). *Immigration to the U.S.: The unfinished story.* Washington, DC: Population Reference Bureau.

Bowerman, M. (1982). Reorganization processes in lexical and syntactic development. In E. Wanner & L. Gleitman (Eds.), *Language acquisition: The state of the art.* Cambridge, England: Cambridge University Press.

Boyce, N. L., & Larson, V. L. (1983). *Adolescents' communication: Development and disorders.* Eau Claire, WI: Thinking Publications.

Bracken, B. A. (1984). *Bracken Basic Concept Scale.* San Antonio, TX: Psychological Corporation.

Braddock, J. H., II, & McPartland, J. M. (1990). Alternatives to tracking. *Educational Leadership, 47*(7), 76–79.

Brannon, L. (1985). Toward a theory of composition. In B. W. McClelland & T. R. Donovan (Eds.), *Perspectives on research and scholarship in composition* (pp. 6–25). New York: Modern Language Corporation of America.

Bransford, J. C., & Johnson, M. K. (1972). Contextual prerequisites for understanding: Some investigations of comprehension and recall. *Journal of Verbal Learning and Verbal Behavior, 11,* 717–726.

Bransford, J. C., & Nitsch, K. E. (1985). Coming to understand things we could not previously understand. In H. Singer & R. B. Ruddell (Eds.), *Theoretical models and processes of reading* (3rd ed., pp. 81–122). Newark, DE: International Reading Association.

Brazelton, T. B. (1973). *Neonatal behavioral assessment scale. Clinics in Developmental Medicine, No. 50,* Philadelphia: J. B. Lippincott.

Brazelton, T. B. (1982). Mother–infant reciprocity. In M. H. Klaus, T. Leger, & M. A. Trause (Eds.), *Maternal attachment and mothering disorders . Pediatric round table: 1* (pp. 49–54). Skillman, NJ: Johnson & Johnson Baby Products Company.

Brazelton, T. B. (1984). *Neonatal behavioral assessment scale (2nd ed.). Clinics in developmental medicine, No. 50.* Philadelphia: J. B. Lippincott.

Brazelton, T. B., Koslowski, B., & Main, M. (1974). The origins of reciprocity: The early mother–infant interaction. In M. Lewis & L. A. Rosenblum (Eds.), *The effect of the infant on its caretaker.* New York: John Wiley.

Breen, C., Haring, T., Pitts-Conway, V., & Gaylord-Ross, R. (1985). The training and generalization of social interaction during breaktime at two job sites in the natural environment. *Journal of the Association for Persons With Severe Handicaps, 10,* 41–50.

Brenneis, D., & Lein, L. (1977). "You fruithead": A sociolinguistic approach to children's dispute settlement. In S. Ervin-Tripp & C. Mitchell-Kernan (Eds.), *Child discourse* (pp. 49–65). New York: Academic Press.

Brinton, B., & Fujiki, M. (1982). A comparison of request–response sequences in the discourse of normal and language-disordered children. *Journal of Speech and Hearing Disorders, 47,* 57–62.

Brinton, B., & Fujiki, M. (1984). Development of topic manipulation skills in discourse. *Journal of Speech and Hearing Research, 27,* 350–358.

Brinton, B., & Fujiki, M. (1989). *Conversational management with language-impaired children: Pragmatic assessment and intervention.* Rockville, MD: Aspen.

Brinton, B., Fujiki, M., Winkler, E., & Loeb, D. F. (1986). Responses to requests for clarification in linguistically normal and language-impaired children. *Journal of Speech and Hearing Disorders, 51,* 370–378.

Britton, B., Glynn, S., & Smith, J. (1985). Cognitive demands of processing expository text: A cognitive workbench model. In B. Britton & J. Black (Eds.), *Understanding expository text.* Hillsdale, NJ: Lawrence Erlbaum.

Britton, J. N. (1970). *Language and learning.* London: Penguin Press.

Britton, J. N. (1979). Learning to use language in two modes. In N. R. Smith & M. B. Franklin (Eds.), *Symbolic functioning in childhood* (pp. 185–197). Hillsdale, NJ: Lawrence Erlbaum.

Bronfenbrenner, U. (1979). Foreword. In P. Chance (Ed.), Learning through play. *Johnson & Johnson Pediatric Round Table Series No. 3* (pp. xv–xx). New York: Gardner Press.

Brooks, D. (1986). Otitis media with effusion and academic attainment. *International Journal of Pediatric Otorhinolaryngology, 12,* 39–47.

Brown, A. L., & Day, J. D. (1983). Macrorules for summarizing texts: The development of expertise. *Journal of Verbal Learning and Verbal Behavior, 22,* 1–14.

Brown, A. L., & Palincsar, A. (1982). Inducing strategic learning from texts by means of informed, self-control training. *Topics in Learning and Learning Disabilities, 2,* 1–17.

Brown, J. B. (1977). *Mind, brain, and consciousness: The neuropsychology of cognition.* New York: Academic Press.

Brown, L., Branston, M. B., Hamre-Nietupski, S., Pumpian, I., Certo, N., & Gruenewald, L. (1979). A strategy for developing chronological age appropriate and functional curricular content for severely handicapped adolescents and young adults. *Journal of Special Education, 13*(1), 81–90.

Brown, L., Nietupski, J., & Hamre-Nietupski, S. (1976). The criterion of ultimate functioning and public school services for severely handicapped students. In M. A. Thomas (Ed.), *Hey, don't forget about me! Education's investment in the severely, profoundly, and multiply handicapped* (pp. 2–15). Reston, VA: Council for Exceptional Children.

Brown, L., Sherbenou, R. J., & Johnsen, S. K. (1985). *Test of nonverbal intelligence: A language-free measure of cognitive ability.* Austin, TX: Pro-Ed.

Brown, R. A. (1958). *Words and things.* New York: Free Press.

Brown, R. A. (1973). *A first language: The early stages.* Cambridge, MA: Harvard University Press.

Brown, R. A. (1977). Introduction. In C. Snow & C. Ferguson (Eds.), *Talking to children.* New York: Cambridge University Press.

Brown, S. F. (Ed.). (1959). *The concept of congenital aphasia from the standpoint of dynamic differential diagnosis.* Washington, DC: American Speech and Hearing Association.

Brown, T. (1985). Foreword. In J. Piaget (T. Brown & K. J. Thampy, Trans.) *The equilibration of cognitive structures: The central problem of intellectual development.* Chicago: University of Chicago Press.

Bruininks, V. L. (1978). Actual and perceived peer status of learning disabled students in mainstream programs. *Journal of Special Education, 12,* 51–58.

Bruner, J. (1968). *Processes of cognitive growth: Infancy (Vol. III, Heinz Werner Lecture Series).* Worcester, MA: Clark University Press.

Bruner, J. (1974/1975). From communication to language—A psychological perspective. *Cognition, 3,* 255–287.

Bruner, J. (1975). The ontogenesis of speech acts. *Journal of Child Language, 2,* 1–19.

Bruner, J. (1977). Early social interaction and language acquisition. In R. Schaffer (Ed.), *Studies in mother–infant interaction* (pp. 271–289). New York: Academic Press.

Bruner, J. (1978). The role of dialogue in language acquisition. In A. Sinclair, R. J. Jarvella, & W. J. M. Levelt (Eds.), *The child's conception of language: Springer series in language and communication* (pp. 242–256). New York: Springer-Verlag.

Bruner, J. (1983). *Child's talk: Learning to use language.* New York: W. W. Norton.

Bruner, J., Oliver, R., & Greenfield, P. (1966). *Studies in cognitive growth.* New York: Wiley.

Bryan, J. H., & Sherman, A. (1980). An observational analysis of classroom behaviors of children with learning disabilities. *Journal of Learning Disabilities, 1,* 23–34.

Bryan, T. (1986). A review of studies on learning disabled children's communicative competence. In R. L. Schiefelbusch (Ed.), *Language competence: Assessment and intervention* (pp. 227–259). Austin, TX: Pro-Ed.

Bullowa, M. (Ed.). (1979). *Before speech: The beginnings of interpersonal communication.* Cambridge, England: Cambridge University Press.

Bunce, B. H., Ruder, K. F., & Ruder, C. C. (1985). Using the miniature linguistic system in teaching syntax: Two case studies. *Journal of Speech and Hearing Disorders, 50,* 247–253.

Burke, C. L. (1980). Reading interview. In B. P. Farr & D. J. Stickler (Eds.), *Reading comprehension: An instructional videotape series resource guide.* Bloomington, IN: Indiana University Press.

Butler, D. (1980). *Cushla and her books.* Boston: Horn Book.

Butler, K. G. (1981). Language processing disorder: Factors in diagnosis and remediation. In R. W. Keith (Ed.), *Central auditory and language disorders in children* (pp. 160–174). San Diego: College-Hill Press.

Butler, K. G. (1984a). From the editor. *Topics in Language Disorders, 4*(2), iv.

Butler, K. G. (1984b). Language processing: Halfway up the down staircase. In G. P. Wallach & K. G. Butler (Eds.), *Language learning disabilities in school-age children* (pp. 60–81). Baltimore, MD: Williams & Wilkins.

Butler, K. G. (Ed.). (1985). From the editor [Special issue: (Language 1 and language 2: Implications for language disorders. *Topics in Language Disorders, 5*(4), iv–vi.

Buttrill, J., Niizawa, J., Biemer, C., Takakashi, C., & Hearn, S. (1989). Serving the language learning disabled adolescent: A strategies-based model. *Language, Speech, and Hearing Services in Schools, 20,* 185–204.

Byrnes, M. (1990). The Regular Education Initiative debate: A view from the field. *Exceptional Children, 56,* 345–349.

Calculator, S. N. (1988). Promoting the acquisition and generalization of conversational skills by individuals with severe disabilities. *Augmentative and Alternative Communication, 4,* 94–103.

Calculator, S. N., & Dollaghan, C. (1982). The use of communicative boards in a residential setting: An evaluation. *Journal of Speech and Hearing Disorders, 47,* 281–287.

Calfee, R., & Chambliss, M. (1988). Beyond decoding: Pictures of expository prose. *Annals of Dyslexia, 38,* 243–257.

Calfee, R., & Curley, R. (1984). Structure of prose in the content areas. In J. Flood (Ed.), *Understanding reading comprehension* (pp. 161–180). Newark, DE: International Reading Association.

Calkins, L. M. (1983). *Lessons from a child: On the teaching and learning of writing.* Portsmouth, NH: Heinemann.

Campbell, S. B. (1985). Hyperactivity in preschoolers: Correlates and prognostic implications. *Clinical Psychology Review, 5,* 405–428.

Campbell, T. F., & Dollaghan, C. A. (1990). Expressive language recovery in severely brain-injured children and adolescents. *Journal of Speech and Hearing Disorders, 55,* 567–581.

Cantwell, D. P., & Baker, L. (1985). Interrelationship of communication, learning, and psychiatric disorders in children. In C. S. Simon (Ed.), *Communication skills and classroom success: Assessment of language-learning disabled students* (pp. 43–61). Austin, TX: Pro-Ed.

Cantwell, D. P., Baker, L., & Mattison, R. E. (1979). The prevalence of psychiatric disorder in children with speech and language disorder: An epidemiologic study. *Journal of the American Academy of Child Psychiatry, 18,* 450–461.

Capper, C. A. (1990). Students with low-incidence disabilities in disadvantaged rural settings. *Exceptional Children, 56,* 338–344.

Capra, F. (1982). *The turning point: Science, society, and the rising culture.* New York: Simon & Schuster.

Carey, S. (1978). The child as word learner. In M. Halle, J. Bresnan, & G. Miller (Eds.), *Linguistic theory and psychological reality* (pp. 264–293). Cambridge, MA: MIT Press.

Carey, S., & Bartlett, E. (1978). Acquiring a single new word. *Papers and Reports in Child Language Development, 15,* 17–29.

Carignan-Belleville, L. (1989). Jason's story: Motivating the reluctant student to write. *English Journal, 78,* 57–60.

Carlson, F. (1982). *Prattle and play: Equipment recipes for nonspeech communication.* Omaha, NE: Meyer Children's Rehabilitation Institute, University of Nebraska Medical Center.

Carnine, D., & Kinder, D. (1985). Teaching low-performing students to apply generative and schema strategies to narrative and expository material. *Remedial and Special Education, 6,* 20–30.

Carpenter, R., Mastergeorge, A., & Coggins, T. (1983). The acquisition of communicative intentions in infants eight to fifteen months of age. *Language and Speech, 26,* 101–116.

Carr, E., Newsom, C. D., & Binkhoff, J. A. (1980). Escape as a factor in the aggressive behavior of two retarded children. *Journal of Applied Behavior Analysis, 13,* 101–117.

Carrow, E. (1973a). *Screening Test of Auditory Comprehension of Language.* Austin, TX: Learning Concepts.

Carrow, E. (1973b). *Test for Auditory Comprehension of Language.* Austin, TX: Teaching Resources.

Carrow-Woolfolk, E. (1988). *Theory, assessment and intervention in language disorders: An integrative approach.* Orlando, FL: Grune & Stratton.

Carta, J. J., Sainato, D. M., & Greenwood, C. R. (1988). Advances in the ecological assessment of classroom instruction for young children with handicaps. In S. L. Odom & M. B. Karnes (Eds.), *Early intervention for infants and children with handicaps* (pp. 217–239). Baltimore, MD: Paul. H. Brookes.

Cartledge, G., Stupay, D., & Kaczala, C. (1988). Testing language in learning disabled and nonlearning disabled Black children: What makes the difference? *Learning Disabilities Research, 3*(2), 101–106.

Casby, M. (1988). Speech-language pathologists' attitudes and involvement regarding language and reading. *Language, Speech, and Hearing Services in Schools, 19,* 352–358.

Casby, M. K., & Ruder, K. F. (1983). Symbolic play and early language development in normal and mentally retarded children. *Journal of Speech and Hearing Research, 26,* 404–411.

Case, R. (1985). *Intellectual development: Birth to adulthood.* Orlando, FL: Academic Press.

Cattell, R. B. (1971). *Abilities: Their structure, growth, and action.* Boston: Houghton Mifflin.

Catts, H. W. (1989). Speech production deficits in developmental dyslexia. *Journal of Speech and Hearing Disorders, 54,* 422–428.

Cazden, C. B. (1972). Preface. In C. Cazden, V. John, & D. Hymes (Eds.), *Functions of language in the classroom.* New York: Teachers College Press, Columbia University.

Cazden, C. B. (1988). *Classroom discourse: The language of teaching and learning.* Portsmouth, NH: Heinemann.

Cazden, C. B., John, V., and Hymes, D. (Eds.). (1972). *Functions of language in the classroom.* New York: Teachers College Press, Columbia University.

Chabon, S. S., & Prelock, P. A. (1989). Strategies of a different stripe: Our response to a zebra question about language and its relevance to the school curriculum. *Seminars in Speech and Language, 10*(3), 241–251.

Chadwick, O., Rutter, M., Brown, G., Shaffer, D., & Traub, M. (1981). A prospective study of children with head injuries: II. Cognitive sequelae. *Psychological Medicine, 11,* 49–61.

Chall, J. S. (1983). *Stages of reading development.* New York: McGraw-Hill.

Chance, P. (1979). *Learning through play: Johnson & Johnson Pediatric Round Table Series No. 3.* New York: Gardner Press.

Chapman, R. (1978). Comprehension strategies in children. In J. Kavanagh & P. Strange (Eds.), *Language and speech in the laboratory, school, and clinic.* Cambridge, MA: MIT Press.

Chapman, R. S., & Miller, J. F. (1980). Analyzing language and communication in the child. In R. L. Schiefelbusch (Ed.), *Nonspeech language and communication* (pp. 159–196). Austin, TX: Pro-Ed.

Chappell, G. E. (1973). Childhood verbal apraxia and its treatment. *Journal of Speech and Hearing Disorders, 38,* 362–368.

Charney, R. (1980). Speech roles and the development of personal pronouns. *Journal of Child Language, 7,* 509–528.

Cheng, L. L. (1989). Service delivery to Asian/Pacific LEP children: A cross-cultural framework. *Topics in Language Disorders, 9* (3), 1–14.

Cherry, R. (1980). *The selective auditory attention test* [SAAT; manual and tape]. St. Louis, MO: Auditec.

Cherry, R., & Kruger, G. (1983). Selective auditory attention abilities of learning disabled and normal achieving children. *Journal of Learning Disabilities, 16,* 202–205.

Chi, J. G., Dooling, E. C., & Gilles, F. H. (1977). Left-right asymmetries of the temporal speech areas of the human fetus. *Archives of Neurology, 34,* 346–348.

Chinn, P., Drew, E., & Logan, D. (1975). *Mental retardation: A life cycle approach.* St. Louis, MO: C. V. Mosby.

Chipman, S., Segal, J., & Glaser, R. E. (Eds.). (1984). *Thinking and learning skills (Volume II): Current research and open questions.* Hillsdale, NJ: Lawrence Erlbaum.

Chollar, S. (1989, April). Conversations with the dolphins. *Psychology Today, 23*(4), 52–57.

Chomsky, N. (1957). *Syntactic structures.* The Hague, The Netherlands: Mouton.

Chomsky, N. (1965). *Aspects of the theory of syntax.* Cambridge, MA: MIT Press.

Chomsky, N. (1968). *Language and mind.* New York: Harcourt, Brace & World.

Chomsky, C. (1969). *The acquisition of syntax in children from 5 to 10.* Cambridge, MA: MIT Press.

Chomsky, N. (1976). On the biological basis of language capacities. In R. W. Rieber (Ed.), *The neuropsychology of language.* New York: Plenum Publishing.

Chomsky, N. (1980). *Rules and representations.* New York: Columbia University Press.

Chomsky, N. (1981). *Lectures on government and binding.* Dordrecht, Holland: Foris.

Churchill, D. W. (1972). The relation of infantile autism and early childhood schizophrenia to developmental language disorders of childhood. *Journal of Autism and Childhood Schizophrenia, 2,* 182–197.

Cirrin, R., & Rowland, C. (1985). Communicative assessment of nonverbal youths with severe/profound mental retardation. *Mental Retardation, 23,* 52–62.

Clark, D. A. (1989). Neonates and infants at risk for hearing and speech–language disorders. *Topics in Language Disorders, 10*(1), 1–12.

Clark, G. N., & Seifer, R. (1985). Assessment of parents' interactions with their developmentally delayed infants. *Infant Mental Health Journal, 6*(4), 214–225.

Clark, T., Morgan, E. C., & Wilson-Vlotman, A. L. (1984). *The INSITE model: A parent centered, in-home, sensory intervention, training and educational program.* Logan, UT: Utah State University.

Clark, T., & Watkins, S. (1985). *SKI*HI curriculum manual: Programming for hearing impaired infants through home intervention.* Logan, UT: Utah State University.

Clarke, C. M., Edwards, J. H., & Smallpiece, V. (1961). 21 trisomy/normal mosaicism in an intelligent child with mongoloid characters. *Lancet, 1,* 1028.

Cleary, L. M. (1988). A profile of Carlos: Strengths of a nonstandard dialect writer. *English Journal, 77*(5), 59–64.

Coggins, T. E., & Carpenter, R. L. (1981). The communicative intention inventory: A system for coding children's early intentional communication. *Applied Psycholinguistics, 2,* 235–252.

Coggins, T. E., Olswang, L. B., & Guthrie, J. (1987). Assessing communicative intents in young children: Low structured or observation tasks? *Journal of Speech and Hearing Disorders, 52,* 44–49.

Cohen, A. L., Torgesen, J. K., & Torgesen, J. L. (1988). Improving speed and accuracy of word recognition in reading disabled children: An evaluation of two computer program variations. *Learning Disability Quarterly, II,* 333–341.

Cole, A. J., Andermann, F., Taylor, L., Olivier, A., Rasmussen, T., Robitaille, Y., & Spire, J.-P. (1988). The Landau-Kleffner syndrome of acquired epileptic aphasia: Unusual clinical outcome, surgical experience, and absence of encephalitis. *Neurology, 38,* 31–38.

Cole, K. N., Mills, P. E., & Dale, P. S. (1989). Examination of test–retest and split-half reliability for measures derived from language samples of young handicapped children. *Language, Speech, and Hearing Services in Schools, 20,* 245–258.

Cole, L. (1989). E Pluribus Pluribus: Multicultural imperatives for the 1990s and beyond. *Asha, 31*(9), 65–70.

Cole, L. & Deal, V. R. (Eds.). (in press). *Communication disorders in multicultural populations.* Rockville, MD: American Speech-Language-Hearing Association.

Coleman, M. (Ed.). (1976). *The autistic syndromes.* New York: American Elsevier.

Collins-Ahlgren, M. (1975). Language development of two deaf children. *American Annals of the Deaf, 120,* 524–539.

Collins, W. A., Wellman, H., Keniston, A. H., & Westby, S. (1978). Age-related aspects of comprehension and inference from a televised dramatic narrative. *Child Development, 49,* 389–399.

Connell, P. J., & Myles-Zitzer, C. (1982). An analysis of elicited imitation as a language evaluation procedure. *Journal of Speech and Hearing Disorders, 47,* 390–396.

Connell, P. J. (1986a). Acquisition of semantic role by language-disordered children: Differences between production and comprehension. *Journal of Speech and Hearing Research, 29,* 366–374.

Connell, P. J. (1986b). Teaching subjecthood to language-disordered children. *Journal of Speech and Hearing Research, 29,* 481–492.

Conners, C. K. (1969). A teacher rating scale for use in drug studies with children. *American Journal of Psychiatry, 126,* 884–888.

Constable, C. M. (1987). Talking with teachers: Increasing our relevance as language interventionists in the schools. *Seminars in Speech and Language, 8*(4), 345–356.

Conti-Ramsden, G. (1990). Maternal recasts and other contingent replies to language-impaired children. *Journal of Speech and Hearing Disorders, 55,* 262–274.

Conti-Ramsden, G., & Friel-Patti, S. (1983). Mothers' discourse adjustments to language-impaired and non-language impaired children. *Journal of Speech and Hearing Disorders, 48,* 360–367.

Cook-Gumperz, J. (1977). Situated instructions. In S. Ervin-Tripp & C. Mitchell-Kernan (Eds.), *Child discourse* (pp. 103–124). New York: Academic Press.

Cooper, C. R. (1976). Tonowanda Middle School's new writing program. *English Journal, 65,* 56–61.

Cooper, C. R. (1977). Holistic evaluation of writing. In C. R. Cooper & L. Odell (Eds.), *Evaluating writing: Describing, measuring, judging* (pp. 3–31). Urbana, IL: National Council of Teachers of English.

Cooper, C. R., & Odell, L. (Eds.). (1977). *Evaluating writing: Describing, measuring, judging.* Urbana, IL: National Council of Teachers of English.

Cooper, D. C., & Anderson-Inman, L. (1988). Language and socialization. In M. A. Nippold (Ed.), *Later language development: Ages nine through nineteen* (pp. 225–245). Austin, TX: Pro-Ed.

Cooper, J. A., & Ferry, P. C. (1978). Acquired auditory verbal agnosia and seizures in childhood. *Journal of Speech and Hearing Disorders, 43,* 176–184.

Cooper, M. M. (1982). Context as vehicle: Implicature in writing. In M. Nystrand (Ed.), *What writers know: The language, process, and structure of written discourse* (pp. 106–129). New York: Academic Press.

Copeland, D. R., Fletcher, J. M., Pfefferbaum-Levine, B., Jaffe, N., Ried, H., & Maor, M. (1985). Neuropsychological sequelae of childhood cancer on long-term survivors. *Pediatrics, 75,* 745–753.

Cornett, R. O. (1967). Cued speech. *American Annals of the Deaf, 112,* 3–13.

Cornett, R. O. (1972). *Cued speech parent training and follow-up program.* Washington, DC: Bureau of Education for the Handicapped, DHEW.

Corrigan, R. (1978). Language development as related to stage six object permanence development. *Journal of Child Language, 5,* 173–190.

Costello, J. (1977). Programmed instruction. *Journal of Speech and Hearing Disorders, 42,* 3–28.

Courchesne, E. (1988). Hypoplasia of cerebellar vermal lobules VI and VII in autism. *New England Journal of Medicine, 318,* 1349–1354.

Crago, M. B. (1990). Development of communicative competence in Inuit children: Implications for speech–language pathology. *Journal of Childhood Communication Disorders, 13,* 73–83.

Crago, M. B., & Cole, E. (1991). Using ethnography to bring children's communicative and cultural worlds into focus. In T. M. Gallagher (Ed.), *Pragmatics of language: Clinical practice issues* (pp. 99–131). San Diego, CA: Singular Publishing Group.

Craig, H. K. (1983). Application of pragmatic language models for intervention. In T. M. Gallagher & C. Prutting (Eds.), *Pragmatic assessment and intervention issues in language* (pp. 101–127). San Diego, CA: College-Hill Press.

Craik, F. I., & Lockhart, R. S. (1972). Levels of processing: A framework for memory research. *Journal of Verbal Learning and Verbal Behavior, 11,* 671–684.

Craik, K. (1943). *The nature of explanation.* Cambridge, England: Cambridge University Press.

Crais, E. (1987). Fast mapping of novel words in oral story context. *Papers and Reports in Child Language Development, 26,* 40–47.

Crais, E. R. (1990). World knowledge to word knowledge. World knowledge and language: Development and disorders. *Topics in Language Disorders, 10*(3), 45–62.

Crary, M. A. (1984). A neurolinguistic perspective on developmental verbal dyspraxia. *Communicative Disorders, 9,* 33–48.

Creaghead, N. A., & Tattershall, S. S. (1985). Observation and assessment of classroom pragmatic skills. In C. S. Simon (Ed.), *Communication skills and classroom success: Assessment of language-learning disabled students* (pp. 105–131). San Diego, CA: College-Hill Press.

Cromer, R. F. (1981). Reconceptualizing language acquisition and cognitive development. In R. L. Schiefelbusch & D. Bricker (Eds.), *Early language: Acquisition and intervention* (pp. 51–138). Baltimore, MD: University Park Press.

Cromer, R. F. (1991). The development of language and cognition: The cognition hypothesis. In R. F. Cromer, *Language and thought in normal and language handicapped children* (pp. 1–54). Cambridge, MA: Basil Blackwell. (Original work published 1974).

Cross, T. G. (1984). Habilitating the language-impaired child: Ideas from studies of parent–child interaction. *Topics in Language Disorders, 4*(4), 1–14.

Crossley, R., & MacDonald, A. (1984). *Annie's coming out.* New York: Viking Penguin.

Crowhurst, M. (1980). Syntactic complexity and teachers' quality ratings of narrations and arguments. *Research in the Teaching of English, 14,* 223–232.

Crystal, D. (1975). *The English tone of voice.* London: Edward Arnold.

Crystal, D. (1979). Prosodic development. In P. Fletcher & M. Garman (Eds.), *Language acquisition* (pp. 33–48). Cambridge, England: Cambridge University Press.

Crystal, D., Fletcher, P., & Garman, M. (1976). *The grammatical analysis of language disability.* London: Edward Arnold.

Cuda, R. A. (1976). *Analysis of speaking rate, syntactic complexity and speaking style of public school teachers.* Unpublished master's thesis, Wichita State University, Wichita, KS.

Cuda, R. A., & Nelson, N. W. (1976, November). *Analysis of teacher speaking rate, syntactic complexity, and hesitation phenomena as a function of grade level.* Paper presented at the annual conference of the American Speech-Language-Hearing Association, Houston.

Culatta, B., Page, J.L., & Ellis, J. (1983). Story retelling as a communicative performance screening tool. *Language, Speech, and Hearing Services in Schools, 14,* 66–74.

Cullinan, B. E. (1989). Literature for young children. In D. S. Strickland & L. M. Morrow (Eds.), *Emerging literacy: Young children learn to read and write* (pp. 35–51). Newark, DE: International Reading Association.

Curtiss, S. (1977). *Genie: A linguistic study of a modern-day "wild child."* New York: Academic Press.

Curtiss, S., Prutting, C. A., & Lowell, E. L. (1979). Pragmatic and semantic development in young children with impaired hearing. *Journal of Speech and Hearing Research, 22,* 534–552.

Dale, P. S. (1980). Is early pragmatic development measurable? *Journal of Child Language, 8,* 1–12.

Dalebout, S. D., Nelson, N. W., Hletko, P. J., & Frentheway, B. (1991). Selective auditory attention and children with attention-deficit hyperactivity disorder: Effects of repeated measurement with and without methylphenidate. *Language, Speech, and Hearing Services in Schools, 22,* 219–227.

Dalton, B. M., & Bedrosian, J. L. (1989). Communicative performance of adolescents with severe speech impairment: Influence of context. *Journal of Speech and Hearing Disorders, 54,* 403–421.

Damico, J. S. (1991). Clinical discourse analysis: A functional approach to language assessment. In C. S. Simon (Ed.), *Communication skills and classroom success: Assessment and therapy methodologies for language and learning disabled students* (pp. 125–148). Eau Claire, WI: Thinking Publications. (Original work published 1985).

Damico, J. S. (1987). Addressing language concerns in the schools: The SLP as consultant. *Journal of Childhood Communication Disorders, 11,* 17–40.

Damico, J. S. (1988). The lack of efficacy in language therapy: A case study. *Language, Speech, and Hearing Services in Schools, 19,* 51–66.

Damico, J. S., & Oller, J.W., Jr. (1980). Pragmatic versus morphological/syntactic criteria for language referrals. *Language, Speech, and Hearing Services in Schools, 11,* 85–94.

Damico, J. S., Oller, J. W., Jr., & Storey, M. E. (1983). The diagnosis of language disorders in bilingual children: Surface-oriented and pragmatic criteria. *Journal of Speech and Hearing Disorders, 48,* 385–394.

Davey, B. (1983). Think aloud: Modeling the cognitive process of reading comprehension. *Journal of Reading, 37,* 104–112.

Davis, G. Z. (1990). Skiing beyond the edge. *Perspectives on Dyslexia, 16*(1), 4.

Davis, J. M., Elfenbein, J., Schum, R., & Bentler, R. A. (1986). Effects of mild and moderate hearing impairments on language, educational, and psychosocial behavior of children. *Journal of Speech and Hearing Disorders, 51,* 53–62.

Davis, K. (1947). Final note on a case of extreme isolation. *American Journal of Sociology, 52,* 432–437.

Davis, W. E. (1989). The Regular Education Initiative debate: Its promises and problems. *Exceptional Children, 55,* 440–446.

Davis, W. E. (1990). Broad perspectives on the Regular Education Initiative: Response to Byrnes. *Exceptional Children, 56,* 349–356.

Deal, V. R., & Rodriguez, V. L. (1987). *Resource guide to multicultural tests and materials in communicative disorders.* Rockville, MD: American Speech-Language-Hearing Association.

DeMyer, M. K. (1975). Research in infantile autism: A strategy and its results. *Biological Psychiatry, 10,* 433–450.

DeMyer, M. K., Barton, S., DeMyer, W. E., Norton, J. A., Allen, J., & Steele, R. (1973). Prognosis in autism: A follow-up study. *Journal of Autism and Childhood Schizophrenia, 3,* 199–246.

DeMyer, M. K., Hingtgen, J. N., & Jackson, R. K. (1981). Infantile autism reviewed: A decade of research. *Schizophrenia Bulletin, 7,* 388–451.

Denckla, M. B. (1972). Clinical syndromes in learning disabilities: The case for "splitting" vs. "lumping." *Journal of Learning Disabilities, 5,* 401–406.

Denckla, M. B., & Rudel, R. G. (1976). Naming of object drawings by dyslexic and other learning disabled children. *Brain and Language, 3,* 1–15.

Denham, C., & Lieberman, A. (Eds.). (1980). *Time to learn.* Washington, DC: National Institute of Education.

Deno, S. L. (1989). Curriculum-based measurement and special education services: A fundamental and direct relationship. In M. R. Shinn (Ed.), *Curriculum-based mea-surement: Assessing special children* (pp. 1–17). New York: Guilford Press.

Deshler, D. D., Alley, G. R., & Carlson, S. C. (1980). Learning strategies: An approach to mainstreaming secondary students with learning disabilities. *Education Unlimited, 2,* 6–11.

Deshler, D. D., Lowrey, N., & Alley, G. R. (1979). Programing alternatives for LD adolescents. *Academic Therapy, 14,* 389–397.

Despain, A. D., & Simon, C. S. (1987). Alternative to failure: A junior high school language development-based curriculum. *Journal of Childhood Communication Disorders, 11,* 139–179.

Deutch, M. (1949). An experimental study of the effects of cooperation and competition upon group process. *Human Relations, 2,* 199–232.

Deutsch, F. (1983). *Child services: On behalf of children.* Monterey, CA: Brooks/Cole Publishing.

De Villiers, J., & De Villiers, P. (1973). A cross-sectional study of the development of grammatical morphemes in child speech. *Journal of Psycholinguistic Research, 2,* 267-268.

Dietrich, K. N., Starr, R. H., & Kaplan, M. G. (1980). Maternal stimulation and care of abused infants. In T. M. Field, S. Goldberg, D. Stern, & A. M. Sostek (Eds.), *High-risk infants and children.* New York: Academic Press.

Dillard, J. L. (1972). *Black English: Its history and usage in the United States.* New York: Random House.

Dobie, R. A., & Berlin, C. I. (1979). Influence of otitis media on hearing and development. *Annals of Otology, Rhinology, and Laryngology, 88*(Suppl. 60), 48–53.

Dodd, B. (1976). The phonological systems of deaf children. *Journal of Speech and Hearing Disorders, 41,* 185–198.

Dollaghan, C. A. (1985). Child meets words: "Fast mapping" in preschool children. *Journal of Speech and Hearing Research, 28,* 449–454.

Dollaghan, C. A. (1987a). Comprehension monitoring in normal and language-impaired children. *Topics in Language Disorders, 7*(2), 45–60.

Dollaghan, C. A. (1987b). Fast mapping in normal and language impaired children. *Journal of Speech and Hearing Disorders, 52,* 218–222.

Dollaghan, C. A., Campbell, T. F., & Tomlin, R. (1990). Video narration as a language sampling context. *Journal of Speech and Hearing Disorders, 55,* 582–590.

Dollaghan, C. A., & Kaston, N. (1986). A comprehension monitoring program for language-impaired children. *Journal of Speech and Hearing Disorders, 51,* 264–271.

Dollaghan, C. A., & Miller, J. (1986). Observational methods in the study of communicative competence. In R. L. Schiefelbusch (Ed.), *Language competence: Assessment and intervention* (pp. 99–129). Austin, TX: Pro-Ed.

Donahue, M., & Bryan, T. (1984). Communicative skills and peer relations of learning disabled adolescents. *Topics in Language Disorders, 4*(2), 10–21.

Donahue, M., Pearl, R., Bryan, T. (1983). Communicative competence in learning disabled children. In K. D. Gadow & I. Bialer (Eds.), *Advances in learning and behavior disabilities* (Vol. 2, pp. 49–84). Greenwich. CT: JAI Press.

Donnellan, A. M., Mirenda, P. L., Mesaros, R. A., & Fassbender, L. L. (1984). Analyzing the communicative functions of aberrant behavior. *JASH (Journal of the Association for Persons With Severe Handicaps), 9,* 202–212.

Donnelly, J. (1991, Summer). Jean Paul keeps on going. *The Advocate, Newletter of the Autism Society of America, 23*(2), 14–15.

Dore, J. (1974). A pragmatic description of early language development. *Journal of Psycholinguistic Research, 4,* 343–350.

Dore, J. (1975). Holophrases, speech acts, and language universals. *Journal of Child Language, 2,* 21–40.

Dore, J. (1986). The development of conversational competence. In R. L. Schiefelbusch (Ed.), *Language competence: Assessment and intervention* (pp. 3–60). Austin, TX: Pro-Ed.

Dorman, C. (1987). Reading disability subtypes in neurologically-impaired students. *Annals of Dyslexia, 37,* 166–188.

Dublinske, S. (1974). Planning for child change in language development/remediation programs carried out by teachers and parents. *Language, Speech, and Hearing Services in Schools, 5,* 225–237.

DuBose, R., Langley, M., & Stass, V. (1977). Assessing severely handicapped children. *Focus on Exceptional Children, 9,* 1–13.

Duchan, J. F. (1983). Language processing and geodesic domes. In T. M. Gallagher & C. Prutting (Eds.), *Pragmatic assessment and intervention issues in language* (pp. 83–99). San Diego, CA: College-Hill Press.

Duchan, J. F. (1984). Clinical interactions with autistic children: The role of theory. *Topics in Language Disorders, 4*(4), 62–71.

Duchan, J. F. (1986). Language intervention through sense-making and fine tuning. In R. L. Schiefelbusch (Ed.), *Language competence: Assessment and intervention* (pp. 187–212). Austin, TX: Pro-Ed.

Duchan, J. F., & Katz, J. (1983). Language and auditory processing: Top down plus bottom up. In E. Z. Lasky & J. Katz (Eds.), *Central auditory processing disorders: Problems of speech, language, and learning* (pp. 31–45). Baltimore, MD: University Park Press.

Dunlea, A. (1989). *Vision and the emergence of meaning: Blind and sighted children's early language.* New York: Cambridge University Press.

Dunn, C., & Newton, L. (1986). A comprehensive model for speech development in hearing-impaired children. *Topics in Language Disorders, 6*(3), 25-46.

Dunn, L. M., & Dunn, L. M. (1981). *Peabody Picture Vocabulary Test—Revised.* Circle Pines, MN: American Guidance Service.

Dunst, C., & Lowe, L. (1986). From reflex to symbol: Describing, explaining, and fostering communicative competence. *Augmentative and Alternative Communication, 2,* 11–18.

Dunst, C., Lowe, L., & Bartholomew, P. (1990). Contingent social responsiveness, family ecology and infant communicative competence. *National Student Speech, Language, and Hearing Association Journal, 17,* 39–49.

Edgar, E. (1987). Secondary programs in special education: Are many of them justifiable? *Exceptional Children, 53,* 555–561.

Edwards, D. (1974). Sensory-motor intelligence and semantic relations in early child grammar. *Cognition, 2,* 395–434.

Egeland, B., & Sroufe, A. (1981). Developmental sequelae of maltreatment in infancy. *New Directions for Child Development, 11,* 77–92.

Ehren, B. J., & Lenz, B. K. (1989). Adolescents with language disorders: Special considerations in providing academically relevant language intervention. *Seminars in Speech and Language, 3,* 193–204.

Ehri, L. (1975). Word consciousness in readers and pre-readers. *Journal of Educational Psychology, 67,* 204–212.

Eichenger, J. (1990). Goal structure effects on social interaction: Nondisabled and disabled elementary students. *Exceptional Children, 56,* 408–416.

Eisenson, J. (1968). Developmental aphasia: A speculative view with therapeutic implications. *Journal of Speech and Hearing Disorders, 33,* 3–13.

Eisenson, J. (1972). *Aphasia in children.* New York: Harper & Row.

Elder, J. L., & Pederson, D. R. (1978). Preschool children's use of objects in symbolic play. *Child Development, 49,* 500–504.

Emig, J. (1971). *The composing processes of twelfth graders (Research Report No. 13)*. Urbana, IL: National Council of Teachers of English.

Emig, J. (1977). Writing as a mode of learning. *College Composition and Communication, 28,* 122–127.

Englert, C. S., & Mariage, T. V. (1991). Making students partners in the comprehension process: Organizing the reading "POSSE." *Learning Disability Quarterly, 14,* 123–138.

Englert, C. S., & Raphael, T. E. (1988). Constructing well-formed prose: Process, structure, and metacognitive knowledge. *Exceptional Children, 54,* 513–527.

Ensher, G. L. (1989). The first three years: Special education perspectives on assessment and intervention. *Topics in Language Disorders, 10*(1), 80–90.

Entus, A. K. (1977). Hemispheric asymmetry in processing of dichotically presented speech and nonspeech stimuli by infants. In S. Segalowitz & F. Gruber (Eds.), *Language development and neurological theory,* (pp. 64–73). New York: Academic Press.

Entwisle, D. R., Forsyth, D. F., & Muuss, R. (1964). The syntagmatic–paradigmatic shift in children's word associations. *Journal of Verbal Learning and Verbal Behavior, 3,* 19–29.

Epstein, H. T. (1974). Phrenoblysis: Special brain and mind growth. II. Human mental development. *Developmental Psychobiology, 7,* 217–224.

Epstein, H. T. (1978). Growth spurts during brain development: Implications for educational policy and practice. In J. S. Chall & A. F. Mirsky (Eds.), *Education and brain yearbook of the N.S.S.E.* Chicago: University of Chicago Press.

Erickson, F. (1977). Some approaches to inquiry in school-community ethnography. *Anthropology and Education Quarterly, 8*(2), 58–69.

Erickson, F., & Schultz, J. (1981). When is a context? Some issues and methods in the analysis of social competence. In J. Green & C. Wallat (Eds.), *Ethnography and language in educational settings* (pp. 147–160). Norwood, NJ: Ablex.

Erickson, J. G. (1981). Communication assessment of the bilingual bicultural child: An overview. In J. G. Erickson & D. R. Omark (Eds.), *Communication assessment of the bilingual bicultural child* (pp. 1–24). Austin, TX: Pro-Ed.

Erickson, J. G., & Omark, D. R. (Eds.). (1981). *Communication assessment of the bilingual bicultural child.* Austin, TX: Pro-Ed.

Erin, J. N. (1990). Language samples from visually impaired four- and five-year olds. *Journal of Childhood Communication Disorders, 13,* 181–191.

Ervin-Tripp, S., & Gordon, D. (1986). The development of requests. In R. L. Schiefelbusch (Ed.), *Language competence: Assessment and intervention* (pp. 61–95). Austin, TX: Pro-Ed.

Ervin-Tripp, S. & Mitchell-Kernan, C. (1977). Introduction. In S. Ervin-Tripp & C. Mitchell-Kernan (Eds.), *Child discourse* (pp. 1–23). New York: Academic Press.

Ewing-Cobbs, L., Fletcher, J. M., & Levin, H. S. (1985). In M. Ylvisaker (Ed.), *Head injury rehabilitation: Children and adolescents* (pp. 71–89). Austin, TX: Pro-Ed.

Ezell, H. K., & Goldstein, H. (1989). Effects of imitation on language comprehension and transfer to production in children with mental retardation. *Journal of Speech and Hearing Disorders, 54,* 49–56.

Ezell, H. K., & Goldstein, H. (1991). Comparison of idiom comprehension of normal children and children with mental retardation. *Journal of Speech and Hearing Research, 34,* 812–819.

Falvey, M. A., Bishop, K. B., Grenot-Scheyer, M., & Coots, J. (1988). Issues and trends in mental retardation. In S. N. Calculator & J. L. Bedrosian (Eds.), *Communication assessment and intervention for adults with mental retardation* (pp. 265–307). Austin, TX: Pro-Ed.

Fasold, R. W., & Wolfram, W. (1970). Some linguistic features of Negro dialect. In R. W. Fasold & R. W. Shuy (Eds.), *Teaching standard English in the inner city* (pp. 41–86). Washington, DC: Center for Applied Linguistics.

Fay, W. H. (1973). On the echolalia of the blind and the autistic child. *Journal of Speech and Hearing Disorders, 38,* 478–489.

Fay, W. H. (1979). Personal pronouns and the autistic child. *Journal of Autism and Developmental Disorders, 9,* 247–260.

Fay, W. H., & Schuler, A. L. (1980). *Emerging language in autistic children.* Baltimore, MD: University Park Press.

Fein, D. (1983). The prevalence of speech and language impairments. *Asha, 25*(2), 37.

Fein, G. (1975). A transformational analysis of pretending. *Developmental Psychology, 11,* 291–296.

Fenson, L., Dale, P. S., Reznick, J. S., Thal, D., Bates, E., Hartung, J. P., Petnick, S., & Reilly, J. S. (1991). *Technical manual for the MacArthur Communicative Development Inventories.* San Diego, CA: San Diego State University Developmental Psychology Laboratory.

Fernald, A. (1989). Intonation and communicative intent in mothers' speech to infants: Is the melody the message? *Child Development, 60,* 1497–1510.

Ferry, P. C. (1981). Neurological considerations in children with learning disabilities. In R. W. Keith (Ed.), *Central auditory and language disorders in children* (pp. 1–10). San Diego, CA: College-Hill Press.

Feuerstein, R. (1979). *The dynamic assessment of retarded performers.* Austin, TX: Pro-Ed.

Feuerstein, R., Rand, Y., & Rynders, J. E. (1988). *Don't accept me as I am: Helping "retarded" people to excel.* New York: Plenum.

Fey, M. E. (1986). *Language intervention with young children.* Needham, MA: Allyn & Bacon.

Fey, M. E., & Leonard, L. B. (1984). Partner age as a variable in the conversational performance of specifically language-impaired and normal-language children. *Journal of Speech and Hearing Research, 27,* 413–423.

Field, T. (1979). Interaction patterns of preterm and term infants. In T. Field, A. M. Sostek, S. Goldberg, & H. Shuman (Eds.), *Infants born at risk: Behavior and development* (pp. 333–356). New York: Spectrum Publications.

Fillmore, C. (1968). The case for case. In E. Bach & R. Harmas (Eds.), *Universals in linguistic theory,* (pp. 1–88). New York: Holt, Rinehart, & Winston.

Fischler, R., Todd, N., & Feldman, C. (1985). Otitis media and language performance in a cohort of Apache Indian children. *American Journal of Diseases of Children, 139,* 355–360.

Fitzgerald, J. (1989). Research on stories: Implications for teachers. In K. D. Muth (Ed.), *Children's comprehension of text* (pp. 2–36). Newark, DE: International Reading Association.

Fletcher, P. (1979). The development of the verb phrase. In P. Fletcher & M. Garman (Eds.), *Language acquisition* (pp. 261–284). New York: Cambridge University Press.

Flexer, C. (1989). Turn on sound: An odyssey of sound field amplification. *Educational Audiology Association Newsletter, 5,* 6.

Flexer, C., Millin, J. P., & Brown, L. (1990). Children with developmental disabilities: The effect of sound field amplification on word identification. *Language, Speech, and Hearing Services in Schools, 21,* 177–182.

Flexer, C., Wray, D., & Ireland, J. (1989). Preferential seating is NOT enough: Issues in classroom management of hearing-impaired students. *Language, Speech, and Hearing Services in Schools, 20,* 11–21.

Flood, J., & Salus, M. W. (1982). Metalinguistic awareness: Its role in language development and its assessment. *Topics in Language Disorders, 2*(4), 56–64.

Flower, L., & Hayes, J. (1980). The dynamics of composing, making plans, and juggling constraints. In L. W. Gregg & E. R. Steinberg (Eds.), *Cognitive processes in writing: An interdisciplinary approach.* Hillsdale, NJ: Erlbaum.

Flynn, G. J. (1990, February/March). Quality education: Community or custody. *Newsletter of the Michigan Society for Autistic Citizens,* pp. 1, 5–6.

Fodor, J. (1983). *The modularity of mind.* Cambridge, MA: MIT Press.

Forrest-Pressley, D. L., & Waller, T. G. (1984). *Cognition, metacognition, and reading.* Cambridge, MA: MIT Press.

Foster, R., Giddan, J., & Stark, J. (1973). *Assessment of Children's Language Comprehension* (2nd ed.). Austin, TX: Learning Concepts.

Fox, C. L. (1980). *Communicating to make friends.* Rolling Hills Estates, CA: B. L. Winch & Assoc.

Fox, C. L. (1989). Peer acceptance of learning disabled children in the regular classroom. *Exceptional Children, 56,* 50–59.

Fox, L., Long, S. H., & Langlois, A. (1988). Patterns of language comprehension deficit in abused and neglected children. *Journal of Speech and Hearing Disorders, 53,* 239–244.

Fraiberg, S. (1977). *Insights from the blind: Comparative studies of blind and sighted infants.* New York: Basic Books.

Fraiberg, S. (1979). Blind infants and their mothers: An examination of the sign system. In *Before speech: The beginning of interpersonal communication* (pp. 149–169). New York: Cambridge University Press.

Fraiberg, S. (1982). Billy: Psychological intervention for a failure-to-thrive infant. In Klaus, M. H., Leger, T., & Trause, M. A. (Eds.), *Maternal attachment and mothering disorders* (pp. 6–14). Skillman, NJ: Johnson & Johnson Baby Products Co.

Frankenburg, W. K., Dodds, J. B., & Fandal, A. W. (1969). *Denver Developmental Screening Test* (manual revised, 1970). Denver, CO: University of Colorado Medical Center.

Frassinelli, L., Superior, K., & Meyers, J. (1983). A consultation model for speech and language intervention. *Asha, 25* (11), 25–30.

Frattali, C., & Lynch, C. (1989). Functional assessment: Current issues and future challenges. *Asha, 31*(4), 70–74.

Frey, W. (1984). Functional assessment in the '80s. In A. Halpern & M. Fuhrer (Eds.), *Functional assessment in rehabilitation* (pp. 11–43). Baltimore, MD: Paul H. Brookes.

Fried-Oken, M. (1987). Terminology in augmentative communication. *Language, Speech, and Hearing Services in Schools, 18,* 188–190.

Friedman, R. J. (1980). The young child who does not talk: Observations on causes and management. *Clinical Pediatrics, 3,* 403–406.

Frith, U. (1980). *Cognitive processes in spelling.* Orlando, FL: Academic Press.

Fry, E. B. (1968). A readability formula that saves time. *Journal of Reading, 11,* 513–516, 575–578.

Frymier, B., & Gansneder, B., (1989). The Phi Delta Kappa study of students at risk. *The Phi Delta Kappan, 71,* 142–147.

Fujiki, M., & Brinton, B. (1984). Supplementing language therapy: Working with the classroom teacher. *Language, Speech, and Hearing Services in Schools, 15,* 98–109.

Fundudis, T., Kolvin, I., & Garside, R. F. (1979). *Speech retarded and deaf children: Their psychological development.* London: Academic Press.

Furth, H. (1966). *Thinking without language: Psychological implications of deafness.* New York: Free Press.

Furuno, S., O'Reilly, A., Hosaka, C. M., Inatsuka, T. T., Allman, T. L., & Zeisloft, B. (1979). *The Hawaii early learning profile (HELP).* Palo Alto, CA: VORT.

Gagné, J-P., Stelmacovich, P., & Yovetich, W. (1991). Reactions to requests for clarification used by hearing-impaired individuals. *The Volta Review, 93,* 129–143.

Galaburda, A. M. (1989). Ordinary and extraordinary brain development: Anatomical variation in developmental dyslexia. *Annals of Dyslexia, 39,* 67–80.

Galaburda, A. M., Corsiglia, J., Rosen, G. D., & Sherman, G. F. (1987). Planum temporale asymmetry: Reappraisal since Geschwind and Levitsky. *Neuropsychologia, 25,* 853–868.

Galaburda, A. M., & Kemper, T. L. (1979). Cytoarchitectonic abnormalities in developmental dyslexia: A case study. *Annals of Neurology, 6,* 94–100.

Gallagher, T. M. (1991). Language and social skills: Implications for assessment and intervention with school-age children. In T. M. Gallagher (Ed.), *Pragmatics of language: Clinical practice issues* (pp. 11–41). San Diego, CA: Singular Publishing Group.

Gallagher, T. M., & Craig, H. K. (1984). Pragmatic assessment: Analysis of a highly frequent repeated utterance. *Journal of Speech and Hearing Disorders, 49,* 368–377.

Gallagher, T. M., & Prutting, C. (Eds.). (1983). *Pragmatic assessment and intervention issues in language.* San Diego, CA: College-Hill Press.

Garbarino, J., & Crouter, A. (1978). Defining the community context of parent–child relations: The correlates of child maltreatment. *Child Development, 49,* 604–606.

Garcia, S. B., & Ortiz, A. A. (1988, June). Preventing inappropriate referrals of language minority students to special education. *New Focus (No. 5), Occasional Papers in Bilingual Education.* Wheaton, MD: The National Clearinghouse for Bilingual Education.

Gardner, H. (1983). *Frames of mind: The theory of multiple intelligences.* New York: Basic Books.

Garnett, K. (1986). Telling tales: Narratives and learning-disabled children. *Topics in Language Disorders, 6*(2), 44–56.

Gates, A. L., & McGinitie, W. E. (1972). *Gates McGinitie Reading Tests.* New York: Columbia University Teacher's College Press.

Gaylord-Ross, R., Haring, T., Breen, C., & Pitts-Conway, V. (1984). The training and generalization of social interaction skills with autistic youth. *Journal of Applied Behavior Analysis, 17,* 229–247.

Geers, A. E., & Moog, J. S. (1987). Predicting spoken language acquisition of profoundly hearing-impaired children. *Journal of Speech and Hearing Disorders, 52,* 84–94.

Geers, A. E., & Moog, J. S. (1989). Factors predictive of the development of literacy in profoundly hearing-impaired adolescents. *The Volta Review, 91,* 69–86.

Geers, A. E., & Schick, B. (1988). Acquisition of spoken and signed English by hearing-impaired children of hearing-impaired or hearing parents. *Journal of Speech and Hearing Disorders, 53,* 136–143.

Gerber, M. M., & Levine-Donnerstein, D. (1989). Educating all children: Ten years later. *Exceptional Children, 56,* 17–27.

Gerber, S. E. (1990). *Prevention: The etiology of communicative disorders in children.* Englewood Cliffs, NJ: Prentice-Hall.

Gerhardt, J. (1989). Monologue as a speech genre. In K. Nelson (Ed.), *Narratives from the crib* (pp. 171–230). Cambridge, MA: Harvard University Press.

German, D. J. (1979). Word finding skills in children with learning disabilities. *Journal of Learning Disabilities, 12*(3), 43–48.

German, D. J. (1982). Word-finding substitutions in children with learning disabilities. *Language, Speech, and Hearing Services in Schools, 13,* 223–230.

German, D. J. (1983). I know it but I can't think of it: Word retrieval difficulties. *Academic Therapy, 18,* 539–545.

German, D. J. (1989). *Revised manual for the Test of Word Finding.* Allen, TX: DLM.

German, D. J. (1991). *The Test of Word Finding in Discourse.* Allen, TX: DLM.

Gibbs, R. W., Jr. (1991). Semantic analyzability in children's understanding of idioms. *Journal of Speech and Hearing Research, 34,* 613–620.

Geschwind, N. (1984). The brain of a learning disabled individual. *Annals of Dyslexia, 34,* 319–327.

Geschwind, N., & Levitsky, W. (1968). Human brain: Left–right asymmetries in temporal speech region. *Science, 161,* 186–187.

Gillespie, S., & Cooper, E. (1973). Prevalence of speech problems in junior and senior high schools. *Journal of Speech and Hearing Research, 16*(4), 739–743.

Gittelman-Klein, R., & Klein, D. (1976). Methylphenidate effects in learning disabilities. *Archives of General Psychiatry, 33,* 655–664.

Gittelman-Klein, R., Klein, D., Abikoff, H., Katz, S., Gloisten, A., & Kates, W. (1976). Relative efficacy of methylphenidate and behavior modification in hyperkinetic children: An interim report. *Journal of Abnormal Child Psychology, 4,* 361–379.

Glanville, B., Best, C., & Levenson, R. (1977). A cardiac measure of cerebral asymmetries in infant auditory perception. *Developmental Psychology, 13,* 54–59.

Gleitman, L. R., & Gleitman, H. (1981). Language. In H. Gleitman (Ed.), *Psychology* (pp. 353–411). New York: W. W. Norton.

Gleitman, L. R., Gleitman, H., & Shipley, E. F. (1972). The emergence of the child as grammarian. *Cognition, 1,* 137–164.

Gleitman, L. R., & Wanner, E. (1982). Language acquisition: The state of the art. In E. Wanner & L. Gleitman (Eds.), *Language acquisition: The state of the art.* Cambridge, England: Cambridge University Press.

Glover, M. E., Preminger, J. L., & Sanford, A. R. (1978). *The early learning accomplishment profile.* Winston-Salem, NC: Kaplan.

Goldgar, D., & Osberger, M. J. (1986). Factors related to academic achievement. In M. J. Osberger (Ed.), Language and learning skills of hearing-impaired students. ASHA *Monographs No. 23,* 87–91. Rockville, MD: American Speech-Language-Hearing Association.

Goldin-Meadow, S., & Feldman, H. (1977). The development of language-like communication without a language model. *Science, 197,* 401–403.

Goldman-Rakic, P. S. (1981). Development and plasticity of primate frontal association cortex. In F. O. Schmidt, F. G. Worden, G. Adelman, & S. G. Dennis (Eds.), *The organization of the cerebral cortex. Proceedings of a neurosciences research program colloquium.* Cambridge, MA: MIT Press.

Goldstein, H. (1985). Enhancing language generalization using matrix and stimulus equivalence training. In S. Warren & A. Rogers-Warren (Eds.), *Teaching functional language* (pp. 225–249). Austin, TX: Pro-Ed.

Goldstein, K. (1948). *Language and language disorders.* New York: Grune & Stratton.

Golin, A. K., & Ducanis, A. J. (1985). *The interdisciplinary team: A handbook for the education of exceptional children.* Rockville, MD: Aspen.

Golinkoff, R., Hirsh-Pasek, K., Cauley, K., & Gordon, L. (1987). The eyes have it: Lexical and syntactic comprehension in a new paradigm. *Journal of Child Language, 14,* 23–45.

Goodglass, H. (1981). The syndromes of aphasia: Similarities and differences in neurolinguistic features. *Topics in Language Disorders, 1*(4), 1–14.

Goodglass, H., & Kaplan, E. (1983). *The assessment of aphasia and related disorders* (2nd ed.) (Manual for The Boston diagnostic aphasia examination, BDAE). Philadelphia: Lea & Febiger.

Goodman, K. S. (1969). Analysis of oral reading miscues: Applied psycholinguistics. *Reading Research Quarterly, 5*(1), 9–30.

Goodman, K. S. (1973a). Analysis of oral reading miscues: Applied psycholinguistics. In F. Smith (Ed.), *Psycholinguistics and reading* (pp. 158–176). New York: Holt, Rinehart & Winston.

Goodman, K. S. (1973b). Psycholinguistic universals in the reading process. In F. Smith (Ed.), *Psycholinguistics and reading* (pp. 21–27). New York: Holt, Rinehart, & Winston.

Goodman, K. S. (1986). *What's whole in whole language?* Portsmouth, NH: Heinemann.

Goodman, Y. M., Watson, D. J., & Burke, C. L. (1987). *Reading miscue inventory: Alternative procedures.* New York: Richard C. Owen Publishers.

Gough, P. B. (1972). One second of reading. In J. F. Kavanagh & I. G. Mattingly (Eds.), *Language by ear and by eye: The relationships between speech and reading* (pp. 331–358). Cambridge, MA: MIT Press.

Gordon, C. J., & Braun, C. (1983). Using story schema as an aid to reading and writing. *The Reading Teacher, 37,* 116–121.

Graves, D. (1978). *Balance the basics: Let them write.* New York: Ford Foundation.

Graves, D. (1983). *Writing: Teachers and children at work.* Portsmouth, NH: Heinemann.

Gray, B., & Ryan, B. (1973). *A language program for the nonlanguage child.* Champaign, IL: Research Press.

Green, J. L., & Wallat, C. (1981). *Ethnography and language in educational settings.* Norwood, NJ: Ablex.

Greenfield, P. M., & Smith, J. H. (1976). *The structure of communication in early language development.* New York: Academic Press.

Greenspan, S. (1985). *First feelings: Milestones in the emotional development of your baby and child.* New York: Viking Penguin.

Greenspan, S. (1988). Fostering emotional and social development in infants with disabilities. *Zero to Three, 8,* 8–18.

Greenspan, S. I., Wieder, S., Nover, R. A., Lieberman, A. F., Lourie, R. S., & Robinson, M. E. (Eds.). (1987). *Infants in multirisk families.* Madison, WI: International Universities Press.

Gregory, M., & Carroll, S. (1978). *Language and situation: Language varieties and their social contexts.* London: Routledge & Kegan Paul.

Grice, H. P. (1975). Logic and conversation. In P. Cole & J. L. Morgan (Eds.), *Syntax and semantics 3: Speech acts* (pp. 41–58). San Diego, CA: Academic Press.

Griffin, K., & Hannah, L. (1960). A study of the results of an extremely short instructional unit in listening. *Journal of Communication, 10,* 135–139.

Grossman, H. (Ed.). (1983). *Classification in mental retardation.* Washington, DC: American Association on Mental Deficiency.

Gualtieri, C. T., Koriath, U., Van Bourgondien, M., & Saleeby, N. (1983). Language disorders in children referred for psychiatric services. *Journal of the American Academy of Child Psychiatry, 22,* 165–171.

Guess, D. (1989). Preface. In E. Siegel-Causey & D. Guess (Eds.), *Enhancing nonsymbolic communication interactions among learners with severe disabilities* (pp. xi–xii). Baltimore, MD: Paul H. Brookes.

Guess, D., & Baer, D. (1973). An analysis of individual differences in generalization between receptive and productive language in retarded children. *Journal of Applied Behavior Analysis, 6,* 311–329.

Guess, D., Sailor, W., & Baer, D. (1974). To teach language to retarded children. In R. Schiefelbusch & L. L. Lloyd (Eds.), *Language perspectives: Acquisition, retardation, and intervention* (pp. 529–533). Baltimore, MD: University Park Press.

Guess, D., Sailor, W., & Baer, D. (1978). Children with limited language. In R. Schiefelbusch (Ed.), *Language intervention strategies* (pp. 101–143). Baltimore, MD: University Park Press.

Guilford, J. P. (1967). *The nature of human intelligence.* New York: McGraw-Hill.

Guralnick, M. J., & Paul-Brown, D. (1977). The nature of verbal interactions among handicapped and nonhandicapped preschool children. *Child Development, 48,* 254–260.

Hagen, J. W., Barclay, C. R., & Schwethelm, B. (1982). In N. Ellis (Ed.), *International review of research in mental retardation* (pp. 1–4). New York: Academic Press.

Hall, P. K., & Tomblin, J. B. (1978). A follow-up study of children with articulation and language disorders. *Journal of Speech and Hearing Disorders, 43,* 227–241.

Halliday, M. A. K. (1975a). Learning how to mean. In E. Lenneberg & E. Lenneberg (Eds.), *Foundations of language development: A multidisciplinary approach* (pp. 239–265). New York: Academic Press.

Halliday, M. A. K. (1975b). *Learning how to mean: Explorations in the development of language.* London: Edward Arnold.

Halliday, M. A. K., & Hasan, R. (1976). *Cohesion in English.* London: Longman.

Hammill, D. D., & Larsen, S. C. (1974). The effectiveness of psycholinguistic training. *Exceptional Children, 40,* 5–14.

Hanline, M. F., & Halvorsen, A. (1989). Parent perceptions of the integration transition process: Overcoming artificial barriers. *Exceptional Children, 55,* 487–493.

Harber, J. (1980). Issues in the assessment of language and reading disorders in learning disabled children. *Learning Disability Quarterly, 3*(4), 20–28.

Harris, A. J. (1983). How many kinds of reading disability are there? *Annual Review of Learning Disabilities, 1,* 50–56.

Harris, D. (1982). Communicative interaction processes involving nonvocal physically handicapped children. *Topics in Language Disorders, 2*(2), 21–37.

Harris, G. A. (1985). Considerations in assessing English language performance of Native American children. *Topics in Language Disorders, 5*(4), 42–52.

Hart, B. (1985). Naturalistic language training techniques. In S. F. Warren & A. K. Rogers-Warren (Eds). *Teaching functional language* (pp. 63–88). Baltimore, MD: University Park Press.

Hart, B., & Risley, T. R. (1968). Establishing the use of descriptive adjectives in the spontaneous speech of disadvantaged preschool children. *Journal of Applied Behavioral Analysis, 1,* 109-120.

Hart, B. & Risley, T. R. (1975). Incidental teaching of language in the preschool. *Journal of Applied Behavioral Analysis, 8,* 411–420.

Hart, B. & Risley, T. R. (1980). In vivo language training: Unanticipated and general effects. *Journal of Applied Behavioral Analysis, 12,* 407–432.

Hart, B., & Risley, T. R. (1986). Incidental strategies. In R. L. Schiefelbusch (Ed.), *Language competence: Assessment and intervention.* San Diego, CA: College-Hill Press.

Hart, B., & Rogers-Warren, A. (1978). Milieu approach to teaching language. In R. L. Schiefelbusch (Ed.), *Language intervention strategies* (pp. 193–235). Baltimore, MD: University Park Press.

Hart, C. (1989). *Without reason: A family copes with two generations of autism.* New York: Harper & Row.

Hart, P. J. (1983). Classroom acoustical environments for children with central auditory processing disorders. In E. Z. Lasky & J. Katz (Eds.), *Central auditory processing disorders: Problems of speech, language, and learning* (pp. 343–352). Austin, TX: Pro-Ed.

Hart, V. (1977). The use of many disciplines with the severely and profoundly handicapped. In E. Sontag & N. Certo (Eds.), *Educational programming for the severely and profoundly handicapped.* Reston, VA: Division on Mental Retardation, Council for Exceptional Children.

Hartup, W. (1983). Peer interaction and the behavioral development of the individual child. In W. Damon (Ed.), *Social personality development: Essays on the growth of the child.* New York: W. W. Norton.

Hartwig, L. J. (1984). Living with dyslexia: One parent's experience. *Annals of Dyslexia, 34,* 313–318.

Hartzell, H. E. (1984). The challenge of adolescence. *Topics in Language Disorders, 4*(2), 1–9.

Hayden, T. L. (1980). The classification of elective mutism. *Journal of the American Academy of Child Psychology, 19,* 118–133.

Hayes, C. W., & Bahruth, R. (1985). Querer Es Poder. In J. T. Hansen, T. Newkirk, & D. Graves (Eds.), *Breaking ground: Teachers relate reading and writing in the elementary school* (pp. 97–108). Portsmouth, NH: Heinemann.

Hayes, J. R., & Flower, L. S. (1980). Identifying the organization of writing processes. In L. Gregg & E. Steinberg (Eds.), *Cognitive processes in writing* (pp. 3–30). Hillsdale, NJ: Lawrence Erlbaum.

Hayes, J. R., & Flower, L. S. (1987). On the structure of the writing process. *Topics in Language Disorders, 7*(4), 19–30.

Haywood, H. C., Towery-Woolsey, J., Arbitman-Smith, R., & Aldridge, A. (1988). Cognitive education with deaf adolescents: Effects of instrumental enrichment. *Topics in Language Disorders, 8*(4), 23–40.

Hazel, J., Schumaker, J., Sherman, J., & Sheldon-Wildgen, J. (1981). *ASSET: A social skills program for adolescents.* Champaign, IL: Research Press.

Heath, S. B. (1982). What no bedtime story means: Narrative skills at home and school. *Language in Society,* 11, 49–76.

Heath, S. B. (1983). *Ways with words: Language, life and work in communities and classrooms.* New York: Cambridge University Press.

Heath, S. B. (1984, November). *Cross cultural acquisition of language.* Paper presented at the annual conference of the American Speech-Language-Hearing Association, San Francisco.

Heath, S. B. (1986). Taking a cross-cultural look at narratives. *Topics in Language Disorders, 7*(1), 84–94.

Hecaen, H. (1976). Acquired aphasia in children and the ontogenesis of hemispheric functional specialization. *Brain and Language, 3,* 114–134.

Hecaen, H. (1983). Acquired aphasia in children: Revisited. *Neuropsychologia, 21,* 581–587.

Heimlich, J. E., & Pittelman, S. D. (1986). *Semantic mapping: Classroom applications.* Newark, DE: International Reading Association.

Hermelin, B., & O'Connor, N. (1967). Remembering of words by psychotic and subnormal children. *British Journal of Psychology, 58,* 213–218.

Hermelin, B., & O'Connor, N. (1970). *Psychological experiments with autistic children.* Oxford: Pergamon.

Hess, L. J., & Fairchild, J. L. (1988). Model, analyse, practise (MAP): A language therapy model for learning-disabled adolescents. *Child Language Teaching and Therapy, 4,* 325–338.

Hier, D., LeMay, M., Rosenberger, P., et al. (1978). Developmental dyslexia. *Archives of Neurology, 35,* 90–92.

Higginbotham, D. J., & Yoder, D. E. (1982). Communication within natural conversational interaction: Implications for severe communicatively impaired persons. *Topics in Language Disorders, 2*(2), 1–19.

Hill, B. P., & Singer, L. T. (1990). Speech and language development after infant tracheostomy. *Journal of Speech and Hearing Disorders, 55,* 15–20.

Hillocks, G., Jr. (1986). *Research on written composition.* Urbana, IL: ERIC Clearinghouse on Reading and Communication Skills.

Hodson, B., & Paden, E. (1983). *Targeting intelligible speech: A phonological approach to remediation.* San Antonio, TX: Pro-Ed.

Hoffman, L. P. (1990). The development of literacy in a school-based program. *Topics in Language Disorders, 10*(2), 81–94.

Hoffman, P. R. (1990). Spelling, phonology, and the speech-language pathologist: A whole language perspective. *Language, Speech, and Hearing Services in Schools, 21,* 238–243.

Hohmann, M., Banet, B., & Weikert, D. P. (1979). *Young children in action: A manual for preschool educators.* Ypsilanti, MI: High/Scope Press.

Holden, M. H., & MacGinitie, W. H. (1972). Children's conceptions of word boundaries in speech and print. *Journal of Educational Psychology, 63,* 551–557.

Hood, L., & Bloom, L. (1979). What, when, and how about why: A longitudinal study of early expressions of causality. *Monographs of the Society for Research in Children Development, 44.*

Horgan, D. (1979). *Nouns: Love 'em or leave 'em.* Address to the New York Academy of Sciences.

Horn, J. L. (1968). Organization of abilities and the development of intelligence. *Psychological Review, 75,* 242–259.

Hoskins, B. (1987). *Conversations: Language intervention for adolescents.* Allen, TX: DLM.

Hoskins, B. (1990). Language and literacy: Participating in the conversation. *Topics in Language Disorders, 10*(2), 46–62.

Hoskins, B., & Nelson, N. W. (1989, August). *Educational design for the future* [workshop]. Monterey, CA.

House, T. D., & House, L. I. (1989, November). *Pragmatic deficits in visually impaired children.* Paper presented at the annual conference of the American Speech-Language-Hearing Association, St. Louis.

Howes, C. (1985). Sharing fantasy: Social pretend play in toddlers. *Child Development, 56,* 1253–1258.

Hresko, W. P., Reid, D. K., & Hammill, D. D. (1981). *The test of early language development* (TELD). Austin, TX: Pro-Ed.

Hubbell, R. D. (1981). *Children's language disorders: An integrated approach.* Englewood Cliffs, NJ: Prentice-Hall.

Hubbell, R. D. (1988). *A handbook of English grammar and language sampling.* Englewood Cliffs, NJ: Prentice Hall.

Hughes, D. L. (1985). *Language treatment and generalization.* San Diego, CA: College-Hill Press.

Hughes, D. L. (1989). Generalization from language therapy to classroom academics. *Seminars, 10*(3), 218–230.

Hughes, D. L., & Carpenter, R. (1983, November). *Effects of two grammar treatment programs on target generalization to spontaneous language.* Paper presented at the Annual Conference of the American Speech-Language-Hearing Association, Cincinnati.

Huisingh, R., Barrett, M., Zachman, L., Blagden, C., & Orman, J. (1990). *The Word Test—R.* East Moline, IL: LinguiSystems.

Hunt, K. W. (1965). *Grammatical structures written at three grade levels.* Urbana, IL: National Council of Teachers of English.

Hunt, K. W. (1970). Syntactic maturity in school children and adults. *Society for Research in Child Development Monographs,* No. 134, *35*(No. 1).

Hunt, K. W. (1977). Early blooming and late blooming syntactic structures. In C. R. Cooper & L. Odell (Eds.), *Evaluating writing: Describing, measuring, judging* (pp. 91–106). Urbana, IL: National Council of Teachers of English.

Hutchinson, D. (1974). *A model for transdisciplinary staff development* (technical report developed as part of the National Collaborative Infant Project). New York: United Cerebral Palsy Association of America.

Huttenlocher, J. (1974). The origins of language comprehension. In R. Solso (Ed.), *Theories in cognitive psychology: The Loyola symposium* (pp. 331–368). New York: Wiley.

Hutter, J. J. (1986). Late effects in children with cancer [Letter to the editor]. *American Journal of Diseases of Children, 140,* 17–18.

Hyman, C. A., Parr, R., & Browne, K. (1979). An observational study of mother–infant interaction in abusing families. *Child Abuse and Neglect, 3,* 241–246.

Hymes, D. (1972a). Introduction. In C. Cazden, V. John, & D. Hymes (Eds.), *Functions of language in the classroom.* New York: Teachers College, Columbia University.

Hymes, D. (1972b). On communicative competence. In J. B. Pride & J. Holmes (Eds.), *Sociolinguistics.* Harmondsworth, England: Penguin.

Hynd, G. W., Marshall, R., & Gonzalez, J. (1991). Learning disabilities and presumed central nervous system dysfunction. *Learning Disability Quarterly, 14,* 283–296.

Idol, L., Nevin, A., & Paolucci-Whitcomb, P. (1986). *Models of curriculum-based assessment.* Rockville, MD: Aspen Publishers.

Idol, L., Paolucci-Whitcomb, P., & Nevin, A. (1986). *Collaborative consultation.* Rockville, MD: Aspen.

Iglesias, A. (1989). My dream. *Asha, 31*(9), 75.

Iglesius, A. (1985). Communication in the home and classroom: Match or mismatch? *Topics in Language Disorders, 5*(4), 29–41.

Ingram, D. (1974). The relationship between comprehension and production. In R. Schiefelbusch & L. Lloyd (Eds.), *Language perspectives—Acquisition, retardation, and intervention* (pp. 313–364). Baltimore, MD: University Park Press.

Ingram, D. (1976). *Phonological disability in children.* New York: American Elsevier.

Ingram, D. (1986). Foreword. In J. R. Muma, *Language acquisition: A functionalist perspective* (pp. xi–xiii). Austin, TX: Pro-Ed.

Irwin, J. W. (1988). Linguistic cohesion and the developing reader/writer. *Topics in Language Disorders, 8*(3), 14–23.

Isaacson, S. (1985). Assessing written language skills. In C. S. Simon (Ed.), *Communication skills and classroom success: Assessment of language-learning disabled students* (pp. 403–425). San Diego, CA: College-Hill Press. Reprinted in C. S. Simon (Ed.). (1991), *Communication skills and classroom success: Assessment and therapy methodologies for language and learning disabled students* (pp. 224–237). Eau Claire, WI: Thinking Publications.

Jakobson, R. (1968). *Child language, aphasia and phonological universals.* The Hague: Mouton.

Jakobson, R., & Halle, M. (1956). *Fundamentals of language.* The Hague: Mouton.

Jaffe, M. B. (1989). Feeding at-risk infants and toddlers. *Topics in Language Disorders, 10*(1), 13–25.

Jagiello, G. M., Fang, J-S., Ducayen, M. B., & Sung, W. K. (1987). Etiology of human trisomy 21. In S. M. Pueschel, C. Tingey, J. E. Rynders, A. C. Crocker, & D. M. Crutcher (Eds.), *New perspectives on Down syndrome* (pp. 23–38). Baltimore, MD: Paul H. Brookes.

James, S. (1989). Assessing children with language disorders. In D. K. Bernstein & E. Tiegerman (Eds.), *Language and communication disorders in children* (2nd ed., pp. 157–207). Columbus, OH: Merrill/Macmillan.

Jenkins, J. R., & Heinen, A. (1989). Students' preferences for service delivery: Pull-out, in-class, or integrated models. *Exceptional Children, 55,* 516–523.

Jenkins, J. R., Odom, S. L., & Speltz, M. L. (1989). Effects of social integration of preschool children with handicaps. *Exceptional Children, 55,* 420–428.

Jenkins, J. R., Speltz, M. L., & Odom, S. L. (1985). Integrating normal and handicapped preschoolers: Effects on child development and social interaction. *Exceptional Children, 52,* 7–17.

Johnson, C. (1985). The emergence of present perfect verb forms: Semantic influences on selective imitation. *Journal of Child Language, 12,* 325–352.

Johnson, D. (1989, September). *Cooperative learning in postsecondary education.* Paper presented at a workshop, Western Michigan University, Kalamazoo.

Johnson, D. J. (1985). Using reading and writing to improve oral language skills. *Topics in Language Disorders, 5*(3), 55–69.

Johnson, D. J., & Myklebust, H. (1967). *Learning disabilities: Educational principles and practices.* New York: Grune & Stratton.

Johnson, D. W., & Johnson, R. (1975). *Learning together and alone.* Englewood Cliffs, NJ: Prentice-Hall.

Johnson, D. W., & Johnson, R. T. (1990). Social skills for successful group work. *Educational Leadership, 47*(4), 29–33.

Johnson, D. W., Johnson, R. T., & Holubec., E. (1988). *Cooperation in the classroom* (revised ed.). Edina, MN: Interaction Book Company.

Johnson, N. S., & Mandler, J. M. (1980). A tale of two structures: Underlying and surface forms in stories. *Poetics, 9,* 51–86.

Johnson, W., Darley, F. L., & Spriestersbach, D. (1952). *Diagnostic methods in speech correction.* New York: Harper & Row.

Johnson-Laird, P. N. (1983). *Mental models: Towards a cognitive science of language, inference, and consciousness.* Cambridge, MA: Harvard University Press.

Johnson-Martin, N., Jens, K. G., & Attermeier, S. M. (1986). *The Carolina curriculum for handicapped infants and infants at risk.* Baltimore, MD: Paul H. Brookes.

Johnston, J. R. (1982a). Interpreting the Leiter IQ: Performance profiles of young normal and language-disordered children. *Journal of Speech and Hearing Research, 25,* 291–296.

Johnston, J. R. (1982b). Narratives: A new look at communication problems in older language-disordered children. *Language, Speech, and Hearing Services in Schools, 13,* 144–155.

Johnston, J. R. (1985). The discourse symptoms of developmental disorders. In T. A. Van Dijk (Ed.), *Handbook of discourse analysis, Vol. 3: Discourse and dialogue* (pp. 79–93). Orlando, FL: Academic Press.

Johnston, J. R., & Kamhi, A. (1984). Syntactic and semantic aspects of the utterances of language impaired children: Can same be less. *Merrill-Palmer Quarterly, 30,* 65–85.

Joint Committee on Infant Hearing. (1991). 1990 position statement. *Asha, 33* (Suppl. 5), 3–6.

Jordon, F. M., Murdoch, B. E., & Buttsworth, D. L. (1991). Closed-head-injured children's performance on narrative tasks. *Journal of Speech and Hearing Disorders, 34,* 572–582.

Jordan, L. S. (1980). Receptive and expressive language problems occurring in combination with a seizure disorder: A case report. *Journal of Communication Disorders, 13,* 295–303.

Just, M. A., & Carpenter, P. A. (1987). *The psychology of reading and language comprehension.* Boston: Allyn & Bacon.

Kagan, J. (1989). The young child at risk. In B. A. Stewart (Ed.), *Partnerships in education: Toward a literate America* (pp. 8–17). *ASHA Reports 17.* Rockville, MD: American Speech-Language-Hearing Association.

Kagan, S. (1990). The structural approach to cooperative learning. *Educational Leadership, 47*(4), 12–15.

Kail, R., & Leonard, L. B. (1986). Word-finding abilities in language-impaired children. *ASHA Monographs Number 25.* Rockville, MD: American Speech-Language-Hearing Association.

Kaiser, A. P., Alpert, C. L., & Warren, S. L. (1987). Teaching functional language: Strategies for intervention. In M. E. Snell (Ed.), *Systematic instruction for persons with severe handicaps* (3rd ed., pp. 247–272). Columbus, OH: Merrill/Macmillan.

Kaiser, A. P., & Warren, S. F. (1988). Pragmatics and generalization. In R. L. Schiefelbusch & L. L. Lloyd (Eds.), *Language perspectives II* (pp. 393–442). Austin, TX: Pro-Ed.

Karlsen, B., & Gardner, E. F. (1984). *Stanford diagnostic reading test* (3rd ed.). San Antonio, TX: The Psychological Corporation.

Kamhi, A. G. (1981). Developmental vs. different theories of mental retardation: A new look. *American Journal of Mental Deficiency, 86,* 1–7.

Kamhi, A. G. (1982). The effect of self-initiated and other-initiated actions on linguistic performance. *Journal of Speech and Hearing Research, 25,* 177–183.

Kamhi, A. G. (1990, June). Unpublished discussion at the 11th Symposium for Research on Child Language Disorders, The University of Wisconsin, Madison.

Kamhi, A. G, & Catts, H. W. (1986). Toward an understanding of developmental language and reading disorders. *Journal of Speech and Hearing Disorders, 51,* 337–347.

Kamhi, A. G., & Catts, H. W. (1989). *Reading disabilities: A developmental language perspective.* Austin, TX: Pro-Ed.

Kamhi, A. G., Catts, H. W., Mauer, D., Apel, K., & Gentry, B. F. (1988). Phonological and spatial processing abilities in language- and reading-impaired children. *Journal of Speech and Hearing Disorders, 53,* 316–327.

Kamhi, A. G., Gentry, B., Mauer, D., & Gholson, B. (1990). Analogical learning and transfer in language-impaired children. *Journal of Speech and Hearing Disorders, 55,* 140–148.

Kamhi, A. G., & Lee, R. F. (1988). Cognition. In M. A. Nippold (Ed.), *Later language development: Ages 9 through 19* (pp. 127–158). Austin, TX: Pro-Ed.

Kamhi, A. G., Minor, J. S., & Mauer, D. (1990). Content analysis and intratest performance profiles on the Columbia and the TONI. *Journal of Speech and Hearing Research, 33,* 375–379.

Kandel, E. R. (1977). Neuronal plasticity and the modification of behavior. In E. R. Kandel (Ed.), *Cellular biology of neurons, Vol. 1: The nervous system* (pp. 1137–1182). Amsterdam: Elsevier.

Kanner, L. (1943). Autistic disturbance of affective contact. *Nervous Child, 2,* 217–250.

Kanter, R. M. (1983). *The change masters: Innovation and entrepreneurship in the American corporation.* New York: Simon & Schuster.

Kaplan, G. K., Fleshman, J. K., Bender, T. R., Baum, C., & Clark, P. (1973). Long-term effects of otitis media; a 10-year cohort study of Alaska Eskimo children. *Pediatrics, 52,* 577–585.

Kaplan, E., & Goodglass, H. (1981). Aphasia-related disorders. In M. T. Sarno (Ed.), *Acquired aphasia* (pp. 303–325). New York: Academic Press.

Kaufman, A. S., & Kaufman, N. L. (1983). *Kaufman Assessment Battery for Children* (K-ABC). Circle Pines, MN: American Guidance Service.

Kawakami, A. J., & Au, K. H. (1986). Encouraging reading and language development in cultural minority children. *Topics in Language Disorders, 6*(2), 71–80.

Kayser, H. (1989). Speech and language assessment of Spanish-English speaking children. *Language, Speech, and Hearing Services in Schools, 20,* 226–244.

Keeler, W. R. (1958). Autistic patterns and defective communication in blind children with retrolental fibroplasia. In P. H. Hoch & J. Subin (Eds.), *Psychopathology of communication* (pp. 64–83). New York: Grune & Stratton.

Keith, R. W. (1977). (Ed.). *Central auditory dysfunction.* New York: Grune & Stratton.

Keith, R. W. (1981). (Ed.),. *Central auditory and language disorders in children.* San Diego, CA: College-Hill Press.

Kekelis, L. S., & Anderson, E. S. (1984). Family communication styles and language development. *Journal of Visual Impairment and Blindness, 78,* 54–65.

Kelford-Smith, A., Thurston, S., Light, J., Parnes, P., & O'Keefe, B. (1989). The form and use of written communication produced by physically disabled individuals using microcomputers. *Augmentative and Alternative Communication, 5,* 115–124.

Kelly, C. A., & Dale, P. S. (1989). Cognitive skills associated with the onset of multiword utterances. *Journal of Speech and Hearing Research, 32,* 645–656.

Kendall, P. C., & Braswell, L. (1985). *Cognitive-behavioral therapy for impulsive children.* New York: Guilford Press.

Kent, L. (1974). *Language acquisition program for the severely retarded.* Champaign, IL: Research Press.

Kent, R., Osberger, M., Netsell, R., & Hustedde, C. (1987). Phonetic development in identical twins differing in auditory function. *Journal of Speech and Hearing Disorders, 52,* 64–75.

Kernan, K. (1977). Semantic and expressive elaboration in children's narratives. In S. Ervin-Tripp & C. Mitchell-Kernan (Eds.), *Child discourse* (pp. 91–102). New York: Academic Press.

King, D. F., & Goodman, K. S. (1990). Whole language: Cherishing learners and their language. *Language, Speech, and Hearing Services in Schools, 21,* 221–227.

King, R. R., Jones, C., & Lasky, E. (1982). In retrospect: A fifteen-year follow-up report of speech-language-disordered children. *Language, Speech, and Hearing Services in Schools, 13,* 24–32.

Kinney, P., Ouellette, T., & Wolery, M. (1989). Screening and assessing sensory functioning. In D. B. Bailey, Jr. & M. Wolery (Eds.), *Assessing infants and preschoolers with handicaps* (pp. 144–165). Columbus, OH: Merrill/Macmillan.

Kinsbourne, M. (1981). The development of cerebral dominance. In S. D. Filskov & T. J. Boll (Eds.), *Handbook of clinical neuropsychology.* New York: John Wiley & Sons.

Kirchner, D. M. (1991). Using verbal scaffolding to facilitate conversational participation and language acquisition in children with prevasive developmental disorders. *Journal of Childhood Communication Disorders, 14,* 81–98.

Kirk, S. A., McCarthy, J. J., & Kirk, W. D. (1968). *The Illinois Test of Psycholinguistic Abilities* (rev. ed.). Urbana, IL: University of Illinois Press.

Kirk, U. (1983). Introduction: Toward an understanding of the neuropsychology of language, reading, and spelling. In U. Kirk (Ed.), *Neuropsychology of language, reading, and spelling* (pp. 3–31). Orlando, FL: Academic Press.

Klecan-Aker, J. S. (1985). Syntactic abilities in normal and language deficient middle school children. *Topics in Language Disorders, 5*(3), 46–54.

Klecan-Aker, J. S. and Hedrick, L. D. (1985). A study of the syntactic language skills of normal school-age children. *Language, Speech, and Hearing Services in Schools, 16,* 187–198.

Klee, T., Schaffer, M., May, S., Membrino, I., & Mougey, K. (1989). A comparison of the age–MLU relation in normal and specifically language-impaired preschool children. *Journal of Speech and Hearing Disorders, 54,* 226–233.

Klein, J., Chase, C., Teele, D., Menyuk, P., & Rosner, B. (1988). Otitis media and the development of speech, language, and cognitive abilities at seven years of age. In D. Lim, C. Bluestone, J. Klein, & J. Nelson (Eds.), *Recent advances in otitis media* (pp. 396–400). Toronto: B. C. Decker.

Klein, M. D., & Briggs, M. H. (1987). Facilitating mother–infant communicative interaction in mothers and high-risk infants. *Journal of Communication Disorders, 10,* 95–106.

Knapczyk, D. (1991). Effects of modeling in promoting generalization of student question asking and question answering. *Learning Disabilities Research & Practice, 6,* 75–82.

Knapp, M. S., Turnbull, B. J., & Shields, P. M. (1990). New directions for educating the children of poverty. *Educational Leadership, 48* (1), 4–8.

Knobloch, H., Stevens, F., & Malone, A. F. (1980). *Manual of developmental diagnosis.* New York: Harper & Row.

Knoll, J. A., & Meyer, L. (1987). Integrated schooling and educational quality: Principles and effective practices. In M. S. Berres & P. Knoblock (Eds.), *Program models for mainstreaming: Integrating students with moderate to severe disabilities* (pp. 41–59). Rockville, MD: Aspen Publishers.

Kochanek, T. T., Kabacoff, R. I., & Lipsitt, L. P. (1990). Early identification of developmentally disabled and at-risk preschool children. *Exceptional Children, 56,* 528–538.

Koegel, R. L., & Traphagen, J. (1982). Selection of initial words for speech training with nonverbal children. In R. L. Koegel, A. Rincover, & A. L. Egel (Eds.), *Educating and understanding autistic children* (pp. 65–77). San Diego, CA: College-Hill Press.

Kolvin, T., & Fundudis, T. (1981). Elective mute children: Psychological development and background factors. *Journal of Child Psychology and Psychiatry, 22,* 219–232.

Konner, M. (1982). *The tangled wing: Biological constraints on the human spirit.* New York: Holt, Rinehart & Winston.

Koppenhaver, D. A., Coleman, P. P., Kalman, S. L., & Yoder, D. E. (1991). The implications of emergent literacy research for children with developmental disabilities. *American Journal of Speech-Language Pathology, 1,* 38–44.

Koppenhaver, D. A., & Yoder, D. E. (1988, October). *Literacy and the augmentative and alternative communication user.* Paper presented at the conference of the International Society for Augmentative and Alternative Communication. Anaheim, CA.

Kovarsky, D. K., & Crago, M. (1991). Toward the ethnography of communication disorders. *The National Student Speech-Language-Hearing Association Journal, 18,* 44–55.

Kramer, C., James, S., & Saxman, J. (1979). A comparison of language samples elicited at home and in the clinic. *Journal of Speech and Hearing Disorders, 44,* 321–330.

Kramer, J. H., Norman, D., Grant-Zawadzki, M., Albin, A., & Moore, I. (1988). Absence of white matter changes on magnetic resonance imaging in children treated with CNS prophylaxis therapy for leukemia. *Cancer, 61,* 928–930.

Krauss, M. W. (1990). New precedent in family policy: Individualized Family Service Plan. *Exceptional Children, 56,* 388–395.

Kuczaj, S., & Maratsos, M. (1975). What children *can* say before they *will*. *Merrill-Palmer Quarterly, 21,* 89–111.

LaBerge, D., & Samuels, S. J. (1987). Toward a theory of automatic information processing in reading. In H. Singer & R. B. Ruddell (Eds.), *Theoretical models and processes of reading* (3rd ed., pp. 689–718). Newark, DE: International Reading Association.

Labov, W. (1966). *The social stratification of English in New York City.* Washington, DC: Center for Applied Linguistics.

Labov, W. (1969). The logic of nonstandard English. In J. E. Alatis (Ed.), *Report of the twentieth annual round table meeting on linguistics and language studies* (pp. 1–43). Washington, DC: Georgetown University Press.

Ladas, H. (1980). Note-taking on lectures: An information-processing approach. *Educational Psychologist, 15,* 44–53.

LaGreca, A., & Mesibov, G. (1981). Facilitating interpersonal functioning with peers in learning disabled children. *Journal of Learning Disabilities, 14,* 197–199.

Lefebvre, M., & Pinard, A. (1972). Apprentisage de la conservation des qualités par une méthode de conflict cognitif. *Canadian Journal of the Behavioral Sciences, 4*(1), 1–12.

Lahey, M. (1988). *Language disorders and language development.* New York: Macmillan.

Lahey, M., & Bloom, L. (1977). Planning a first lexicon: Which words to teach first. *Journal of Speech and Hearing Disorders, 42,* 340–350.

Lakoff, G. (1987). *Women, fire, and dangerous things: What categories reveal about the mind.* Chicago: The University of Chicago Press.

Lamphear, V. S. (1985). The impact of maltreatment on children's psychosocial adjustment: A review of the research. *Child Abuse and Neglect, 9,* 251–263.

Landau, W. M., & Kleffner, F. R. (1957). Syndrome of acquired aphasia with convulsive disorder in children. *Neurology, 7,* 523–530.

Langer, J. (1982). Facilitating text processing: The elaboration of prior knowledge. In J. Langer & M. T. Smith-Burke (Eds.), *Reader meets author/Bridging the gap.* Newark, DE: International Reading Association.

Larson, V. L., & McKinley, N. L. (1987). *Communication assessment and intervention strategies for adolescents.* Eau Claire, WI: Thinking Publications.

Lasky, E. Z., & Cox, L. C. (1983). Auditory processing and language interaction: Evaluation and intervention strategies. In E. Z. Lasky & J. Katz (Eds.), *Central auditory processing disorders: Problems of speech, language, and learning* (pp. 243–268). Needham, MA: Allyn & Bacon.

Lasky, E. Z., & Katz, J. (Eds.). (1983). *Central auditory processing disorders: Problems of speech, language, and learning.* Needam, MA: Allyn & Bacon.

Lasky, E. Z., & Klopp, K. (1982). Parent-child interactions in normal and language-disordered children. *Journal of Speech and Hearing Disorders, 47,* 7–18.

Lasky, E., & Tobin, H. (1973). Linguistic and nonlinguistic competing message effects. *Journal of Learning Disabilities, 6,* 46–53

Laughton, J., & Hasenstab, M. S. (1986). *The language learning process.* Rockville, MD: Aspen.

Launer, P. B., & Lahey, M. (1981). Passages: From the fifties to the eighties in language assessment. *Topics in Language Disorders, 1*(3), 11–29.

Lazar, R. T., Warr-Leeper, G. A., Nicholson, C. B., & Johnson, S. (1989). Elementary school teachers' use of multiple meaning expressions. *Language, Speech, and Hearing Services in Schools, 20,* 420–430.

Lederberg, A. (1980). The language environment of children with language delays. *Journal of Pediatric Psychology, 5,* 141–159.

Lee, L. L. (1966). Developmental sentence types: A method for comparing normal and deviant syntactic development. *Journal of Speech and Hearing Disorders, 31,* 311–330.

Lee, L. L. (1974). *Developmental sentence analysis.* Evanston, IL: Northwestern University Press.

Leiter, R. G. (1959). Part I of the manual for the 1948 revision of the Leiter International Performance Scale. *Psychological Service Center Journal, 11,* 1–72.

Lenneberg, E. H. (1967). *Biological foundations of language.* New York: Wiley.

Leonard, L. B. (1972). What is deviant language? *Journal of Speech and Hearing Disorders, 37,* 427–446.

Leonard, L. B. (1973). The role of intonation in recall of various linguistic stimuli. *Language and Speech, 16,* 327–335.

Leonard, L. B. (1980). The speech of language-disabled children. *Bulletin of the Orton Society, 30,* 141–152.

Leonard, L. B. (1987). Is specific language impairment a useful construct? In S. Rosenberg (Ed.), *Advances in applied psycholinguistics, Vol. 1: Disorders of first language acquisition* (pp. 1–39). New York: Cambridge University Press.

Leonard, L. B. (1991). Specific language impairment as a clinical category. *Language, Speech, and Hearing Services in Schools, 22,* 66–68.

Leonard, L. B., & Fey, M. E. (1991). Facilitating grammatical development: The contributions of pragmatics. In T. M. Gallagher (Ed.), *Pragmatics of language: Clinical practice issues* (pp. 333–355). San Diego, CA: Singular.

Leonard, L. B., & Loeb, D. F. (1988). Government binding theory and some of its applications: A tutorial. *Journal of Speech and Hearing Research, 31,* 515–524.

Leonard, L. B., Schwartz, R., Chapman, K., Rowan, L., Prelock, P., Terrell, B., Weiss, A., & Messick, C. (1982). Early lexical acquisition in children with specific language disorder. *Journal of Speech and Hearing Research, 25,* 554–564.

Leonard, L. B., Schwartz, R., Folger, M., & Wilcox, M. (1978). Some aspects of child phonology in imitative and spontaneous speech. *Journal of Child Language, 5,* 403–415.

Leonard, L. B., Steckol, K. F., & Panther, K. M. (1983). Returning meaning to semantic relations: Some clinical applications. *Journal of Speech and Hearing Disorders, 48,* 25–36.

Levi, G., Capozzi, F., Fabrizi, A., & Sechi, E. (1982). Language disorders and prognosis for reading disabilities in developmental age. *Perceptual and Motor Skills, 54,* 1119–1122.

Levin, H. S., & Eisenberg, H. M. (1979). Neuropsychological impairment after closed head injury in children and adolescents. *Journal of Pediatric Psychology, 4,* 389–402.

Levin, H. S., Ewing-Cobbs, L., & Benton, A. L. (1984). Age and recovery from brain damage: A review of clinical studies. In S. W. Scheff (Ed.), *Aging and recovery of function in the central nervous system* (pp. 169–205). New York: Plenum Publishing.

Levine, M. (1987). *Developmental variation and learning disorders.* Cambridge, MA: Educators Publishing Service.

Levinson, S. (1983). *Pragmatics.* Cambridge: Cambridge University Press.

Levitt, H., McGarr, N., & Geffner, D. (1988). Development of language and communication skills in hearing-impaired children. *ASHA Monographs* (No. 26).

Rockville, MD: American Speech-Language-Hearing Association.

Liberman, A. M., Cooper, F. S., Shankweiler, D. P., & Studdert-Kennedy, M. (1967). Perception of the speech code. *Psychological Review, 74,* 431–461.

Liberman, I. Y., & Liberman, A. M. (1990). Whole language vs. code emphasis: Underlying assumptions and their implications for reading instruction. *Annals of Dyslexia, 40,* 51–76.

Liberman, I. Y., Shankweiler, D., Liberman, A. M., Fowler, C., & Fischer, F. W. (1977). Phonetic segmentation and recording in the beginning reader. In S. S. Reber & D. Scarborough (Eds.), *Toward a psychology of reading* (pp. 201–225). Hillsdale, NJ: Erlbaum.

Liebergott, J. W., Bashir, A. S., & Schultz, M. C. (1984). Dancing around and making strange noises: Children at risk. In A. Holland (Ed.), *Language disorders in children* (pp. 37–56). San Diego, CA: College-Hill Press.

Lieberman, I., & Shankweiler, D. (1985). Phonology and problems of learning to read and write. *Remedial and Special Education, 6,* 8–17.

Lieven, E. V. M. (1984). Interactional style and children's language learning. *Topics in Language Disorders, 4*(4), 15–23.

Light, J. (1988). Interaction involving individuals using augmentative and alternative communication systems: State of the art and future directions. *Augmentative and Alternative Communication, 4,* 66–82.

Light, J., Collier, B., & Parnes, P. (1985a). Communicative interaction between young nonspeaking physically disabled children and their primary caregivers: Part I—Discourse patterns. *Augmentative and Alternative Communication, 1,* 74–83.

Light, J., Collier, B., & Parnes, P. (1985b). Communicative interaction between young nonspeaking physically disabled children and their primary caregivers: Part II—Communicative function. *Augmentative and Alternative Communication, 1,* 98–107.

Light, J., Collier, B., & Parnes, P. (1985c). Communicative interaction between young nonspeaking physically disabled children and their primary caregivers: Part III—Modes of communication. *Augmentative and Alternative Communication, 1,* 125–133.

Light, J., Kelford-Smith, A., & McNaughton, D. (1990, August). *The literacy experiences of preschoolers who use augmentative and alternative communication systems.* Paper presented at the biennial meeting of the International Society for Augmentative and Alternative Communication, Stockholm, Sweden.

Liles, B. Z. (1985). Cohesion in the narratives of normal and language-disordered children. *Journal of Speech and Hearing Research, 28,* 123–133.

Lindamood, C. H., & Lindamood, P. C. (1969). *Auditory discrimination in depth.* Austin, TX: DLM Teaching Resources.

Linder, T. W. (1990). *Transdisciplinary play-based assessment* (TPBA). Baltimore, MD: Paul H. Brookes.

Lindfors, J. W. (1987). *Children's language and learning* (2nd ed.). Needham Heights, MA: Allyn & Bacon

Ling, D. (1976). *Speech and the hearing-impaired child: Theory and practice.* Washington, DC: A. G. Bell.

Ling, D. (Ed.). (1984a). *Early intervention for hearing impaired children: Oral options.* Austin, TX: Pro-Ed.

Ling, D. (Ed.). (1984b). *Early intervention for hearing impaired children: Total communication options.* Austin, TX: Pro-Ed.

Ling, D., & Clarke, B. R. (1975). Cued speech: An evaluative study. *American Annals of the Deaf, 120,* 480–488.

Ling, D., & Clarke, B. R. (1976). The effects of using cued speech: A follow-up study. *Volta Review, 78,* 23–34.

Ling, D., & Ling, A. H. (1978). Aural habilitation: The foundations of verbal learning in hearing-impaired children. Washington, DC: A. G. Bell Assocation for the Deaf.

Lipsky, D. K. & Gartner, A. (Eds.). (1989). *Beyond separate education: Quality education for all.* Baltimore, MD: Paul H. Brookes Publishing.

Lloyd, J. (1980). Academic instruction and cognitive behavior modification: The need for attack strategy training. *Exceptional Education Quarterly, 1,* 53–63.

Loban, W. D. (1963). The language of elementary school children. *NCTE Research Report No. 1.* Urbana, IL: National Council of Teachers of English.

Loban, W. D. (1976). *Language development: Kindergarten through grade twelve.* Urbana, IL: National Council of Teachers of English.

Longhurst, T. M. (Ed.). (1974). *Linguistic analysis of children's speech: Readings.* New York: MSS Information Corporation.

Lovaas, O. I. (1987). Behavioral treatment and normal educational and intellectual functioning in young autistic children. *Journal of Consulting and Clinical Psychology, 55,* 3–9.

Lovaas, O. I., Schaeffer, B., & Simmons, J. Q. (1965). Experimental studies in childhood schizophrenia: Building social behavior in autistic children by use of electric shock. *Journal of Experimental Research in Personality, 1,* 99–109.

Love, R. J., & Webb, W. G. (1986). *Neurology for the speech-language pathologist.* Stoneham, MA: Butterworth Publishers.

Lowe, M., & Costello, A. (1976). *Manual for Symbolic Play Test.* London: National Foundation of Educational Research.

Lucariello, J. (1990). Freeing talk from the here-and-now: The role of event knowledge and maternal scaffolds. *Topics in Language Disorders, 10*(3), 14–29.

Lucas, E. V. (1980). *Semantic and pragmatic language disorders: Assessment and remediation.* Rockville, MD: Aspen.

Lund, N. J., & Duchan, J. F. (1988). *Assessing children's language in naturalistic contexts* (2nd ed.). Englewood Cliffs, NJ: Prentice-Hall.

Lundsteen, S. W. (1979). *Listening: Its impact at all levels on reading and the other language arts.* Urbana, IL: National Council of Teachers of English.

Luterman, D. (1979). *Counseling parents of hearing impaired children.* Boston, MA: Little, Brown.

Lyman, H. (1986). *Test scores and what they mean* (4th ed.). Englewood Cliffs, NJ: Prentice-Hall.

Lynch, M. P., Eilers, R. E., Oller, D. K., & Cobo-Lewis, A. (1989). Multisensory speech perception by profoundly hearing-impaired children. *Journal of Speech and Hearing Disorders, 54,* 57–67.

Lynch-Fraser, D., & Tiegerman, E. (1987). *Baby signals.* New York: Walker and Company.

Lyon, S., & Lyon, G. (1980). Team functioning and staff development: A role release approach to providing integrated educational services for severely handicapped students. *JASH (Journal of the Association for Persons with Severe Handicaps), 5*(3), 250–263.

Mabbett, B. (1990). The New Zealand story. *Educational Leadership, 47*(6), 59–61.

MacDonald, J. (1989). *Becoming partners with children: From play to conversation.* San Antonio, TX: Special Press.

MacKeith, R. C., & Rutter, M. (1972). A note on the prevalence of language disorders in young children. In M. Rutter & J. A. M. Martin (Eds.), *The child with delayed speech. Clinics in developmental medicine.* (No. 43, pp. 48–51). London: Heineman Medical Books.

MacMurray, J. (1961). *Persons in relation.* London: Faber.

MacWhinney, B. (1987). The competition model. In B. MacWhinney (Ed.), *Mechanisms of language acquisition* (pp. 249–308). Hillsdale, NJ: Lawrence Erlbaum.

Magnotta, O. H. (1991). Looking beyond tradition. *Language, Speech, and Hearing Services in Schools, 22,* 150–151.

Mahoney, T. M., & Eichwald, J. G. (1987). The ups and "Downs" of high-risk screening: The Utah statewide program. *Seminars in Hearing, 8*(2), 155–163.

Mandler, J., & Johnson, N. L. (1977). Remembrance of things parsed: Story structure and recall. *Cognitive Psychology, 9,* 111–191.

Manis, F. R., Szeszulski, P. A., Holt, L. K., & Graves, K. (1988). A developmental perspective on dyslexic subtypes. *Annals of Dyslexia, 38,* 139–153.

Mantovani, J. F., & Landau, W. M. (1980). Acquired aphasia with convulsive disorder: Course and prognosis. *Neurology, 30,* 524–529.

Mardell, C., & Goldenberg, D. (1975). *The Developmental Indicators for the Assessment of Learning (DIAL).* Chicago, IL: Childcraft Education.

Mardell-Czudnowski, C., & Goldenberg, D. (1984). Revision and restandardization of a preschool screening test: DIAL becomes DIAL-R. *Journal of the Division for Early Childhood, 11,* 238–246.

Mardell-Czudnowski, C., & Goldenberg, D. (1990). *Developmental Indicators for the Assessment of Learning—Revised (DIAL-R).* Circle Pines, MN: AGS.

Markus, D. (1988, November). Out of the shadows. *Parenting, 1988,* 113–114.

Marin-Padilla, M. (1975). Neuron differences in mental retardation. In D. Bergsma (Ed.), *Morphogenesis and malformation of the face and brain.* New York: Allen R. Liss.

Marshall, J. C. (1979). Language acquisition in a biological frame of reference. In P. Fletcher & M. Garman (Eds.), *Language acquisition* (pp. 437–453). Cambridge, England: Cambridge University Press.

Marston, D. B. (1989). A curriculum-based measurement approach to assessing academic performance: What it is and why do it. In M. R. Shinn (Ed.), *Curriculum-based measurement: Assessing special children* (pp. 18–78). New York: Guilford Press.

Martin Luther King Junior Elementary School Children et al. v. Ann Arbor School District Board, Civil Action No. 7–71861, 451 F. Supp. 1324 (1978), 463 F. Supp. 1027 (1978) and 473 F. Supp. 1371 (1979, E. D. Detroit, Michigan).

Martin, V. E. (1974). Consulting with teachers. *Language, Speech, and Hearing Services in Schools, 5,* 176–179.

Marvin, C. A. (1987). Consultation services: Changing roles for SLPs. *Journal of Childhood Communication Disorders, 11,* 1–15.

Marvin, C. A. (1990). Problems in school-based speech-language consultation and collaboration services: Defining the terms and improving the process. *Best Practices in School Speech–Language Pathology, 1,* 37–47.

Marx, M. H., & Hillix, W. A. (1979). *Systems and theories in psychology.* New York: McGraw-Hill.

Marzano, R., Hagerty, P., Valencia, S., & DiStefano, P. (1987). *Reading diagnosis and instruction: Theory into practice.* Englewood Cliffs, NJ: Prentice-Hall.

Mason, J. (1980). When do children begin to read: An exploration of four-year-old children's letter and word reading competencies. *Reading and Research Quarterly, 15,* 203–227.

Massaro, D. W. (1973). Perception of letters, words, and nonwords. *Journal of Experimental Psychology, 100,* 349–353.

Matarazzo, J. D. (1972). *Wechsler's measurement and appraisal of adult intelligence.* Baltimore, MD: Williams & Wilkins.

Matsuyama, U. K. (1983). Can story grammar speak Japanese? *The Reading Teacher, 36,* 666–669.

Mattis, S. (1978). Dyslexia syndromes: A working hypothesis that works. In A. L. Benton & D. Pearl (Eds.), *Dyslexia: An appraisal of current knowledge.* New York: Oxford University Press.

Mattis, S., French, J. H., & Rapin, I. (1975). Dyslexia in children and young adults: Three independent neuropsychological syndromes. *Developmental Medicine and Child Neurology, 17,* 150–163.

Mautner, T. S. (1984). Dyslexia—My "invisible handicap." *Annals of Dyslexia, 34,* 299–311.

Maxon, A., & Brackett, D. (1987). The hearing-impaired child in regular schools. *Seminars in Speech and Language, 8*(4), 393–413.

Maxwell, D. L. (1984). The neurology of learning and language disabilities: Developmental considerations. In G. P. Wallach & K. G. Butler (Eds.), *Language learning disabilities in school-age children* (pp. 35–59). Baltimore, MD: Williams & Wilkins.

Maxwell, S. E., & Wallach, G. P. (1984). The language-learning disabilities connection: Symptoms of early language disability change over time. In G. P. Wallach & K. G. Butler (Eds.), *Language learning disabilities in school-age children* (pp. 15–34). Baltimore, MD: Williams & Wilkins.

McCalla, J. L. (1985). A multidisciplinary approach to identification and remedial intervention for adverse late effects of cancer therapy. *Nursing Clinics of North America, 20,* 117–129.

McCarthy, D. A. (1930). The language development of the pre-school child. *University of Minnesota Institute of Child Welfare Monograph Series IV.* Minneapolis, MN: University of Minnesota Press.

McCarthy, D.A. (1954). Language development in children. In L. Carmichael (Ed.), *Manual of child psychology* (pp. 492–630). New York: Wiley.

McCauley, R. J., & Swisher, L. (1984). Psychometric review of language and articulation tests for preschool children. *Journal of Speech and Hearing Disorders, 49,* 34–42.

McCauley, R. J., & Swisher, L. (1987). Are maltreated children at risk for speech or language impairment? An unanswered question. *Journal of Speech and Hearing Disorders, 52,* 301–303.

McClelland, J., Rumelhart, D., & PDP Research Group. (1986). *Parallel distributed processing: Explorations in the microstructure of cognition* (Vol. 2). Cambridge, MA: Bradford Books.

McClure, E., Mason, J., & Williams, J. (1983). Sociocultural variables in children's sequencing of stories. *Discourse Processes, 6,* 131–143.

McConkey, R. (1984). The assessment of representational play: A springboard for language remediation. In D. Mueller (Ed.), *Remediating children's language: Behavioral and naturalistic approaches (pp. 113–134).* Austin, TX: Pro-Ed.

McCormick, L. (1990a). Developing objectives. In L. McCormick & R. L. Schiefelbusch (Eds.), *Early language intervention: An introduction* (2nd ed., pp. 181–214). Columbus, OH: Merrill/Macmillan.

McCormick, L. (1990b). Intervention processes and procedures. In L. McCormick & R. L. Schiefelbusch (Eds.), *Early language intervention: An introduction* (2nd ed., pp. 216–260). Columbus, OH: Merrill/Macmillan.

McCormick, L. (1990c). Extracurricular roles and relationships. In L. McCormick & R. L. Schiefelbusch (Eds.), *Early language intervention: An introduction* (2nd ed., pp. 262–301). Columbus, OH: Merrill/Macmillan.

McCormick, L., & Goldman, R. (1979). The transdisciplinary model: Implications for service delivery and personnel preparation for the severely and profoundly handicapped. *AAESPH Review, 4*(2), 152–161.

McCormick, L. & Schiefelbusch, R. L. (Eds.). (1990). *Early language intervention: An introduction* (2nd ed.). Columbus, OH: Merrill/Macmillan.

McCormick, M. C. (1989). Long-term follow-up of infants discharged from neonatal intensive care units. *Journal of the American Medical Association, 261,* 1767–1772.

McCune-Nicolich, L. (1981). Toward symbolic functioning: Structure of early pretend games and potential parallels with language. *Child Development, 52,* 785–797.

McCune-Nicolich, L., & Fenson, L. (1984). Methodological issues in studying pretend play. In T. D. Yawkey & A. D. Pelligrini (Eds.), *Child's play: Developmental and applied* (pp. 81–104). Hillsdale, NJ: Lawrence Erlbaum.

McDermott, R. P. (1977). Social relations as contexts for learning in school. *Harvard Educational Review, 47,* 198–213.

McGee, L. M., & Richgels, D. J. (1990). *Literacy's beginnings: Supporting young readers and writers.* Needham Heights, MA: Allyn & Bacon.

McKenzie, R. G. (1991). Content area instruction delivered by secondary learning disabilities teachers: A national survey. *Learning Disability Quarterly, 14,* 115–122.

McKinley, N. L., & Lord-Larson, V. (1985). Neglected language-disordered adolescent: A delivery model. *Language, Speech, and Hearing Services in Schools, 16,* 2–15.

McKirdy, L. S., & Blank, M. (1982). Dialogue in deaf and hearing preschoolers. *Journal of Speech and Hearing Research, 25,* 487–499.

McLean, J. E., & Snyder-McLean, L. K. (1978). *A transactional approach to early language training: Derivation of a model system.* Columbus, OH: Merrill/Macmillan.

McNeill, D. (1966). Developmental psycholinguistics. In F. Smith & G. Miller (Eds.), *The genesis of language* (pp. 15–84). Cambridge, MA: MIT Press.

McNeill, D. (1970). *The acquisition of language: The study of developmental psycholinguistics.* New York: Harper & Row.

Mehan, H. (1979). *Learning lessons: Social organization in the classroom.* Cambridge, MA: Harvard University Press.

Meier, R. P. (1991). Language acquisition by deaf children. *American Scientist, 79*(1), 60–70.

Menyuk, P. (1964). Comparison of grammar of children with functionally deviant and normal speech. *Journal of Speech and Hearing Research, 7,* 109–121.

Menyuk, P. (1968). Children's learning and reproduction of grammatical and nongrammatical phonological sequences. *Child Development, 39,* 849–959.

Mercer, J. R. (1973). *Labeling the mentally retarded.* Berkeley: University of California Press.

Mercer, J. R., & Denti, L. (1989). Obstacles to integrating students in a "two-roof" elementary school. *Exceptional Children, 56,* 30–38.

Mercer, J. R., & Lewis, J. P. (1975). *System of multicultural pluralistic assessment. Technical manual.* Unpublished manuscript. University of California at Riverside.

Meyer, B. J. F. (1975). *The organization of prose and its effects on memory.* Amsterdam: North Holland.

Miedzianik, D. (1990, Spring). I hope some lass will want me after reading all this. *The Advocate* (newsletter of the Autism Society of America), *22*(1), 7.

Miller, B. L. (1988). *Effects of intervention on the ability of students with hearing impairments to write personal narrative stories.* Unpublished master's thesis, Western Michigan University, Kalamazoo, MI.

Miller, G. A., & Gildea, P. M. (1987). How children learn words. *Scientific American, 257,* 94–99.

Miller, J. F. (1981). *Assessing language production in children: Experimental procedures.* Needham Heights, MA: Allyn & Bacon.

Miller, J. F. (1987). Language and communication characteristics of children with Down syndrome. In S. M. Pueschel, C. Tingey, J. E. Rynders, A. C. Crocker, & D. M. Crutcher (Eds.), *New perspectives on Down syndrome* (pp. 233–262). Baltimore, MD: Paul H. Brookes.

Miller, J. F., Campbell, T. F., Chapman, R. S., & Weismer, S. E. (1984). Language behavior in acquired childhood aphasia. In A. Holland (Ed.), *Language disorders in children* (pp. 57–99). San Diego, CA: College-Hill Press.

Miller, J. F., & Chapman, R. S. (1981). The relation between age and mean length of utterance in morphemes. *Journal of Speech and Hearing Research, 24,* 154–161.

Miller, J. F., & Chapman, R. (1986). *Systematic analysis of language transcripts (SALT)* [computer program; A. Nockerts, Programmer]. Madison, WI: Language Analysis Laboratory, Waisman Center on Mental Retardation and Human Development.

Miller, J. F., Chapman, R., Branston, M. B., & Reichle, J. (1980). Language comprehension in sensorimotor stages V and VI. *Journal of Speech and Hearing Research, 23,* 284–311.

Miller, L. (1978). Pragmatics and early childhood language disorders: Communicative interactions in a half-hour sample. *Journal of Speech and Hearing Disorders, 43,* 419–436.

Miller, L. (1989). Classroom-based language intervention. *Language, Speech, and Hearing Services in Schools, 20,* 153–169.

Miller, L. (1990). *The smart profile: A qualitative approach for describing learners and designing instruction.* Austin, TX: Smart Alternatives.

Mills, A. E. (Ed.). (1983). *Language acquisition in the blind child: Normal and deficient.* San Diego, CA: College-Hill.

Milosky, L. M. (1987). Narratives in the classroom. *Seminars in Speech and Language, 8*(4), 329–343.

Milosky, L. M. (1990). The role of world knowledge in language comprehension and language intervention. *Topics in Language Disorders, 10*(3), 1–13.

Minskoff, E. (1982). Sharpening language skills in secondary LD students. *Academic Therapy, 18*(1), 53–60.

Minuchin, P. (1985). Families and individual development: Provocations from the field of family therapy. *Child Development, 56,* 289–302.

Mire, S. P., & Chisholm, R. W. (1990). Functional communication goals for adolescents and adults who are severely and moderately mentally handicapped. *Language, Speech, and Hearing Services in Schools, 21,* 57–58.

Mirenda, P., & Locke, P. A. (1989). A comparison of symbol transparency in nonspeaking persons with intellectual disabilities. *Journal of Speech and Hearing Disorders, 54,* 131–140.

Mirenda, P., & Santogrossi, J. (1985). A prompt-free strategy to teach pictorial communication system use. *Augmentative and Alternative Communication, 1,* 143–150.

Mishler, E. G. (1979). Meaning in context: Is there any other kind? *Harvard Educational Review, 49,* 1–19.

Moeller, M. P. (1989, November). *Strategies for enhancing hearing parent's sign communication with deaf children.* Paper presented at the Annual Convention of the American Speech-Language-Hearing Association, St. Louis.

Moeller, M. P., Osberger, M. J., & Eccarius, M. (1986). Cognitively based strategies for use with hearing-impaired students with comprehension deficits. *Topics in Language Disorders, 6*(4), 37–50.

Molfese, D., Freeman, R., & Palermo, D. (1975). The ontogeny of brain lateralization for speech and non-speech stimuli. *Brain and Language, 2,* 356–368.

Montague, M., Graves, A., & Leavell, A. (1991). Planning, procedural facilitation, and narrative composition of Junior High students with learning disabilities. *Learning Disabilities Research & Practice, 6,* 219–224.

Moon, M. S., Diambra, T., & Hill, M. (1990). An outcome-oriented vocational process for students with severe handicaps. *Teaching Exceptional Children, 23*(1), 47–50.

Moores, D. (1969). Cued speech: Some practical and theoretical considerations. *American Annals of the Deaf, 114,* 23–27.

Moran, M. R. (1987). Individualized objectives for writing instruction. *Topics in Language Disorders, 7*(4), 42–54.

Moran, M. R. (1988). Rationale and procedures for increasing the productivity of inexperienced writers. *Exceptional Children, 54,* 552–558.

Morgan, D., & Guilford, A. (1984). *Adolescent Language Screening Test* (ALST). Tulsa, OK: Modern Educational Corp.

Morley, M. E. (1972). *The development and disorders of speech in childhood.* London: Churchill Livingstone.

Morris, C. (1946). *Foundation of the theory of signs. International encyclopedia of unified science.* Chicago: University of Chicago Press.

Morris, N.T., and Crump, W. D. (1982). Syntactic and vocabulary development in the written language of learning disabled and non-disabled students at four age levels. *Learning Disability Quarterly, 5,* 163–172.

Morris, S. E. (1981). Communication/interaction development at mealtimes for the multiply handicapped child: Implications for the use of augmentative communication systems. *Language, Speech, and Hearing Services in Schools, 12,* 216–232.

Morris, S. E. (1982). *Prespeech assessment scale.* Clifton, NJ: J. A. Preston.

Morris, S. E., & Klein, M. D. (1987). *Pre-feeding skills.* Tucson, AZ: Communication Skill Builders.

Moses, K. L. (1985). Infant deafness and parental grief: Psychosocial early intervention. In F. Powell, T. Finitzo-Hieber, S. Friel-Patti, & D. Henderson (Eds.), *Education of the hearing impaired child* (pp. 85–102). Austin, TX: Pro-Ed.

Mroczkowski, M. M. (1988). Self–contained language classes for kindergartners—Nine years of data. *Seminars in Speech and Language, 9,* 329–339.

Mulac, A., & Tomlinson, C. (1977). Generalization of an operant remediation program for syntax with language delayed children. *Journal of Communication Disorders, 10,* 231–243.

Mulligan, M., Guess, D., Holvoet, J., & Brown, F. (1980). The individualized curriculum sequencing model: Implications from research on massed, distributed, or spaced trial training. *JASH (Journal for the Association for Persons with Severe Handicaps), 5,* 325–336.

Muma, J. (1978). *Language handbook: Concepts, assessment, intervention.* Englewood Cliffs, NJ: Prentice-Hall.

Muma, J. (1983). Speech-language pathology: Emerging clinical expertise in language. In T. M. Gallagher & C. Prutting (Eds.), *Pragmatic assessment and intervention issues in language* (pp. 195–214). San Diego, CA: College-Hill Press.

Murray-Seegert, C. (1989). *Nasty girls, thugs, and humans like us: Social relations between severely disabled and nondisabled students in high school.* Baltimore, MD: Paul H. Brookes.

Musselwhite, C. R. (1986). *Adaptive play for special needs children.* Austin, TX: Pro-Ed.

Muth, K. D. (1989). *Children's comprehension of text.* Newark, DE: International Reading Association.

Myklebust, H. R. (1954). *Auditory disorders in children.* New York: Grune & Stratton.

Myklebust, H. R. (1957). Aphasia in children—Diagnosis and training. In L. E. Travis (Ed.), *Handbook of speech pathology and audiology* (pp. 514–530). Englewood Cliffs, NJ: Prentice-Hall.

Myklebust, H. R. (1964). *The psychology of deafness* (2nd ed.). New York: Grune & Stratton.

National Assessment of Educational Progress. (1980). Writing achievement, 1969–1979: Results from the Third National Writing Assessment. Denver, CO: Author. (ERIC Document Reproduction Service Nos. ED 196 043, ED 196 044).

National Joint Committee on Learning Disabilities. (1985). *Learning disabilities and the preschool child.* (A position paper of the National Joint Committee on Learning Disabilities, February 10, 1985). Baltimore MD: The Orton Dyslexia Society.

National Joint Committee on Learning Disabilities. (1991). Learning disabilities: Issues on definition (A position paper of the National Joint Committee on Learning Disabilities). *ASHA, 33*(Suppl. 5), 18–20.

Neisworth, J. T., & Bagnato, S. J. (1988). Assessment in early childhood special education: A typology of dependent measures. In S. L. Odom & M. B. Karnes (Eds)., *Early intervention for infants and children with handicaps* (pp. 23–50). Baltimore, MD: Paul H. Brookes.

Nelson, K. (1973). Structure and strategy in learning to talk. *Monographs of the Society for Research in Child Development, 38.*

Nelson, K. (1985). *Making sense: The acquisition of shared meaning.* New York: Academic Press.

Nelson, K. (1986). *Event knowledge: Structure and function in development.* Hillsdale, NJ: Lawrence Erlbaum.

Nelson, K. (Ed.). (1989). *Narratives from the crib.* Cambridge, MA: Harvard University Press.

Nelson, K., Benedict, H., Gruendel, J., & Rescorla, L. (1977). *Lessons from early lexicons.* Paper presented at the biennial meeting of the Society for Research in Child Development, New Orleans.

Nelson, N. W. (1981a). An eclectic model of language intervention for disorders of listening, speaking, reading, and writing. *Topics in Language Disorders, 1*(2), 1–23.

Nelson, N. W. (1981b). Tests and materials in speech and language screening. *Seminars in Speech, Language, and Hearing, 2,* 11–36.

Nelson, N. W. (1984). Beyond information processing: The language of teachers and textbooks. In G. P. Wallach & K. G. Butler (Eds.), *Language learning disabilities in school-age children* (pp. 154–178). Baltimore, MD: Williams & Wilkins.

Nelson, N. W. (1985). Teacher talk and child listening—Fostering a better match. In C. S. Simon (Ed.), *Communication skills and classroom success: Assessment of language-learning disabled students* (pp. 65–102). San Diego, CA: College-Hill Press. Reprinted in C. S. Simon (Ed.). (1991), *Communication skills and classroom success: Assessment and therapy methodologies for language and learning disabled students* (pp. 78–103). Eau Claire, WI: Thinking Publications.

Nelson, N. W. (1986). Individual processing in classroom settings. *Topics in Language Disorders, 6*(2), 13–27.

Nelson, N. W. (1988a). The nature of literacy. In M. A. Nippold (Ed.), *Later language development: Ages nine through nineteen* (pp. 11–28). Austin, TX: Pro-Ed.

Nelson, N. W. (1988b). *Planning individualized speech and language intervention programs* (2nd ed.). Tucson, AZ: Communication Skill Builders.

Nelson, N. W. (1988c). Reading and writing. In M. A. Nippold (Ed.), *Normal language development: Ages nine through nineteen* (pp. 97–126). Austin, TX: Pro-Ed.

Nelson, N. W. (1989a). Language intervention in school settings. In D. K. Bernstein & E. Tiegerman (Eds.), *Language and communication disorders in children* (2nd ed.), (pp. 417–468). Columbus, OH: Merrill/Macmillan.

Nelson, N. W. (1989b). Curriculum-based language assessment and intervention. *Language, Speech, and Hearing Services in Schools, 20,* 170–184.

Nelson, N. W. (1990). Only relevant practices can be best. *Best Practices in School Speech-Language Pathology, 1,* 15–27.

Nelson, N. W. (in press-a). Curriculum-based language assessment and intervention across the grades. In G. P. Wallach & K. G. Butler (Eds)., *Language learning disabilities in school-age children and adolescents: Some underlying principles and applications.* Columbus, OH: Merrill/Macmillan.

Nelson, N. W. (in press-b). Targets of curriculum-based language assessment. *Best Practices in School Speech-Language Pathology, 2.*

Nelson, N. W., & Friedman, K. K. (1988). *Development of the concept of story in narratives written by older children.* Unpublished paper. Kalamazoo, MI: Western Michigan University.

Nelson, N. W., & Gillespie, L. (1991). *Analogies for thinking and talking.* Tucson, AZ: Communication Skill Builders.

Nelson, N. W., & Hyter, Y. D. (1990a). *Black English Sentence Scoring: Development and use as a tool for non-biased assessment.* Unpublished manuscript.

Nelson, N. W., & Hyter, Y. D. (1990b, November). *How to use Black English Sentence Scoring.* Short course presented at the Annual Conference of the American Speech-Language-Hearing Association, Seattle, WA.

Nelson, N. W., & Schwentor, B. A. (1990). Reading and writing. In D. R. Beukelman & K. M. Yorkston (Eds.), *Communication disorders following traumatic brain injury: Management of cognitive, language, and motor impairments* (pp. 191–249). Austin, TX: Pro-Ed.

Nelson, N. W., Silbar, J. C., & Lockwood, E. L. (1981, November). *The Michigan decision-making strategy for determining appropriate communicative services for physically and/or mentally handicapped children.* Paper presented at the annual conference of the American Speech-Language-Hearing Association, Los Angeles.

Nelson, N. W., & Snyder, T. [Programmer]. (1990). *Planning individualized speech and language intervention programs: Software version* (rev. ed.) [Computer program]. Tucson, AZ: Communication Skill Builders.

Newborg, J., Stock, J. R., Wnek, L., Guidubaldi, J., & Svinicki, J. (1984). *The Battelle Developmental Inventory.* Allen, TX: DLM.

Newcomer, P. L., & Hammill, D. D. (1988). *Test of Language Development—2 Primary.* Austin, TX: Pro-Ed.

Newhoff, M. (1986, Fall). Attentional deficit—What it is, what it is not. *The Clinical Connection,* pp. 10–11.

Newhoff, M. (1990). Attention deficit hyperactivity disorder: Defining our role. *The Clinical Connection, 1st Quarter,* 10–12.

Newman, P., Creaghead, N. A., & Secord, W. (1985). *Assessment and remediation of articulatory and phonological disorders.* Columbus, OH: Merrill/Macmillan.

Newport, E. L., & Ashbrook, E. (1977). The emergence of semantic relations in American Sign Language. *Papers and Reports on Child Language Development, 13,* 16–21.

Newton, L. (1985). Linguistic environment of the deaf child: A focus on teachers' use of nonliteral language. *Journal of Speech and Hearing Research, 28,* 336–344.

Ninio, A. (1983). Joint book reading as a multiple vocabulary acquisition device. *Developmental Psychology, 19,* 445–451.

Ninio, A., & Bruner, J. S. (1978). The achievements and antecedents of labelling. *Journal of Child Language, 5,* 1–16.

Nippold, M. A. (1985). Comprehension of figurative language in youth. *Topics in Language Disorders, 5*(3), 1–20.

Nippold, M. A. (1986). Verbal analogical reasoning in children and adolescents. *Topics in Language Disorders, 6*(4), 51–63.

Nippold, M. A. (1988a). Figurative language. In M. A. Nippold (Ed.), *Later language development: Ages nine through nineteen* (pp. 179–210). Austin, TX: Pro-Ed.

Nippold, M. A. (1988b). Introduction. In M. A. Nippold (Ed.), *Later language development: Ages nine through nineteen* (pp. 1–10). Austin, TX: Pro-Ed.

Nippold, M. A. (Ed.). (1988c). *Later language development: Ages nine through nineteen*. Austin, TX: Pro-Ed.

Nippold, M. A. (1988d). The literate lexicon. In M. A. Nippold (Ed.), *Later language development: Ages nine through nineteen* (pp. 29–47). Austin, TX: Pro-Ed.

Nippold, M. A. (1988e). Verbal reasoning. In M. A. Nippold (Ed.), *Later language development: Ages nine through nineteen* (pp. 159–177). Austin, TX: Pro-Ed.

Nippold, M. A. (1991). Evaluating and enhancing idiom comprehension in language-disordered students. *Language, Speech, and Hearing Services in Schools, 22,* 100–106.

Nippold, M. A., Erskine, B. A., & Freed, D. B. (1988). Proportional and functional analogical reasoning in normal and language-impaired children. *Journal of Speech and Hearing Disorders, 53,* 440–448.

Nippold, M. A., & Fey, S. H. (1983). Metaphoric understanding in preadolescents having a history of language acquisition difficulties. *Language, Speech, and Hearing Services in Schools, 14,* 171–180.

Nippold, M. A., Leonard, L. B., & Anastopoulos, A. (1982). Development in the use and understanding of polite forms in children. *Journal of Speech and Hearing Research, 25,* 193–202.

Nippold, M. A., & Martin, S. T. (1989). Idiom interpretation in isolation versus context: A developmental study with adolescents. *Journal of Speech and Hearing Research, 32,* 59–66.

Nisbett, R. E., & Wilson, T. D. (1977). The halo effect: Evidence for unconscious alteration of judgements. *Journal of Personality and Social Psychology, 35,* 250–256.

Norlin, P. F. (1986). Familiar faces, sudden strangers: Helping families cope with the crisis of aphasia. In R. Chapey (Ed.), *Language intervention strategies in adult aphasia* (pp. 174–186). Baltimore, MD: Williams & Wilkins.

Norman, J. B. (1983, November). *A holistic treatment approach to elective mutism.* Paper presented at the Annual Conference of the American Speech-Language-Hearing Association, Cincinnati.

Norris, J. A. (1988). Using communication strategies to enhance reading acquisition. *The Reading Teacher, 47,* 668–673.

Norris, J. A. (1989). Providing language remediation in the classroom: An integrated language-to-reading intervention method. *Language, Speech, and Hearing Services in Schools, 20,* 205–218.

Norris, J. A., & Bruning, R. H. (1988). Cohesion in the narratives of good and poor readers. *Journal of Speech and Hearing Research, 53,* 416–424.

Norris, J. A., & Damico, J. S. (1990). Whole language in theory and practice: Implications for language intervention. *Language, Speech, and Hearing Services in Schools, 21,* 212–220.

Norris, J. A., & Hoffman, P. R. (1990a). Comparison of adult-initiated vs. child-initiated interaction styles with handicapped pre-language children. *Language, Speech, and Hearing Services in Schools, 21,* 28–36.

Norris, J. A., & Hoffman, P. R. (1990b). Language intervention within naturalistic environments. *Language, Speech, and Hearing Services in Schools, 21,* 72–84.

Northcott, W. H. (Ed.). (1977). *Curriculum guide: Hearing impaired children—birth to three years—and their parents* (rev. ed.). Washington, DC: A. G. Bell Association for the Deaf.

Northern, J. L., & Downs, M. P. (1984). *Hearing in children* (3rd ed.). Baltimore, MD: Williams & Wilkins.

Nye, C., & Montgomery, J. K. (1989, Spring). Identification criteria for language disordered children: A national survey. *Hearsay* (Journal of the Ohio Speech and Hearing Association), pp. 26–33.

Nystrand, M. (Ed.). (1982). *What writers know: The language, process, and structure of written discourse.* New York: Academic Press.

O'Brien, M. A., & O'Leary, T. S. (1988). Evolving to the classroom model: Speech-language service for the mentally retarded. *Seminars in Speech and Language, 9,* 355–366.

O'Connor, L., & Eldredge, P. (1981). *Communication disorders in adolescence: Program planning, diagnostics, and practical remediation techniques.* Springfield, IL: Charles C. Thomas.

Odell, L. (1981). Defining and assessing competence in writing. In C. R. Cooper (Ed.), *The nature and measurement of competency in English* (pp. 95–138). Urbana, IL: National Council of Teachers of English.

Odom, S. L., & Karnes, M. B. (Eds.). (1988). *Early intervention for infants and children with handicaps*. Baltimore, MD: Paul H. Brookes.

Odom, S. L., & Warren, S. F. (1988). Early childhood education in the year 2000. *Journal of the Division for Early Childhood, 12,* 262–273.

O'Donnell, K. J., & Oehler, J. M. (1989). Neurobehavioral assessment of the newborn infant. In D. B. Bailey, Jr. & M. Wolery (Eds.), *Assessing infants and preschoolers with handicaps* (pp. 167–201). Columbus, OH: Merrill/Macmillan.

O'Donnell, R C., Griffin, W. J., and Norris, R. D. (1967). *Syntax of kindergarten and elementary school children: A transformational analysis.* (Research Rep. No. 8). Champaign, IL: National Council of Teachers of English.

Office of Special Education and Rehabilitative Services, United States Department of Education (1989, Summer). Community integration: The next step. *OSERS News in Print!,* p. 1.

Oller, D. K. (1978). Infant vocalization and the development of speech. *Allied Health and Behavioral Sciences, 1,* 523–549.

Oller, D. K. (1980). The emergence of sounds of speech in infancy. In G. Yeni-Komshian, J. F. Kavanagh, & C. A. Ferguson (Eds.), *Child phonology: Production* (Vol. 1, pp. 93–112). New York: Academic Press.

Oller, D. K., Eilers, R., Bull, D., & Carney, A. (1985). Prespeech vocalizations of a deaf infant: A comparison with normal metaphonological development. *Journal of Speech and Hearing Research, 28,* 47–63.

Oller, D. K., Jensen, H., & Lafayette, R. (1978). The relatedness of phonological processes of a hearing impaired child. *Journal of Communication Disorders, 11,* 97–105.

Olson, C., & Bennett, C. W. (1987a, March). *Regional differences in receptive and expressive vocabulary skills of normal children.* Paper presented at the meeting of the Speech and Hearing Association of Virginia, Roanoke, VA.

Olson, C., & Bennett, C. W. (1987b, March). *Referential semantic analysis: Test–retest reliability.* Paper presented at the meeting of the Speech and Hearing Association of Virginia, Roanoke, VA.

Olswang, L., & Carpenter, R. (1978). Elicitor effects on the language obtained from language-impaired children. *Journal of Speech and Hearing Disorders, 43,* 76–88.

Olswang, L. B., & Carpenter, L. B. (1982a). The ontogenesis of agent: Cognitive notion. *Journal of Speech and Hearing Research, 25,* 297–306.

Olswang, L. B., & Carpenter, L. B. (1982b). The ontogenesis of agent: Linguistic expression. *Journal of Speech and Hearing Research, 25,* 306–314.

O'Neil, W. (1990). Dealing with bad ideas: Twice is less. *English Journal, 79*(4), 80–88.

O'Neill, T. J. (1987). Foreword: The person comes first. In S. M. Pueschel, C. Tingey, J. E. Rynders, A. C. Crocker, & D. M. Crutcher (Eds.), *New perspectives on Down syndrome* (pp. xviii–xix). Baltimore, MD: Paul H. Brookes.

Ornitz, E., & Ritvo, E. (1976). The syndrome of autism: A critical review. *The American Journal of Psychiatry, 133,* 609–621.

Orr, E. W. (1987). *Twice as less: Black English and the performance of Black students in mathematics and science.* New York: W. W. Norton.

Orton, S. (1937). *Reading, writing, and speech problems in children.* New York: W. W. Norton.

Osberger, M. J. (1986). Introduction. In M. J. Osberger (Ed.), *Language and learning skills of hearing-impaired students* (pp. 3–5). ASHA Monographs No. 23. Rockville, MD: American Speech-Language-Hearing Association.

Osgood, C. E. (1967). The nature of meaning. In J. P. DeCecco (Ed.), *The psychology of language, thought, and instruction* (pp. 156–164). New York: Holt, Rinehart & Winston.

Osgood, C. E. (1968). Toward a wedding of insufficiencies. In T. R. Dixon & D. L. Horton (Eds.), *Verbal behavior and general behavior theory* (pp. 495–519). Englewood Cliffs, NJ: Prentice-Hall.

Osgood, C. E., & Miron, M. S. (1963). *Approaches to the study of aphasia.* Urbana, IL: University of Illinois Press.

Osofsky, J. D. (1990). Risk and protective factors for teenage mothers and their infants. *Newsletter of the Society for Research in Child Development, Winter,* 1–2.

Owens, R. E., Jr. (1988). *Language development: An introduction* (2nd ed.). Columbus, OH: Merrill/Macmillan.

Owens, R. E., Jr. (1989). Mental retardation: Difference or delay? In D. K. Bernstein & E. Tiegerman (Eds.), *Language and communication disorders in children* (2nd ed.) (pp. 229–297). Columbus, OH: Merrill/Macmillan.

Owens, R. E., Jr. (1992). *Language development: An introduction* (3rd ed.). Columbus, OH: Merrill/Macmillan.

Padgett, S. Y. (1988). Speech- and language-impaired three and four year olds: A five year follow-up study. In R. L. Masland & M. W. Masland (Eds.), *Preschool prevention of reading failure* (pp. 52–77). Parkton, MD: York Press.

Page, J. L., & Stewart, S. R. (1985). Story grammar skills in school-age children. *Topics in Language Disorders, 5*(2), 16–30.

Paley, V. G. (1981). *Wally's stories: Conversations in the kindergarten.* Cambridge, MA: Harvard University Press.

Palin, M. W., Mordecal, D. R., & Palmer, C. B. (1985). Lingquest 1: Language sample analysis software. [Computer program]

Palincsar, A. S., & Brown, D. (1984). Reciprocal teaching of comprehension-fostering and comprehension-monitoring activities. *Cognition and instruction, 1,* 117–175.

Palincsar, A. S., & Brown, D. (1987). Enhancing instructional time through attention to metacognition. *Journal of Learning Disabilities, 20,* 66–75.

Palincsar, A. S., & Ransom, K. (1988). From the mystery spot to the thoughtful spot: The instruction of metacognitive strategies. *The Reading Teacher, 41,* 784–789.

Panagos, J. M., & Prelock, P. A. (1982). Phonological constraints on the sentence productions of language-disordered children. *Journal of Speech and Hearing Research, 25,* 171–177.

Pang, D. (1985). In M. Ylvisaker (Ed.), *Head injury rehabilitation: Children and adolescents* (pp. 3–70). Austin, TX: Pro-Ed.

Papanicolaou, A. C., DiScenna, A., Gillespie, L., & Aram, D. M. (1990). Probe evoked potential findings following unilateral left hemisphere lesions in children. *Archives of Neurology, 47,* 562–566.

Parker, F. (1986). *Linguistics for non-linguists.* Boston: College-Hill.

Pascual-Leone, J. (1969). *Cognitive development and cognitive style.* Unpublished doctoral dissertation, University of Geneva.

Pascual-Leone, J. (1984). Attentional, dialectic, and mental effort. In M. L. Commons, F. A. Richards, & C. Armon (Eds.), *Beyond formal operations.* New York: Plenum.

Patterson, F. G. (1978). The gestures of a gorilla: Language acquisition by another pongid. *Brain and Language, 12,* 72–97.

Paul, L. (1985). Programming peer support for functional language. In Warren, S. F., & Rogers-Warren, A. K. (Eds). *Teaching functional language* (pp. 289–307). Baltimore, MD: University Park Press.

Paul, R. (1981). In J. Miller (Ed.). *Assessing language production in children: Experimental procedures.* Needham Heights, MA: Allyn & Bacon.

Paul, R. (1990). Comprehension strategies: Interactions between world knowledge and the development of sentence comprehension. *Topics in Language Disorders, 10*(3), 63–75.

Pease, D. M., Gleason, J. B., & Pan, B. A. (1989). Gaining meaning: Semantic development. In J. B. Gleason (Ed.), *The development of language* (2nd ed., pp. 101–134). Columbus, OH: Merrill/Macmillan.

Pehrsson, R. S., & Denner, P. R. (1988). Semantic organizers: Implications for reading and writing. *Topics in Language Disorders, 8*(3), 24–37.

Perera, K. (1984). *Children's writing and reading.* London: Blackwell.

Peters, A. (1977). Does the whole equal the sum of the parts? *Language, 53,* 560–573.

Peterson, C., & McCabe, A. (1983). *Developmental psycholinguistics: Three ways of looking at a child's narrative.* New York: Plenum.

Philips, S. U. (1983). *The invisible culture.* New York: Longman.

Piaget, J. (1926). *The language and thought of the child.* London: Routledge & Kegan Paul.

Piaget, J. (1952). *The origins of intelligence in children.* New York: International Universities Press.

Piaget, J. (1962). *Play, dreams, and imitation in childhood.* London: Routledge & Kegan Paul.

Piaget, J. (1964). Development and learning. In R. E. Ripple & V. N. Rockcastle (Eds.), *Piaget rediscovered* (pp. 7–20). Ithaca, NY: Cornell School of Education Press.

Piaget, J. (1969). *Psychology of intelligence.* Totowa, NJ: Littlefield, Adams.

Piaget, J. (1970). Piaget's theory. In P. H. Mussen (Ed.), *Carmichael's manual of child psychology* (3rd ed., Vol. 1, pp. 703–732). New York: Wiley.

Piaget, J. (1977). The mission of the idea. In H. H. Gruber & J. J. Vonèche (Eds. and Trans.), *The essential Piaget.* New York: Basic Books.

Piaget, J., & Inhelder, B. (1971). *Mental imagery in the child.* London: Routledge & Kegan Paul.

Piccolo, J. (1987). Expository text structure: Teaching and learning strategies. *The Reading Teacher, 40,* 838–847.

Pickering, M., & Kaelber, P. (1978). The speech-language pathologist and the classroom teacher: A team approach to language development. *Language, Speech, and Hearing Services in Schools, 9,* 43–49.

Pidek, C. (1987). *The assignment notebook.* Schaumburg, IL: Communication Concepts.

Pinker, S. (1984). *Language learnability and language development.* Cambridge, MA: Cambridge University Press.

Pinker, S. (1987). The bootstrapping problem in language acquisition. In B. MacWhinney (Ed.), *Mechanisms of language acquisition* (pp. 399–441). Hillsdale, NJ: Lawrence Erlbaum.

Pitcher, E. G., & Prelinger, E. (1963). *Children tell stories: An analysis of fantasy.* New York: International Universities Press.

Polani, P. E., Briggs, J. H., Ford, C. E., Clarke, C. M., & Berg, J. M. (1960). A mongol girl with 46 chromosomes. *Lancet, 1,* 1028.

Pollack, D. (1984). An acoupedic program. In D. Ling (Ed.), *Early intervention for hearing impaired children: Oral options* (pp. 181–254). Austin, TX: Pro-Ed.

Poyadue, F. (1979). *Visiting parents: Peer counselling training manual.* San Jose, CA: Parents Helping Parents (535 Race St., Suite 20).

Prather, E., Beecher, S., Stafford, M., & Wallace, E. (1980). *Screening Test of Adolescent Language* (STAL). Seattle, WA: University of Washington Press.

Prather, E., Hedrick, D., & Kern, C. (1975). Articulation development in children aged two to four years. *Journal of Speech and Hearing Disorders, 40,* 179–191.

President's Committee on Mental Retardation. (1978). *Mental retardation: The leading edge.* Washington, DC: U.S. Government Printing Office, Pub. No. (OHDS) 79–21018.

Pressley, M., & Harris, K. R. (1990). What we really know about strategy instruction. *Education Leadership, 48*(1), 31–34.

Prizant, B. M. (1983). Language acquisition and communicative behavior in autism: Toward an understanding of the "whole" of it. *Journal of Speech and Hearing Disorders, 48,* 296–307.

Prizant, B. M. (1984). Assessment and intervention of communicative problems in children with autism. *Communication Disorders, 9,* 127–142.

Prizant, B. M. (1987). Theoretical and clinical implications of echolalic behavior in autism. In T. L. Layton (Ed.), *Language and treatment of autistic and developmentally disordered children* (pp. 65–88). Springfield, IL: Charles C. Thomas.

Prizant, B. M., Audet, L. R., Burke, G. M., Hummel, L. J., Maher, S. R., & Theadore, G. (1990). Communication disorders and emotional/behavioral disorders in children and adolescents. *Journal of Speech and Hearing Disorders, 55,* 179–192.

Prizant, B. M., & Duchan, J. F. (1981). The functions of immediate echolalia in autistic children. *Journal of Speech and Hearing Disorders, 46,* 241–249.

Prizant, B. M., & Rydell, P. J. (1984). Analysis of functions of delayed echolalia in autistic children. *Journal of Speech and Hearing Research, 27,* 183–192.

Prizant, B. M., & Wetherby, A. M. (1990). Toward an integrated view of early language and communication development and socioemotional development. *Topics in Language Disorders, 10*(4), 1–16.

Proctor, A. (1989). Stages of normal noncry vocal development: A protocol for assessment. *Topics in Language Disorders, 10*(1), 26–42.

Prutting, C. A. (1982). Pragmatics as social competence. *Journal of Speech and Hearing Disorders, 47,* 123–134.

Prutting, C. A., Gallagher, T., & Mulac, A. (1975). The expressive portion of the NSST compared to a spontaneous language sample. *Journal of Speech and Hearing Disorders, 40,* 40–68.

Prutting, C. A., & Kirchner, D. M. (1987). A clinical appraisal of the pragmatic aspects of language. *Journal of Speech and Hearing Disorders, 52,* 105–119.

Public Law 94–142. (1977, August). Implementation of Part B of the Education of the Handicapped Act. *Federal Register.*

Public Law 99–372. (1986, October). The Handicapped Children's Protection Act of 1986. *Federal Register.*

Public Law 99–457. (1986, October). Education of Handicapped Amendments of 1986. *Federal Register.*

Public Law 101–476. (1990, October). Individuals with Disabilities Education Act. *Federal Register.*

Pueschel, S. M. (1987). Health concerns in persons with Down syndrome. In S. M. Pueschel, C. Tingey, J. E. Rynders, A. C. Crocker, & D. M. Crutcher (Eds.), *New perspectives on Down syndrome* (pp. 113–148). Baltimore, MD: Paul H. Brookes.

Purves, A. (1981). Competence in reading. In C. R. Cooper (Ed.), *The nature and measurement of competency in English* (pp. 65–94). Urbana, IL: National Council of Teachers of English.

Quigley, S. P., & Paul, P. V. (1984). *Language and deafness.* Austin, TX: Pro-Ed.

Quigley, S. P., Power, D. J., & Steinkamp, M. W. (1977). The language structure of deaf children. *The Volta Review, 79,* 73–84.

Quigley, S. P., Smith, N. L., & Wilbur, R. B. (1974). Comprehension of relativized sentences by deaf students. *Journal of Speech and Hearing Research, 17,* 325–341.

Ramey, C. T., Trohanis, P. L., & Hostler, S. L. (1982). An introduction. In C. T. Ramey & P. L. Trohanis (Eds.), *Finding and educating high-risk and handicapped infants.* San Antonio, TX: Pro-Ed.

Randall, D., Rynell, J., & Curwen, M. (1974). A study of language development in a sample of three-year-old children. *British Journal of Disorders of Communication, 9,* 3.

Raphael, T. E. (1982). Question–answer strategies for children. *The Reading Teacher, 36,* 186–190.

Raphael, T. E. (1986). Teaching question–answer relationships, revisited. *The Reading Teacher, 39,* 516–522.

Raphael, T. E., & Pearson, P. D. (1982). *The effects of metacognitive strategy awareness training on students' question answering behavior* (Tech. Rep. No. 238). Urbana: University of Illinois, Center for the Study of Reading.

Rapin, I., & Allen, D. A. (1983). Developmental language disorders: Nosologic consideration. In U. Kirk (Ed.), *Neuropsychology of language, reading, and spelling* (pp. 155–184). Orlando, FL: Academic Press.

Rapin, I., Mattis, S., Rowan, A. J., & Golden, G. G. (1977). Verbal auditory agnosia in children. *Developmental Medicine and Child Neurology, 19,* 192–207.

Rapport, M., Stoner, G., DuPaul, G., Birmingham, B., & Tucker, S. (1985). Methylphenidate in hyperactive children: Differential effects of dose on academic, learning and social behavior. *Journal of Abnormal Child Psychology, 13,* 227–244.

Ray, H., Sarff, L. S., & Glassford, J. E. (1984, Summer/Fall). Sound field amplification: An innovative educational intervention for mainstreamed learning disabled students. *The Directive Teacher,* pp. 18–20.

Records, N. L., Tomblin, J. B., & Freese, P. R., (1992). The quality of life of young adults with histories of specific language impairment. *American Journal of Speech-Language Pathology, 1*(2), 44–53.

Reed, V. A. (1986). Language disordered adolescents. In V. A. Reed (Ed.), *An introduction to children with language disorders* (pp. 228–249). New York: Macmillan.

Rees, N. (1973). Auditory processing factors in language disorders: The view from Procrustes' bed. *Journal of Speech and Hearing Disorders, 38,* 304–315.

Rees, N. (1981). Saying more than we know: Is auditory processing disorder a meaningful concept? In R. Keith (Ed.), *Central auditory and language disorders in children* (pp. 94–120). San Diego, CA: College-Hill Press.

Rescorla, L. (1989). The language development survey: A screening tool for delayed language in toddlers. *Journal of Speech and Hearing Disorders, 54,* 587–599.

Rescorla, L., & Manzella, L. (1990, June). *Toddlers with specific expressive language delay (SELD): Language outcome at age 3.* Paper presented at the 11th annual Symposium for Research on Child Language Disorders, Madison, WI.

Restak, R. M. (1979). *The brain: The last frontier.* New York: Warner Books.

Reveron, W. W. (in press). Issues in nondiscriminatory assessment of minority populations. In L. T. Cole (Ed.), *Training manual on communication disorders in multicultural populations.* Rockville, MD: American Speech-Language-Hearing Association.

Reynolds, M. C., & Wang, M. C. (1983). Restructuring "special" school programs: A position paper. *Policy Studies Review, 2*(1), 189–212.

Rice, M. L. (1980). *Cognition to language: Categories, word meanings, and training.* Baltimore, MD: University Park Press.

Rice, M. L. (1983). Contemporary accounts of the cognition/language relationship: Implications for speech-language clinicians. *Journal of Speech and Hearing Disorders, 48,* 347–359.

Rice, M. L., Buhr, J. C., & Nemeth, M. (1990). Fast mapping word-learning abilities of language-delayed preschoolers. *Journal of Speech and Hearing Disorders, 55,* 33–42.

Rice, M. L., Sell, M. A., & Hadley, P. A. (1990). The Social Interactive Coding System (SICS): An on-line, clinically relevant descriptive tool. *Language, Speech, and Hearing Services in Schools, 21,* 2–14.

Rich, H. L., & Ross, S. M. (1989). Students' time on learning tasks in special education. *Exceptional Children, 55,* 508–515.

Richardson, J. S., & Morgan, R. F. (1990). *Reading to learn in the content areas.* Belmont, CA: Wadsworth.

Richardson, K., Calnan, M., Essen, J. & Lambert, L. (1976). The linguistic maturity of 11-year-olds: Some analysis of the written composition of children in the National Development Study. *Journal of Child Language, 3,* 99–115.

Richgels, D., McGee, L. M., Lomax, R., & Sheard, C. (1987). Awareness of four text structures: Effects on recall of expository text. *Reading Research Quarterly, 22,* 177–196.

Rie, E., & Rie, H. (1977). Recall, retention and ritalin. *Journal of Consulting and Clinical Psychology, 45,* 967–972.

Rie, H., Rie, E., & Stewart, S. (1976). Effects of methylphenidate on underachieving children. *Journal of Consulting and Clinical Psychology, 44,* 250–260.

Rief, L. (1990). Finding the value in evaluation: Self-assessment in a middle school classroom. *Educational Leadership, 47*(6), 24–29.

Rimland, B. (1964). *Infantile autism.* Norwalk, CT: Appleton-Century-Crofts.

Ripich, D. N., & Griffith, P. L. (1985, November). *Story structure, cohesion and propositions in learning disabled children.* Paper presented at the meeting of the American Speech-Language-Hearing Association, Washington, DC.

Ritvo, E. R., & Freeman, B. J. (1978). National Society for Autistic Children definition of the syndrome of autism. *Journal of Autism and Childhood Schizophrenia, 8,* 162–167.

Robbins, A. M. (1986). Facilitating language comprehension in young hearing-impaired children. *Topics in Language Disorders, 6*(3), 12–24.

Roberts, J., Burchinal, M., Collier, A. Ramey, C., Koch, M., & Henderson, F. (1989). Otitis media in early childhood and cognitive, academic, and classroom performance of the school-aged child. *Pediatrics, 83,* 477–485.

Roberts, J. E., & Crais, E. R. (1989). Assessing communication skills. In D. B. Bailey, Jr., & M. Wolery (Eds.), *Assessing infants and preschoolers with handicaps* (pp. 339–389). Columbus, OH: Merrill/Macmillan..

Roberts, J. E., Sanyal, M., Burchinal, M., Collier, A. M., Ramey, C. T., & Henderson, F. W. (1986). Otitis media in early childhood and its relationship to later verbal and academic performance. *Pediatrics, 78,* 423–430.

Robinson, F. P. (1970). *Effective study.* New York: Harper & Row.

Roeser, R. J. (1988). Cochlear implants and tactile aids for the profoundly deaf student. In R. J. Roeser & M. P. Downs (Eds.), *Auditory disorders in school children* (pp. 260–280). New York: Thieme Medical Publishers.

Roeser, R. J., & Downs, M. P. (Eds.). (1988). *Auditory disorders in school children.* New York: Thieme Medical Publishers.

Rogers, S. J., D'Eugenio, D. B., Brown, S. L., Donovan, C. M., & Lynch, E. W. (1981). *Early Intervention Developmental Profile.* Ann Arbor: University of Michigan Press.

Rogers-Warren, A., & Warren, S. (1980). Mands for verbalization: Facilitating the display of newly-taught language. *Behavior Modification, 4,* 361–382.

Rohwer, W. D., Jr., & Dempster, F. N. (1977). Memory development and educational processes. In R. V. Kail & J. W. Hagen (Eds.), *Perspectives on the development of memory and cognition* (pp. 407–435). Hillsdale, NJ: Lawrence Erlbaum.

Romski, M. A. (1989, May). Two decades of language research with great apes. *Asha, 31,* 81–82,38.

Romski, M. A., Sevcik, R. A., & Pate, J. L. (1988). Establishment of symbolic communication in persons with severe retardation. *Journal of Speech and Hearing Disorders, 53,* 94–107.

Rosen, C. D., & Gerring, J. P. (1986). *Head trauma: Educational reintegration.* Austin, TX: Pro-Ed.

Rosenbek, J. C., & Wertz, R. T. (1972). A review of 50 cases of developmental apraxia of speech. *Language, Speech, and Hearing Services in Schools, 3,* 23–33.

Rosenberg, J. B., & Lindblad, M. B. (1978). Behavior therapy in a family context: Treating elective mutism. *Family Process, 17,* 77–82.

Rosenthal, R., & Jacobson, L. (1968). *Pygmalion in the classroom: Teacher expectation and pupils' intellectual development.* New York: Holt, Rinehart & Winston.

Rosenzweig, M. R., & Bennett, E. L. (1976). Enriched environments: Facts, factors, and fantasies. In L. Petrinovitch & J. L. McGaugh (Eds.), *Knowing, thinking, and believing* (pp. 179–213). New York: Plenum.

Ross, G. S. (1982). Language functioning and speech development of six children receiving tracheostomy in infancy. *Journal of Communication Disorders, 15,* 95–111.

Ross, M. (1977). Definitions and descriptions. In J. Davis (Ed.), *Our forgotten children: Hard-of-hearing pupils in the schools.* Minneapolis, MN: National Support Systems Project and Division of Personnel Preparation, Bureau of Education for the Handicapped, Department of Health, Education, and Welfare.

Ross, M. (1978). Classroom acoustics and speech intelligibility. In J. Katz (Ed.), *Handbook of clinical audiology* (pp. 469–478). Baltimore, MD: Williams & Wilkins.

Ross, M. (1982). *Hard of hearing children in regular schools.* Englewood Cliffs, NJ: Prentice-Hall.

Ross, M., & Calvert, D. R. (1973). The semantics of deafness. In W. H. Northcott (Ed.), *The hearing impaired child in a regular classroom* (pp. 13–17). Washington, DC: A. G. Bell.

Roth, F. P., & Cassatt-James, E. L. (1989). The language assessment process: Clinical implications for individuals with severe speech impairments. *Augmentative and Alternative Communication, 5,* 165–172.

Roth, F. P., & Clark, D. M. (1987). Symbolic play and social participation abilities of language-impaired and normally developing children. *Journal of Speech and Hearing Disorders, 52,* 17–29.

Roth, F. P., & Perfetti, C. A. (1980). A framework for reading, language comprehension, and language disability. *Topics in Language Disorders, 1*(1), 15–27.

Roth, F. P., & Spekman, N. J. (1984). Assessing the pragmatic abilities of children: Part I. Organizational framework and assessment parameters. *Journal of Speech and Hearing Disorders, 49,* 2–11.

Roth, F. P., & Spekman, N. J. (1986). Narrative discourse: Spontaneously generated stories of learning-disabled and normally achieving students. *Journal of Speech and Hearing Disorders, 51,* 8–23.

Roth, F. P., & Spekman, N. J. (1989). Higher-order language processes and reading disabilities. In A. G. Kamhi & H. W. Catts (Eds.), *Reading disabilities: A developmental language perspective* (pp. 159–197). Austin, TX: Pro-Ed.

Ruben, D. (1988, November). Triumph of the heartland: How two mothers and their disabled sons made their Iowa town a beacon for the nation. *Parenting,* pp. 120–126.

Rubin, D. L. (1982). Adapting syntax in writing to varying audiences as a function of age and social cognitive ability. *Journal of Child Language, 9,* 497–510.

Rubin, D. L. (1984). The influence of communicative context on stylistic variation in writing. In A. Pelligrini & T. Yawkey (Eds.), *The development of oral and written language in social contexts* (pp. 213–231). Norwood, NJ: Ablex.

Rubin, D. L. (1987). Divergence and convergence between oral and written communication. *Topics in Language Disorders, 7*(4), 1–18.

Ruder, K., Bunce, B., & Ruder, C. (1984). Language intervention in a preschool/ classroom setting. In L. McCormick & R. Schiefelbusch (Eds.), *Early language intervention: An introduction* (pp. 267–297). Columbus, OH: Merrill/Macmillan.

Rueda, R. (1989). Defining mild disabilities with language-minority students. *Exceptional Children, 56,* 121–128.

Rumelhart, D. E. (1975). Notes on a schema for stories. In D. G. Bobrow & A. Collins (Eds.), *Representation and understanding: Studies in cognitive science* (pp. 211–236). New York: Academic Press.

Rumelhart, D. E., & McClelland, J. L. (1981). Interactive processing through spreading activation. In A. M. Lesgold & C. A. Perfetti (Eds.), *Interactive processes in reading* (pp. 37–60). Hillsdale, NJ: Lawrence Erlbaum.

Russell, W. K., Quigley, S. P., & Power, D. J. (1976). *Linguistics and deaf children.* Washington, DC: A. G. Bell Association for the Deaf.

Rutter, M. (1965). Speech disorders in a series of autistic children. In A. W. Franklin (Ed.), *Children with communication problems.* London: Plenum.

Rutter, M. (1983). Cognitive deficits in the pathogenesis of autism. *Journal of Child Psychology and Psychiatry, 24,* 513–531.

Rutter, M., Graham, P. J., & Yule, W. (1970). *A neuropsychiatric study in childhood. Clinics in developmental medicine* (No. 35/36). London: S.I.M.P. with Heinemann.

Rutter, M., Tizard, J., & Whitmore, K. (Eds.). (1970). *Education, health, and behavior.* London: Longmans Green.

Rynders, J. E. (1987). History of Down syndrome: The need for a new perspective. In S. M. Pueschel, C. Tingey, J. E. Rynders, A. C. Crocker, & D. M. Crutcher (Eds.), *New perspectives on Down syndrome* (pp. 1–17). Baltimore, MD: Paul H. Brookes.

Saber, D., & Hutchinson, T. A. (1990). *User norms software.* Chicago, IL: Riverside Publishing Company.

Sameroff, A., & Chandler, M. (1975). Reproductive risk and the continuum of caretaking causality. In F. Horowitz (Ed.), *Review of child development research* (Vol. 4, pp. 187–244). Chicago, IL: University of Chicago Press.

Sameroff, A., & Fiese, B. (1990). Transactional regulation and early intervention. In S. Meisels & P. Shonkoff (Eds.), *Early intervention: A handbook of theory, practice, and analysis.* New York: Cambridge University Press.

Sandler, A., Coren, A., & Thurman, S. (1983). A training program for parents of handicapped preschool children: Effects upon mother, father, and child. *Exceptional Children, 49,* 355–357.

Sanford, A. R., & Zelman, J. G. (1981). *The Learning Accomplishment Profile.* Winston-Salem, NC: Kaplan.

Sapir, E. (1949). *Language.* New York: Harcourt, Brace, & World.

Sarachan-Deily, A. B., Hopkins, C., & DeVivo, S. (1983). Correlating the DIAL and the BTBC. *Language, Speech, and Hearing Services in Schools, 14,* 54–59.

Sarff, L., Ray, H., & Bagwell, C. (1981). Why not amplification in every classroom? *Hearing Aid Journal, 34*(10), 11, 47–52.

Sattler, J. M. (1988). *Assessment of Children* (3rd ed.). San Diego: Jerome M. Sattler, Publisher.

Satz, P., & Bullard-Bates, C. (1981). Acquired aphasia in children. In M. T. Sarno (Ed.), *Acquired aphasia* (pp. 399–426). New York: Academic Press.

Satz, P., & Morris, R. (1981). Learning disability subtypes: A review. In F. J. Pirozzolo & M. C. Wittrock (Eds.), *Neuropsychological and cognitive processes in reading* (pp. 109–141). New York: Academic Press.

Sawyer, D. J., Dougherty, C., Shelly, M., & Spaanenburg, L. (1985). Auditory segmenting performance and reading acquisition. In C. S. Simon (Ed.), *Communication skills and classroom success: Assessment of language-learning disabled students* (pp. 375–400). San Diego, CA: College-Hill Press.

Scarborough, H. S., & Dobrich, W. (1985). Illusory recovery from language delay. *Proceedings of the Symposium on Research in Child Language Disorders, 6,* 90–99.

Scarborough, H. S., & Dobrich, W. (1990). Development of children with early language delay. *Journal of Speech and Hearing Disorders, 33,* 70–83.

Schaeffer, A. L., Zigmond, N., Kerr, M. M., & Farra, H. E. (1990). Helping teenagers develop school survival skills. *Teaching Exceptional Children, 23*(1), 6–9.

Schaffer, R. (1977). *Mothering.* Cambridge, MA: Harvard University Press.

Schein, E. (1978). The role of the consultant: Content expert or process facilitator? *Personnel and Guidance Journal, 6,* 339–343.

Scherer, N. J., & Olswang, L. B. (1989). Using structured discourse as a language intervention technique with autistic children. *Journal of Speech and Hearing Disorders, 54,* 383–394.

Schery, T. K. (1985). Correlates of language development in language disordered children. *Journal of Speech and Hearing Disorders, 50,* 73–83.

Schickedanz, J. A. (1989). The place of specific skills in preschool and kindergarten. In D. S. Strickland & L. M. Morrow (Eds.), *Emerging literacy: Young children learn to read and write* (pp. 96–106). Newark, DE: International Reading Association.

Schiff-Myers, N. (1983). From pronoun reversals to correct pronoun usage: A case study of a normally developing child. *Journal of Speech and Hearing Disorders, 48,* 394–402.

Schildroth, A. N., & Karchmer, M. A. (Eds.). (1986). *Deaf children in America.* Austin, TX: Pro-Ed.

Schirmer, B. R. (1989). Framework for using a language acquisition model in assessing semantic and syntactic development and planning instructional goals for hearing-impaired children. *The Volta Review, 91,* 87–94.

Schlesinger, I. M. (1981). Semantic assimilation in the development of relational categories. In H. Whitaker & H. A. Whitaker (Eds.), *Studies in neurolinguistics* (pp. 1–58). New York: Academic Press.

Schlesinger, H. S., & Meadow, K. P. (1972). *Sound and sign: Childhood deafness and mental health.* Berkeley: University of California Press.

Schopler, E., & Mesibov, G. B. (Eds.). (1985). *Communication problems in autism.* New York: Plenum.

Schopler, E., & Mesibov, G. (Eds.). (1986). *Social behavior in autism.* New York: Plenum.

Schory, M. E. (1990). Whole language and the speech-language pathologist. *Language, Speech, and Hearing Services in Schools, 21,* 206–211.

Schreibman, L. (1988). *Developmental Clinical Psychology and Psychiatry. Vol. 15: Autism.* Newbury Park, CA: Sage Publications.

Schuler, A. L., & Goetz, C. (1981). The assessment of severe language disabilities: Communicative and cognitive considerations. *Analysis and Intervention in Developmental Disabilities, 1,* 333–346.

Schumaker, J. B., & Deshler, D. D. (1984). Setting demand variables: A major factor in program planning for the LD adolescent. *Topics in Language Disorders, 4*(2), 22–40.

Schumaker, J. B., Deshler, D., Alley, G., & Warner, M. (1983). Toward the development of an intervention model for learning disabled adolescents: The University of Kansas Institute. *Exceptional Education Quarterly, 4,* 45–74.

Schumaker, J. B., Deshler, D. D., Alley, G. R, Warner, M. M., & Denton, P. H. (1982). Multipass: A learning strategy for improving reading comprehension. *Learning Disability Quarterly, 5,* 295–304.

Schumaker, J. B., Sheldon-Wildgen, J., & Sherman, J. A. (1980). *An observational study of the academic and social behaviors of learning disabled adolescents in the regular classroom* (Research Rep. No. 22). Lawrence, KS: University of Kansas Institute for Research in Learning Disabilities.

Schwartz, L., & McKinley, N. K. (1984). *Daily communication: Strategies for the language disordered adolescent.* Eau Claire, WI: Thinking Publications.

Schwartz, R., & Leonard, L. (1982). Do children pick and choose? An examination of phonological selection and avoidance in early lexical acquisition. *Journal of Child Language, 9,* 319–336.

Schwartz, R., & Leonard, L. (1984). Words, objects, and actions in early lexical acquisition. *Journal of Speech and Hearing Research, 27,* 119–127.

Scinto, L. (1986). *Written language and psychological development.* Boston, MA: Academic Press.

Scott, C. M. (1984, November). *What happened in that: Structural characteristics of school children's narratives.* Paper presented at the Annual Convention of the American Speech-Language-Hearing Association, San Francisco.

Scott, C. M. (1988a). A perspective on the evaluation of school children's narratives. *Language, Speech, and Hearing Services in Schools, 19,* 67–82.

Scott, C. M. (1988b). Producing complex sentences. *Topics in Language Disorders, 8*(2), 44–62.

Scott, C. M. (1988c). Spoken and written syntax. In M. A. Nippold (Ed.), *Later language development: Ages nine through nineteen* (pp. 49–95). Austin, TX: Pro-Ed.

Scott, C. M. (1989). Problem writers: Nature, assessment, and intervention. In A. G. Kamhi & H. W. Catts (Eds.), *Reading disabilities: A developmental language perspective* (pp. 303–344). Austin, TX: Pro-Ed.

Scribner, S., & Cole, M. (1978). Literacy without schooling: Testing for intellectual effects. *Harvard Educational Review, 48,* 448–461.

Scribner, S., & Cole, M. (1980). Literacy without schooling: Testing for intellectual effects. In M. Wolf, M. K. McQuillan, & E. Radwin (Eds.), *Thought and language/Language and reading* (pp. 382–395). Reprint Series No. 14. Cambridge: Harvard Educational Review. (Original work published 1978)

Scruggs, T. E., & Mastropieri, M. A. (1990). Mnemonic instruction for students with learning disabilities: What it is and what it does. *Learning Disability Quarterly, 13,* 271–280.

Searle, J. R. (1969). *Speech acts.* Cambridge, England: Cambridge University Press.

Searle, J. R. (1975). Indirect speech acts. In P. Cole & J. L. Morgan (Eds.), *Syntax and semantics 3: Speech acts* (pp. 59–82). New York: Academic Press.

Searle, J. R. (1976). The classification of illocutionary acts. *Language in Society, 5,* 1–24.

Seashore, H. G. (1955). Methods of expressing test scores. *Test Service Bulletin,* No. 48. Reprinted in W. A. Mehrens (Ed.). (1976). *Readings in Measurement and evaluation in education and psychology* (pp. 65–72). New York: Holt, Rinehart & Winston.

Section 504 of the Rehabilitation Act of 1973, as amended, 29 U.S.C. 794. Regulations last published in *Federal Register, 45* (92), May 9, 1980.

Seidel, U. P., Chadwick, O., & Rutter, M. (1975). Psychological disorders in crippled children with and without brain damage. *Developmental Medicine and Child Neurology, 17,* 563–573.

Seidenberg, P. L. (1988). Cognitive and academic instructional intervention for learning disabled adolescents. *Topics in Language Disorders, 8*(3), 56–71.

Seidenberg, P. L., & Bernstein, D. K. (1986). The comprehension of similes and metaphors by learning-disabled and nonlearning-disabled children. *Language, Speech, and Hearing Services in Schools, 17,* 219–229.

Semel, E. (1976). *Semel auditory processing program.* Chicago, IL: Follett.

Semel, E., & Wiig, E. H. (1980). *Clinical Evaluation of Language Functions: Advanced Level Screening (CELF).* Columbus, OH: Merrill/Macmillan.

Semel, E., Wiig, E. H., & Secord, W. (1987). *Clinical Evaluation of Language Fundamentals—Revised.* San Antonio, TX: The Psychological Corporation.

Shaffer, D. (1985). *Developmental psychology.* Monterey, CA: Brooks/Cole.

Shaffer, D., Bijur, P., Chadwick, O. F. D., & Rutter, M. (1980). Head injury and later reading disability. *Journal of the American Academy of Child Psychiatry, 19,* 592–610.

Shapiro, N. Z., & Anderson, R. (1985). Toward an ethics and etiquette for electronic mail. National Science Foundation Report. Cited in "Stop reading my e-mail!" (1988, November 28) *Academic Technology, 1,* (3).

Shepard, N. T., Davis, J. M., Gorga, M. P., & Stelmachowicz, P. G. (1981). Characteristics of hearing-impaired children in the public schools: Part I—Demographic data. *Journal of Speech and Hearing Disorders, 46,* 123–129.

Shinn, M. R. (Ed.). (1989). *Curriculum-based measurement: Assessing special children.* New York: Guilford Press.

Shriberg, L. D., & Kwiatkowski, J. (1982a). Phonological disorders I: A diagnostic classification system. *Journal of Speech and Hearing Disorders, 47,* 226–241.

Shriberg, L. D., & Kwiatkowski, J. (1982b). Phonological disorders II: A conceptual framework for management. *Journal of Speech and Hearing Disorders, 47,* 242–256.

Shriberg, L. D., & Kwiatkowski, J. (1982c). Phonological disorders III: A procedure for assessing severity of involvement. *Journal of Speech and Hearing Disorders, 47,* 256–270.

Siegel, G. M., Cooper, M., Morgan, J. L., & Brenneise-Sarshad, R. (1990). Imitation of intonation by infants. *Journal of Speech and Hearing Research, 33,* 9–15.

Siegel-Causey, E., Ernst, B., & Guess, D. (1987). Elements of nonsymbolic communication and early interactional processes. In M. Bullis (Ed.), *Communication development in young children with deaf blindness: Literature review III* (pp. 57–102). Monmouth, OR: Deaf-Blind Communication Skills Center.

Siegel-Causey, E., & Guess, D. (1989). *Enhancing nonsymbolic communication interactions among learners with severe disabilities.* Baltimore, MD: Paul H. Brookes.

Silliman, E. R. (1987). Individual differences in the classroom performance of language-impaired students. *Seminars in Speech and Language, 8*(4), 357–375.

Silliman, E. R., & Lamanna, M. L. (1986). Interactional dynamics of turn disruption: Group and individual effects. *Topics in Language Disorders, 6*(2), 28–43.

Silliman, E. R., & Wilkinson, L. C. (1991). *Communicating for learning: Classroom observation and collaboration.* Gaithersburg, MD: Aspen Publishers.

Silva, P. A. (1980). The prevalence, stability and significance of language delay in preschool children. *Developmental Medicine and Child Neurology, 22,* 768–777.

Silva, P. A., Kirkland, C., Simpson, A., Stewart, I., & Williams, S. (1982). Some developmental and behavioral problems associated with bilateral otitis media with effusion. *Journal of Learning Disabilities, 15,* 417–421.

Simmons, A. A. (1962). A comparison of type-token ratios of spoken and written language of deaf and hearing children. *Volta Review, 64,* 417–421.

Simon, C., & Fourcin, A. J. (1978). Cross-language study of speech pattern learning. *Journal of the Acoustical Society of America, 63,* 925–935.

Simon, C. S. (1977). Cooperative programming: A partnership between the learning disabilities teacher and the speech-language pathologist. *Language, Speech, and Hearing Services in Schools, 8,* 188–200.

Simon, C. S. (1985). Teaching logical thinking and discussion skills. In C. S. Simon (Ed.), *Communication skills and classroom success: Therapy methodologies for language-learning disabled students* (pp. 219–237). San Diego, CA: College-Hill.

Simon, C. S. (1987). Out of the broom closet and into the classroom: The emerging SLP. *Journal of Childhood Communication Disorders, 11,* 41–66.

Simons, R. (1987). *After the tears: Parents talk about raising a child with a disability.* Orlando, FL: Harcourt, Brace, Jovanovich.

Singer, H., & Ruddell, R. B. (Eds.). (1985). *Theoretical models and processes of reading* (3rd ed.). Newark, DE: International Reading Association.

Singer, S., & Singer, J. (1977). *Partners in play.* New York: Harper & Row.

Sitnick, V. N., Rushmer, N., & Arpan, R. (1982). *Parent–infant communication: A program of clinical and home training for parents and hearing impaired infants* (rev. ed.). Portland, OR: IHR Publications, Good Samaritan Hospital and Medical Center.

Skarakis-Doyle, E., MacLellan, N., & Mullin, K. (1990). Nonverbal indicants of comprehension monitoring in language-disordered children. *Journal of Speech and Hearing Disorders, 55,* 461–467.

Skarakis-Doyle, E., & Mullin, K. (1990). Comprehension monitoring in language-disordered children: A preliminary investigation of cognitive and linguistic factors. *Journal of Speech and Hearing Disorders, 55,* 700–705.

Skinner, B. F. (1957). *Verbal behavior.* Norwalk, CT: Appleton-Century-Crofts.

Skinner, B. F. (1983). *A matter of consequences.* New York: Albert A. Knopf.

Skinner, M. W. (1978). The hearing of speech during language acquisition. *Otolaryngology Clinics of North America, 11,* 631–650.

Slater, W. H., & Graves, M. F. (1989). Research on expository text: Implications for teachers. In K. D. Muth (Ed.), *Children's comprehension of text* (pp. 140–166). Newark, DE: International Reading Association.

Slavin, R. E. (1983). *Cooperative learning.* New York: Longman.

Slingerland, B. H. (1981). Specific language disability: Some general characteristics. In the *Slingerland multi-sensory approach to language arts for specific language disability children in the primary grades.* Cambridge, MA: Educators Publishing Service.

Sloan, C. (1986). *Treating auditory processing difficulties in children.* Austin, TX: Pro-Ed.

Sloane, H., & MacAulay, B. (Eds.). (1968). *Operant procedures in remedial speech and language training.* Boston, MA: Houghton Mifflin.

Slobin, D. (1979). *Psycholinguistics* (2nd ed.). Glenview, IL: Scott, Foresman.

Smith v. Robinson, 104 S. Ct. 3457 (1984).

Smith, C. (1970). An experimental approach to children's linguistic competence. In J. Hayes (Ed.), *Cognition and the development of language* (pp. 109–135). New York: Wiley.

Smith, F. (1973). *Psycholinguistics and reading.* New York: Holt, Rinehart & Winston.

Smith, F. (1975). *Comprehension and learning: A conceptual framework for teachers.* New York: Holt, Rinehart & Winston.

Smith, P. L., & Friend, M. (1986). Training learning disabled adolescents in a strategy for using text structure to aid recall of instructional prose. *Learning Disabilities Research, 2,* 38–44.

Smitherman, G. (1985). "What go round come round": King in perspective. In C. K. Brooks (Ed.), *Tapping potential: English and language arts for the Black learner.* Urbana, IL: National Council of Teachers of English.

Snow, C. E. (1977a). The development of conversation between mothers and babies. *Journal of Child Language, 4,* 1–22.

Snow, C. E. (1977b). Mothers' speech research: From input to interaction. In C. E. Snow & C. A. Ferguson (Eds.), *Talking to children: Language input and acquisition* (pp. 31–49). Cambridge, England: Cambridge University Press.

Snow, C. E. (1983). Literacy and language: Relationships during the preschool years. *Harvard Educational Review, 53* (2), 165–189.

Snow, C. E. (Ed.). (1984). Language development and disorders in the social context [Special issue] *Topics in Language Disorders, 4*(4).

Snow, C. E. (1991). Diverse conversational contexts for the acquisition of various language skills. In J. Miller (Ed.), *Research on child language disorders* (pp. 105–124). Austin, TX: Pro-Ed.

Snow, C. E., & Ferguson, C. (1977). *Talking to children.* New York: Cambridge University Press.

Snow, C. E., & Ninio, A. (1986). The contracts of literacy: What children learn from learning to read books. In W. Teale & E. Sulzby (Eds.), *Emergent literacy: Writing and reading* (pp. 116–138). Norwood, NJ: Ablex.

Snyder, L. S., & Downey, D. C. (1983). Pragmatics and information processing. *Topics in Language Disorders, 4*(1), 75–86.

Snyder, L. S., & Downey, D. M. (1991). The language–reading relationship in normal and reading-disabled children. *Journal of Speech and Hearing Research, 34,* 129–140.

Sparks, S. N. (1984). *Birth defects and speech–language disorders.* Austin, TX: Pro-Ed.

Sparks, S. N. (1989a). Assessment and intervention with at-risk infants and toddlers: Guidelines for the speech–language pathologist. *Topics in Language Disorders, 10*(1), 43–56.

Sparks, S. N. (1989b). Speech and language in maltreated children: Response to McCauley and Swisher (1987). *Journal of Speech and Hearing Disorders, 54,* 124–126.

Sparks, S. N., Clark, M. J., Erickson, R. L., & Oas, D. B. (1990). *Infants at risk for communication disorders: The professional's role with the newborn.* Tucson, AZ: Communication Skill Builders.

Spearman, C. E. (1923). *The nature of intelligence and the principles of cognition.* London: Macmillan.

Spearman, C. E. (1927). *The abilities of man.* New York: Macmillan.

Springer, S. P., & Deutsch, G. (1985). *Left brain, right brain* (rev. ed.). New York: W. H. Freeman.

Squire, J. R. (1964). *The responses of adolescents while reading four short stories* (NCTE Res. Rep. No. 2). Urbana, IL: National Council of Teachers of English.

Squire, J. R. (Ed.). (1987). *The dynamics of language learning: Research in reading and English.* Urbana, IL: ERIC Clearinghouse on Reading and Communication Skills.

Staats, A. (1971). Linguistic-mentalistic theory versus an explanatory S-R learning theory of language development. In D. Slobin (Ed.), *The ontogenesis of grammar.* (pp. 103–150) New York: Academic Press.

Stainback, S., & Stainback, W. (1988). *Understanding and conducting qualitative research.* Reston, VA: The Council for Exceptional Children.

Stainback, W., Stainback, S., Courtnage, L., & Jaben, T. (1985). Facilitating mainstreaming by modifying the mainstream. *Exceptional Children, 52,* 144–152.

Stampe, D. (1969). The acquisition of phonetic representation. In R. I. Binnick, A. Davison, G. M. Greene, & J. L. Morgan (Eds.), *Papers from the fifth regional meeting, Chicago Linguistic Society.* Chicago, IL: Chicago Linguistic Society.

Stanovich, K. E. (1985). Explaining the variance in reading ability in terms of psychological processes: What have we learned? *Annals of Dyslexia, 35,* 67–96.

Stanovich, K. E. (1986). Explaining the variance in reading ability in terms of psychological processes: What have we learned? *Annals of Dyslexia, 35,* 67–96.

Stanovich, K. E. (1988). The right and wrong places to look for the cognitive locus of reading disability. *Annals of Dyslexia, 38,* 154–177.

Stark, R. E., Bernstein, L. E., Condino, R., Bender, M., Tallal, P., & Catts, H. (1984). Four-year follow-up study of language impaired children. *Annals of Dyslexia, 34,* 49–68.

Stark, R. E., & Tallal, P. (1981). Selection of children with specific language deficits. *Journal of Speech and Hearing Disorders, 46,* 114–122.

Statewide Project for the Deaf. (1982). *Developmental language centered curriculum for hearing impaired children: Stage 0.* Austin, TX: Texas Education Agency, Resource Center and Publications.

Stauffer, R. G. (1975). *Directing the reading–thinking process.* New York: Harper & Row.

Steckol, K. F., Leonard, L. B. (1981). Sensorimotor development and the use of prelinguistic performatives. *Journal of Speech and Hearing Research, 24,* 262–268.

Stein, N., & Glenn, C. (1979). An analysis of story comprehension in elementary school children. In R. Freedle (Ed.), *New directions in discourse processing* (Vol. 2, pp. 53–120). Norwood, NJ: Ablex.

Stephens, M. I., & Montgomery, A. A. (1985). A critique of recent relevant standardized tests. *Topics in Language Disorders, 5*(3), 21–45.

Stern, D. (1985). *The interpersonal world of the infant.* New York: Basic Books.

Sternberg, L. (1982). Communication instruction. In L. Sternberg & G. L. Adams (Eds.), *Educating severely and profoundly handicapped students* (pp. 209–241). Rockville, MD: Aspen.

Sternberg, L., Battle, C., & Hill, J. (1980). Prelanguage communication programming for the severely and profoundly handicapped. *JASH* (Journal of the Association for Persons With Severe Handicaps), *5,* 224–233.

Sternberg, L., McNerney, C. D., & Pegnatore, L. (1985). Developing co-active imitative behaviors with profoundly mentally handicapped students. *Education and Training of the Mentally Retarded, 20,* 260–267.

Sternberg, L., & Owens, A. (1984). Establishing pre-language signalling behaviour with profoundly mentally handicapped students: A preliminary investigation. *Journal of Mental Deficiency Research, 29,* 81–93.

Sternberg, L., Pegnatore, L., & Hill, C. (1983). Establishing interactive communication behaviors with profoundly mentally handicapped students. *JASH* (Journal of the Association for Persons With Severe Handicaps), *8,* 39–46.

Sternberg, L., Ritchey, H., Pegnatore, L., Wills, L., & Hill, C. (1986). *A curriculum for profoundly handicapped students.* Rockville, MD: Aspen.

Sternberg, R. J. (1979). The nature of mental abilities. *American Psychologist, 34,* 214–230.

Sternberg, R. J. (1981). The nature of intelligence. *New York University Education Quarterly, 12,* 10–17.

Sternberg, R. J. (1985). *Beyond IQ: A Triarchic theory of human intelligence.* New York: Cambridge University Press.

Sternberg, R. J. (1988). *The triarchic mind.* New York: Viking.

Sternberg, R. J., Okagaki, L., & Jackson, A. S. (1990). Practical intelligence for success in school. *Educational Leadership, 48*(1), 35–39.

Stewart, S. R. (1985). Development of written language proficiency: Methods for teaching text structure. In C. Simon (Ed.), *Communication skills and classroom success: Therapy methodologies for language–learning disabled students* (pp. 341–361). San Diego, CA: College-Hill. Reprinted in C. S. Simon (Ed.). (1991), *Communication skills and classroom success: Assessment and therapy methodologies for language and learning disabled students* (pp. 419–432). Eau Claire, WI: Thinking Publications.

Stickler, K. R. (1987). *Guide to analysis of language transcripts.* Eau Claire, WI: Thinking Publications.

Stockman, I. J., & Vaughn-Cooke, F. B. (1986). Implications of semantic category research for the language assessment of nonstandard speakers. *Topics in Language Disorders, 6* (4), 15–25.

Stoel-Gammon, C. (1987). Phonological skills of 2-year-olds. *Language, Speech, and Hearing Services in Schools, 18,* 323–329.

Stoel-Gammon, C. (1988). Prelinguistic vocalizations of hearing-impaired and normally hearing subjects: A comparison of consonantal inventories. *Journal of Speech and Hearing Disorders, 53,* 302–315.

Stoel-Gammon, C., & Otomo, K. (1986). Babbling development of hearing-impaired and normally hearing subjects. *Journal of Speech and Hearing Disorders, 51,* 33–41.

Stokes, T. F., & Baer, D. M. (1977). An implicit technology of generalization. *Journal of Applied Behavioral Analysis, 10,* 349–367.

Stremel-Campbell, K., & Campbell, C. R. (1985). Training techniques that may facilitate generalization. In S. F. Warren & A. K. Rogers-Warren (Eds.), Teaching functional language (pp. 251–285). Austin, TX: Pro-Ed.

Strickland, D. S., & Taylor, D. (1989). Family storybook reading: Implications for children, families, and curriculum. In D. S. Strickland & L. M. Morrow (Eds.), *Emerging literacy: Young children learn to read and write* (pp. 27–34). Newark, DE: International Reading Association.

Strominger, A. Z., & Bashir, A. S. (1977, November). *Longitudinal study of language-delayed children.* Paper presented at the annual convention of the American Speech-Language-Hearing Association, Chicago.

Strong, W. (1986). Creative approaches to sentence combining. *Theory and research into practice (TRIP).* Urbana, IL: ERIC Clearinghouse on Reading and Communication Skills.

Sturm, J. M. (1990). *Teacher and student discourse variables in academic communication.* Unpublished masters thesis, Western Michigan University, Kalamazoo, MI.

Sturm, J. M., & Nelson, N. W. (1989, November 19). *Mediated language and cognitive intervention for post-leukemia encephalopathy—Sarah's story.* Poster presentation at the Annual Conference of the American Speech-Language-Hearing Association, St. Louis.

Suritsky, S. K., & Hughes, C. A. (1991). Benefits of notetaking: Implications for secondary and postsecondary students with learning disabilities. *Learning Disability Quarterly, 14,* 7–18.

Sussman, H. M. (1989, May). A bird brain approach to language. *Asha, 31,* 83–86.

Sutter, J. C., & Johnson, C. J. (1988, November). *Production of later acquired verb forms: An issue of oral vs. literate language.* Paper presented at the American Speech-Language-Hearing Association Convention, New Orleans.

Sutter, J. C., & Johnson, C. J. (1990). School-age children's metalinguistic awareness of grammaticality in verb form. *Journal of Speech and Hearing Research, 33,* 84–95.

Sutton, A. C. (1989). The social-verbal competence of AAC users. *Augmentative and Alternative Communication, 5,* 150–164.

Sutton-Smith, B. (1986). The development of fictional narrative performances. *Topics in Language Disorders, 7*(1), 1–10.

Swisher, L., & Demetras, M. J. (1985). The expressive language characteristics of autistic children compared with mentally retarded or specific language-impaired children. In E. Schopler & G. B. Mesibov (Eds.), *Communication problems in autism* (pp. 147–162). New York: Plenum.

Swoger, P. A. (1989). Scott's gift. *English Journal, 78,* 61–65.

Szkeres, S. F., Ylvisaker, M., & Holland, A. L. (1985). Cognitive rehabilitation therapy: A framework for intervention. In M. Ylvisaker, M. (Ed.), *Head injury rehabilitation: Children and adolescents* (pp. 219–246). Austin, TX: Pro-Ed.

Taff, T. G. (1990). Success for the unsuccessful. *Educational Leadership, 48* (1), 71–72.

Tager-Flusberg, H. (1985). Putting words together: Morphology and syntax in the preschool years. In J. B. Gleason (Ed.), *The development of language* (pp. 135–171). Columbus, OH: Merrill/Macmillan.

Tager-Flusberg, H. (1989). Putting words together: Morphology and syntax in the preschool years. In J. B. Gleason (Ed.), *The development of language* (2nd. ed., pp. 135–165). Columbus, OH: Merrill/Macmillan.

Tallal, P. (1980). Auditory temporal processing, phonics, and reading disabilities in children. *Brain and Language, 9,* 182–198.

Tallal, P. (1988). Developmental language disorders. In J. F. Kavanagh & T. J. Truss, Jr. (Eds.), *Learning disabilities: Proceedings of the National Conference* (pp. 181–272). Parkton, MD: York Press.

Tallal, P., & Piercy, M. (1973). Developmental aphasia: Impaired rate of non-verbal processing as a function of sensory modality. *Neuropsychologia, 11,* 389–398.

Tallal, P., & Piercy, M. (1975). Developmental aphasia: The perception of brief vowels and extended stop consonants. *Neuropsychologia, 13,* 69–74.

Tallal, P., & Piercy, M. (1978). Defects of auditory perception in children with developmental dysphasia. In N. A. Wyke (Ed.), *Developmental dysphasia* (pp. 63–84). San Diego, CA: Academic Press.

Tallal, P., & Stark, R. (1976). Relation between speech perception and speech production impairment in children with developmental dysphasia. *Brain and Language, 3,* 305–317.

Tallal, P., Stark, R., Kallman, C., & Mellits, D. (1981). A reexamination of some nonverbal perceptual abilities of language-impaired and normal children as a function of age and sensory modality. *Journal of Speech and Hearing Research, 24,* 351–357.

Tamaroff, M., Miller, D. R., Murphy, M. L., Salwen, R., Ghavini, F., & Nir, Y. (1982). Immediate and long-term posttherapy neuropsychologic performance in children with acute lymphoblastic leukemia treated without central nervous system radiation. *The Journal of Pediatrics, 101,* 524–529.

Tannen, D. (1982). *Spoken and written language: Exploring orality and literacy.* Norwood, NJ: Ablex.

Tateyama-Sniezek, K. M. (1990). Cooperative learning: Does it improve the academic achievement of students with handicaps? *Exceptional Children, 56,* 426–437.

Tattershall, S. (1987). Mission impossible: Learning how a classroom works before it's too late! *Journal of Childhood Communication Disorders, 11,* 181–184.

Taylor, B. M., & Beach, R. W. (1984). The effects of text structures instruction on middle grade students' comprehension and production of expository text. *Reading Research Quarterly, 19,* 134–146.

Taylor, D. (1983). *Family literacy: Young children learning to read and write.* Portsmouth, NH: Heinemann.

Taylor, D., & Dorsey-Gaines, C. (1987). *Growing up literate: Learning from inner city families.* Portsmouth, NH: Heinemann.

Taylor, O. L. (1972). An introduction to the historical development of Black English. *Language, Speech, and Hearing Services in Schools, 3*(4), 5–15.

Taylor, O. L. (1985). *Nature of communication disorders in culturally and linguistically diverse populations.* Austin, TX: Pro-Ed.

Taylor, O. L. (Ed.). (1986). *Nature of communication disorders in culturally and linguistically diverse populations.* San Diego, CA: College-Hill Press.

Taylor, O. L. (in press). Clinical practice as a social occasion. In L. Cole & V. R. Deal (Eds.), *Communication disorders in multicultural populations.* Rockville, MD: American Speech-Language-Hearing Association.

Taylor, O. L., & Payne, K. T. (1983). Culturally valid testing: A proactive approach. *Topics in Language Disorders, 3*(3), 8–20.

Taylor, O. L., Stroud, V., Moore, E., Hurst, C., & Williams, R. (1969). Philosophies and goals of ASHA Black Caucus. *Asha, 11,* 216–218.

Templin, M. (1957). *Certain language skills in children.* Minneapolis, MN: University of Minnesota Press.

Templin, M., & Darley, F. (1960). *The Templin-Darley Test of Articulation.* Iowa City, IA: University of Iowa, Iowa City Bureau of Educational Research.

Terrell, B. Y., Schwartz, R. G., Prelock, P. A., & Messick, C. K. (1984). Symbolic play in normal and language-impaired children. *Journal of Speech and Hearing Research, 27,* 424–429.

Terrell, S. L., & Terrell, F. (1983). Distinguishing linguistic differences from disorders: The past, present, and future of nonbiased assessment. *Topics in Language Disorders, 3* (3), 1–7.

Tharp, R. G., & Gallimore, R. (1988). *Rousing minds to life: Teaching, learning, and schooling in social context.* New York: Cambridge Press.

Thatcher, V. S. (Ed.). (1980). *The new Webster Encyclopedic dictionary of the English language.* Chicago: Consolidated Book Publishers.

Thomas, C., Englert, C. S., & Morsink, C. (1984). Modifying the classroom program in language. In C. V. Morsink (Ed.), *Teaching special needs students in regular classrooms* (pp. 239–276). Boston, MA: Little, Brown.

Thorndike, E. L. (1917). Reading as reasoning: A study of mistakes in paragraph reading. *Journal of Educational Psychology, 8,* 323–332.

Thorndike, R. L., Hagen, E. P., & Sattler, J. M. (1986). *Stanford-Binet Intelligence Scale—Revised.* Chicago: Riverside.

Thorndyke, P. W. (1977). Cognitive structures in comprehension and memory of narrative discourse. *Cognitive Psychology, 9,* 77–110.

Tibbits, D. (1982). *Language disorders in adolescents.* Lincoln, NE: Cliff Notes.

Tiegerman, E. (1989). Autism: Learning to communicate. In D. Bernstein & E. Tiegerman (Eds.), *Language and communication disorders in children* (2nd ed., pp. 298–338). Columbus, OH: Merrill/Macmillan.

Tiegerman, E., & Siperstein, M. (1984). Individual patterns of interaction in the mother–child dyad: Implications for parent intervention. *Topics in Language Disorders, 4*(4), 50–61.

Tierney, R. J. (1990). Redefining reading comprehension. *Educational Leadership, 47*(6), 37–42.

Tierney, R. J., & Cunningham, J. W. (1984). Research on teaching reading comprehension. In P. D. Pearson (Ed.), *Handbook of reading research* (pp. 609–655). New York: Longman.

Timothy W. v. Rochester School District, 875 F. 2d 954 (1st Cir. New Hampshire 1989).

Timothy W. v. Rochester School District, 110 S. Ct. 519, 493 U. S. 983 (1989).

Tindal, G., & Parker, R. (1991). Identifying measures for evaluating written expression. *Learning Disabilities Research and Practice, 6,* 211–218.

Tizard, B., Philips, J., & Plewis, J. (1976). Play in preschool centers: Play measures and their relation to age, sex and IQ. *Journal of Child Psychology and Psychiatry, 17,* 251–264.

Tjossem, T. D. (1976). Early intervention: Issues and approaches. In T. D. Tjossem (Ed.), *Intervention strategies for high risk infants and young children.* Austin, TX: Pro-Ed.

Tomblin, J. B. (1983). An examination of the concept of disorder in the study of language variation. *Proceedings from the Symposium on Research in Child Language Disorders, 4,* 81–109.

Tomblin, J. B. (1989, November). *Comments on causation in specific language disorders.* Paper presented at the annual convention of the American Speech-Language-Hearing Association, St. Louis.

Tomblin, J. B., Freese, P., & Records, N. (1990, June). *Language, cognition, and social characteristics of young adults with histories of developmental language disorder.* Paper presented at the symposium for research on child language disorders, Madison, WI.

Tonjes, M. J., & Zintz, M. V. (1987). *Teaching reading thinking study skills in content classrooms.* Dubuque, IA: William C. Brown.

Torgesen, J. K. (1982). The learning disabled child as an interactive learner: Educational implications. *Topics in Learning and LD, 2,* 45–52.

Torgesen, J. K., & Licht, B. G. (1983). The learning disabled child as an inactive learner: Retrospect and prospects. In J. D. McKinney & L. Feagans (Eds.), *Current topics in learning disabilities* (pp. 3–31). Norwood, NJ: Ablex Publishing.

Torgesen, J. K., & Torgesen, J. L. (1985). WORDS [Computer program]. Tallahassee: Florida State University.

Trapani, C. (1990). *Transition goals for adolescents with learning disabilities.* Boston, MA: Little, Brown.

Trevarthen, C. (1974). Prespeech in communication of infants with adults. *Journal of Child Language 1,* 335–337.

Tronick, E. (1989). Emotions and emotional communication in infants. *American Psychologist, 44,* 112–119.

Tronick, E., Als, H., & Adamson, L. (1979). Structure of early face-to-face communicative interactions. In M. Bullowa (Ed.), *Before speech.* New York: Cambridge University Press.

Trout, M., & Foley, G. (1989). Working with families of handicapped infants and toddlers. *Topics in Language Disorders, 10*(1), 57–67.

Tucher, A. (Ed.). (1990). *Bill Moyers: A world of ideas (II): Public opinions from private citizens.* New York: Doubleday.

Tucker, J. A. (1985). Curriculum-based assessment: An introduction. *Exceptional Children, 52,* 199–204.

Turner, R. G. (1990, September). Recommended guidelines for infant hearing screening: Analysis. *Asha, 32,* 57–61, 66.

Tyack, D. L. (1981). Teaching complex sentences. *Language, Speech, and Hearing Services in Schools, 12,* 49–56.

Tyack, D. L., & Gottsleben, R. H. (1977). *Language sampling, analysis, and training: A handbook for teachers and clinicians.* Palo Alto, CA: Consulting Psychologists Press.

Tyack, D. L., & Gottsleben, R. H. (1986). Acquisition of complex sentences. *Language, Speech, and Hearing Services in Schools, 17,* 160–174.

U.S. Department of Health, Education, and Welfare. (1969). *Minimal brain dysfunction in children.* (Public Health Service Publication No. 2015). Washington, DC: U.S. Government Printing Office.

U.S. Department of Health and Human Services. (1981). *Study findings of the National Study of the Incidence and Severity of Child Abuse and Neglect* [DHHS Publication No. (OHDS) 82–30325]. Washington, DC: U.S. Government Printing Office.

Vail, P. L. (1987). *Smart kids with school problems: Things to know and ways to help.* New York: E. P. Dutton.

van Dijk, J. (1965). The first steps of the deaf/blind child toward language. *Proceedings of the conference on the deaf/blind, Refsnes, Denmark.* Boston, MA: Perkins School for the Blind.

van Dijk, T., & Kintsch, W. (1978). Cognitive psychology and discourse: Recalling and summarizing stories. In W. U. Dressler (Eds.), *Current trends in textlinguistics* (pp. 61–80). New York: Walter de Druyter.

Vanderheiden, G. C., & Lloyd, L. L. (1986). Communication systems and their components. In S. W. Blackstone (Ed.), *Augmentative communication: An introduction* (pp. 49–161). Rockville, MD: American Speech-Language-Hearing Association.

Vanderheiden, G. C., & Yoder, D. E. (1986). Overview. In S. W. Blackstone (Ed.), *Augmentative communication: An introduction* (pp. 1–28). Rockville, MD: American Speech-Language-Hearing Association.

van der Lely, H. K. J., & Harris, M. (1990). Comprehension of reversible sentences in specifically language-impaired children. *Journal of Speech and Hearing Disorders, 55,* 101–117.

Van Dongen, R., & Westby, C. E. (1986). Building the narrative mode of thought through children's literature. *Topics in Language Disorders, 7*(1), 70–83.

Vane, J. (1975). Vane Evaluation of Language Scale. *Archives of Behavioral Sciences, 49,* 3–33.

van Kleeck, A. (1984). Metalinguistic skills: Cutting across spoken and written language and problem-solving abilities. In G. P. Wallach & K. G. Butler (Eds.), *Language learning disabilities in school-age children* (pp. 128–153). Baltimore, MD: Williams & Wilkins.

van Kleeck, A. (1990). Emergent literacy: Learning about print before learning to read. *Topics in Language Disorders, 10*(2), 25–45.

Vaughn, S., McIntosh, R., & Spencer-Rowe, J. (1991). Peer rejection is a stubborn thing: Increasing peer acceptance of rejected students with learning disabilities. *Learning Disabilities Research and Practice, 6,* 83–88.

Vaughn-Cooke, F. B. (1983). Improving language assessment in minority children. *Asha, 25*(9), 29–34.

Vaughn-Cooke, F. B. (1989). Speech–language pathologists and educators: Time to strengthen the partnership. In B. A. Stewart (Ed.), *ASHA Reports No. 17, Partnerships in education: Toward a literate America* (pp. 67–72). Rockville, MD: American Speech-Language-Hearing Association.

Vavra, E. (1987). Grammar and syntax: The student's perspective. *English Journal, 76*(6), 42–48.

Vellutino, F. (1979). *Dyslexia: Theory and research.* Cambridge, MA: MIT Press.

Vellutino, F. R., & Schub, M. J. (1982). Assessment of disorders in formal school language: Disorders in reading. *Topics in Language Disorders, 2*(4), 20–33.

Venezky, R. L. (1970). *The structure of English orthography.* The Hague, The Netherlands: Mouton.

Vernon, M. (1969). Sociological and psychological factors associated with hearing loss. *Journal of Speech and Hearing Research, 12,* 541–563.

Vygotsky, L. S. (1962). E. Hanfmann & G. Vakar (Eds. & Trans.), *Thought and language.* Cambridge, MA: MIT Press. (Original work published 1934)

Vygotsky, L. S. (1967). Play and its role in the mental development of the child. *Soviet Psychology, 5,* 6–18.

Vygotsky, L. S. (1978). *Mind in society: The development of higher psychological processes.* Cambridge, MA: Harvard University Press.

Wada, J. A. (1977). Prelanguage and functional asymmetry of the infant brain. *Annals of the New York Academy of Sciences, 299,* 370–379.

Wada, J. A., Clark, R., & Hamm, A. (1975). Cerebral hemispheric asymmetry in humans. *Archives of Neurology, 32,* 239–246.

Wallach, G. P. (1984). Later language learning: Syntactic structures and strategies. In G. P. Wallach & K. G. Butler (Eds.), *Language learning disabilities in school-age children* (pp. 82–102). Baltimore, MD: Williams & Wilkins.

Wallach, G. P. (1989). Current research as a map for language intervention in the school years. *Seminars in Speech and Language, 10*(3), 205–217.

Wallach, G. P. (1990). Magic Buries Celtics: Looking for broader interpretations of language learning and literacy. *Topics in Language Disorders, 10*(2), 63–80.

Wallach, G. P., & Miller, L. (1988). *Language intervention and academic success.* Austin, TX: Pro-Ed.

Wanat, P. (1983). Social skills: An awareness program with learning disabled adolescents. *Journal of Learning Disabilities, 16,* 35–38.

Wang, M. C., & Reynolds, M. C. (1985). Avoiding the "Catch 22" in special education reform. *Exceptional Children, 51*, 497–502.

Warren, D. H. (1984). *Blindness and early childhood development.* New York: Academic Foundation for the Blind.

Warren, S. F. (1988). A behavioral approach to language generalization. *Language, Speech, and Hearing Services in Schools, 19*, 292–303.

Warren, S. F., & Bambara, L. M. (1989). An experimental analysis of milieu language intervention: Teaching the action–object form. *Journal of Speech and Hearing Disorders, 54*, 448–461.

Warren, S. F., & Kaiser, A. P. (1986). Incidental language teaching: A critical review. *Journal of Speech and Hearing Disorders, 51*, 291–299.

Warren, S. F., McQuarter, R. J., & Rogers-Warren, A. K. (1984). The effects of mands and models on the speech of unresponsive language-delayed preschool children. *Journal of Speech and Hearing Disorders, 49*, 43–52.

Warren, S. F., & Rogers-Warren, A. K. (1983). A longitudinal analysis of language generalization among adolescents with severely handicapping conditions. *JASH* (Journal of the Association for Persons With Severe Handicaps), *8*(4), 18–31.

Warren, S. F., & Rogers-Warren, A. K. (Eds). (1985). *Teaching functional language.* Baltimore, MD: University Park Press.

Wasserman, G. A., Green, A., & Allen, R. (1983). Going beyond abuse: Maladaptive patterns of interaction in abusing mother-infant pairs. *Journal of the American Academy of Child Psychiatry, 22*, 245–252.

Watson, B. U., Sullivan, P. M., Moeller, M. P., & Jensen, J. K. (1982). Nonverbal intelligence and English language ability in deaf children. *Journal of Speech and Hearing Disorders, 47*, 199–204.

Watson, L., Lord, C., Schaffer, B., & Schopler, E. (1989). *Teaching spontaneous communication to autistic and developmentally handicapped children.* New York: Irvington Publishers.

Watzlawick, P., Beavin, J. H., & Jackson, D. D. (1967). *Pragmatics of human communication.* New York: W. W. Norton.

Weaver, C. (1982). Welcoming errors as signs of growth. *Language Arts, 59*, 438–444.

Weber-Olsen, M., Putnam-Sims, P., & Gannon, J. D. (1983). Elicited imitation and the *Oral Language Sentence Imitation Screening Test* (OLSIST): Content or context? *Journal of Speech and Hearing Disorders, 48*, 368–378.

Wechsler, D. (1967). *Wechsler Preschool and Preprimary Scale of Intelligence.* San Antonio, TX: Psychological Corporation.

Wechsler, D. (1974). *Wechsler Intelligence Scale for Children–Revised.* San Antonio, TX: Psychological Corporation.

Wechsler, D. (1981). *Wechsler Adult Intelligence Scale— Revised.* San Antonio, TX: Psychological Corporation.

Weicker, L. (1989). "Testimony on ADA," *Word From Washington,* pp. 17–18.

Weiner, B. (1979). A theory of motivation for some class-room experiences. *Journal of Educational Psychology, 71*, 3–25.

Weiner, B. (1980). The role of affect in rational (attribu-tional) approaches to human motivation. *Educational Researcher, 9*, 4–11.

Weiner, P. S. (1985). The value of follow-up studies. *Topics in Language Disorders, 5*(3), 78–92.

Weiss, A. L. (1986). Classroom discourse and the hearing-impaired child. *Topics in Language Disorders, 6* (3), 60–70.

Wells, G. (1986). *The meaning makers: Children learning language and using language to learn.* Portsmouth, NH: Heinemann.

Wepman, J. M., Jones, L. V., Bock, R. D., & van Pelt, D. (1960). Studies in aphasia: Background and theoretical formulations. *Journal of Speech and Hearing Disorders, 25*, 323–332.

Werner, H., & Kaplan, E. (1950). The acquisition of word meanings: A developmental study. *Monographs of the Society of Research in Child Development, 15* (Serial No. 51).

Werner, E. O., & Kresheck, J. D. (1983). *Structured Photographic Expressive Language Test—II* (SPELT-II). Sandwich, IL: Janelle Publications, Inc.

West, J., & Weber, J. (1973). A phonological analysis of the spontaneous language of a four-year-old hard-of-hearing child. *Journal of Speech and Hearing Disorders, 38*, 25–35.

Westby, C. E. (1980). Assessment of cognitive and lan-guage abilities through play. *Language, Speech, and Hearing Services in Schools, 11*, 154–168.

Westby, C. E. (1982). *Cognitive and linguistic aspects of children's narrative development* [Audiotape journal]. New York: Grune & Stratton, Vol. 7, no. 1.

Westby, C. E. (1984). Development of narrative language abilities. In G. P. Wallach & K. G. Butler (Eds.), *Language learning disabilities in school-age children* (pp. 103–127). Baltimore, MD: Williams & Wilkins.

Westby, C. E. (1988). Children's play: Reflections of social competence. *Seminars in Speech and Language, 9*, 1–14.

Westby, C. E. (1989). Assessing and remediating text comprehension problems. In A. G. Kamhi & H. W. Catts (Eds.), *Reading disabilities: A developmental language perspective* (pp. 199–259). Austin, TX: Pro-Ed.

Westby, C. E. (1990). Ethnographic interviewing: Asking the right questions to the right people in the right ways. *Journal of Childhood Communication Disorders, 13,* 101–111.

Westby, C. E. (1991). Learning to talk—Talking to learn: Oral–literate language differences. In C. S. Simon (Ed.). *Communication skills and classroom success: Assessment and therapy methodologies for language and learning disabled students* (pp. 334–355). Eau Claire, WI: Thinking Publications. (Original work published 1985)

Westby, C. E. (1991, October 4). Understanding classroom texts. Presented as part of an audioteleconference on steps to developing and achieving language based curriculum in the classroom, originating from the American Speech-Language-Hearing Association, Rockville, MD.

Wetherby, A. M., Cain, D., Yonclas, D., & Walker, V. (1988). Analysis of intentional communication of normal children from the prelinguistic to the multi-word stage. *Journal of Speech and Hearing Research, 31,* 240–252.

Wetherby, A. M., & Prizant, B. M. (1990). *Communication and symbolic behavior scales* (CSBS). San Antonio, TX: Special Press.

Wetherby, A. M., & Prutting, B. M. (1984). Profiles of communicative and cognitive-social abilities in autistic children. *Journal of Speech and Hearing Research, 27,* 364–377.

Wetherby, A. M., Yonclas, D. G., & Bryan, A. A. (1989). Communication profiles of preschool children with handicaps: Implications for early identification. Journal of *Speech and Hearing Disorders, 54,* 148–158.

Wetherby, B., & Striefel, S. (1978). Application of a miniature linguistic system on matrix-training procedures. In R. L. Schiefelbusch (Ed.), *Language intervention strategies* (pp. 317–356). Austin, TX: Pro-Ed.

Wexler, K. (1982). A principle theory for language acquisition. In E. Wanner & L. Gleitman (Eds.), *Language acquisition: The state of the art.* Cambridge: Cambridge University Press.

Whitaker, H., & Whitaker, H. A. (1981). *Studies in neurolinguistics.* New York: Academic Press.

White, S. H. (1980). Cognitive competence and performance in everyday environments. *Bulletin of the Orton Society, 30,* 29–45.

White, S. J., & White, R. E. C. (1984). The deaf imperative: Characteristics of maternal input to hearing-impaired children. *Topics in Language Disorders, 4*(4), 38–49.

Whiteman, M. F. (Ed.). (1981). *Writing: The nature, development, and teaching of written communication: Volume 1, Variation in writing: Function and linguistic-cultural differences.* Hillsdale, NJ: Lawrence Erlbaum.

Wieder, S., & Findikoglu, P. (1987). The infant center: A developmentally based environment to support difficult lives. In S. I. Greenspan, S. Wieder, R. A. Nover, A. F. Lieberman, R. S. Lourie, & M. E. Robinson (Eds.), *Infants in multirisk families: Case studies in preventive intervention* (pp. 23–37). Clinical infant reports series of the National Center for Clinical Infant Programs. Madison, WI: International Universities Press.

Wieder, S., & Greenspan, S. I. (1987). Staffing, process, and structure of the clinical infant development program. In S. I. Greenspan, S. Wieder, R. A. Nover, A. F. Lieberman, R. S. Lourie, & M. E. Robinson (Eds.), *Infants in multirisk families: Case studies in preventive intervention* (pp. 9–21). Clinical infant reports series of the National Center for Clinical Infant Programs. Madison, WI: International Universities Press.

Wiener, F. D., Lewnau, L. E., & Erway, E. (1983). Measuring language competency in speakers of Black American English. *Journal of Speech and Hearing Disorders, 48,* 76–84.

Wiig, E. H. (1982). *Let's talk: Developing prosocial communication skills.* Columbus, OH: Merrill/Macmillan.

Wiig, E. H. (1984). Language disabilities in adolescents: A question of cognitive strategies. *Topics in Language Disorders, 4*(2), 41–58.

Wiig, E. H. (1989, May). The interpretation of CELF-R results: A process. *CELF-R Update 2, 2,* 8–10.

Wiig, E. H., & Semel, E. M. (1976). *Language disabilities in children and adolescents.* Columbus, OH: Merrill/Macmillan.

Wiig, E. H., & Semel, E. M. (1980). *Language assessment and intervention for the learning disabled.* Columbus, OH: Merrill/Macmillan.

Wiig, E. H., & Semel, E. M. (1984). *Language assessment and intervention for the learning disabled* (2nd ed.). Columbus, OH: Merrill/Macmillan.

Wilbur, R. B. (1976). The linguistics of manual languages and manual systems. In L. Lloyd (Ed.), *Communication assessment and intervention strategies* (pp. 423–500). Austin, TX: Pro-Ed.

Wilbur, R. B. (1977). An explanation of deaf children's difficulty with certain syntactic structures of English. *Volta Review, 79,* 85–91.

Wilcox, M. J. (1989). Delivering communication-based services to infants, toddlers, and families: Approaches and models. *Topics in Language Disorders, 10*(1), 68–79.

Wilkins, R. (1985). A comparison of elective mutism and emotional disorders in children. *British Journal of Psychiatry, 146,* 198–203.

Wilkinson, L. C., & Milosky, L. M. (1987). School-age children's metapragmatic knowledge of requests and responses in the classroom. *Topics in Language Disorders, 7*(2), 61–70.

Wilkinson, L. C., Milosky, L. M., & Genishi, C. (1986). Second language learners' use of requests and responses in elementary classrooms. *Topics in Language Disorders, 6*(2), 57–70.

Will, M. (1986). *Educating students with learning problems: A shared responsibility.* A report to the Secretary. Office of Special Education and Rehabilitative Services. Washington, DC: Dept. of Education.

Willeford, J. A., & Burleigh, J. M. (1985). *Handbook of central auditory processing disorders in children.* Orlando, FL: Grune & Stratton.

Williams, J. P. (1988). Identifying main ideas: A basic aspect of reading comprehension. *Topics in Language Disorders, 8*(3), 1–13.

Wing, L. (1983). Social and interpersonal needs. In E. Schopler & G. B. Mesibov (Eds.), *Autism in adolescents and adults* (pp. 337–354). New York: Plenum.

Winitz, H. (1973). Problem solving and the delay of speech as strategies in the teaching of language. *Asha, 15,* 583–586.

Winograd, P., & Niquette, G. (1988). Assessing learned helplessness in poor readers. *Topics in Language Disorders, 8* (3), 38–55.

Wixson, K., Boskey, A., Yochum, M., & Alverman, D. (1984). An interview for assessing students' perceptions of classroom reading tasks. *The Reading Teacher, 37,* 348.

Wolery, M. (1989). Child find issues and screening. In D. B. Bailey, Jr., & M. Wolery (Eds.), *Assessing infants and preschoolers with handicaps* (pp. 119–143). Columbus, OH: Merrill/Macmillan.

Wolff, P. H. (1963). Observations on the early development of smiling. In B. M. Foss (Ed.), *Determinants of infant behaviour* (Vol. 2, pp. 113–138). London: Metheun; New York: Wiley.

Wolff, S., & Barlow, A. (1979). Schizoid personality in childhood. *Journal of Child Psychology and Psychiatry, 20,* 29–46.

Wolfram, W. (1979). *Speech pathology and dialect differences.* Arlington, VA: Center for Applied Linguistics.

Wolfram, W. (1983). Test interpretation and sociolinguistic differences. *Topics in Language Disorders, 3*(3), 21–34.

Wolfram, W., Williams, R., & Taylor, O. L. (1972, November). *Dialectal bias of language assessment instruments.* Short course presented at the annual meeting of the American Speech and Hearing Association, San Francisco.

Wolfus, B., Moskovitch, M., & Kinsbourne, M. (1980). Subgroups of language development. *Brain and Language, 10,* 152–171.

Wong, B. Y., & Jones, W. (1982). Increasing metacomprehension in learning disabled and normally achieving students through self-questioning training. *Learning Disability Quarterly, 5,* 228–240.

Wong, B. Y. L., Wong, R., Darlington, D., & Jones, W. (1991). Interactive teaching: An effective way to teach revision skills to adolescents with learning disabilities. *Learning Disabilities Research and Practice, 6,* 117–127.

Wood, B. S. (1976). *Children and communication: Verbal and nonverbal language development.* Englewood Cliffs, NJ: Prentice-Hall.

Wood, P. (1980). Appreciating the consequences of disease: The classification of impairments, disabilities, and handicaps. *The World Health Organization Chronicle, 34,* 376–380.

Woodcock, R., & Johnson, M. B. (1989). *Woodcock-Johnson Psycho-Educational Battery–Revised.* Allen, TX: DLM.

Woodruff, G., & McGonigel, M. J. (1988). Early intervention team approaches: The transdisciplinary model. In J. B. Jordan, J. J. Gallagher, P. L. Hutinger, & M. B. Karnes (Eds.), *Early childhood special education: Birth to three* (pp. 163–182). Reston, VA: Council for Exceptional Children and the Division for Early Childhood.

Worster-Drought, C. (1971). An unusual form of acquired aphasia in children. *Developmental Medicine and Child Neurology, 13,* 563–571.

Wurman, R. S. (1989). *Information anxiety.* New York: Doubleday.

Yell, M. L, & Espin, C. A. (1990). The Handicapped Children's Protection Act of 1986: Time to pay the piper? *Exceptional Children, 56,* 396–407.

Ylvisaker, M. (Ed.). (1985). *Head injury rehabilitation: Children and adolescents.* Austin, TX: Pro-Ed.

Ylvisaker, M., & Szekeres, S. F. (1986). Management of the patient with closed head injury. In R. Chapey (Ed.), *Language intervention strategies in adult aphasia* (pp. 474–490). Baltimore, MD: Williams & Wilkins.

Yoder, D. (1980). Communication systems for nonspeech children. *New Directions in the Exceptional Child, 2,* 63–78.

Yoder, P. J. (1989). Maternal question use predicts later language development in specific-language-disordered children. *Journal of Speech and Hearing Disorders, 54,* 347–355.

Yoshida, R. K. (1983). Are multidisciplinary teams worth the investment? *School Psychology Review, 12,* 127–143.

Yoshinago-Itano, C., & Downey, D. M. (1986). A hearing-impaired child's acquisition of schemata: Something's missing. *Topics in Language Disorders, 7*(1), 45–57.

Yoss, K. A., & Darley, F. L. (1974). Developmental apraxia of speech in children with defective articulation. *Journal of Speech and Hearing Research, 17,* 399–416.

Ysseldyke, J. E., & Algozzine, B. (1982). *Critical issues in special and remedial education.* Boston: Houghton Mifflin.

Ysseldyke, J. E., Thurlow, M., Graden, J., Wesson, C.,

Algozzine, B., & Deno, S. (1983). Generalizations from five years of research on assessment and decision-making: The University of Minnesota Institute. *Exceptional Education Quarterly, 4,* 75–93.

Zametkin, A. J., & Rapoport, J. L. (1987). Neurobiology of attention deficit disorder with hyperactivity: Where have we come in 50 years? *Journal of American Academy of Child and Adolescent Psychiatry, 26,* 676–686.

Zinkus, P., & Gottlieb, M. (1980). Patterns of perceptual and academic deficits related to early chronic otitis media. *Pediatrics, 66,* 246–253.

Zwitman, D., & Sonderman, J. (1979). A syntax program designed to present base linguistic structures to language-disordered children. *Journal of Communication Disorders, 2,* 323–335.

Author Index

Abikoff, H., 113
Abrams, J. C., 80
Ackerman, B. P., 478
Adamson, L., 283
Adler, S., 411
Aitchison, J., 26
Albin, A., 120
Aldridge, A., 436
Algozzine, B., 167, 192, 215
Algozzine, K. M., 167
Allen, D. A., 81, 86, 91–92, 106, 109, 135
Allen, J. P. B., 41
Allen, R. E., 140, 142, 143
Alley, G. R., 210, 440
Allman, T. L., 328
Alpert, C. L., 293
Als, H., 263, 282, 283
Alter, K. S., 353
Alverman, D., 418
Amochaev, A., 261
Anastopoulos, A., 368
Anders, P. L., 462
Anderson, E. S., 131
Anderson, G. M., 182, 192, 245, 443
Anderson, R., 33
Anderson, R. C., 460
Anderson-Inman, L., 74, 403, 404
Andreasen, N. C., 143, 145
Andrews, J. F., 441
Apel, K., 93, 194
Applebee, A. N., 48, 246, 357, 383, 415, 428, 429, 430, 431, 460
Aram, D. M., 80, 81, 91, 116, 117, 118, 120, 194, 219, 233, 235n
Arbitman-Smith, R., 436
Aronson, E., 176
Arpan, R., 282
Arwood, E., 212
Asch, A., 481
Ashbrook, E., 29
Attermeier, S. M., 282, 288
Au, K. H., 436
Augoustinos, M., 140

Augustine, D. K., 176
Austin, J. L., 46
Aylward, E. H., 223, 226

Baer, D., 200, 204, 376
Bagnato, S. J., 266
Bagwell, C., 363
Bahruth, R., 453
Bailey, D. B., Jr., 14, 262, 266, 267, 328, 329
Baker, L., 112, 113, 114–115, 143, 144, 145, 148, 448
Baldwin, D. A., 303
Baldwin, J. M., 68–70
Baltaxe, C. A. M., 146, 287
Bambara, L. M., 313, 314n
Banet, B., 175
Baratz, J. C., 35
Barber, P. A., 267, 268
Barbero, G., 139, 140
Barclay, C. R., 441
Barkley, R. A., 115
Barlow, A., 145
Barnard, K., 138
Barnes, A., 11
Baroff, G. S., 98, 102, 103, 138
Barrett, M., 360
Barrie-Blackley, S., 230
Bartholomew, P., 283
Bartlett, E., 380
Bashir, A. S., 79, 80, 215, 216, 260, 395
Bass, P. M., 112
Bates, E., 65, 66, 67, 72, 205, 209, 210, 213, 264n, 297, 317, 355, 365, 376
Bateson, M., 29, 47, 290
Battle, C., 290
Bayley, N., 328
Beach, R. W., 462
Bean, C., 33
Beavin, J. H., 264
Bedrosian, J. L., 296, 297
Beecher, S., 399
Behr, S. K., 267

Beitchman, J. H., 144, 222
Bellack, A. A., 183
Bellugi, U., 29
Benedict, H., 307, 308–309
Benigni, L., 72, 209, 317
Bennett, C. W., 353
Bennett, E. L., 60
Benson, D. F., 26
Bentler, R. A., 126, 130
Benton, A. L., 116
Berg, J. M., 81
Berk, L. E., 436
Berko, J., 50
Berlin, C. I., 124
Berlin, L., 437
Bernstein, B. B., 338
Bernstein, D. K., 478, 480
Bertalanffy, L. von, 18
Bess, F. H., 123, 126, 129
Best, C., 59
Bettelheim, B., 110
Beukelman, D. R., 1, 8, 10, 12, 15, 24, 138, 168, 219, 239, 240, 245, 268–269, 270n, 307, 389, 396, 397
Bickerton, D., 34
Biemer, C., 182
Bijur, P., 117
Biklen, D., 236, 256, 485
Binkhoff, J. A., 201
Birmingham, B., 113
Bishop, D. V. M., 80, 81, 223, 233, 235n, 237
Bishop, K. B., 484
Bivens, J. A., 436
Bjorkland, B., 228
Bjorklund, D., 228
Blackstone, S., 13, 14
Blagden, C., 360
Blager, F. B., 140, 141, 143
Blaney, N., 176
Blank, M., 125, 337, 363, 364n, 380, 437, 470
Bliss, L. S., 372
Bloom, B. S., 444, 445

Bloom, L., 27, 35, 62, 82, 140, 196, 197, 198, 206, 213, 216, 231, 232, 247, 307, 312, 375, 376
Bloome, D., 452
Bock, R. D., 206, 207*n*
Boder, E., 423
Bodner-Johnson, B., 458
Boehm, A. E., 329, 360
Bohannon, J. N., III, 57, 204
Bond, D. J., 81
Boothroyd, A., 123
Bos, C. S., 448, 462
Boskey, A., 418
Botvin, G. J., 429, 430, 431, 459, 460
Bouvier, L. F., 33
Bowerman, M., 62
Boyce, N. L., 445
Bracken, B. A., 360
Brackett, D., 439
Braddock, J. H., II, 329
Brannon, L., 469
Bransford, J. C., 460, 469
Braswell, L., 113
Braun, C., 384
Brazelton, T. B., 138, 141, 142, 263, 282, 283, 292
Breen, C., 483–484
Brenneis, D., 32, 456, 457
Brenneise-Sarshad, R., 292
Bretherton, I., 66, 72, 205, 209, 210, 317
Briggs, J. H., 81
Briggs, M. H., 281
Brinton, B., 172, 173, 354, 357, 370, 371*n*, 451
Britton, B., 446
Britton, J. N., 48, 336, 357, 419
Broca, P. P., 58
Bronfenbrenner, U., 318
Brooks, D., 124
Brown, A. L., 448, 449, 464
Brown, D., 467
Brown, F., 203
Brown, F. R., III, 226
Brown, G., 117
Brown, J. B., 145
Brown, L., 217, 218*n*, 363, 484, 485
Brown, R. A., 206, 230, 308, 310, 312, 314, 346, 348*n*, 373
Brown, S. F., 86
Brown, S. L., 328
Brown, T., 70
Browne, K., 142
Bruininks, V. L., 455
Bruner, J., 61, 73–74, 110, 132, 141, 246, 303, 304*n*, 415, 446
Bruning, R. H., 382, 384, 462
Bruskin, C., 470
Bryan, A. A., 260, 281
Bryan, J. H., 455
Bryan, T., 90, 370, 454, 456
Buhr, J. C., 380

Bull, D., 285
Bullard-Bates, C., 116
Bullowa, M., 29, 292
Bunce, B., 179, 311, 312
Burke, C. L., 418, 421
Burleigh, J. M., 208
Bush, G., 160
Buswell, B., 185
Butler, D., 383
Butler, K. G., 33, 206, 209, 398
Buttrill, J., 182, 210
Buttsworth, D. L., 459
Byrnes, M., 162

Cain, D., 284
Calculator, S. N., 134, 297
Calfee, R., 428*n*, 431, 432*n*
Calkins, L. M., 387, 462
Calvert, D. R., 123
Camaioni, L., 72, 209, 264*n*, 297, 317
Campbell, C. R., 311
Campbell, S. B., 111
Campbell, T. F., 118, 232, 237
Cantwell, D. P., 112, 113, 114–115, 143, 144, 145, 148
Capozzi, F., 80
Capper, C. A., 183, 184*n*
Capra, F., 18, 20
Carey, S., 380
Carignan-Belleville, L., 448–449
Carlson, F., 321
Carlson, S. C., 210
Carney, A., 285
Carnine, D., 384
Carpenter, L. B., 313
Carpenter, P. A., 450
Carpenter, R., 204, 231, 284, 297
Carr, E., 201
Carroll, S., 338
Carrow, E., 331
Carrow-Woolfolk, E., 194, 205–206
Carta, J. J., 267
Casby, M., 171, 317
Case, R., 69–70, 71, 72, 211
Cassatt-James, E. L., 134
Cattell, R. B., 102
Catts, H. W., 88, 93, 194, 386, 418
Cauley, K., 310
Cazden, C. B., 26–27, 74, 246, 330, 336–337, 383, 415, 427, 428*n*, 439, 452
Chabon, S. S., 440
Chadwick, O., 117, 136
Chall, J. S., 386
Chambliss, M., 431, 432*n*
Chance, P., 318, 321
Chandler, M., 283
Chandley, A. C., 81
Chang, L. L., 227, 228
Chapman, R. S., 118, 310, 339, 342, 344, 350, 353, 376

Chappell, G. E., 135
Charney, R., 133
Chase, C., 124
Cherry, R., 113, 189
Chi, J. G., 58
Chinn, P., 98, 99
Chipman, S., 445
Chisholm, R. W., 391, 485
Chomsky, C., 394
Chomsky, N., 41–42, 49, 58, 61, 62, 66, 127, 197, 198, 206, 230, 348, 349, 373
Churchill, D. W., 109
Clark, D. A., 260
Clark, D. M., 365
Clark, G. N., 281
Clark, R., 58
Clark, T., 282
Clarke, B. R., 309
Clarke, C. M., 81
Cleary, L. M., 34–35
Clegg, M., 144, 222
Cobo-Lewis, A., 309
Coggins, T. E., 284, 294, 295, 296*n*
Cohen, A. L., 478
Cole, A. J., 92, 118
Cole, E., 403–404
Cole, K. N., 231
Cole, L., 33
Cole, M., 29, 337
Coleman, M., 106
Coleman, P. P., 29, 485
Collier, B., 297
Collins, W. A., 384
Collins-Ahlgren, M., 29
Connell, P. J., 232, 372, 376, 378
Conners, C. K., 111
Constable, C. M., 399–400, 407
Conti-Ramsden, G., 18, 362
Cook-Gumperz, J., 337, 338
Cooper, C. R., 422, 423, 469
Cooper, D. C., 74, 403, 404
Cooper, E., 398
Cooper, F. S., 36
Cooper, J. A., 118
Cooper, M., 292
Cooper, M. M., 337
Cooper, W. E., 33
Coots, J., 484
Copeland, D. R., 120
Coren, A., 177
Cornett, R. O., 309
Corrigan, R., 72, 209
Corsiglia, J., 58
Costello, A., 365
Costello, J., 200
Courchesne, E., 109
Courtnage, L., 14, 170
Cox, L. C., 209
Crago, M., 54, 219, 343, 403–404
Craig, H. K., 200, 212, 213, 300–301
Craik, F. I., 464

Craik, K., 65
Crais, E. R., 278, 306, 341, 379, 380, 475–476, 477
Crary, M. A., 135
Creaghead, N. A., 37, 417, 418n
Cromer, R. F., 206, 213
Cross, T. G., 18, 19, 315, 316, 334
Crossley, R., 256, 485
Crouter, A., 140
Crowhurst, M., 469
Crystal, D., 31, 32, 342, 347–348, 349
Cuda, R. A., 74, 452
Culatta, B., 331, 332–333
Cullinan, B. E., 382
Cunningham, J. W., 449
Curley, R., 428n
Curtiss, S., 125, 140, 141
Curwen, M., 222

Dale, P. S., 231, 297, 317, 355
Dalebout, S. D., 113
Dalton, B. M., 296, 297
Damico, J. S., 1, 15, 16–17, 18, 24, 165, 174, 193, 228, 234, 239, 330, 386
Darley, F. L., 135, 230
Darlington, D., 438
Davey, B., 418
Davis, G. Z., 225
Davis, J. M., 126, 129, 130, 131
Davis, K., 140
Davis, W. E., 162
Day, J. D., 464
Demetras, M. J., 106, 107–108
Dempster, F. N., 445–446
DeMyer, M. K., 106, 109, 234, 235
Denckla, M. B., 94, 381
Denham, C., 182
Denner, P. R., 431, 432, 477
Deno, S., 192, 413
Denti, L., 167
Denton, P. H., 440
Deshler, D. D., 210, 440
Despain, A. D., 168, 182
D'Eugenio, D. B., 328
Deutsch, F., 140
Deutsch, G., 194
De Villiers, J., 346, 348n
De Villiers, P., 346, 348n
DeVivo, S., 329
Diambra, T., 484
Dietrich, K. N., 142
Dillard, J. L., 34
DiScenna, A., 120
DiStefano, P., 444
Dobie, R. A., 124
Dobrich, W., 80, 81, 193, 223, 235n
Dodd, B., 125
Dodds, J. B., 328
Dollaghan, C. A., 232, 237, 297, 355, 357, 358, 377–378, 380, 450
Donahue, M., 90, 454, 456

Donnellan, A. M., 201, 204, 298–300
Donnelly, J., 484, 486
Donovan, C. M., 328
Dooling, E. C., 58
Dore, J., 47, 73, 74–75, 297, 355, 368–369
Dorman, C., 136, 138
Dorsey-Gaines, C., 317
Dougherty, C., 209
Downey, D. C., 208
Downey, D. M., 420, 459
Downs, M. P., 123, 124, 125, 127, 128n, 237
Drew, E., 98
Dublinske, S., 172, 173
DuBose, R., 278
Ducanis, A. J., 215
Ducayen, M. B., 81
Duchan, J. F., 200, 201, 204, 206, 207–208, 209, 230, 234, 294, 301, 341, 342, 343, 345, 346, 347, 355, 391–392, 478, 480
Dunlea, A., 132
Dunn, C., 125
Dunn, L. M., 130
Dunst, C., 282, 283
DuPaul, G., 113

Eccarius, M., 125
Edgar, E., 484
Edmundson, A., 80, 81, 223, 233, 235n, 237
Edwards, D., 312
Edwards, J. H., 81
Egeland, B., 140, 142
Ehren, B. J., 398, 440, 442
Ehri, L., 418
Eichenger, J., 175
Eilers, R., 285, 309
Einstein, A., 389
Eisenson, J., 115
Ekelman, B. L., 80, 116, 117, 120, 194, 233, 235n
Elder, J. L., 318
Eldredge, P., 399
Elfenbein, J., 126, 130
Ellis, J., 331, 332–333
Emig, J., 418, 419, 448
Englert, C. S., 463–464, 467, 468n
Ensher, G. L., 260
Entus, A. K., 59
Entwisle, D. R., 475
Epstein, H. T., 60
Erickson, F., 23, 452
Erickson, J. G., 227, 228, 229
Erin, J. N., 131–132, 133
Ernst, B., 292, 295
Erskine, B. A., 390
Ervin-Tripp, S., 46, 52, 366, 368, 369, 452
Erway, E., 227

Espin, C. A., 158
Ewing-Cobbs, L., 116, 120
Ezell, H. K., 312, 480

Fabrizi, A., 80
Fairchild, J. L., 455, 456
Falvey, M. A., 484
Fandal, A. W., 328
Fang, J-S., 81
Farra, H. E., 442
Fasold, R. W., 34, 373–374
Fassbender, L. L., 201
Fay, W. H., 107, 132, 301
Fein, D., 398
Fein, G., 322
Feldman, C., 124
Feldman, H., 127
Fenson, L., 318
Ferguson, C., 73, 74, 75
Fernald, A., 31
Ferry, P. C., 118, 195
Feuerstein, R., 100, 102, 246, 409, 436, 445
Fey, M. E., 91, 92, 93n, 169–170, 177–178, 179–180, 198, 200, 213, 217, 219, 245, 247, 252, 296, 341, 342, 355–356, 358, 360–361, 366, 368n, 373, 374n, 378, 379, 452
Fey, S. H., 480
Field, T., 260
Fiese, B., 259, 325
Fiess, K., 375
Fillmore, C., 45
Findikoglu, P., 266
Fischer, F. W., 418
Fischler, R., 124
Fitzgerald, J., 428n, 429
Fletcher, J. M., 116
Fletcher, P., 342, 347–348
Flexer, C., 363, 365
Flood, J., 416, 417n
Flower, L. S., 418, 448
Flynn, G. J., 14
Fodor, J., 210
Folger, M., 322
Folkins, J. W., 33
Ford, C. E., 81
Forrest-Pressley, D. L., 440, 449
Forsyth, D. F., 475
Foster, R., 310
Fourcin, A. J., 59
Fowler, C., 418
Fox, C. L., 175, 455
Fox, L., 140, 142, 147
Fraiberg, S., 131, 132, 134, 141
Frankenburg, W. K., 328
Frassinelli, L., 172, 174
Frattali, C., 250
Freed, D. B., 390
Freeman, B., 103, 129
Freeman, R., 59

Freese, P., 146, 435
French, J. H., 136
Frentheway, B., 113
Frey, W., 10, 13, 156
Friedman, K. K., 430n, 431
Friedman, R. J., 147
Fried-Oken, M., 263, 265n
Friel-Patti, S., 18
Friend, M., 462
Frith, U., 422
Fry, E. B., 424
Frymier, B., 398
Fujiki, M., 172, 173, 354, 357, 370, 371n, 451
Fundudis, T., 145, 233
Furth, H., 130
Furuno, S., 328

Gagné, J-P., 455
Galaburda, A. M., 58, 95, 96
Gallagher, T., 213, 232, 300–301, 455, 456
Gallimore, R., 448
Gannon, J. D., 232
Gansneder, B., 398
Garbarino, J., 140
Garcia, S. B., 228
Gardner, H., 72, 103, 198, 408, 443
Gardner, R. W., 33
Garman, M., 342, 347–348
Garnett, K., 459
Garrett, K., 389
Garside, R. F., 233
Gartner, A., 480
Gaylord-Ross, R., 483–484
Geers, A. E., 126, 127, 236, 237, 362, 435
Geffner, D., 123
Genishi, C., 452–453
Gentry, B., 93, 194, 390
Gerber, M. M., 150n
Gerber, S. E., 123, 133, 151, 395, 396
German, D. J., 381, 382n
Gerring, J. P., 118, 122
Geschwind, N., 10, 26, 58, 59n, 95
Gholson, B., 390
Giddan, J., 310
Gildea, P. M., 475
Gilles, F. H., 58
Gillespie, L., 117, 120, 194, 390
Gillespie, S., 398
Gittelman, R., 113
Gittelman-Klein, R., 113
Glanville, B., 59
Glaser, R. E., 445
Glassford, J. E., 363
Gleason, J. B., 304, 309
Gleitman, H., 140
Gleitman, L. R., 62, 140
Glenn, C., 357, 460
Glover, M. E., 328

Glynn, S., 446
Goetz, C., 299, 480–482
Golden, G. G., 118
Goldenberg, D., 329
Goldgar, D., 236
Goldin-Meadow, S., 127
Goldman, R., 215
Goldman-Rakic, P. S., 62
Goldstein, H., 311n, 312, 480
Goldstein, K., 122
Golin, A. K., 215
Golinkoff, R., 310
Gonzales, J., 95
Goodglass, H., 40, 88, 194
Goodman, K. S., 49, 385, 386, 420, 421n, 424
Goodman, Y. M., 421, 422
Gordon, C. J., 384
Gordon, D., 366, 368, 369, 452
Gordon, L., 310
Gorga, M. P., 130
Gottlieb, M., 124
Gottsleben, R. H., 342, 347, 349, 375
Gough, P. B., 206
Graden, J., 192
Graham, P. J., 222
Grant-Zawadzki, M., 120
Graves, A., 461
Graves, D., 387, 419
Graves, K., 94–95
Graves, M. F., 428n
Gray, B., 177, 198, 200, 251, 378
Green, A., 142
Green, J. L., 22, 23, 229
Greenfield, P., 297, 446
Greenspan, S., 14, 268, 282, 292
Greenwood, C. R., 267
Gregory, M., 338
Grenot-Scheyer, M., 484
Grice, H. P., 48
Griffin, K., 183
Griffith, P. L., 384
Grossman, H., 98, 101, 102
Gruber, K. D., 176
Gruendel, J., 308–309
Gualtieri, C. T., 144, 146
Guess, D., 100, 200, 203, 204, 290, 292, 293, 295n, 305, 306n, 376
Guidubaldi, J., 328
Guilford, A., 399
Guilford, J. P., 102
Guralnick, M. J., 174
Guthrie, J., 294, 296n

Hadley, P. A., 356
Hagen, J. W., 441, 445
Hagerty, P., 444
Haien, J., 361
Hall, N. E., 219
Hall, P. K., 80, 235n
Halle, M., 36

Halliday, M. A. K., 47, 295, 297, 355, 460, 473
Halvorsen, A., 185–186
Hamm, A., 58
Hammill, D. D., 196, 206, 359
Hamre-Nietupski, S., 484
Hanline, M. F., 185–186
Hannah, L., 183
Hanson, L. R., 176
Harber, J., 91
Haring, T., 483–484
Harris, A. J., 94
Harris, D., 297
Harris, G. A., 227–228
Harris, K. R., 440, 441
Harris, M., 376
Hart, B., 179, 205, 212, 213, 296, 362
Hart, C., 273
Hart, P. J., 209
Hart, V., 214
Hartup, W., 455
Hartwig, L. J., 10, 12
Hartzell, H. E., 394, 396, 402n
Hasan, R., 460, 473
Hasenstab, M. S., 375
Hayden, T. L., 145
Hayes, C. W., 453
Hayes, J. R., 418, 448
Haywood, H. C., 436, 445
Hazel, J., 454
Hearn, S., 182
Heath, S. B., 227, 316, 317, 334, 429, 459
Hecaen, H., 116, 120
Hedrick, D., 322
Hedrick, L. D., 469
Heimlich, J. E., 477, 479n
Heinen, A., 165, 183, 185
Hermelin, B., 109, 110, 301
Hess, L. J., 455, 456
Hier, D., 95
Hietko, P. J., 113
Higginbotham, D. J., 30
Hill, B. P., 284
Hill, J., 290, 291n
Hill, M., 484
Hillix, W. A., 147
Hillocks, G., Jr., 426
Hingtgen, J. N., 235
Hirsh-Pasek, K., 310
Hodson, B., 245
Hoffman, L. P., 167, 168, 192, 245
Hoffman, P. R., 212, 239, 247, 269, 279–280, 294, 295–296, 317, 318, 363, 378
Hohmann, M., 175
Holden, M. H., 418
Holland, A. L., 118
Holt, L. K., 94–95
Holubec, E., 176
Holvoet, J., 203

Hood, L., 232, 375, 376
Hopkins, C., 329
Horgan, D., 308
Horn, J. L., 102
Hosaka, C. M., 328
Hoskins, B., 52, 149, 171, 173, 177, 396, 437, 451, 454, 461
Hostler, S. L., 260
House, L. I., 132, 133, 134
House, T. D., 132, 133, 134
Howes, C., 318, 321, 335
Hubbell, R. D., 179, 230, 231, 344
Hughes, C. A., 464, 465
Hughes, D. L., 177, 178, 179, 204, 439
Huisingh, R., 360
Hunt, K. W., 345–346, 347, 425, 472
Huntington, G. S., 262
Hurst, C., 35, 226
Hustedde, C., 285
Hutchinson, D., 215
Hutchinson, T. A., 217, 333
Huttenlocher, J., 307, 308
Hutter, J. J., 120
Hyman, C. A., 142
Hyman, R. T., 183
Hymes, D., 355
Hynd, G. W., 95
Hyter, Y. D., 227, 352, 373

Idol, L., 21, 22, 172, 226, 413, 414
Iglesias, A., 53, 404
Inatsuka, T. T., 328
Ingram, D., 38, 66, 307
Ireland, J., 365
Irwin, J. W., 473n, 474, 475n
Isaacson, S., 422

Jaben, T., 14, 170
Jackson, A. S., 441, 444n
Jackson, D. D., 264
Jackson, R. K., 235
Jacobson, L., 189
Jaffe, M. B., 284–285, 287–288, 289
Jagiello, G. M., 81
Jakobson, R., 36
James, C., 353
James, S., 231, 232
Jarrico, S., 423
Jenkins, J. R., 165, 171, 174, 183, 185
Jens, K. G., 282, 288
Jensen, H., 124
Jensen, J. K., 130
Johnsen, S. K., 217, 218n
Johnson, C. J., 375, 376
Johnson, D. J., 94, 206, 339, 435, 443
Johnson, D. L., 376
Johnson, D. W., 7, 22, 176, 215, 381
Johnson, M. B., 408
Johnson, M. K., 460
Johnson, N. L., 460
Johnson, N. S., 357

Johnson, R., 7, 22, 215
Johnson, R. T., 176
Johnson, S., 452, 480
Johnson, W., 230
Johnson-Laird, P. N., 65–66
Johnson-Martin, N., 282, 288
Johnston, J. R., 217, 357, 372, 391
Joiner, C. W., 35
Jones, C., 80, 235n
Jones, L. V., 206, 207n
Jones, W., 438, 449–450
Jordan, F. M., 459
Jordan, L. S., 118
Just, M. A., 450

Kabacoff, R. I., 327
Kaelber, P., 172, 173
Kagan, J., 145–146
Kagan, S., 176–177
Kail, R., 381
Kaiser, A. P., 205, 212, 213, 293, 362
Kallman, C., 96
Kalman, S. L., 29, 485
Kamhi, A. G., 71, 72, 88, 93, 100, 194, 217, 218, 372, 375, 386, 390, 418
Kandell, E. R., 60
Kanner, L., 103, 106, 108, 110
Kanter, R. M., 23–24
Kaplan, E., 40, 88, 194, 475
Kaplan, G. K., 124
Kaplan, M. G., 142
Karchmer, M. A., 126, 236
Karnes, M. B., 14
Kaston, N., 377–378, 450
Katz, J., 206, 208
Kaufman, A. S., 223
Kaufman, N. L., 223
Kawakami, A. J., 436
Keeler, W. R., 132
Keith, R. W., 195, 206, 208
Kekelis, L. S., 131
Kelford-Smith, A., 29, 137, 485
Kelly, C. A., 317
Kemper, T. L., 95
Kendall, P. C., 113
Keniston, A. H., 384
Kent, L., 201
Kent, R., 285
Kern, C., 322
Kernan, K., 429, 431
Kerns, G. M., 267
Kerr, M. M., 442
Kinder, D., 384
King, D. F., 386
King, R. R., 80, 235n
Kinney, P., 261
Kinsbourne, M., 81, 95
Kintsch, W., 427, 460
Kirchner, D. M., 47, 205, 363
Kirk, S. A., 196, 206, 224
Kirk, U., 140, 141, 196

Kirk, W. D., 196, 224
Kirkland, C., 124
Klecan-Aker, J. S., 469
Klee, T., 344
Kleffner, F. R., 118
Klein, D., 113
Klein, J., 124
Klein, M. D., 281, 289
Kliebard, H. M., 183
Klima, E., 29
Klopp, K., 18, 334
Knapczyk, D., 465, 467
Knapp, M. S., 435–436
Knibbs, C., 167
Knobloch, H., 328, 329
Knoll, J. A., 14
Knott, G., 452
Kochanek, T. T., 327
Koegel, R. L., 287, 322
Kolven, I., 233
Kolvin, T., 145
Koppenhaver, D. A., 29, 137, 485
Koriath, U., 144, 146
Koslowski, B., 292
Kovarsky, D. K., 219
Kramer, C., 231
Kramer, J. H., 120
Krauss, M. W., 158
Kresheck, J. D., 360
Kruger, G., 113
Kuczaj, S., 232
Kwiatkowski, J., 379

LaBerge, D., 448
Labov, W., 35
Ladas, H., 464
Lafayette, R., 124
LaGreca, A., 454
Lahey, M., 35, 82, 196, 197, 198, 199, 206, 213, 216, 220, 222, 231, 247, 307, 341, 351, 375, 376, 407, 429, 461
Lakoff, G., 83
Lamanna, M. L., 452, 453
Lamphear, V. S., 140
Landau, W. M., 118
Lange, U., 389
Langer, J., 246, 415, 443, 449
Langley, M., 278
Langlois, A., 140, 142
Larsen, S. C., 196, 206
Larson, V. L., 177, 178, 398, 399, 400, 401, 402n, 403, 440, 445, 465
Lasky, E., 18, 80, 113, 206, 208, 209, 235n, 334
Laughton, J., 375
Launer, P. B., 197, 407
Lazar, R. T., 452, 480
Leavell, A., 461
Lederberg, A., 97
Lee, L. L., 197, 206, 227, 341, 342, 345, 346, 347, 348, 349, 350, 352, 372

Lee, R. F., 71, 72
Lefebvre, M., 71
Lein, L., 32, 456, 457
Leiter, R. G., 217
Lenneberg, E. H., 58
Lenz, B. K., 398, 440, 442
Leonard, L. B., 18, 19, 33, 41, 42–43, 62, 85, 89–91, 96–97, 108, 198, 211, 217, 219, 307, 311, 322, 334, 348, 358, 368, 376, 381, 452
Lester, B. M., 263, 282
Levenson, R., 59
Levi, G., 80
Levin, H. S., 116
Levine, M., 113
Levine-Donnerstein, D., 150n
Levinson, S., 46
Levitsky, W., 58, 59n, 95
Levitt, H., 123, 130
Lewis, J. P., 103
Lewnau, L. E., 227
Liberman, A. M., 36, 387, 418, 424
Liberman, I. Y., 387, 418, 424
Licht, B. G., 441
Liebergott, J. W., 260
Lieberman, A., 182
Lieberman, I., 194
Lieven, E. V. M., 317
Lifter, K., 375
Light, J., 29, 134, 137, 138–139, 297, 485
Lightbown, P., 232
Liles, B. Z., 462
Lindamood, C. H., 209
Lindamood, P. C., 209
Lindblad, M. B., 145
Linder, T. W., 211, 213, 269, 276–277, 294, 318
Lindfors, J. W., 326, 336, 339, 453, 456–457
Ling, A. H., 130
Ling, D., 129–130, 285–287, 309
Lipsitt, L. P., 327
Lipsky, D. K., 480
Lloyd, H., 145
Lloyd, J., 210
Lloyd, L. L., 305
Loban, W. D., 346, 353, 406, 425
Locke, P. A., 305
Lockhart, R. S., 464
Lockwood, E. L., 269, 271n, 272n, 275n, 331
Loeb, D. F., 41, 42–43, 62, 198, 370
Logan, D., 98
Lomax, R., 431
Long, S. H., 140, 142, 342
Longhurst, T. M., 230
Lord, C., 251, 252n
Lord-Larson, V., 446–447
Lovaas, O. I., 109, 236, 254
Love, R. J., 60, 95

Lowe, L., 282, 283
Lowe, M., 365
Lowell, E. L., 125
Lowrey, N., 440
Lucariello, J., 288, 314–315
Lucas, E. V., 211
Luick, T., 13
Lund, N. J., 230, 234, 294, 341, 342, 343, 345, 346, 347, 355, 478, 480
Luterman, D., 160
Lyman, H., 226
Lynch, C., 250
Lynch, E. W., 328
Lynch, M. P., 309
Lynch-Fraser, D., 283
Lyon, G., 215
Lyon, S., 215

Mabbett, B., 386
MacAulay, B., 200
MacDonald, A., 256, 485
MacDonald, J., 282, 284, 292, 293, 306–307
MacGinitie, W. H., 418
MacKeith, R. C., 80
MacLellan, N., 377
MacMurray, J., 75
MacWhinney, B., 65, 66, 67, 205, 209
Magnotta, O. H., 399
Mahan, H., 427
Main, M., 292
Malone, A. F., 328, 329
Mandler, J., 357, 460
Manis, F. R., 94–95
Mantovani, J. F., 118
Manzella, L., 135–136
Maratsos, M., 232
Mardell, C., 329
Mardell-Czudnowski, C., 329
Mariage, T. V., 467, 468n
Marin-Padilla, M., 82
Markman, E. M., 303
Markus, D., 14
Marshall, J. C., 58, 59, 60
Marshall, R., 95
Marston, D. B., 226
Martin, H. P., 140, 141
Martin, S. T., 480
Martin, V. E., 172, 173
Marvin, C. A., 172
Marx, M. H., 147
Marzano, R., 444
Mason, J., 249, 429, 441
Massaro, D. W., 418
Mastergeorge, A., 284
Mastropieri, M. A., 446
Matarazzo, J. D., 130
Matsuyama, U. K., 429
Mattis, S., 118, 136
Mattison, R. E., 112, 113
Mauer, D., 93, 194, 217, 390

Mautner, T. S., 10–12, 15
Maxon, A., 439
Maxwell, D. L., 60
Maxwell, S. E., 17, 80, 233, 395
May, S., 344
McCabe, A., 384, 429
McCalla, J. L., 120
McCarthy, D. A., 230, 341
McCarthy, J. J., 196, 224
McCauley, R. J., 140, 358–359, 407
McClelland, J., 66, 208, 209
McClure, E., 429
McConkey, R., 318
McConnell, F., 126
McCormick, L., 200, 201, 202, 204, 214, 215
McCormick, M. C., 262
McCune-Nicolich, L., 317, 318
McDermott, R. P., 336
McGarr, N., 123
McGee, L. M., 316, 317, 387, 428, 431
McGonigel, M. J., 215
McIntosh, R., 455
McKenzie, R. G., 440
McKinley, N. K., 445, 446
McKinley, N. L., 177, 178, 398, 399, 400, 401, 402n, 403, 440, 446–447, 465
McKirdy, L. S., 125
McLean, J. E., 247, 248n
McNaughton, D., 485
McNeill, D., 49, 58, 61
McNerney, C. D., 290
McPartland, J. M., 329
McQuarter, R. J., 296, 363
Meadow, K. P., 130
Meier, R. P., 29
Mellits, D., 96
Membrino, I., 344
Menyuk, P., 89, 124, 232
Mercer, J. R., 98, 103, 167
Mesaros, R. A., 201
Mesibov, G. B., 107, 110, 454, 455
Messick, C., 318
Meyer, B. J. F., 431
Meyer, L., 14
Meyers, J., 172, 174
Miedzianik, D., 106
Miller, B. L., 460–461
Miller, G. A., 475
Miller, J. F., 82, 118, 230, 231, 232, 310, 339, 341, 342, 344, 345, 346, 349, 350, 353, 355, 357, 358
Miller, L., 17, 18, 165, 174, 238, 408, 443, 462
Millin, J. P., 363
Mills, A. E., 131
Mills, P. E., 231
Milosky, L. M., 354–355, 417, 452–453, 458, 460
Minor, J. S., 217
Minskoff, E., 454

Minuchin, P., 18, 19
Mire, S. P., 391, 485
Mirenda, P., 1, 8, 10, 12, 15, 24, 168,
  201, 204–205, 219, 239, 240, 245,
  268–269, 270n, 300, 305, 397
Miron, M. S., 206
Mishler, E. G., 9, 20, 240
Mitchell-Kernan, C., 52
Moeller, M. P., 125, 129, 130, 316
Molfese, D., 59
Montague, M., 461
Montgomery, A. A., 394, 399, 407, 408
Moog, J. S., 126, 127, 236, 237, 435
Moon, M. S., 484
Moore, E., 35, 226
Moore, I., 120
Moores, D., 309
Moran, M. R., 420, 422, 423, 472, 474
Mordecai, D. R., 342
Morgan, D., 399
Morgan, E. C., 282
Morgan, J. L., 292
Morley, M. E., 80
Morris, C., 73
Morris, R., 94, 219
Morris, S. E., 287, 288, 289, 293
Morsink, C. V., 167
Moses, K. L., 131
Moskovitch, M., 81
Mougey, K., 344
Mroczkowski, M. M., 182
Mulac, A., 177, 232
Mulligan, M., 203
Mullin, K., 377
Muma, J., 212
Murdoch, B. E., 459
Murray-Seegert, C., 177, 238–239, 480,
  482–483
Musselwhite, C. R., 230, 321
Muuss, R., 475
Myklebust, H. R., 94, 126, 130, 206,
  339, 381, 443
Myles-Zitzer, C., 232

Nair, R., 144, 222
Nation, J. E., 80, 81, 91, 194, 233, 235n
Neisworth, J. T., 266
Nelson, K., 75–76, 132, 290, 292, 303,
  306, 307, 308–309, 344, 357, 382
Nelson, N. W., 17, 18, 44, 74, 75, 113,
  117, 122, 148, 167, 168, 173, 182,
  192, 195, 198, 209, 212, 226, 227,
  241, 243n, 245, 252, 253, 269, 271n,
  272n, 275n, 281, 283, 290, 291n,
  300, 308, 309, 318, 327, 330, 331,
  337, 338n, 352, 360, 363, 373, 374,
  375, 377n, 384, 387, 390, 408, 409,
  410n, 411n, 412n, 413, 414, 415,
  416n, 428n, 430n, 431, 435, 443,
  445, 448, 452, 456, 462, 465, 466n,
  472, 474, 476, 477, 478

Nemeth, M., 380
Netsell, R., 285
Nevin, A., 21, 226, 413, 414
Newborg, J., 328
Newcomer, P. L., 359
Newhoff, M., 111
Newman, P., 37
Newport, E. L., 29
Newsom, C. D., 201
Newton, L., 125, 480
Nicholson, C. B., 452, 480
Nietupski, J., 484
Niizawa, J., 182
Ninio, A., 132, 316
Nippold, M. A., 75, 368, 390, 394,
  395n, 399, 407, 440, 445, 474, 475,
  478, 479–480
Niquette, G., 97–98
Nisbett, R. E., 15
Nitsch, K. E., 469
Norlin, P. F., 18
Norman, D., 120
Norman, J. B., 145, 147
Norris, J. A., 174, 212, 239, 247, 269,
  279–280, 294, 295–296, 317, 318,
  363, 378, 382, 384, 386, 462
Northcott, W. H., 282
Northern, J. L., 123, 124, 127, 128n,
  237
Nystrand, M., 448

O'Brien, M. A., 164, 171, 174
O'Connor, L., 399
O'Connor, N., 109, 110, 301
Odell, L., 422, 447
Odom, S. L., 14, 171, 260
O'Donnell, K. J., 263
Oehler, J. M., 263
Okagaki, L., 441, 444n
O'Keefe, B., 29, 137
O'Leary, T. S., 164, 171, 174
Oliver, J. M., 140
Oliver, R., 446
Oller, D. K., 124, 285, 309
Oller, J. W., Jr., 228, 330
Olson, C., 353
Olswang, L. B., 231, 294, 296n, 313
Omark, D. R., 229
O'Neil, W., 405
O'Neill, T. J., 84
O'Reilly, A., 328
Orman, J., 360
Ornitz, E., 236
Orr, E. W., 405
Ortiz, A. A., 228
Orton, S., 88
Osberger, M., 125, 236, 285
Osgood, C. E., 206
Osofsky, J. D., 140, 142, 143
Otomo, K., 285
Ouellette, T., 261

Owens, A., 290, 291n
Owens, R. E., Jr., 27, 30, 72, 100, 101,
  102, 283, 285, 292, 302, 303, 304n, 309

Paden, E., 245
Padgett, S. Y., 80
Page, J. L., 331, 332–333, 429n, 460
Palermo, D., 59
Paley, V. G., 390
Palin, M. W., 342
Palincsar, A. S., 449, 467
Palmer, C. B., 342
Pan, B. A., 304, 309
Panagos, J. M., 379
Pang, D., 120
Panther, K. M., 311
Paolucci-Whitcomb, P., 21, 172
Papanicolaou, A. C., 120
Parker, F., 26, 39, 43, 44–45, 211
Parker, R., 422
Parnes, P., 29, 137, 297
Parr, R., 142, 143
Pascual-Leone, J., 71
Pate, J. L., 288
Patel, P. G., 144, 222
Paul, L., 174
Paul, P. V., 127, 130
Paul, R., 350, 376–377
Paul-Brown, D., 174
Payne, K. T., 33, 154, 216, 226, 227
Pearl, R., 90
Pearson, P. D., 450
Pease, D. M., 304, 305, 309
Pederson, D. R., 318
Pegnatore, L., 290, 291n
Pehrsson, R. S., 431, 432, 477
Perera, K., 384
Perfetti, C. A., 385
Peters, A., 108
Peterson, C., 384, 429
Philips, S. U., 334
Piaget, J., 60, 67–72, 102, 210, 211,
  317, 322, 365, 423–424
Piccolo, J., 462
Pickering, M., 172, 173
Pidek, C., 240
Piercy, M., 96, 206
Pinard, A., 71
Pinker, S., 62, 317
Pitcher, E. G., 426
Pittelman, S. D., 477, 479n
Pitts-Conway, V., 483–484
Polani, P. E., 81
Pollack, D., 129
Power, D. J., 124, 126
Poyadue, F., 54
Prather, E., 322, 399
Prelinger, E., 426
Prelock, P. A., 318, 379, 440
Preminger, J. L., 328
Pressley, M., 440, 441

Prizant, B. M., 28, 108, 143, 144, 145, 146, 148, 149, 264, 269, 276, 277–278, 279n, 281, 283, 292, 294, 301, 302n, 304, 308, 355
Proctor, A., 285, 286n
Prutting, B. M., 278
Prutting, C. A., 46, 47, 125, 213, 232
Pueschel, S. M., 82
Purves, A., 447
Putnam-Sims, P., 232

Quigley, S. P., 124, 125, 126, 127, 130

Ramey, C. T., 260
Rand, Y., 100, 436
Randall, D., 222
Ransom, K., 449
Raphael, T. E., 450, 463–464
Rapin, I., 81, 86, 91–92, 106, 109, 118, 135, 136
Rapoport, J. L., 113
Rapport, M., 113
Ray, H., 363, 364
Records, N., 146, 435
Reed, V. A., 394, 398
Rees, N., 96, 196, 206
Rescorla, L., 135–136, 223, 304, 308–309
Restak, R. M., 61, 141
Reveron, W. W., 226–227
Reynolds, M. C., 189, 192
Rice, M. L., 211, 356, 380
Rich, H. L., 182
Richardson, S. O., 23, 32, 154
Richgels, D. J., 316, 317, 387, 428, 431
Rie, E., 113
Rie, H., 113
Rief, L., 414
Rimland, B., 109
Ripich, D. N., 384
Risley, T. R., 205, 212, 213, 296, 362
Ritchey, H., 291n
Ritvo, E., 103, 236
Robbins, A. M., 125
Roberts, J., 124, 278, 341
Robinson, F. P., 450
Roeser, R. J., 123, 125
Rogers, S. J., 328
Rogers-Warren, A. K., 204, 205, 212, 296, 363
Rogister, S. H., 230
Rohwer, W. D., Jr., 445–446
Romski, M. A., 288, 305, 306
Rose, S. A., 437
Rosen, C. D., 118, 122
Rosen, G. D., 58
Rosenbek, J. C., 135
Rosenberg, J. B., 145
Rosenthal, R., 189
Rosenzweig, M. R., 60
Rosner, B., 124

Ross, G. S., 284
Ross, M., 123, 209
Ross, S. M., 182
Roth, F. P., 134, 297, 298n, 355, 356n, 365, 384, 385, 426, 428, 429, 459
Rowan, A. J., 118
Ruben, D., 13, 14
Rubin, D. L., 419, 420, 469
Ruddell, R. B., 206
Rudel, R. G., 381
Ruder, C. C., 179, 311
Ruder, K. F., 179, 311, 317
Rueda, R., 220
Rumelhart, D. E., 66, 208, 209, 357, 460
Rushmer, N., 282
Russell, W. K., 126
Rutter, M., 80, 109, 110, 112, 113, 117, 136, 222
Ryan, B., 177, 198, 200, 251, 378
Rydell, P. J., 28, 301, 355
Rynders, J. E., 81, 82, 100, 436
Rynell, J., 222

Saber, D., 217, 333
Sailor, W., 200, 204
Sainato, D. M., 267
Saleeby, N., 144, 146
Salus, M. W., 416, 417n
Sameroff, A., 259, 283, 325
Samuels, S. J., 448
Sandler, A., 177
Sanford, A. R., 328
Santogrossi, J., 204–205, 300
Sapir, E., 58
Sarachan-Deily, A. B., 329
Sarff, L. S., 363, 364
Sattler, J. M., 111, 112, 115
Satz, P., 94, 116
Sawyer, D. J., 209, 424
Saxman, J., 231
Scarborough, H. S., 80, 81, 193, 223, 235n
Schaeffer, A. L., 442
Schaeffer, B., 109
Schaffer, B., 251, 252n
Schaffer, M., 344
Schaffer, R., 283
Schein, E., 172
Scherer, N. J., 313
Schery, T. K., 234, 235n
Schick, B., 362
Schickedanz, J. A., 388n
Schiefelbusch, R. L., 204
Schiff-Myers, N., 133
Schildroth, A. N., 126, 236
Schirmer, B. R., 313–314
Schlesinger, H. S., 130
Schlesinger, I. M., 127
Schopler, E., 107, 110, 251, 252n, 455
Schory, M. E., 386

Schreibman, L., 105, 106, 107, 108–109, 110, 234
Schub, M. J., 332
Schuler, A. L., 107, 299, 480–482
Schultz, J., 452
Schultz, M. C., 260
Schum, R., 126, 130
Schumaker, J. B., 210, 440, 442, 450, 454
Schwartz, L., 445, 446
Schwartz, R., 307, 318, 322
Schwentor, B. A., 117, 122
Schwethelm, B., 441
Scinto, L., 426
Scott, C. M., 383–384, 426, 462, 469, 470, 471n, 474
Scribner, S., 29, 337
Scruggs, T. E., 446
Searle, J. R., 46, 47
Seashore, H. G., 216
Sechi, E., 80
Secord, W., 37, 223
Segal, J., 445
Seidel, U. P., 136
Seidenberg, P. L., 450–451, 480
Seifer, R., 281
Sell, M. A., 356
Semel, E. M., 17, 209, 223, 359, 381, 399, 454, 476
Sevcik, R. A., 288
Shaffer, D., 71–72, 117
Shankweiler, D., 36, 194, 418
Shapiro, N. Z., 33
Sheard, C., 431
Sheldon-Wildgen, J., 442, 454
Shelly, M., 209
Shepard, N. T., 130
Sherbenou, R. J., 217, 218n
Sherman, A., 455
Sherman, G. F., 58
Sherman, J., 442, 454
Shinn, M. R., 226
Shortz, C., 178
Shriberg, L. D., 379
Siegel, G. M., 292
Siegel-Causey, E., 100, 290, 292, 293, 295n, 305, 306n
Sikes, J., 176
Silbar, J. C., 269, 271n, 272n, 275n, 331
Silliman, E. R., 440, 441, 452, 453
Silva, P. A., 80, 124
Simeonsson, R. J., 262, 266, 267
Simmons, A. A., 126
Simmons, J. Q., 109, 146, 287
Simon, C. S., 59, 168, 174, 182, 445
Simons, R., 158n, 160, 170
Simpson, A., 124
Sinclair, J. S., 129
Singer, H., 206
Singer, J., 321

Singer, L. T., 284
Singer, S., 321
Siperstein, M., 316
Sitnick, V. N., 282
Skarakis-Doyle, E., 377
Skinner, B. F., 62, 63, 64, 200, 206
Skinner, M. W., 124
Slater, W. H., 428n
Slavin, R. E., 176
Slingerland, B. H., 88
Sloan, C., 209
Sloane, H., 200
Slobin, D., 28, 35, 49, 61, 248–249
Smallpiece, V., 81
Smith, C., 232
Smith, F., 7, 114, 214
Smith, F. L., Jr., 183
Smith, J., 446
Smith, J. H., 297
Smith, N. L., 125
Smith, P. L., 462
Smitherman, G., 35
Snapp, M., 176
Snow, C. E., 14, 73, 74, 75, 246, 316,
  317, 403
Snyder, L., 66, 72, 205, 208, 209, 210,
  420
Snyder, T., 281, 360
Snyder-McLean, L. K., 247, 248n
Sonderman, J., 177
Spaanenburg, L., 209
Sparks, S. N., 123, 139, 140, 262, 263,
  266, 268, 282
Spearman, C. E., 102
Spekman, N. J., 297, 298n, 355, 356n,
  384, 426, 428, 429, 459
Speltz, M. L., 171
Spencer-Rowe, J., 455
Spriestersbach, D., 230
Springer, S. P., 194
Squire, J. R., 425, 426, 427
Sroufe, A., 140, 142
Staats, A., 63
Stafford, M., 399
Stainback, S., 14, 170, 229
Stainback, W., 14, 170, 192, 229
Stampe, D., 37
Stanovich, K. E., 94, 136, 418
Stark, J., 310
Stark, R. E., 80, 86, 96, 206, 219, 233,
  235n
Starr, R. H., 142
Stass, V., 278
Steckol, K. F., 211, 311
Stein, N., 357, 460
Steinkamp, M. W., 124
Stelmachowicz, P. G., 130
Stelmacovich, P., 455
Stephan, C., 176
Stephens, M. I., 394, 399, 407, 408
Sternberg, L., 290, 291n

Sternberg, R. J., 102, 103, 441, 442,
  443, 444n, 445
Stevens, F., 328, 329
Stewart, I., 124
Stewart, S., 113
Stewart, S. R., 389, 429n, 460
Stickler, K. R., 342
Stock, J. R., 328
Stockman, I. J., 311, 312, 354
Stoel-Gammon, C., 285, 322
Stokes, T. F., 204
Stoner, G., 113
Storey, M. E., 228
Stremel-Campbell, K., 311
Strickland, D. S., 383, 428
Striefel, S., 312
Strong, W., 471, 472, 473
Stroud, V., 35, 226
Studdert-Kennedy, M., 36
Sturm, J. M., 51, 74, 169, 195, 330,
  339, 374, 425, 452
Sullivan, P. M., 130
Sung, W. K., 81
Superior, K., 172, 174
Suritsky, S. K., 464, 465
Sussman, H. M., 49
Sutter, J. C., 375, 376
Sutton, A. C., 134
Sutton-Smith, B., 429, 430, 431, 459,
  460
Svinicki, J., 328
Swisher, L., 106, 107–108, 140,
  358–359
Swoger, P. A., 454, 478
Szeszulski, P. A., 94–95
Szkeres, S. F., 118, 441

Taff, T. G., 406
Tager-Flusberg, H., 308, 375
Takakashi, C., 182
Tallal, P., 86, 96, 206, 216, 219
Tamaroff, M., 120
Tannen, D., 337
Tateyama-Sniezek, K. M., 176
Tattershall, S. S., 417, 418n, 441–442
Taylor, B. M., 462
Taylor, D., 228, 317, 383, 428
Taylor, O. L., 30, 33, 34, 35, 154, 216,
  226, 227
Telle, D., 124
Templin, M., 230, 353
Terrell, B. Y., 318
Terrell, F., 35, 91, 227, 239
Terrell, S. L., 35, 91, 227, 239
Tharp, R. G., 448
Thatcher, V. S., 214
Thorndyke, P. W., 357
Thurlow, M., 192
Thurman, S., 177
Thurston, S., 29, 137
Tibbits, D., 399

Tice, R., 307, 389
Tiegerman, E., 283, 293, 316
Tierney, R. J., 418, 419, 449
Tindal, G., 422
Tizard, J., 112, 113
Tjossem, T. D., 260
Tobin, H., 113
Todd, N., 124
Tomblin, J. B., 80, 146, 147, 219, 235n,
  435
Tomlin, R., 232
Tomlinson, C., 177
Tonjes, M. J., 444
Torgesen, J. K., 210, 441, 478
Torgesen, J. L., 478
Towery-Woolsey, J., 436
Trapani, C., 404, 407
Traphagen, J., 287, 322
Traub, M., 117
Trevarthen, C., 29
Trohanis, P. L., 260
Tronick, E., 263, 282, 283
Tucker, J. A., 226, 413
Tucker, S., 113
Turnbull, A. P., 267
Turner, R. G., 260
Tyack, D. L., 342, 347, 349, 375

Vail, P. L., 113–114
Valencia, S., 444
Van Bourgondien, M., 144, 146
Van Buren, P., 41
Vanderheiden, G. C., 263, 265n,
  305
van der Lely, H. K. J., 376
van Dijk, J., 290, 291n
van Dijk, T., 427, 460
Van Dongen, R., 460
van Kleeck, A., 75, 199, 200, 249, 316,
  317, 424
van Pelt, D., 206, 207n
Vaughn, S., 455
Vaughn-Cooke, F. B., 217, 227, 311,
  312, 354
Vavra, E., 472
Vellutino, F., 194, 332
Venezky, R. L., 418
Vernon, M., 130
Volterra, V., 72, 209, 264n, 297, 317
Vygotsky, L. S., 74, 246–247, 317, 365,
  415, 423–424, 436, 448

Wada, J. A., 58, 59
Walker, V., 284
Wallace, E., 399
Wallach, G. P., 17, 80, 233, 376, 395,
  440, 441, 462
Wallat, C., 22, 23, 229
Waller, T. G., 440, 449
Wanat, P., 454
Wang, M. C., 189, 192

Wanner, E., 62
Warner, M., 210, 440
Warren, D. H., 131, 133
Warren, S. F., 186, 204, 205, 212, 213, 260, 293, 296, 313, 314n, 362, 363
Warren-Leubecker, A., 57, 204
Warr-Leeper, G. A., 452, 480
Wasserman, G. A., 140, 142, 143
Watkins, S., 282
Watson, B. U., 130
Watson, D. J., 421
Watson, L., 251, 252n
Watzlawick, P., 264, 298
Weaver, C., 469
Webb, W. G., 60, 95
Weber, J., 124
Weber-Olsen, M., 232
Wechsler, D., 111, 226
Weicker, L., 14
Weikert, D. P., 175
Weiner, B., 97
Weiner, D. S., 435
Weismer, S. E., 118
Wellman, H., 384
Wells, G., 53, 61, 62, 63, 199, 290, 292, 315, 330, 335–336, 382
Wepman, J. M., 206, 207n
Werner, E. O., 360
Werner, H., 61, 475
Wertz, R. T., 135
Wesson, C., 192
West, J., 124
Westby, C. E., 53, 54, 318, 320n, 335, 357, 366, 367n, 382, 383, 384, 418, 419, 426, 428, 429, 430, 431, 443, 445, 450, 460, 461, 462, 463n, 470
Westby, S., 384

Wetherby, A. M., 260, 269, 276, 277–278, 279n, 281, 283, 284, 294, 300, 304
Wetherby, B., 312
Wexler, K., 62
Whitaker, H., 26
Whitaker, H. A., 26, 116
White, R. E. C., 259, 315
White, S. H., 51, 244
White, S. J., 259, 315, 437
Whiteman, M. F., 337
Whitmore, K., 112
Wieder, S., 266, 268
Wiener, F. D., 227
Wiess, A. L., 125
Wiig, E. H., 17, 80, 223, 381, 399, 446, 447n, 454, 474–475, 476
Wilbur, R. B., 124, 125, 309
Wilcox, M., 249, 322
Wilkins, R., 146
Wilkinson, L. C., 417, 452–453
Will, M., 11, 161
Willeford, J. A., 208
Williams, J., 429, 464, 465
Williams, R., 35, 226
Williams, S., 124
Wills, L., 291n
Wilson, E. O., 61
Wilson, T. D., 15
Wilson-Vlotman, A. L., 282
Wing, L., 106
Winitz, H., 376, 448
Winkler, E., 370
Winograd, P., 97–98
Wixson, K., 418
Wnek, L., 328
Wolery, M., 14, 261, 262
Wolff, P. H., 292

Wolff, S., 145
Wolfram, W., 34, 226, 227, 352, 373–374
Wolfus, B., 81
Wong, B. Y., 438, 449–450
Wong, R., 438
Wood, B. S., 29
Wood, P., 8, 10, 13, 156
Woodcock, R., 408
Woodruff, G., 215
Worster-Drought, C., 118
Wray, D., 365
Wurman, R. S., 6, 214

Yell, M. L., 158
Ylvisaker, M., 118, 122, 441, 460
Yochum, M., 418
Yoder, D. E., 29, 30, 134, 137, 262, 263, 265n, 485
Yoder, P. J., 362
Yonclas, D., 260, 281, 284
Yorkston, K. M., 396
Yoshida, R. K., 215
Yoshinago-Itano, C., 459
Yoss, K. A., 135
Yovetich, W., 455
Ysseldyke, J. E., 192
Ysseldyke, J. R., 215
Yule, W., 222

Zachman, L., 360
Zametkin, A. J., 113
Zeisloft, B., 328
Zelman, J. G., 328
Zigmond, N., 442
Zinkus, P., 124
Zintz, M. V., 444
Zwitman, D., 177

Subject Index

AAC devices. *See* Augmentative and alternative communication devices
AAMD (American Association on Mental Deficiency), 98
ABNQ. *See* "Almost but not quite"
ABR (auditory brain stem response), 261
Abstract meanings, 474–480
Abuse, 3, 139–143
Accommodation, 69
Accountability, 253–254
Acquiescence, 16–17
Acquired brain injury, 3, 115–123
  age of child and, 120
  central processing factors in, 115–123
  contributing factors in, 119–122
  features of language and cognition with, 117
  focal, 116
  stimulus-response-reinforcement factors and, 121–122
  traumatic, 116–118, 395–396, 459–460
Acquisition components, of information processing, 102
Acquisition of Syntax in Children From 5 to 10, The (Chomsky), 394
Active conversationalists, 356
Activities of daily living (ADLs), 250, 333, 400, 401
Activity language, 306
Adaptation, 70
Adaptive techniques, 283
Adaptors, 30
ADD. *See* Attention-deficit disorder
ADHD. *See* Attention-deficit hyperactivity disorder
ADLs. *See* Activities of daily living
Adolescence. *See* Later stages of language acquisition
Adolescent Language Screening Test (ALST), 399
Adolescent pregnancy, 140–141, 142, 143

African Americans, 30, 33. *See also* Black English Vernacular
After the Tears (Simons), 160
Age
  chronological, 216, 220
  joint reference and, 303, 304
  language, 216–217, 221
  mental, 114, 155, 216, 217, 221
Agent, 313
Agentive, 45
Agnosia, 92, 118–119, 121
AIDS, 260
Alcohol abuse, 151
"Almost but not quite" (ABNQ), 250, 260, 325, 327, 338, 394, 397
ALST (Adolescent Language Screening Test), 399
Alternation rules, 52
Alternative school programs, 406
Ambiguity, lexical and syntactic, 43
American Association on Mental Deficiency (AAMD), 98
American Psychiatric Association, 104. *See also Diagnostic and Statistical Manual of Mental Disorders, Third Edition—Revised*
American Sign Language (ASL), 29
American Speech-Language-Hearing Association (ASHA), 27, 28n
  Committee on Amplification for the Hearing Impaired, 365
  Committee on Language, Speech, and Hearing Services in Schools, 164, 173, 180, 181n, 216
  Joint Committee on Infant Hearing, 261
Amnesia, 116, 118
Amplification of speech, 363–365
Anaphora, 45
Antonymy, 44
Aphasia
  congenital, 86, 115
  with epilepsy (Landau syndrome), 87, 118–119, 121

APIB (Assessment of Preterm Infant Behavior), 263
APR (auropalpebral response), 261
Apraxia, 135, 137
Arguments, 456, 457
Artifacts
  analysis of, 414
  gathering, 233
ASA (Autism Society of America), 202n, 256
ASHA. *See* American Speech-Language-Hearing Association
Asian Americans, 33
ASL (American Sign Language), 29
ASS (Assigning Structural Stage), 346–347, 350
Assertive acts, 356
Assessment, 4, 188–244
  bias in, 226–229
  contextually based assessment, 407, 413–415
  culture and, 226–229, 334–335, 404–406
  curriculum-based, 226, 232–233, 413–415, 416, 433
  determining eligibility for service, 219–233
  diagnosing disorder, 215–219
  dynamic, 409
  in early stages. *See under* Early stages of language acquisition
  establishing prognosis, 233–238
  formal
    in early stages, 279–280
    informal vs., 279–280
    in later stages, 407–409
    in middle stages, 358–360
  gathering baseline data, 242–244
  informal, 229–233
    in early stages, 278–281
    formal vs., 279–280
    in later stages, 409–433
    in middle stages, 341–358

Assessment, *continued*
  in later stages. *See under* Later
    stages of language acquisition
  in middle stages. *See under* Middle
    stages of language acquisition
  outlining parameters of impairment,
    disability, and handicap, 238–240
  play-based, 211, 276–277
  process-oriented, 278–279
  selecting goals, 240–242, 243
  sequence of questions in, 188–194
  serial, 262
  starter questions for, 410
  steps in, 190–191
  team contributions to, 214–215
  theoretical perspectives, 194–214
    behaviorist theories, 200–205
    biological maturation theories,
      194–196
    cognitivist theories, 209–211
    information processing theories,
      205–209
    linguistic theories, 196–200
    social interaction theories, 211–213
Assessment of Children's Language
  Comprehension, 310
Assessment of Preterm Infant Behavior
  (APIB), 263
Assigning Structural Stage (ASS),
  346–347, 350
Assimilation, 38
Association for Individuals with Severe
  Handicaps (TASH), 256
Asymmetries, cerebral, 58–59
Attention, 7, 283
Attentional deficit, 114
Attention-deficit disorder (ADD), 161
Attention-deficit hyperactivity disorder
  (ADHD), 3, 110–115
  central processing factors in,
    110–115, 145
  contributing factors in, 112–115
  defined, 110–111
  describing disability, 240
  diagnostic criteria for, 111–112
  drugs with, 196
  psychiatric disorders and, 145, 148
Attention training, 201
Attorney's fees, 158
Auditory brain stem response (ABR),
  261
Auditory language-learning context,
  363–365
Auditory problems. *See* Hearing
  impairment
Augmentative and alternative
  communication (AAC), 265
Augmentative and alternative
  communication (AAC) devices
  in early stages, 263–265, 268,
    273–276

mainstreaming and, 245
  selective reinforcement and, 138
  social interaction and, 138–139
  speech and, 29, 33, 99–100, 134, 268
  written language and, 29, 136–137
Auropalpebral response (APR), 261
Autism, 273
  central processing factors in, 103–110
  contributing factors in, 108–110
  defined, 103–105
  development of language, speech,
    and communication with, 107
  diagnostic criteria for, 104–105
  peer tutoring and, 483–484
  prognosis of language disorder with,
    234–236
  semantic relations and, 313
  speech and, 27, 287
  unconventional language and, 28
Autism Society of America (ASA), 202*n*,
  256
Autoclitic behavior, 64

Baby Signals (Lynch-Fraser and
  Tiegerman), 283
Background information, 408
Baseline data, 242–244
Base morphemes, 30
Battelle Developmental Inventory, 328
Bayley Scales of Infant Development,
  328
BBCS (Bracken Basic Concept Scale), 360
Behavior
  autoclitic, 64
  changing, 192
  echoic verbal, 64
  feeding, 287–289
  intraverbal, 64
  vocal and phonological, 284–287
Behavioral adaptation, 70
Behavioral problems, 3, 143–149
Behavioral state communication,
  282–283
Behaviorism, 3, 62–65. *See also*
  Stimulus-response-reinforcement
  factors
  contributions of, 200–203
  limitations of, 203–205
  strategies used in, 201–203
BESS (Black English Sentence Scoring),
  227, 352, 373
BEV. *See* Black English Vernacular
Bias
  in assessment, 226–229
  in evaluation and eligibility
    determination, 154–155
  therapist, 15–16
Bilingualism, 33–34, 452–453
Binding theory, 42
Biological maturation
  abuse and, 141

acquired brain injury and, 119–120
attention-deficit hyperactivity disorder
  and, 112–113
autism and, 108–109
hearing impairment and, 126–127
mental retardation and, 101–102
neglect and, 141
physical impairment and, 137
psychiatric disorders and, 145–146
specific language disability and, 95
theories, 3, 57–61
  contributions of, 194–196
  limitations of, 196
visual impairment and, 132–133
Biological risks, 260
Birth weight, low, 260, 263
Black English Sentence Scoring (BESS),
  227, 352, 373
Black English Vernacular (BEV), 34–35,
  40, 226, 350, 352, 373–374, 405,
  419, 420
Blindness, 131–134
Blissymbols, 137
Bloom's taxonomy, 444–445
Boder Test of Reading–Spelling
  Patterns, 423
Body language, 30
Boehm Test of Basic Concepts (BTBC),
  329, 360
Bounding theory, 42
Bound morphemes, 27–28, 39, 40
Bracken Basic Concept Scale (BBCS),
  360
Brain
  asymmetries in, 58–59
  chemistry of, 145–146
  development of, 58–61
  hemispheres of, 40, 59
  weight of, 59–60
Brain damage. *See also* Acquired brain
  injury
  to Broca's area, 39, 40
  minimal, 86
  neuropsychology and, 26
  prognosis of language disorder with,
    237
  to Wernicke's area, 39–40
Brain dysfunction, minimal, 86
Broca's area of brain, 39, 40, 42, 194
BTBC (Boehm Test of Basic Concepts),
  329, 360
Bureaucratic policies and procedures,
  18. *See also* Public policy

Care, early sensing of, 282
Care centers, acute and long-term, 406
Caregivers, techniques used by, 283
*Carolina Curriculum for Handicapped
  Infants and Infants at Risk*
  (Johnson-Martin, Jens, and
  Attermeier), 288

Case grammar, 45
Caseload sizes, 180, 181
Case theory, 42
Cataphora, 45
Categorization, 82–85
Causation, 78–151
  central processing factors, 85–123
  elusiveness of cause, 79–82
  emotional factors, 139–149
  environmental factors, 139–149
  hearing impairment, 123–131
  mixed factors and changes over time,
    149–150
  neglect and abuse, 139–143
  patterns of, 18–19
  physical impairment, 134–139
  speech motor control, 134–139
  visual impairment, 131–134
CBA. *See* Curriculum-based
  assessment
CBM (curriculum-based measurement),
  413
CELF-R (Clinical Evaluation of Language
  Fundamentals—Revised), 223,
  359, 399
Central nervous system
  development of, 58–61
  model of levels of function in, 207
Central processing factors, 85–123
  in acquired brain injury, 115–123
  in attention-deficit hyperactivity
    disorder, 110–115, 145
  in autism, 103–110
  in mental retardation, 98–103
  in specific language disability, 85–98
Central processing skills, 413
Cerebral asymmetries, 58–59
Cerebrovascular accidents (CVAs), 115,
  116, 119, 120
Chaining, 203
Change
  expectations for, 402
  relevant, 250
Charting, 251, 252
Child-centered mode, 212
Child-directed play, 174–175
Child Discourse (Ervin-Tripp and
  Mitchell-Kernan), 52
Child-Find programs, 262–263, 327
Children
  neglect and abuse of, 3, 139–143
  older children with early-stage
    abilities, 268–276
  scheduling preferences of, 183–185
Chromosomal defects, 81
Chronological age (CA), 216, 220
Circular reactions, 69
Clarity, of speech, 322–323, 401
Classical conditioning, 63
Classrooms
  as assessment settings, 267, 336–340

conversation in, 451–454
  regular, 168–169
  routines and rules of, 418
  special, 166–168
Clinical Evaluation of Language Fundamentals—Revised (CELF-R), 223,
  359, 399
Cluster reduction, deletion, or
  substitution, 38
Cocaine, 260
Code learning, 73
Cogitative knowledge, 70
Cognition factors
  in acquired brain injury, 122
  in attention-deficit hyperactivity
    disorder, 114–115
  in autism, 110
  hearing impairment and, 130
  in mental retardation, 102–103
  neglect and abuse, 142
  physical impairment and, 138–139
  psychiatric disorders and, 148
  in specific language disability, 97
  visual impairment and, 133
Cognitive development, stages of,
  68–69, 71–72
Cognitive rehabilitation therapy, 122
Cognitivism, 3, 67–72, 209–210
Cohesion, 473–474, 475
Collaborative consultation, 2, 17, 21–22
Comments, defined, 296
Communicating to Make Friends (Fox),
  175
Communication, 29–33
  behavioral state, 282–283
  defined, 29
  nonlinguistic, 30, 47
  nonsymbolic, 290, 294–295
  paralinguistic, 30–33, 47
  reasons for, 53
  as social interaction, 51–54
Communication aids. *See* Augmentative
  and alternative communication
  devices
Communication and Symbolic Behavior
  Scales (CSBS), 277–278, 304
Communication needs model, 8, 10–12
Communication processes model, 8–10
Communication units, 425
Communicative reading strategies
  (CRS), 212
Compensation, 325
Competence
  developing edge of, 244
  in discourse, 451–468
  identifying aspects of, 341
  language, 49
Competitive goals, 22
Competitiveness, 17
Complex sentences, 350–351, 374–375
Componential operations, 443

Compound sentences, 350–351
Comprehension
  informal assessment of, 232–233
  reading, 449–450
  of routines and events by infants,
    290–292
Concepts, acquisition of, 379–382
Concrete operations stage of cognitive
  development, 69
Conditioning, 63
Conscious megacognitive strategies,
  413
Consonants
  assimilation between, 38
  final consonant deletion, 38
Construct-related evidence,
  224
Consultants, roles of, 172–174. *See
  also* Providers
Consultation
  collaborative, 2, 17, 21–22
  recognizing need for, 401
Content–form constructions, complex,
  371–379
Content-related evidence, 224
Content variables, 350–355
Content words, 39, 40
Context(s)
  acute-care center, 406
  alternative school programs, 406
  auditory language-learning, 363–365
  in early-stage assessment and
    intervention, 266–267
  higher education, 406–407
  home and family, 169–170, 403–404
  importance of, 52
  in later-stage assessment and
    intervention, 400–407, 435–439
  long-term care center, 406
  in middle-stage assessment and
    intervention, 334–340
  modifying, 435–439
  social, 170–171, 404
  variation in, 48
  vocational, 171, 406–407
Contextually based assessment, 407,
  413–415
Contextual operations, 443
Control
  executive, 440–441
  speech motor, 134–139
  techniques for, 283
  topic, 47
Control theory, 42
Conversation. *See also* Discourse
  in classrooms, 451–454
  defined, 451
  expanding purposes of, 366–371
  in families, 457–458
  with peers, 454–457
  requirements for, 403

Conversational discourse, 411, 426, 427–428
Conversationalists, active and passive, 356
Conversation rules, 52
Convulsive disorder, with aphasia, 87, 118–119
Co-occurrence rules, 52
Cooperative goal setting, 2, 17, 22, 215
Cooperative learning, peers in, 176–177
Coreference, 45
Creativity, 361
Criteria
  diagnostic, 104–105, 111–112
  discrepancy, 216–219
  exit, 252–253
  referral, 329–331
Criterion-referenced testing, 226
Criterion-related evidence, 224
CRS (communicative reading strategies), 212
CSBS (Communication and Symbolic Behavior Scales), 277–278, 304
Cuing, 202
Culture
  differences in, 53–54, 399
  in later-stage assessment, 404–406
  methodology and, 22–23, 399
  in middle-stage assessment, 334–335
  multicultural perspectives in assessment, 226–229
  narrative discourse and, 429
  socialization and, 403–404
  specific language disability and, 91
Culture-fair language tests, 227
Curriculum, practical intelligence, 444
Curriculum-based assessment (CBA), 226, 232–233, 413–415, 416, 433
Curriculum-based language intervention, mediational discourse in, 436–438
Curriculum-based measurement (CBM), 413
CVAs (cerebrovascular accidents), 115, 116, 119, 120
Cytomegalovirus, 260

Danger signals, 328
Data
  baseline, 242–244
  charting, 251, 252
Dative, 45
Deafness. See Hearing impairment
Deafness Management Quotient (DMQ), 237
Decentering, 318
Decision(s), false-negative and false-positive, 224, 262
Decision-making model, 253, 269–276, 331
Decoding, 354–355

Deep structures (D-structures), 41, 42
Deficit theory of language variation, 405
Deixis, 45
Delivery. See Service delivery
Denasalization, 38
Dendritic arborization, 60
Denver Developmental Screening Test, 328
Derivational morphemes, 40
Developmental Indicators of the Assessment of Learning (DIAL), 329
Developmental Sentence Scoring (DSS) system, 227, 348
Diabetes, 133
Diagnosis, of language disorders, 215–219. See also Assessment
Diagnostic and Statistical Manual of Mental Disorders, Third Edition—Revised (DSM-III-R)
  on attention-deficit disorder, 110–111
  on autism, 104–105
  on psychiatric disorders, 143, 144
  on specific language disability, 86, 87
Diagnostic criteria
  for ADHD, 111–112
  for autism, 104–105
DIAL (Developmental Indicators of the Assessment of Learning), 329
Dialects, 34–35. See also Black English Vernacular
Dialogue journals, 453–454
Difference theory of language variation, 405
Dimensional stage of development, 71
Disability. See also Profound disabilities; Specific language disability
  counting, 398
  defined, 1, 10, 156
  defining, 10–12
  describing, 240
  learning, 86, 87, 149, 150
  multiple, 331–333, 400, 401
  new categories of, 161
  reading, 86, 87
Discourse
  competence in, 451–468
  conversational, 411, 426, 427–428
  expository, 357–358, 411, 426, 431–433, 461–468
  mediational, 436–438
  narrative, 411, 426, 428–431, 458–461
  of teachers, 362–363, 364
Discourse knowledge, 423
Discrepancy criteria, 216–218
Discrimination training, 202–203
Disputes, 456, 457
Distance, and communication, 30
DMQ (Deafness Management Quotient), 237

Down's syndrome, 81–82, 84, 100, 281. See also Mental retardation
Drugs
  abuse of, 151, 260
  with ADHD, 196
DSM-III-R. See Diagnostic and Statistical Manual of Mental Disorders, Third Edition—Revised
DSS (Developmental Sentence Scoring) system, 227, 348
D-structures, 41, 42
Dynamic assessment, 409
Dyslexia. See also Specific language disability
  adolescents with, 396–397
  brain injury and, 96
  characteristics of, 88
  defined, 10
  example of, 12
  as label, 87
  phonological skills and, 94–95

Early Intervention Developmental Profile, 328
Early language delay (ELD), 80–81
Early Learning Accomplishment Profile, 328
Early stages of language acquisition, 258–323
  AAC devices in, 263–265, 268, 273–276
  assessment, 266–281
    contexts for, 266–267
    family systems approach to, 267–268
    formal, 279–280
    informal, 278–281
    models for older children, 268–276
    strategies for, 276–281
    tools for, 276–278
  intervention, 281–323
    clarity of speech, 322–323
    combining words, 310–314
    comprehension of routines and events, 290–292
    feeding behaviors and needs, 287–289
    imitation, 292–293
    intentionality, 293–302
    literacy, 316–317
    parents' role in, 314–316
    play and, 317–322
    reciprocation, 292
    scaffolding, 293, 313
    semantics in, 310–314
    symbols, 302–309
    vocal and phonological behavior, 284–287
  later stages vs., 395
  problem identification in, 259–265

Ebonics, 226. *See also* Black English Vernacular
Echoic verbal behavior, 64
Echolalia, 301–302
Eclectic practice, 214
"Ecological and Student Repertoire Inventories" (Brown et al.), 485
Ecological thinking, 1–2, 19–20
Educable mentally retarded, 99
Education
    free appropriate public education (FAPE), 153
    higher, 406–407
    inclusive, 162
    reeducation, 259
Education for All Handicapped Children Act of 1975 (PL 94–142), 153–157
    on dialect differences, 35
    on least restrictive environment, 13–14
    problem identification and, 327, 329, 331, 398
    on program duration, 183
    on termination of special programs, 253
Education of Handicapped Act Amendments of 1986 (PL 99–457), 158–160
    early-stage problems and, 189, 261
    intermediate policy and, 163
    on least restrictive environment, 14
    problem identification and, 327
    on program duration, 183
EEGs (electroencephalograms), 120
Elaborative techniques, 283
ELD (early language delay), 80–81
Electroencephalograms (EEGs), 120
Elementary school students. *See also* Middle stages of language acquisition
    language learning and use in classroom, 336–340
    referral criteria for, 329–331
Elicited samples, 231–232
Eligibility determination
    assessment and, 219–233
    bias and, 154–155
Emblems, 30
Emerging literacy, 382–385
Emotional development, and socialization, 103
Emotional factors, 139–149
Emotional problems, 3, 143–149, 150
Empiricist theories, 57
Encephalopathy secondary to infection or irradiation, 119
Encoding, 354–355
English
    Black English Vernacular (BEV), 34–35, 40, 226, 350, 352, 373–374, 405, 419, 420

    standard, 40, 226, 373–374
Entailment, 44
Environmental factors, 139–149
Environmental risks, 260
Epilepsy, aphasia with, 87, 118–119, 121
Equal opportunity, 480–484
Equivalent scores, 221–222
Ethnographic methodology, 2, 22–23
Evaluation
    bias in, 154–155
    multidisciplinary approach to, 154–156
    periodic reevaluation, 157
Event knowledge, 290–292
Exclusionary criteria, 218–219
Executive control strategies, 440–441
Exit criteria, 252–253
Experiencer, 45
Experiential operations, 443
Expertise, diverse, 22
Expository discourse, 357–358, 411, 426, 431–433
Expository texts, 461–468
Extension, 44
Eyeblink response, 261
Eye contact, 30

Facial expression, 30
Facilitative techniques, 283
Factitive, 45
Fading, 202
Failure, factors contributing to, 15–18
Failure-to-thrive syndrome, 139
False-negative decision, 224, 262
False-positive decision, 224, 262
Family. *See also* Parents
    as assessment setting, 266, 403–404
    conversation in, 457–458
    Individualized Family Service Plans for, 158, 159–160, 183, 193
    as intervention setting option, 169–170
    life cycle of, 267
    roles and relationships in service delivery, 177–180
Family Rights and Privacy Act, 153
Family systems approach, to early-stage assessment, 267–268
FAPE (free appropriate public education), 153
Fast mapping, 380–381
Federal policy, 153–162
Federal Register, 153
Feeding behavior, of infants, 287–289
Feeding tubes, 284–285, 287–288
Figurative language, 478–480
Figurative schemes, 71
Focal acquired brain injury, 116
Follow-up, importance of, 17–18
Formal assessment. *See under* Assessment

Formal operations stage of cognitive development, 69, 71
Fragmentation fallacy, 15
Free appropriate public education (FAPE), 153
Free morphemes, 30
Frication, 38
Fronting, 38
Functional capabilities, 397
Functional meanings, 307
Functional responses, 204
Function words, 39

Garbles, 346
Gastrostomy tube, 285, 287–288
GB (government-binding) theory, 41–43, 62, 198
Genetic counseling, 151
Gesell Development Schedules, 328, 329
Gestalt Closure, 223
g factor, 102–103
Gliding, 38
Goal setting, 240–242, 243
    competitive, 22
    cooperative, 2, 17, 22, 215
    individualistic, 22
    in middle-stage intervention, 390–392
    shifting focus of, 241–242
Government-binding (GB) theory, 41–43, 62, 198
Government policy. *See* Public policy
Government theory, 42
Grammar
    case, 45
    in linguistic theories of language acquisition, 62
    phrase structure, 41
    story, 357, 429
    syntax vs., 40–41
    transformational generative, 41, 62, 198
    universal, 41, 62
Grammar schemata, 357
Grammatical morphemes, 39–40
Graphophonemic knowledge, 423

Habit formation, 69–70
Halo effect, 15
Handicap(s)
    defined, 1, 13, 155–156, 159
    describing, 240
    multidisciplinary evaluation and determination of, 154–156
Handicapped Children's Protection Act of 1986 (PL 99–372), 157–158
Hard-of-hearing, 124. *See also* Hearing impairment
Hawaii Early Learning Profile, 328
Hawthorne effect, 175
Head Start, 27, 327, 335

Health and Human Services, U.S.
    Department of, 139
Hearing impairment, 123–131
    conversing with family and, 458
    conversing with peers and, 456
    defined, 123
    in Down's syndrome children, 82
    equal opportunity and, 481
    identifying, 261
    in infants, 261
    language acquisition and, 29
    language disorders and, 123–131
    measurement of, 123, 128
    prognosis of language disorder with,
        236–237
    speech amplification and, 363–365
    speech and, 27
    subtypes of, 123–124
    written language problems with, 126
Helplessness, learned, 448
High/Scope Preschool Cognitive
    Curriculum, 175
Hispanic Americans, 33–34, 452–453
History information, 341, 408
Holistic thinking, 20
Home. See also Family
    assessment in, 266
    as intervention setting option,
        169–170
    language in home vs. school, 337,
        338
    shift to school in middle stages,
        335–336
Homeostasis, 19, 20, 266
Hospital-based assessment, 266, 406
Hyperactive disorder, 3. See also
    Attention-deficit hyperactivity
    disorder
Hyperbole, 478
Hyperkinesis. See Attention-deficit
    hyperactivity disorder
Hyponymy, 44

Iconic sign, 305
IDEA. See Individuals with Disabilities
    Education Act of 1990
Idiomatic language, 480
IEPs. See Individualized Education
    Plans
IFSPs. See Individualized Family Service
    Plans
Illinois Test of Psycholinguistic Abilities,
    196
Illocutionary act, 46–47
Illocutionary stage of language
    acquisition, 263, 264
Illusory recovery, 80–81
Illustrators, 30
Imitation, 201, 292–293
Impairment(s)
    defined, 1, 8, 156

defining, 8–9
describing, 239–240
types of, 3
Implicature, 48
Inactive learners, 441
Incidental teaching, 205, 362–363
Inclusive education, 162
Independence, fostering, 484–486
Index, 305
Indirect speech act, 47
Individual differences, 237
Individualized Education Plans (IEPs),
    153, 156–157
    content of, 157, 161
    for individuals age 16 or older, 396
    mass screenings and, 398
    meetings concerning, 156–157, 230
    parents and, 156–157, 177, 178
    in progress measurement, 193
Individualized Family Service Plans
    (IFSPs), 158, 159–160, 183, 193
Individualized Transition Plans (ITPs),
    484
Individuals with Disabilities Education
    Act of 1990 (IDEA) (PL 101–476),
    153, 160–161. See also
    Education for All Handicapped
    Children Act of 1975
    on Child-Find programs, 262–263
    evaluation requirements of, 223
    follow-up monitoring under, 193–194
    on least restrictive environment, 14
    on parental participation, 177
    review of service delivery plan under,
        193
    state policy and, 162
    on transitional services, 407
Infant(s)
    assessment of. See under Early
        stages of language acquisition
    communication by, 282–284
    comprehension of routines and
        events by, 290–292
    family life cycle and, 267
    feeding behavior of, 287–289
    handicapped, 159
    imitation by, 292–293
    intervention with. See under Early
        stages of language acquisition
    intubation of, 284–285, 287–288
    low birth weight, 260, 263
    premature, 260–261
    risk identification in , 260–263
    sensing of care and safety by, 282
    techniques used with, 283
    vocal and phonological behavior of,
        284–287
Infant center of clinic, as assessment
    setting, 266–267
Infant Scale of Nonverbal Interaction,
    280, 295

Inference, 475
Inflectional morphemes, 40
Informal assessment. See under
    Assessment
Information, history, 341, 408
Information Anxiety (Wurman), 6
Information processing
    abuse and, 142
    acquired brain injury and, 122
    attention-deficit hyperactivity disorder
        and, 113–114
    autism and, 109–110
    components of, 102
    hearing impairment and, 129–130
    mental retardation and, 102
    neglect and, 142
    physical impairment and, 138
    psychiatric disorders and, 148
    specific language disability and,
        96–97
    theories, 3, 65–67
        contributions of, 205–206
        limitations of, 206–209
    visual impairment and, 133
Initiating techniques, 283
Injunctive relief, 157
Innateness, 66
Instructions, failure to understand, 401
Integration, 14, 162, 168–169
Integrative approaches, 24
Intelligence, g factor in, 102–103. See
    also Cognition factors;
    Cognitivism; IQ
Intentionality, 293–302
Interactions, adult-initiated vs. child-
    initiated, 280. See also Social
    interaction(s)
Interactive teaching, 438. See also
    Mediated learning
Interdisciplinary teams, 215
Intermediate policy, 162–163
Internal Work Experience (IWE),
    482–483
Interpretive approach to multiword
    utterances, 311
Intervention, 4, 244–254
    accountability in, 253–254
    contexts for, 192, 266–267, 334–340,
        400–407, 435–439
    designing and implementing
        intervention plan, 244–249
    in early stages. See under Early
        stages of language acquisition
    exit criteria for, 252–253
    failure of, 15–18
    identifying need for, 263–265
    in later stages. See under Later
        stages of language acquisition
    in middle stages. See under Middle
        stages of language acquisition
    monitoring progress during, 249–252

purpose of, 8
remediation vs., 325
sequence of questions in, 188–194
skill-based, 396
steps in, 190–191
strategy-based, 396
team contributions to, 214–215
terminating, 193, 252–253
theoretical perspectives guiding,
    194–214
  behaviorist, 200–205
  biological maturation, 194–196
  cognitivist, 209–211
  information processing, 205–209
  linguistic, 196–200
  social interaction, 211–213
for word-finding impairments,
    381–382
Intervention setting options, 165–171
home and family contexts, 169–170
pullout rooms, 165–166
regular classrooms, 168–169
social contexts, 170–171
special classrooms
  in regular buildings, 167–168
  in special buildings, 166–167
vocational contexts, 171
Interviewing, 229–230
Intonation, 31, 33
Intraverbal behavior, 64
Intrinsic knowledge, 2
Intubation, 284–285, 287–288
"Invitation-by-success," 399
IQ
  in diagnosis of language disorders,
    86, 94, 147, 217, 219
  in diagnosis of mental retardation, 98.
    See also Mental retardation
  in eligibility determination, 220
  performance, 223
  verbal, 223
ITPs (Individualized Transition Plans), 484
IWE (Internal Work Experience), 482–483

Jobs. *See* Work
Joint reference, 73–74, 303, 304
Judgments of degree, 219
Judgments of kind, 219

Kaufman Assessment Battery for
    Children (K-ABC), 223
Knowledge
cogitative, 70
event, 290–292
intrinsic, 2
metalinguistic, 2
semiotic-operational, 70
Knowledge structures, 412–413, 423

Labels, 3, 83–84, 87
LAD (language acquisition device), 58,
    61, 95

Landau syndrome, 87, 118–119, 121
Language, 27–28
acquisition of, 26–27, 263, 264. *See
    also* Language acquisition
    theories
activity, 306
body, 30
communication and, 29–33
defined, 27, 28
in elementary school, 336–340
figurative, 478–480
in home vs. school, 337, 338
idiomatic, 480
metalinguistic, 389
metapragmatic, 389
multidisciplinary perspectives on,
    26–27
nature of, 33–51
speech and, 28–29
subcomponents of, 35–48
unconventional use of, 27–28
whole, 386–387
Language acquisition device (LAD), 58,
    61, 95
Language acquisition theories, 56–77
behaviorism, 3, 62–65, 200–205
biological maturation, 3, 57–61,
    194–196
clinical implications of, 75–77
cognitivism, 3, 67–72, 209–211
information processing, 3, 65–67,
    205–209
linguistic rule induction, 3, 61–62,
    196–200
social interactionism, 3, 72–75,
    211–213
Language age (LA), 216–217, 221
Language assessment, remediation,
    and screening procedures
    (LARSP), 347–348
Language competence, 49
Language content abilities, 397
Language content variables, 350–355
Language delay
in autism, 106–108
with hearing impairment, 124–126
language disorder vs., 48
in mental retardation, 100–101
in specific language disability, 88–91
Language Development Survey (LDS),
    304
Language difference
in autism, 106–108
with hearing impairment, 124–126
language disorder vs., 189
in mental retardation, 100–101
in specific language disability, 88–91
Language disorders. *See also specific
    disorders*
categorizing, 82–85
causative factors. *See* Causation

defined, 79–80, 215–216
defining and diagnosing, 215–219
finding problems related to, 188–189
identifying
  in early stages, 259–265
  in later stages, 397–400
  in middle stages, 327–333
language delay vs., 48
language difference vs., 189
prevention of, 151
specific, 3, 85–98
Language form abilities, 397
Language form variables, 346–352
Language rules, assessing knowledge
    of, 48–51
Language sampling
in later stages, 410–411
in middle stages, 341–358
Language specialist. *See also* Providers
recognizing need for consultation
    with, 401
roles of, 172–174
Language use variables, 350–352,
    355–358
LARSP (language assessment,
    remediation, and screening
    procedures), 347–348
*Later Language Development: Ages
    Nine Through Nineteen* (Nippold),
    394
Later stages of language acquisition,
    393–486
adolescent pregnancy in, 140–141,
    142, 143
assessment, 400–434
  contexts for, 400–407, 435–439
  contextually based, 407, 413–415
  culture in, 404–406
  of discourse events, 411, 426–433
  formal, 407–409
  informal, 409–433
  of linguistic units, 411, 424–426
  miscue analysis, 420–422
  starter questions for, 410
  strategies for, 407–433
  thinking language analysis,
    423–424
  tools for, 407–433
  of written language samples,
    422–423
earlier stages vs., 395
general expectations for change in,
    402
intervention, 434–486
  developing abstract and nonliteral
    meanings, 474–480
  developing discourse competence,
    451–468
  encouraging syntactic-semantic
    developments, 468–474
  fostering metaskills, 440–451

Later stages of language acquisition,
continued
   learning strategies models,
     440–441
   modifying contexts for, 435–439
   with severely disabled young
     adults, 480–486
   skill-based, 396
   strategy-based, 396
   needs of individuals with multiple and
     severe disabilities, 400
   prevention in, 395–396
   problem identification in, 397–400
   recognizing need for consultation in,
     401
   referral in, 399–400, 401
   screening in, 398–399
   work experience and, 396
LDS (Language Development Survey),
   304
Learned helplessness, 448
Learners, inactive, 441
Learning
   cooperative, 176–177
   mediated, 246–247, 435–439
Learning disabilities, 86, 87, 149, 150.
   See also Specific language
   disability
*Learning Disabilities: Educational
   Principles and Practices* (Johnson
   and Myklebust), 206
Learning strategies models, 440–441
Least restrictive environment (LRE),
   13–14, 153, 338
LEP (limited English proficiency), 226
Leukemia, 119
Lexical and syntactic ambiguity, 43
Lexical and syntactic synonymy, 43–44
Lexical morphemes, 39
Lexical selection rules, 47
Lexicon, 379–381, 474–478
LF (logical form) rules, 42, 43
Limited English proficiency (LEP), 226
Linguistic reference, 44
Linguistic rule-induction theories, 3,
   61–62
   contributions of, 196–198
   limitations of, 198–200
Linguistics
   defined, 26
   psycholinguistics vs., 49–50
Linguistic sense, 43–44
Linguistic system factors
   abuse and, 141
   in acquired brain injury, 120–121
   in attention-deficit hyperactivity
     disorder, 113
   in autism, 109
   hearing impairment and, 127, 129
   in mental retardation, 102
   neglect and, 141

   physical impairment and, 137
   psychiatric disorders and, 146–147
   in specific language disability, 95–96
   visual impairment and, 133
Linguistic units, 411, 424–426
Liquid replacement, 38
Literacy. *See also* Reading; Written
   language
   early-stage intervention and, 316–317
   emerging, 382–385
   middle-stage intervention and,
     382–389
Literate lexicon, 474–478
Local policy, 163
Locative, 45
Locutionary act, 46
Locutionary stage of language
   acquisition, 263, 264
Logical form (LF) rules, 42, 43
Log notes, 251
LRE (least restrictive environment),
   13–14, 153, 338

MA. *See* Mental age
Magnetic resonance image (MRI), 121
Mainstreaming, 14, 162, 168–169, 245
Mand, 64
Mand-model strategy, 205
Manner, maxim of, 48
Manual of Developmental Diagnosis,
   328, 329
MAP approach, 455, 456
Mapping, 211
   fast, 380–381
   semantic, 477–478, 479
*Martin Luther King Elementary School
   Children et al.* v. *Ann Arbor
   School District Board*, 35, 405
Mazes, 346
Meaning(s)
   abstract, 474–480
   functional, 307
   multiple, 43
   nonliteral, 474–480
   referential, 307
   referents and, 304–305
"Meaning in Context: Is There Any
   Other Kind?" (Mishler), 9
Mean length of utterance (MLU)
   in defining disorder, 216
   in early stages, 316
   incidental teaching and, 363
   language sampling and, 344, 345,
     346
   in later stages, 411, 425
   physical impairment and, 136
   specific language disability and, 89, 90
Measurement. *See also* Assessment
   curriculum-based, 413
   of early-stage abilities, needs, and
     accomplishments, 266–281

   of later-stage needs and abilities,
     400–434
   of middle-stage abilities, needs, and
     accomplishments, 334–360
Mediated learning, 246–247, 435–439
Mediational discourse, 436–438
Memory
   improving, 445–446, 447
   metamemory, 447
   short-term, 203, 445–446, 472
Mental age (MA), 114, 155, 216, 217,
   221
Mental retardation, 3, 98–103
   central processing factors in, 98–103
   contributing factors in, 101–103
   defined, 98
   Down's syndrome, 81–82, 84, 100, 281
   emotions and, 103
   functional communication goals with,
     391
   levels of, 98–100
   in middle stages, 326
   semantic relations and, 313
   statistics on, 150
Metacognition, 7, 210, 412, 413
Metacognitive abilities, 418
Metacognitive strategies, 443–450
Metacomponents, of information
   processing, 102
Metalinguistic abilities, 416–417
Metalinguistic language, 389
Metalinguistics, 2, 199–200
   awareness of, 375–376
   in later-stage assessment, 411,
     415–418
Metalinguistic strategies, 446–450
Metamemory, 447
Metaphors, 478–479
Metapragmatic abilities, 417
Metapragmatic language, 389
Metapragmatic strategies, 441–443
Metaskills, fostering, 440–451
Metatextual abilities, 417–418
Metatextual strategies, 446–450
Metathesis, 39
Michigan Decision-Making Model, 253,
   269–276, 331
Middle stages of language acquisition,
   324–392
   assessment, 334–360
     contexts for, 334–340
     culture in, 334–335
     formal, 358–360
     informal, 341–358
     strategies for, 340–358
     tools for, 340–358
   intervention, 360–392
     acquiring words and concepts,
      379–382
     complex content–form
      constructions, 371–379

early stages of learning to read, 385–387
early stages of learning to write, 387–389
emerging literacy, 382–385
enhancing auditory language-learning context, 363–365
expanding conversational purposes, 366–371
goals for older students, 390–392
parents' role in, 360–362
phonological development, 379
storytelling, 382–385
symbolic play, 365–366, 367
teacher discourse, 362–363, 364
later stages vs., 395
needs of individuals with multiple and severe disabilities, 331–333
problem identification in, 325–333
referral in, 329–331, 341
shift from home to school in, 335–336
Milieu approach to semantic relations, 313, 314
Minimal brain dysfunction, 86
Minimal pairs, 36
Minorities. See also specific minority groups
bilingualism and, 33–34, 452–453
cultural differences of, 53–54
in school population, 33
Miscue analysis, 420–422, 438–439
MLU. See Mean length of utterance
Mnemonic instruction, 446
Modal auxiliaries, 372–373
Modeling, 201, 205
Modularity, 66, 210
Modular models of language proficiency, 15
Monterey language program, 378
Morphemes
base, 30
bound, 27–28, 39, 40
defined, 39
derivational, 40
free, 30
grammatical, 39–40
inflectional, 40
learning in written language, 470–472
lexical, 39
Morphogenesis, 19
Morphology, 39–40, 346–348
autism and, 108
hearing impairment and, 125
mental retardation and, 101
Motor system. See Peripheral sensory and motor system factors
MRI (magnetic resonance image), 121
Multidisciplinary teams, 214–215
Multipass strategy, 450
Multiple meaning, 43

Mutism, elective, 145, 146
Myelination, 60

Narrative discourse, 411, 426, 428–431, 458–461
Narratives from the Crib (Nelson), 76
Nasogastric tube, 285
National Center for Child Abuse, 140
National Conference on Learning Disabilities, 219
National Joint Committee on Learning Disabilities, 87
Native Americans
nonlinguistic communication of, 30
in school population, 33
Nativist theories, 57
Naturalistic observation, 244
Naturalistic samples, 230–231
Nature of Explanation, The (Craik), 65
Nature vs. nurture
in behaviorism, 65
in brain development, 60–61
NBAS (Neonatal Behavioral Assessment Scale), 263
Needs
identifying, 10–12
model of, 8, 10–12
Negative reinforcers, 201
Neglect, 3, 139–143
Neonatal Behavioral Assessment Scale (NBAS), 263
NEP (non-proficient) child, 226
Nervous system. See Central nervous system
NES (non-English speaking) child, 226
Neurolinguists, 26
Neuronal growth patterns, 60
Neuropsychologists, 26
Neutralization, 38
Noncommunicators, 356
Non-English speaking (NES) child, 226
Nonlinguistic communication, 30, 47
Nonliteral meanings, 474–480
Non-proficient (NEP) child, 226
Nonsymbolic communication, 290, 294–295
Note passing, 457
Note taking, 464–467

Objectives, 45
accomplishment of, 251–252
short-term, 243
Object symbolism, 318
Observation
naturalistic, 244
onlooker, 230, 414
participant, 230, 414–415
Observation of Communicative Interactions (OCI), 280–281
Office of Special Education and Rehabilitation Services, 162

OME (otitis media with effusion), 124
Onlooker observation, 230, 414
Operant conditioning, 63
Operative schemes, 71
Organization, 354, 357, 449
Orton Dyslexia Society, 88
Otitis media with effusion (OME), 124
Overextensions, 308
Overlap, 44

Paralinguistic communication, 30–33, 47
Parallel-distributed processing (PDP) models, 66, 208–209
Paraphrase, 44
Parent(s). See also Family
in early-stage assessment, 267–268
in early-stage intervention, 314–316
Individualized Education Plans and, 156–157, 177, 178
language intervention, roles in, 177–180, 314–316, 360–362
in middle-stage assessment, 334–335
in middle-stage intervention, 360–362
notification of, 153–154, 156, 157
reactions to handicapped child, 160
scheduling preferences of, 185–186
sensitivity to, 179–180
Parent-Infant Interaction Scale, 281
Participant mode, 336
Participant observation, 230, 414–415
Participation
opportunities for, 12–15
parental, 177
social, 168
social conversational, 92–93
Participation model, 8, 12–15, 270
Passive conversationalists, 356
Pathogenesis, 81
PDP (parallel-distributed processing) models, 66, 208–209
Peabody Picture Vocabulary Test—Revised (PPVT-R), 130
Peers
conversing with, 454–457
in cooperative learning relationships, 176–177
in later-stage assessment, 404
in middle-stage assessment, 335
percentage of school day spent with, 184
in social interaction relationships, 174–176, 335
tutoring by, 483–484
Percentile scores, 221
Performance components, of information processing, 102
Performance IQ, 223
Performatives, 46
Peripheral processing skills, 413

Peripheral sensory and motor system factors, 123–139
  hearing impairment, 123–131
  physical impairment, 134–139
  speech motor control, 134–139
  visual impairment, 131–134
Perlocutionary act, 47
Perlocutionary stage of language acquisition, 263, 264
PF (phonetic form) rules, 42
Phasing techniques, 283
Phenomenology, 2, 20–21
Phonemes, 36
Phonetic form (PF) rules, 42
Phonological development, 94–95, 379
Phonological simplification processes, 38
Phonologic-syntactic syndrome, 91, 135
Phonology, 36–39, 379
  hearing impairment and, 125
  infants and, 284–287
  mental retardation and, 101
  in middle stages, 379
  specific language disability and, 90
Phonotactic rules, 37
Phrase structure grammar (PSG), 41
Physical distance, 30
Physical impairment
  equal opportunity and, 481
  language disorders and, 134–139
PIQ (performance IQ), 223
Pitch direction and range, 31
Plans. See also Individualized Education Plans
  for family service, 158, 159–160, 183, 193
  for intervention, 244–249
  for transition, 484
Play
  child-directed, 174–175
  in early-stage intervention, 317–322
  peer interaction and, 335
  social relations in, 318
  symbolic, 318, 319–320, 365–366, 367
Play-based assessment, 211, 276–277
Politeness, 368, 401
Positive reinforcers, 201
POSSE strategy, 467, 468
Post-traumatic amnesia (PTA), 116, 118
PPVT-R (Peabody Picture Vocabulary Test—Revised), 130
Pragmatic functions, 370–371
Pragmatic knowledge, 423
Pragmatics, 45–48
  autism and, 108
  hearing impairment and, 125
  mental retardation and, 101
  specific language disability and, 90
Predicating expression, 46
Pregnancy, adolescent, 140–141, 142, 143

Prekindergarten screening, 329
Preoperational thought, 68–69
Prereading plan (PREP), 443
Preschool screening, 327–329
Pre-Speech Assessment Scale (PSAS), 289
Prevention, 151
  primary, 395–396
  secondary, 395, 396
  tertiary, 395, 396
Primary contours, 31
Primary prevention, 395–396
Prior knowledge, 423
Problem identification. See also Assessment
  in early stages, 259–265
  in later stages, 397–400
  in middle stages, 327–333
Processing skills, 413
Process-oriented assessment, 278–279
Profound disabilities
  equal opportunity and, 480–484
  example of, 326
  functional communication goals with, 391
  intentionality and, 297–300
  later-stage needs of individuals with, 400, 401, 480–486
  limited expression with, 300–302
  middle-stage needs of individuals with, 331–333
  symbol learning by, 305–306
Prognosis, 233–238
Progressive assimilation, 38
Progress monitoring, 249–252
Prompting, 202
Prosody, 31–33
Protoconversations, 47
Prototype, 44, 83
Providers
  forms of communicative expressions, 306
  qualifications of, 160
  recognizing need for consultation with, 401
  roles and relationships in service delivery, 172–174
Proxemics, 30
PSAS (Pre-Speech Assessment Scale), 289
PSG (phrase structure grammar), 41
Psychiatric disorders, 143–149
Psycholinguistics
  defined, 26
  information processing theories and, 206
Psycholinguists, vs. linguists, 49–50
Psychometric scatter, 86
Psychosis, 105
PTA (post-traumatic amnesia), 116, 118

Public Law 94–142. See Education for All Handicapped Children Act of 1975
Public Law 99–372. See Handicapped Children's Protection Act of 1986
Public Law 99–457. See Education of Handicapped Act Amendments of 1986
Public Law 101–476. See Individuals with Disabilities Education Act of 1990
Public policy, 4, 153–164
  federal, 153–162
  intermediate, 162–163
  local, 163
  state, 162
Pullout rooms, 165–166
Punishment, 201–202
Purpose
  clarity of, 249
  of intervention, 8
"Pygmalion effect," 189

Quality, maxim of, 48
Quantity, maxim of, 48
Questions
  for assessment, 410
  importance of, 6–8
  in mediated learning, 436–437
  in multipass strategy, 450
  sequence of, 188–194

Reading
  early learning about, 316–317
  improving with metacognition, 449–450
  mediated, 438–439
  middle-stage intervention and, 385–387
Reading disability, 86, 87. See also Specific language disability
Reciprocation, 292
Redefinition, 259
Reeducation, 259
Reevaluation, periodic, 157
Reference, 44–45
Referent, 44, 304–305
Referential meanings, 307
Referential Semantic Analysis (RSA), 353–354
Referral
  criteria for, 329–331
  in later stages, 399–400, 401
  in middle stages, 329–331, 341
  reasons for, 341, 401, 408
Referring expression, 46
Regressive assimilation, 38
Regular Education Initiative (REI), 11, 161–162
Regulators, 30
Rehabilitation, Comprehensive Services and Developmental Disabilities Amendments of 1978, 153

Rehabilitation Act of 1973, 153
REI (Regular Education Initiative), 11, 161–162
Reinforcement. *See* Stimulus-response-reinforcement factors
Reinforcement schedules, 201
Reinforcement strategies, 201, 204
Relation, maxim of, 48
Relational stage of development, 71
Relevant component approach to multiword utterances, 311
Reliability, 225–226
Relief, types of, 157–158
Remediation, 259, 325
Repeated trials, 203
Representational stage of cognitive development, 68
Requests, 296, 366–368
Resolution on Abusive Treatment and Neglect, 202
Response generalization, 203
Responsive acts, 356
Retardation. *See* Mental retardation
Retention components, of information processing, 102
Retinitis pigmentosa, 133
Rhythms, speech, 32
Risk(s)
  biological, 260
  environmental, 260
  established, 260
  identifying in infants, 260–263
Rosenthal effect, 15
RSA (Referential Semantic Analysis), 353–354
Rubella, 133
Rules
  alternation, 52
  conversation, 52
  language, 48–51
  logical form, 42, 43
  questionnaire regarding, 418
  violation of, 401, 442

Safety, early sensing of, 282
SALT (Systematic Analysis of Language Transcripts) program, 339, 353
Samples, 251, 341–358
  analyzing, 342, 346–358
  elicited, 231–232
  gathering, 343–344
  for later-stage assessment, 410–411
  naturalistic, 230–231
  recording, 344–345
  transcribing, 345–346
  written, 422–423
Sarcasm, 31
Scaffolding, 246–247, 293, 313, 364, 380, 384, 436, 464
Scheduling, 180–186
  children's preferences in, 183–185

flexible, 18
  parents' preferences in, 185–186
  program duration, 183
  reinforcement, 201
  session frequency, 180–182
  session length, 182–183
Schema, 70
Schizophrenia, 105
School(s). *See also* Classrooms
  alternative, 406
  beginning, 385–390
  higher education, 406–407
  language in school vs. home, 337, 338
  shift from home to, 335–336
  transition to work from, 484
Scores
  equivalent, 221–222
  percentile, 221
  reliability of, 225–226
  standard, 220, 221, 222–223
Screening, 262. *See also* Assessment
  in later stages, 398–399
  prekindergarten, 329
  preschool, 327–329
  story retelling as tool for, 331, 332–333, 344
Screening Test of Auditory Comprehension of Language (STACL), 331
Screening Tests of Adolescent Language (STAL), 399
SE. *See* Standard English
Secondary prevention, 395, 396
Segmentalism, 24
SELD (specific expressive language delay), 136
Selective Auditory Attention Test, 189
Selective reinforcement, 138
Self, concept of, 74–75
Semantic knowledge, 423
Semantic mapping, 477–478, 479
Semantic-pragmatic syndrome without autism, 92
Semantic reference, 44
Semantics, 43–44
  autism and, 108
  in early stages, 310–314
  hearing impairment and, 125
  in later stages, 468–474
  mental retardation and, 101
  in middle stages, 354
  specific language disability and, 90
Semiotic-operational knowledge, 70
Sense groups, 31
Sensorimotor stage of cognitive development, 68, 71
Sensory system. *See* Peripheral sensory and motor system factors
Sentence(s)
  acquisition of, 64

combining, 472–473
  complex, 350–351, 374–375
  compound, 350–351
  in later stages, 470–473
Sentence-level analysis, 424–426
Sequential rules, 52
Serial assessment, 262
Service(s)
  eligibility for. *See* Eligibility determination
  special
    need for, 192
    qualifying for, 189
    termination of, 253
Service delivery, 4, 164–186
  caseload sizes, 180, 181
  duration of, 183
  family roles and relationships in, 177–180
  intervention setting options for, 165–171
  peer roles and relationships in, 174–177
  provider roles and relationships in, 172–174
  public policy influences on, 153–164
    federal, 153–162
    intermediate, 162–163
    local, 163
    state, 162
  scheduling variables in, 180–186
  of transition services, 161
Sessions
  frequency of, 180–182
  length of, 182–183
Severe disabilities. *See* Profound disabilities
Severe expressive syndrome with good comprehension, 91
Shaping, 202
Short-term memory (STM), 203, 445–446, 472
Short-term storage space (STSS), 71
Siblings, interaction with, 335. *See also* Family
SICS (Social Interactive Coding System), 356–357
Similes, 478–479
Simplification processes, 38
Skill-based intervention, 396
Slang, 480
SLI (specific language impairment), 96–97
SLP (Spoken Language Predictor) index, 237
Smart Profile, The (Miller), 408, 443
Smith v. *Robinson*, 158
Social contexts for intervention, 170–171, 404
Social conversational participation, levels of, 92–93

Social interaction(s). *See also* Peers
  AAC devices and, 138–139
  abuse and, 142–143
  acquired brain injury and, 122
  attention-deficit hyperactivity disorder
      and, 115
  autism and, 110
  communication as, 51–54
  hearing impairment and, 131
  mental retardation and, 103
  neglect and, 142–143
  peers in, 174–176, 335
  peer tutoring and, 483–484
  physical impairment and, 138–139
  psychiatric disorders and, 148–149
  specific language disability and,
      97–98
  visual impairment and, 133–134
Social interactionism, 3, 72–75
  contributions of, 211–213
  limitations of, 213
Social Interactive Coding System
      (SICS), 356–357
Socialization
  culture and, 403–404
  emotions and, 103
Social participation, 168
Social relations, in play, 318
Social rules, violation of, 401
Sociolinguistics, 26–27, 52
Sound-level analysis, 424
Speakers, effective, 453
Special classrooms, 166–168
Specific expressive language delay
      (SELD), 136
Specific language disability, 3
  central processing factors in, 85–98
  contributing factors in, 95–98
  culture and, 91
  deviant vs. delayed language, 88–91
  identifying, 85–88
  subtypes of, 91–95
Specific language impairment (SLI), 96–97
Spectator mode, 336
Speech
  AAC devices and, 29, 33, 99–100,
      134, 268
  amplification of, 363–365
  autism and, 27, 287
  clarity of, 322–323, 401
  infantile, 89
  language and, 28–29
  processing model of, 411–413
  prosodic devices in, 31–33
  rhythms in, 32
  statistics on impairments, 149, 150
Speech acts, 46–48
Speech event rules, 52
Speech motor control, 134–139
SPELT-II (Structured Photographic Ex-
      pressive Language Test—II), 360

Spoken Language Predictor (SLP) index,
      237
S-structures, 42
STACL (Screening Test of Auditory
      Comprehension of Language),
      331
STAL (Screening Tests of Adolescent
      Language), 399
Standard deviation, 221, 222, 223
Standard English (SE), 40, 226, 373–374
Standard scores, 220, 221, 222–223
State policy, 162
State representations, 71
Stereotypes, 44
Stimulus clustering, 64
Stimulus generalization, 64, 203
Stimulus-response-reinforcement factors
  abuse and, 141–142
  in acquired brain injury, 121–122
  in attention-deficit hyperactivity
      disorder, 113
  in autism, 109
  hearing impairment and, 129
  in mental retardation, 102
  neglect and, 141–142
  physical impairment and, 137–138
  psychiatric disorders and, 147–148
  in specific language disability, 96
  visual impairment and, 133
STM (short-term memory), 203,
      445–446, 472
Story grammar, 357, 429
Story retelling, 331, 332–333, 344
Storytelling, 382–385, 428–431,
      458–461
Strategies
  behavioral, 201–203
  communicative reading, 212
  conscious metacognitive, 413
  for early-stage assessment, 276–281
  executive control, 440–441
  importance of, 7
  in language sample analysis, 342
  for later-stage assessment, 407–433
  learning strategies models, 440–441
  mand-model, 205
  mediated learning, 246–247, 435–439
  metacognitive, 443–450
  metalinguistic, 446–450
  metapragmatic, 441–443
  metatextual, 446–450
  for middle-stage assessment,
      340–358
  multipass, 450
  POSSE, 467, 468
  reinforcement, 201, 204
  time delay, 205
  word-creation, 387, 388
Strategy-based intervention, 396
Strokes (cerebrovascular accidents),
      115, 116, 119, 120

Structured Photographic Expressive
      Language Test—II (SPELT-II),
      360
STSS (short-term storage space), 71
Studying, 464–467
Stylistic variation, 47
Subjecthood, 371–372
Substance abuse, 151
Substitution processes, 38
Subsystems, 19–20
Summarizing, 464–467, 468
Suprasegmental devices, 31–33
Supreme Court, U.S., 158
Surface structures (S-structures), 42
Surveying, 450
Syllable(s)
  tonic, 31
  unstressed syllable deletion, 38
Syllable-level analysis, 424
Syllable structure processes, 38
Symbol(s)
  Blissymbols, 137
  in early stages, 302–309
  inability to read, 401
  object symbolism, 318
Symbolic play, 365–366, 367
Symbolic Play Scale, 318, 319–320,
      366, 367
Symbolic Play Test, 365
Synonymy, 43–44
Syntactic ambiguity, 43
Syntactic knowledge, 423
Syntactic-pragmatic syndrome, 91–92
Syntactic-semantic relationships, 45
Syntactic Structures (Chomsky), 62–63
Syntactic synonymy, 424
Syntagmatic words, 475
Syntax, 40–43
  in analyzing language form variables,
      348–350
  autism and, 106–108
  hearing impairment and, 125
  in later stages, 468–474
  mental retardation and, 101
  specific language disability and, 90
Systematic Analysis of Language
      Transcripts (SALT) program, 339,
      353
System theory, 1, 18–20

Tact, 65
TASH (Association for Individuals with
      Severe Handicaps), 256
TAT (teacher assistance team), 228
Taxonomy, 444–445
TBI. *See* Traumatic brain injury
Teacher(s)
  discourse of, 362–363, 364
  expectations of, 442
Teacher assistance team (TAT), 228
Teaching

incidental, 205, 362–363
interactive, 438
Teams
  effective use of, 214–215
  teacher assistance, 228
Temperament, and brain chemistry,
    145–146
Temporally displaced talk, 314
Termination
  exit criteria for, 252–253
  of intervention, 193, 252–253
Tertiary prevention, 395, 396
Testing. *See also specific tests*
  criterion-referenced, 226
  culture-fair, 227
  for formal assessment in later stages,
    407–409
Test of Language Development—2
    Primary (TOLD-2 P), 359
Test of Nonverbal Intelligence (TONI),
    217
Test validity, 223–229
TGG (transformational generative
    grammar), 41, 62, 198
Theories. *See also* Language acquisition
    theories
  empiricist, 57
  government-binding, 41–43, 62
  of language variation, 405
  nativist, 57
  system, 1, 18–20
Therapist bias, 15–16
Θ-theory, 42
Thinking
  ecological, 1–2, 19–20
  higher order, 443–446
  holistic, 20
Thinking language analysis, 423–424
Thought and Language (Vygotsky),
    74
Time delay strategy, 205
Timing, 66
Timothy W. v. *Rochester School
    District*, 161
Toddlers. *See also* Early stages of
    language acquisition
  handicapped, 159
  identifying risk in, 260–263
TOLD-2 P (Test of Language
    Development—2 Primary), 359
Tone units, 31
TONI (Test of Nonverbal Intelligence),
    217
Tonic syllables, 31
Tools
  for early-stage assessment, 276–278
  for later-stage assessment, 407–433
  for middle-stage assessment, 340–358
Topic control rules, 47

Topics and topic organization, 354
TPBA (Transdisciplinary Play-Based
    Assessment), 211, 276–277
Trainable mentally retarded, 99
Transdisciplinary Play-Based
    Assessment (TPBA), 211,
    276–277
Transdisciplinary teams, 215
Transfer components, of information
    processing, 102
Transformational generative grammar
    (TGG), 41, 62, 198
Transition services, 161, 407, 484
Transparent sign, 305
Traumatic brain injury (TBI), 116–118.
    See also Acquired brain injury
  in adolescence, 395–396, 459–460
  narrative discourse and, 459–460
Trials, repeated, 203
Trisomy 21, 81
True narratives, 430, 431
TTR (type/token ratio), 353
Tuition reimbursement relief, 157–158
T-units, 425, 426, 452, 472
Turn-taking rules, 47
Tutoring, peer, 483–484
Type/token ratio (TTR), 353

UG (universal grammar), 41, 62
Underextensions, 308
Universal grammar (UG), 41, 62
Usher syndrome, 133
Utterances, segmentation of, 346, 347.
    See also Mean length of
    utterance

Vai culture, 29
Validity, 223–229
Vectorial stage of development, 71
Verb(s), 372–374
Verbal auditory agnosia, 92, 121
Verbal Behavior (Skinner), 62–63
Verbal IQ, 223
Verbal noncommunicators, 356
VIQ (verbal IQ), 223
Visual impairment, 131–134
Vocabulary Tool Box, 307
Vocalization, 38, 284–287. *See also*
    Speech
Vocational contexts for intervention,
    171, 406–407. *See also* Work
Vowels, 38

WAIS-R (Wechsler Adult Intelligence
    Scale—Revised), 147
Warm Springs Indian Community
    (Oregon), 334
Wechsler Adult Intelligence Scale—
    Revised (WAIS-R), 147

Wechsler Intelligence Scale for
    Children—Revised (WISC-R),
    111, 223, 226
Wernicke's area of brain, 39–40, 194
Whole language, 386–387
WISC-R (Wechsler Intelligence Scale
    for Children—Revised), 111, 223,
    226
Woodcock-Johnson Psycho-Educational
    Battery—Revised, 408
Word(s)
  abstract meanings of, 474–480
  acquisition of, 64, 379–382, 474–478
  combining, 310–314
  content, 39, 40
  in early stages, 303–314
  first, 306–308
  function, 39
  in later stages, 474–480
  in middle stages, 379–382
  nonliteral meanings of, 474–480
  referents and meanings and,
    304–305
  syntagmatic, 475
Word blindness, 88
Word-creation strategies, 387, 388
Word deafness, 92
Word-finding impairments, intervention
    for, 381–382
Word-level analysis, 424
Work
  adolescents with learning disabilities
    and, 396
  Internal Work Experience program,
    482–483
  as intervention setting option, 171
  transition from school to, 484
World Health Organization, 8, 156
World knowledge, 423
Writing paranoia, 449
Written language
  AAC devices and, 29, 136–137
  analyzing samples of, 422–423
  early-stage intervention and, 316–317
  expository, 461–468
  hearing impairment and, 126
  in home vs. school, 337, 338
  in later stages, 468–474
  middle-stage intervention and,
    382–385, 387–389
  note passing, 457
  physical impairment and, 136–137
  processing model of, 411–413
  writing process intervention models
    and, 448–449

Zone of proximal development, 246
Zones of significance, 408, 409–410,
    439, 472

ISBN 0-675-21203-0

9 780675 212038